FOURTH EDITION

Physical Activity & Health

An Interactive Approach

Jerome E. Kotecki
Ball State University
Muncie, Indiana

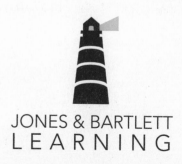

JONES & BARTLETT
LEARNING

World Headquarters
Jones & Bartlett Learning
5 Wall Street
Burlington, MA 01803
978-443-5000
info@jblearning.com
www.jblearning.com

Jones & Bartlett Learning books and products are available through most bookstores and online booksellers. To contact Jones & Bartlett Learning directly, call 800-832-0034, fax 978-443-8000, or visit our website, www.jblearning.com.

Substantial discounts on bulk quantities of Jones & Bartlett Learning publications are available to corporations, professional associations, and other qualified organizations. For details and specific discount information, contact the special sales department at Jones & Bartlett Learning via the above contact information or send an email to specialsales@jblearning.com.

Production Credits

Chief Executive Officer: Ty Field
President: James Homer
SVP, Editor-in-Chief: Michael Johnson
SVP, Chief Marketing Officer: Alison M. Pendergast
Publisher: William Brottmiller
Associate Acquisitions Editor: Megan R. Turner
Editorial Assistant: Sean Coombs
Production Editor: Jessica Steele Newfell
Senior Marketing Manager: Jennifer Stiles

Production Services Manager: Colleen Lamy
Online Products Manager: Dawn Mahon Priest
VP, Manufacturing and Inventory Control: Therese Connell
Composition: Publishers' Design and Production Services, Inc.
Cover Design: Scott Moden
Director of Photo Research and Permissions: Amy Wrynn
Cover Images: © Peter Hurley Studio/Chicago
Printing and Binding: Courier Companies
Cover Printing: Courier Companies

To order this product, use ISBN: 978-1-284-02587-3

Library of Congress Cataloging-in-Publication Data
Kotecki, Jerome Edward.
  Physical activity and health / by Jerome E. Kotecki. — 4th ed.
    p. cm.
  Includes bibliographical references and index.
  ISBN 978-1-4496-4633-2 — ISBN 1-4496-4633-6
1. Exercise. 2. Physical fitness. 3. Health. I. Title.
  RA781.K763 2013
    613.7'1—dc23
        2012035156

6048

Printed in the United States of America
17 16 15 14 13   10 9 8 7 6 5 4 3 2 1

Brief Contents

Contents

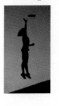
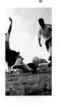

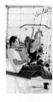
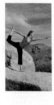
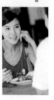
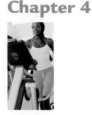
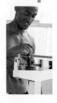

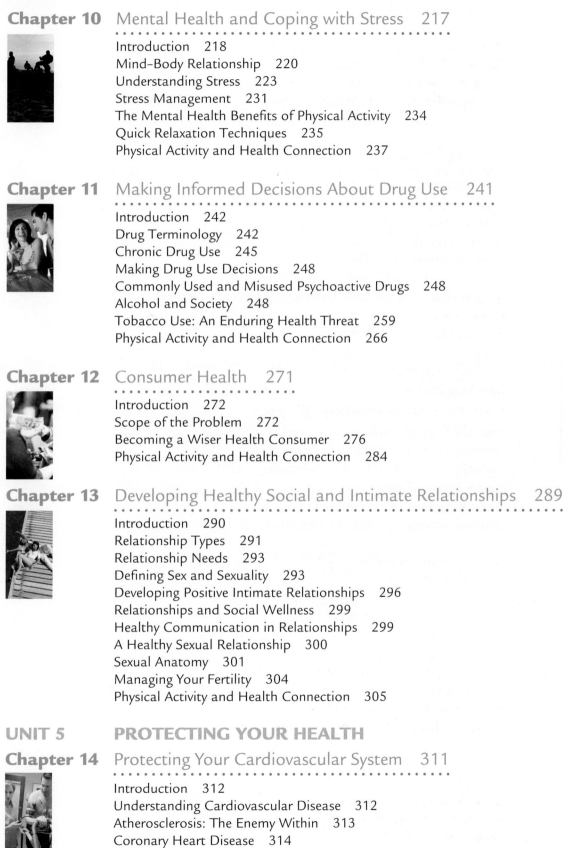

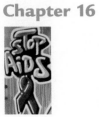

Preface

To the Student

Physical Activity & Health: An Interactive Approach, Fourth Edition serves as a valuable text to understand the workings of the complex systems within the human body and the multidimensional components of human health. This text presents scientific evidence on the relationship between physical activity and health in a readable and understandable format. Filled with information, guidance, recommendations, and practical applications, it prepares you to identify the aspects of personal behavior that, with modification, can improve your overall health. With engaging features that address self-assessment and changing health habits, *Physical Activity & Health* charts a path, putting you in control and allowing you to decide what to do, how to do it, and when to do it. With its assistance, you will know where you are heading, the best way to get there, and the ways to travel without getting lost or running into detours. This pathway will better allow your behaviors to come naturally into alignment with your sense of what is best to create optimal health and happiness.

To the Instructor

Physical Activity & Health: An Interactive Approach, Fourth Edition consists of 16 chapters that clearly and systematically cover the core essentials of a physical fitness and personal health course. These interesting and informative chapters engage students with a variety of instructive elements that assist and encourage readers in assuming control over their health and well-being. Valuable chapter features include short scenarios and key concepts listed at the beginning of each chapter and marginal definitions for key terms and concepts placed throughout each chapter. Every chapter concludes with a chapter summary that reinforces chapter concepts, offers critical thinking questions, and reiterates the connection between physical activity and health. Each chapter's content is richly illustrated with supporting tables, illustrations, and original photos to aid in the reader's understanding and retention of the material.

    Physical Activity & Health uses a distinct interactive approach to support the belief that students have more control over their lives and well-being than anything or anyone else. This text equips students with the information, skills, and practical know-how to gain control of their health, and it enables them to decide what to do and how and when to do it. By reading the chapters carefully and making an honest effort to complete the activities and assessments provided in the accompanying manual, students will gain the confidence and competence to make responsible decisions and take fitting action to improve their health.

    Physical Activity & Health: An Interactive Approach, Fourth Edition is an essential course text that offers expert knowledge in a synthesized manner that is readable and understandable to its intended audience. This is an adaptable book that fits nicely into a lecture/physical activity format, and it easily accommodates a variety of physical activity, fitness, wellness, and personal health courses. The content is carefully constructed to be meaningful to college students from all academic disciplines. It is a versatile text that has been implemented in large four-year universities, small community colleges, and other institutions of higher education.

New to This Edition
. . . .

Although the format of this edition is similar to the previous edition, much has changed. First, I have thoroughly revised and updated the content in each chapter, including tables, illustrations, and photos. Throughout the text, photographs depicting common exercises have been replaced with brand-new, original phtographs using the latest equipment. Second, when possible, I made the changes requested by the reviewers of the previous edition of this text.

Chapter 1 includes expanded coverage related to epidemiology, risk factors, and protective factors. A new validated visual graphic developed specifically for Chapter 3 is the "My Physical Activity and Exercise Pyramid." This graphic effectively integrates the *Physical Activity Guidelines for Americans* and the American College of Sports Medicine (ACSM) exercise guidelines for obtaining optimal health and fitness, thereby increasing the fluidity of understanding between each set of recommendations. New features for the chapters related to the building blocks of fitness—Chapters 4, 5, and 6—also include the updated 2011 ACSM exercise guidelines.

Chapter 7 includes the latest dietary information including the revised *Dietary Guidelines for Americans*, the MyPlate Food Guidance System, and expanded coverage of Acceptable Macronutrient Distribution Ranges (AMDRs). The revision of Chapter 8 includes new details on body fat distribution—specifically abdominal obesity—and its association with destructive metabolic abnormities.

Chapter 12, which is focused on consumer health, has been completely rewritten. Health fraud, common marketing techniques, the need for health literacy, becoming a wiser health consumer, surfing the Web for health information, locating reliable health organizations, and understanding the health care system are succinctly described and explained.

New to Chapter 13 are sections on developing a healthy sexual relationship and managing fertility. The integration of this information makes this topic more coherent.

The unit related to major diseases—Chapters 14, 15, and 16—has been revised to further enhance the students' understanding of the basic mechanisms of these diseases, including how they relate to lifestyle and how their onset can be delayed or prevented.

Acknowledgments

The author's writing is only one portion of the work that goes into the development and production of a textbook. Many other people work long hours with a shared goal: to produce a visually appealing, error-free, up-to-date, high-quality product for students. I would like to acknowledge the dedication and hard work of these individuals—for without them this project never would have been realized.

First, this text could not have been published without the efforts of the Health Science team at Jones & Bartlett Learning. I would like to extend my sincere appreciation to Megan Turner, associate acquisitions editor; Sean Coombs, editorial assistant; Jessica Newfell, production editor; Amy Wrynn, director of rights and photo research; and Jennifer Stiles, senior marketing manager. They did an extraordinary job of keeping the revision process on schedule by providing constant technical support, guidance, and encouragement.

Second, I asked Doug Strange, MA, assistant athletic director for campus athletics/strength and conditioning at Lehigh University, to supervise the resistance and stretching exercise photo shoot for this fourth edition of *Physical Activity & Health*. Doug instructed the students and advised the photography team so this edition could include updated photos to illustrate proper exercise form and technique that clearly convey the unique qualities of this text. His expertise and never-ending enthusiasm was deeply valued. I thank Doug for his professional dedication to the book and his personal commitment to the health of students with whom he works on a daily basis.

Third, I would like to express my appreciation to the Lehigh University students and staff who participated in the photo shoot for this edition. This includes Raquel Antoine, Eric Chuanroong, Scott Emeigh, Phil Gertner, Carol Ham, Joanne Hoffman, Chad Kusko, Sarah Minardi, Alex Peluso, Tobi Showunmi, James Feindt, and Emilee Strange.

Fourth, I would like to express my appreciation to those professionals who took the time and effort to review and provide their expert knowledge, thoughtful critiques, and constructive suggestions to make this edition stronger:

- Karen K. Dennis, MS, Illinois State University
- Carol Friesen, PhD, RD, Ball State University
- Nicole Fernandes, PhD, RD, Ball State University
- Stacie M. Humm, MS, HFS, Boston University
- John Janowiak, PhD, Appalachian State University
- Susan J. Massad, HSD, Framingham State University
- Douglas W. Strange, MA, HFI, CSCS, Lehigh University
- Jagdish Khubchandani, PhD, MPH, CHES, Ball State University
- Anne M. Roubal, MS, University of Wisconsin

Special Acknowledgments

First, I am deeply grateful to those who continue to teach me on a daily basis: my students. The way in which they embrace learning—by being intellectually curious and inquisitive— provides a feedback loop that helps keep me focused on my own research and on investigating the latest findings in health research to expand my perspicacity as a professor.

Second, I am fortunate to work with administrators who maintain that a well-written textbook, based on expert knowledge, reflects an important faculty contribution when it comes to the scholarship of teaching and learning. I appreciate the support of Dr. Michael Maggiotto, dean of the College of Sciences and Humanities, Dr. Terry King, provost and vice president for Academic Affairs, and Dr. Jo Ann Gora, president, of Ball State University.

Third, I would like to extend my gratitude to my mentors. Thank you to Dr. James Stewart, my undergraduate advisor, for having faith in my abilities and encouraging me to stretch myself intellectually; and to Dr. John Seffrin, Dr. Mohammad Torabi, Dr. Morgan Pigg, and Dr. Budd Stalnaker, my graduate advisors, for your expertise and high standards and for guiding me on a path of enlightenment during my years at Indiana University and beyond.

Finally, I wish to thank my friends and family for their continued support and love. They allowed me the time and energy to focus my passion and write this book.

Features of This Text

Physical Activity & Health: An Interactive Approach, Fourth Edition incorporates a number of engaging pedagogical features to aid in the student's understanding and retention of the material.

Each chapter starts with **What's the Connection?** This short scenario profiles a college student who wants to change a specific behavior that is relevant to that chapter's content. At the end of the chapter, **Making the Connection** shows what the student has learned about the behavior he or she wants to change and the action(s) that should be taken to change that behavior.

what's the connection?

Finding her way to classes. Learning to schedule time for studying. Meeting new people and making friends. These are just a few of Destiny's experiences during the first weeks of her first year at college. Destiny spends lots of time in the library, and when she isn't studying or going to classes she is working as a part-time receptionist at the university bookstore. With all these commitments, Destiny is finding it difficult to stay physically active; as a matter of fact, her daily routine requires very little physical activity. In high school, Destiny was physically ... walked or rode her bike to ... continues, Destiny notices ... hargic—she is not as ener- ... attributes these feelings to ... hange in environment, and to

making the connection

Destiny realizes that she is in college to learn and do well academically. Her midterm grades are fine, but she doesn't like feeling tired all the time. After reading this chapter, Destiny realizes that she must take more responsibility for how she is feeling. She surmises that the lack of physical activity in her life may be contributing to her worn-out feeling and begins to think of ways she can find time to become more physically active while still maintaining other positive aspects of college life.

Each chapter also begins with a **Concepts** list that identifies the content and skills that should be mastered in the chapter. Students should review the concepts before reading the chapter to use the concepts effectively.

concepts

1. The health benefits of muscle-strengthening activities are well documented.

2. Skeletal muscles move and support the skeleton.

3. Skeletal muscle is made up of thousands of cylindrical muscle fibers.

4. Resistance training is essential for improving the health-related components of physical fitness—muscular strength and endurance.

5. Muscle-strengthening activities are recommended on 2 or more days a week for both adults and older adults.

Stress is a natural process, and understanding its effects can help you use it to your own advantage.

These **Key Concepts** are referenced in the chapter with a numbered icon, allowing students to quickly find the information when reviewing the chapter.

concept connections

① Many of us are concerned about our present and future health. We feel that we have some control over our health through our lifestyle or behaviors—things we can do or not do—that will promote health and prevent disease. However, the actions of far too many of us do not produce the good health we desire. As a college student, you face many health choices— choices that can affect you in the "here-and-now" and for the rest of your life. You are responsible for learning and implementing the best choices regarding your health. It is a responsibility only you can own.

② Wellness is conceptualized as a complex interaction and integration of the seven dimensions of health, each based on a dynamic level of functioning oriented toward maximizing our potential and based on self-responsibility. When a person makes a conscious decision to work toward these enhanced aspects of health, well-being or wellness is identified. Halbert Dunn (1967) first wrote about the upper limits of health in his book *High Level Wellness*. Dunn saw wellness as a dynamic process of change and growth that was largely determined by the decisions we make about how to live our lives.

③ A healthy lifestyle is a recurring pattern of health-promoting and disease-preventing behaviors undertaken to achieve wellness. It is a way of life based on the idea that our chances of self-fulfillment are increased or decreased directly by our level of health. Further, it can decrease significantly the risk of disease and increase the chances of living a high quality of life into the later decades of life.

④ A self-change approach assumes that human beings can manage their lifestyle change and learn to control environmental factors that are detrimental to health. It puts you in control of your health and permits you to determine what to do, how, and when to do it. A self-help approach requires planning, time and effort, and, most important, the development of special lifestyle skills.

At the end of each chapter, **Concept Connections** reinforce important concepts with a brief narrative following each original concept. This emphasizes what students have learned by carefully reading the chapter and works as an excellent review tool.

Physical Activity and Health Connection
. . . .

Sexual behavior is an instinctive form of physical intimacy. It is most often performed for the purpose of expressing affection and enjoying yourself. When we decide to have sexual contact, we want it to be satisfying for ourselves and our partner. Regular physical activity makes us feel more energized and makes us look and feel better about ourselves—which has a positive influence on our sex lives. We also need to understand what responsibilities our sexual behavior entails for both ourselves and our partner when it comes to our physical health. Looking after our physical health involves behaving in ways that reduce or eliminate the possibility of being infected with a sexually transmitted infection.

The **Physical Activity and Health Connection** section reinforces and summarizes the connection between physical activity and health in relation to the topics discussed at the end of each chapter.

At the beginning of each chapter is a listing of the corresponding exercises in *Activities & Assessment Manual, Fourth Edition*. These chapter-specific exercises assist students in better understanding themselves and in making informed health behavior changes. Instructors may assign these as homework assignments or students may undertake them on their own.

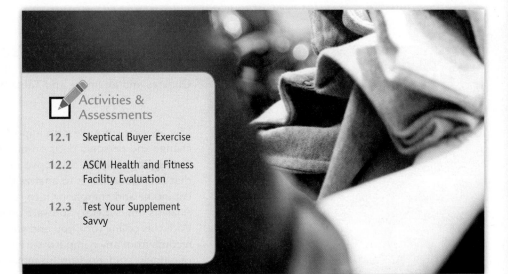

Activities & Assessments

12.1 Skeptical Buyer Exercise

12.2 ASCM Health and Fitness Facility Evaluation

12.3 Test Your Supplement Savvy

This text has a website (**go. jblearning.com/kotecki4e**) that offers interactive flashcards, practice quizzes, an anatomy review, Web exercises, self-assessments, and much more. Bookmark this website for use throughout the course!

Physical Activity & Health *An Interactive Approach*

FOURTH EDITION

Jerome E. Kotecki

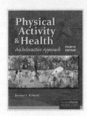

Home

Student Resources

Anatomical Review

Behavior Change Contract

Interactive Crossword Puzzles

Interactive Flashcards

Interactive Glossary

Physical Activity and Nutrition Journals

Practice Quizzes

Self-Assessments

Web Exercises

Web Links

Welcome to the Companion Website dedicated to the text, *Physical Activity and Health, Fourth Edition*. We are pleased to provide these online resources to support classroom education.

Student Resources

Anatomical Review
This Anatomical Review will help you study human anatomy to improve your understanding of how it relates to physical activity and health. Drag each label to its corresponding part and click submit to check your answers.

Behavior Change Contract
Use this Behavioral Change Contract to write down what you want to change about your behavior. When you commit in writing, you increase the likelihood that you will accomplish it.

Interactive Crossword Puzzles
These Interactive Crossword Puzzles will help you review important concepts and terms from your textbook.

Interactive Flashcards
These Interactive Flashcards will guide you through the key definitions vital to your understanding of important topics.

Interactive Glossary
With this Interactive Glossary, you have the power to search or browse all the key terms within your textbook, in three different ways: by term, alphabetically, or by chapter number.

Physical Activity and Nutrition Journals
These Journaling activities help you keep track of your diet and exercise and show the progress you are making.

Practice Quizzes
These Practice Quizzes test your knowledge of the important concepts in each chapter and provide an explanation for each answer.

Self-Assessments
These links direct you to interactive Self-Assessments on key topics

Web Exercises
Web Exercises are web links accompanied by an exercise for you to complete on each site. Each exercise helps you apply the information you are learning.

Web Links
The following are a list of reliable Web Links organized by chapter. These links can be used to research additional information on selected topics discussed in your textbook.

Supplements

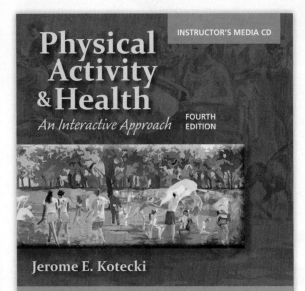

The **Instructor's Media CD** is a comprehensive teaching resource available to adopters of this text. It includes PowerPoint Lecture Outlines and an Image and Table Bank.

Diet analysis software is an important component of the behavioral change and personal decision-making focus of a nutrition course. **EatRight Analysis**, developed by ESHA Research, provides software that enables students to analyze their diets by calculating their nutrient intake and comparing it to recommended intake levels. EatRight Analysis offers dietary software online at **EatRight.jblearning.com**. With this online tool, you and your students can access personal records from any computer with Internet access. Through a variety of reports, students learn to make better choices regarding their diet and activity habits.

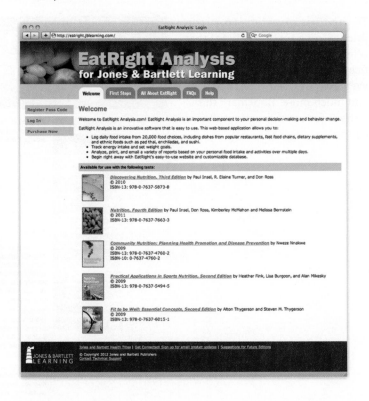

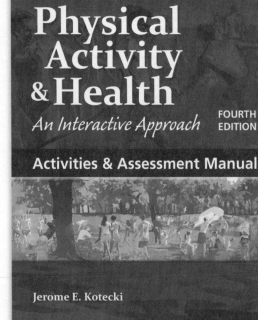

The *Activities & Assessment Manual* provides a practical framework for your students to individually apply the concepts outlined in *Physical Activity & Health: An Interactive Approach, Fourth Edition*. An important step in applying this knowledge is starting with a baseline assessment of each student's current health, fitness status, and daily habits. To assist, the author has put together more than 70 science-based health and fitness activities and assessments that examine each student's current status and measure what he or she is doing now. Completing each activity and assessment will help students identify the aspects of their personal behavior that with modification can improve their overall health. The manual is available as both a print option and an online option as an Express PDF.

About the Author

Jerome E. Kotecki is a professor of Health Science in the Department of Physiology and Health Science at Ball State University. Dr. Kotecki earned his doctorate in health education and his master's degree in exercise science from Indiana University. Dr. Kotecki has published more than 40 scientific research papers on the prevention, arrest, and reversal of the most common chronic diseases facing Americans today. He has authored or coauthored multiple textbooks on the importance of healthy lifestyle habits to enhance the multidimensional components of human health and prevent cardiovascular disease, diabetes, cancer, and other chronic conditions. An experienced teacher and researcher, he is devoted to helping students adopt and maintain healthy lifestyles. Dr. Kotecki has been recognized for his contributions to the scholarship of teaching and learning by his department, college, and university. When he is not writing or teaching, he is an avid fitness participant and enjoys cycling, resistance training, running, mountain biking, hiking, and yoga.

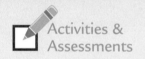

Activities &
Assessments

The Physical Activity and Health Connection

what's the connection?

Finding her way to classes. Learning to schedule time for studying. Meeting new people and making friends. These are just a few of Destiny's experiences during the first weeks of her first year at college. Destiny spends lots of time in the library, and when she isn't studying or going to classes she is working as a part-time receptionist at the university bookstore. With all these commitments, Destiny is finding it difficult to stay physically active; as a matter of fact, her daily routine requires very little physical activity. In high school, Destiny was physically active in club sports and either walked or rode her bike to school every day. As the semester continues, Destiny notices that she feels more and more lethargic—she is not as energetic as she used to be. Destiny attributes these feelings to being away from home, to the change in environment, and to studying a lot.

concepts

1. Many of us are concerned about our present and future health.

2. Wellness is conceptualized as a complex interaction and integration of the seven dimensions of health, each based on a dynamic level of functioning oriented toward maximizing our potential and based on self-responsibility.

3. A healthy lifestyle is a recurring pattern of health-promoting and disease-preventing behaviors undertaken to achieve wellness.

4. A self-change approach assumes that human beings can manage their lifestyle change and learn to control environmental factors that are detrimental to health.

5. No medicinal treatment in current or prospective use holds as much promise for sustained health as a regular program of physical activity.

6. Current physical activity guidelines call attention to the health-related benefits of regular moderate physical activity that do not meet the traditional exercise/physical fitness guidelines.

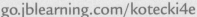

go.jblearning.com/kotecki4e
The website for this book is a great source for supplementary physical health information for both students and instructors. Visit **go.jblearning.com/kotecki4e** to find a variety of useful tools for learning, thinking, and teaching.

The first wealth is health.
          —Ralph Waldo Emerson

Introduction

Almost everyone wants good health. Nationwide polls indicate that we consider good health as one of the most important determinants of our quality of life. It is a precious resource and one of our most prized possessions, but it is often taken for granted until it is lost.

Many of us feel that we have some control over our health through our lifestyle or behaviors—things we can do or not do—that will promote health and prevent disease. However, the actions of far too many of us do not produce the good health we desire. As a college student, you face many health choices—choices that can affect you in the "here-and-now" and for the rest of your life. Too many of you do not know the best possible answers on how to maintain or improve your health or you lack the necessary lifestyle skills to implement these optimal choices. By reading this text, you have taken an important step toward becoming more informed about your health. This text provides you with the information, skills, and practical know-how to develop and maintain a healthy lifestyle. You are responsible for learning and implementing the best choices regarding your health. It is a responsibility only you can own.

This chapter provides an understanding of the concepts of health and physical activity. It explores the inseparable relationship between health and physical activity when it comes to achieving and maintaining a high quality of life (FIGURE 1.1).

Health, Wellness, and Lifestyle

The concept of health is diverse and has been viewed in a number of ways over the last century. This section identifies three different perceptions of health over the last 100 years: (1) health as an absence of disease, (2) health as a holistic concept, and (3) health as wellness.

In the early twentieth century, health was viewed as the absence of disease. If you were not sick or physically ill, you were naturally healthy. If you were ill or had evidence of disease, the best way to restore health was to have a medical doctor cure or treat the disease through medicine. This medical model approach has two important limitations. First, restoring health through medicine, drugs, or surgery in an attempt to treat disease was the primary viewpoint, rather than prevention of the disease. Still many people today maintain this attitude: "Here I am, Doctor, with all my worn-out parts—fix me up." Even as today's scientists explore the frontiers of biomedicine, they keep confirming the truism that health is easier to preserve than it is to repair.

Second, viewing health as the direct opposite of physical disease does not take into account that human beings are multidimensional. One can be free of physical symptoms or disease and still not enjoy a full and satisfying life. All aspects of a person (e.g., thoughts, emotions, beliefs, values, relationships, passions) affect that person's functioning. Further, these individual aspects affect one another. For example, a

Many of us are concerned about our present and future health.

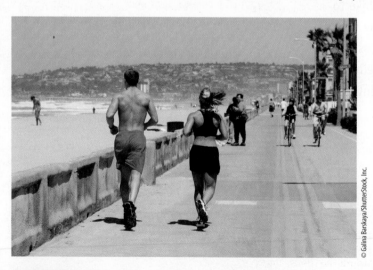
© Galina Barskaya/ShutterStock, Inc.

FIGURE 1.1 Relationship Between Health and Physical Activity. Regular physical activity is an essential lifestyle behavior for promoting health.

college student who is not passionate about his chosen major may experience boredom and pessimism (intellectual and emotional dimensions). A sense of uselessness (spiritual dimension) may develop that causes others to avoid him (social dimension). This increases the student's emotional stress or level of despair and can lead him to drop out of college.

It was not until 1948—at the World Health Organization (WHO), an international entity—that the term *health* was defined to recognize the whole person. WHO defined **health** in its constitution as "a state of complete physical, mental, and social well-being and not merely the absence of disease or infirmity" (WHO, 1948). This still widely used definition recognizes that any meaningful description of health must include the multidimensional aspects of human life and must be positive (i.e., not merely addressing the absence of disease or infirmity). Even so, the definition has been criticized over the years for its flaws. Many feel it is too idealistic in its expectations for complete well-being, which remains as elusive as it is positive, and it is too static in viewing health as a state rather than a dynamic or ever-changing process that requires constant effort and activity to preserve. Others see the dimensions cited in the definition as inadequate to capture each of the variations of health.

Subsequently, in 1986, the original WHO definition was modified and health was redefined more broadly "as less of an abstract state and more as means to an end which can be expressed in functional terms as a resource which permits people to lead an individually, socially, and economically productive life. Health is a resource for everyday life, not the object of living. It is a positive concept emphasizing social and personal resources as well as physical capabilities" (WHO, 1986, p. 1).

The evolution of the contemporary concept of health into a wellness concept reflects the idea that health is dynamic and requires the sense that a person is actively working toward functioning at a higher level. To achieve greater levels of health, you have to make a deliberate choice to assume personal responsibility for the process. When a person makes a conscious decision to work toward these enhanced aspects of health, well-being or wellness is identified. Halbert Dunn (1967) first wrote about the upper limits of health in his book *High Level Wellness*. Dunn saw **wellness** as a dynamic process of change and growth that was largely determined by the decisions we make about how to live our lives.

Expanding on the three dimensions of health cited in the WHO definition, the contemporary view includes seven dimensions of health: physical, intellectual, emotional, social, spiritual, occupational, and environmental factors (**FIGURE 1.2**).

Dimensions of Health

- *Physical health* refers to the overall condition of the organ systems of the body (cardiovascular, respiratory, skeletal, muscular, digestive, nervous, endocrine, immune, reproductive, urinary, and integumentary).
- *Intellectual health* refers to the use of our mental capacities. The characteristics include having a mind that is open to new ideas and concepts. Intellectual health includes expanding our decision-making capacity and then being willing to take action. This can be accomplished by processing information using higher-order thinking skills through synthesizing, analyzing, applying, and evaluating information.
- *Emotional health* is the ability to express feelings appropriately. Thoughts cause feelings. We can look at the same event in different ways—in an optimistic way or a pessimistic way. People who manage their own feelings well and deal with them effectively are more likely to live content and productive lives. These people generally manifest the qualities of optimism, self-esteem, and trust. Emotional health is the sense of well-being that we obtain from feeling capable, courageous, worthy, respected, appreciated, and loved.

Health Considered less of an abstract state and more as a means to an end, which can be expressed in functional terms as a resource that permits people to lead an individually, socially, and economically productive life. Health is a resource for everyday life, not the object of living. It is a positive concept emphasizing social and personal resources as well as physical capabilities.

Wellness A complex interaction and integration of the seven dimensions of health, each based on a dynamic level of functioning oriented toward maximizing one's potential and based on self-responsibility.

Wellness is conceptualized as a complex interaction and integration of the seven dimensions of health, each based on a dynamic level of functioning oriented toward maximizing our potential and based on self-responsibility.

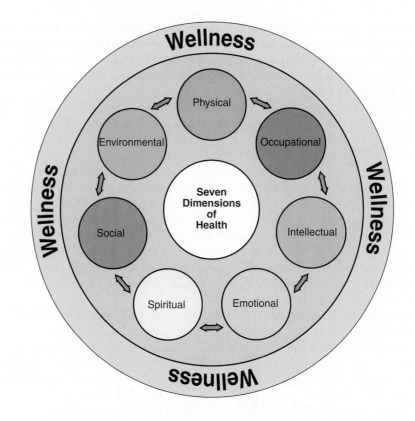

FIGURE 1.2 **Concept of Health as Wellness.** The contemporary view of health contains seven dimensions. Wellness is conceptualized as a complex interaction and integration of these seven dimensions. It is your responsibility to respect and honor each of the seven dimensions of health uniformly.

- *Social health* refers to having the ability to interact effectively with other people and have meaningful/caring relationships. Socially healthy persons behave in ways to help and assist others. They accomplish this by understanding and respecting differences in various social groups based on their age, ethnicity, personality characteristics, beliefs, education, religion, and sexual orientation. Social health is the sense of well-being that we obtain from having intellectually interesting and emotionally compassionate relationships with friends and family (**FIGURE 1.3**).

- *Spiritual health* pertains to the soul or spirit. *Soul* or *spirit* can be defined as the inspiring principle or dominating influence in a person's life. Spiritual health is the belief that we are a part of a larger scheme of life and that our lives have purpose. Spirituality provides meaning and direction in life. Selflessness, compassion, a passion for living, faith, a sense of right and wrong, ethics, and morals are important components of spiritual health. Spiritual health is a sense of well-being that we obtain from having an awareness and appreciation for the life force that moves us.

- *Career or occupational health* pertains to our chosen vocation in life. People spend most of their life at work. It is therefore essential that we choose work that is satisfying intrinsically and extrinsically. It means choosing the kind of work that makes the best use of our abilities and gives a sense of accomplishment. It includes being able to earn a living and contribute to society.

- *Environmental health* refers to everything around us and includes the impact of natural and human-made environments on our health. It includes

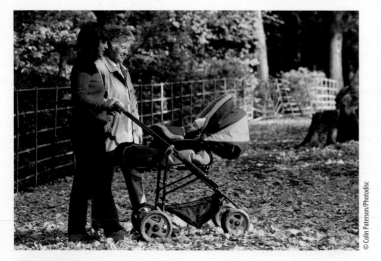

FIGURE 1.3 **Social Health.** Walks through the park with friends and family can enhance social and physical health.

working to preserve ecosystems and the biodiversity of the planet. It also means adapting the human-made environment to reduce the risk of suffering from intentional and unintentional injuries and communicable and noncommunicable diseases.

Each of these seven dimensions, or component parts, of health—all interacting in a synergistic way—allow us to assume higher levels of functioning that can lead to more productive and satisfying lives. One of the best descriptors of this complex mixture of factors that are dependent on each other is **quality of life**. Quality of life is a subjective measure that reflects our levels of fulfillment, satisfaction, happiness, and feeling good about ourselves despite any limitations we may have. For example, it is not essential that individuals satisfy the traditional definition of good health to rate themselves high in terms of wellness. For instance, many people with chronic diseases or disabilities report high levels of satisfaction within each of the seven dimensions of health. Similarly, people who are symptom or disease free or completely able may not necessarily give themselves high scores in all seven aspects of health.

Health is a continually changing process; it changes from day to day, week to week, month to month, and year to year. **FIGURE 1.4** illustrates the concept of the multidimensional aspects of health as a continuum: from high-level functioning at one end to disability, limitation, and premature death at the other end. Moving from the neutral point or center (where there is no discernable disease) to the left indicates a progressive worsening of health resulting from inappropriate and undesirable adaptation by the body, or *diseases of maladaptation* or **pathogenesis**. This includes asymptomatic disease, symptomatic disease, disability limitation, and finally the absence of functioning or premature death. Moving to the right of the neutral point indicates not only an absence of disease but also increasing levels of health and optimal functioning, or **salutogenesis**.

Everyone falls on the continuum somewhere. Most young adults are likely to be found in the center. However, by becoming more aware of what you can become, you can take steps to improve your own wellness—because moving from adolescence to young adulthood provides you increasing control over your lifestyle choices. A goal of wellness is not being perfect in each dimension, but rather managing and balancing the dimensions in such a way as to maximize your quality of life and self-fulfillment based on your daily challenges.

Quality of life A subjective measure that reflects our levels of fulfillment, satisfaction, happiness, and feeling good about ourselves despite any limitations we may have.

Pathogenesis The origination and development of a disease.

Salutogenesis An approach focusing on factors that support human health and well-being rather than on factors that cause disease.

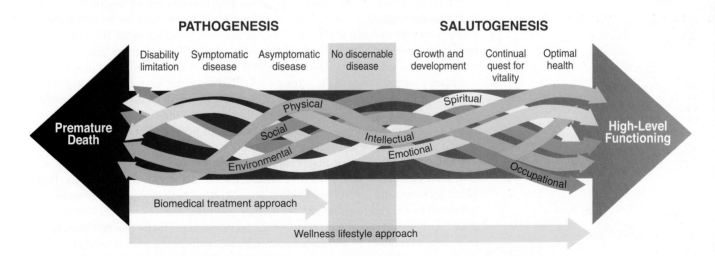

FIGURE 1.4 **The Dimensions of Health and Wellness.** The continuum allows you to visualize the seven interrelated dimensions of health and wellness and biomedical treatment approaches to health and disease.

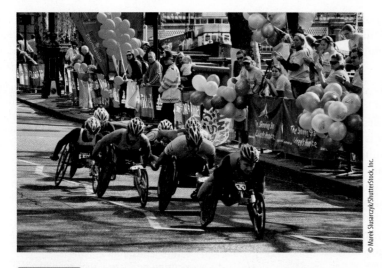

© Marek Slusarczyk/ShutterStock, Inc.

FIGURE 1.5 **Wellness and Medical Approaches to Health.**
A wellness lifestyle approach to health can be utilized at any point on the health continuum, including for individuals with differing degrees of disability or disease. In such cases, the goal is to move above physical or mental limitations to live a richer, fuller life.

Epidemiology The study of factors affecting the health and illness of populations; serves as the basic science for public health and preventive medicine.

Risk factor An exposure that in some way increases the chance of getting a certain disease.

Protective factor An exposure that in some way decreases the chance of getting a certain disease.

The continuum also is a way to visualize the wellness and medical approaches to health. As discussed earlier, the biomedical treatment approach to health attempts to bring individuals to the neutral point where signs, symptoms, and disability are alleviated. The biomedical treatment approach to health, however, is not designed to take people past the neutral point to higher levels of growth and functioning. Only you can decide to do that for yourself. Conversely, individuals, including individuals with differing degrees of disease or disability, can use the wellness lifestyle approach to health at any point on the continuum. Wellness does not assume you live free of disease or disability or some other limitation (**FIGURE 1.5**). The motivation to improve quality of life within the framework of your own unique capabilities is important to achieving wellness.

It is important to recognize that the wellness approach to health is not intended to replace the biomedical treatment approach but rather to work in combination with it. Modern medical treatment is a great thing, but there is a problem with it: people expect too much from it. Promoting healthy lifestyles has become increasingly important in recent years as the epidemiological evidence of the association between behavior and disease continues to grow (Alpert, 2009; King, Mainous, Carnemolla, & Everett, 2009).

Epidemiology is the study of factors affecting the health and illness of populations, and it serves as the basic science for public health and preventive medicine. It is a highly quantitative discipline based on principles of statistics and research studies. The purpose of the studies is to investigate the relationships between various characteristics of people and the occurrence of specific health outcomes across time. Epidemiological studies assist scientists in sorting through many factors and identifying those that are most highly associated with a specific health outcome, which then provides the foundation and logic for creating interventions made in the interest of preventing disease and promoting health (Centers for Disease Control and Prevention [CDC], 2012a).

To fully appreciate the impact of various determinants on our health, it's essential to understand the terms *risk factor* and *protective factor*. Both are based on the probability that an event will occur. In epidemiology, these terms are most often used to express that a particular outcome will occur following a particular exposure utilizing statistical analysis. The term **risk factor** means an exposure that in some way increases a person's chance for getting a certain disease; for example, smoking is a specific health behavior that is proven to be associated with an increased susceptibility to developing lung cancer. **Protective factors** decrease the chance of getting a certain disease. Some examples of protective factors for preventing cancer are getting regular physical activity, maintaining a healthy weight, and eating a nutritious diet.

Unhealthy lifestyles are major contributing factors to many chronic medical conditions, including cardiovascular disease, cancer, diabetes mellitus, obesity, high blood pressure, and high blood lipids (CDC, 2012c). These diseases are generally not cured by medication, and neither do they just disappear (Kotecki & Clayton, 2003). Despite the major advances in medical research, medicine has not been able to restore individuals to health. It merely helps us cope better with serious and often debilitating conditions. So, while we continue to be in awe of the advances in medical technology, we must recognize that this is not *restorative* health care. Only the human body, when it is kept fit, has its own restorative capacities.

A **healthy lifestyle** is a way of life based on the idea that our chances of self-fulfillment are increased or decreased directly by our level of health. Further, a healthy lifestyle can decrease significantly the risk of disease and increase the chances of living a high quality of life into the later decades of life. Or, as this author likes to say, "It is to allow us to die young as late as possible."

It is important to mention that although your daily choices are the most important determinants of your well-being, health is the culmination of many interacting factors. Besides lifestyle behaviors, heredity and human biology, social circumstances, environment, and medical care play key roles in disease and premature death (McGinnis, 2003). **FIGURE 1.6** shows the extent to which human longevity is affected by these factors along with lifestyle decisions.

Heredity refers to the transfer of biological characteristics from natural parents to offspring. Each of us has a cellular design that dictates shape and size and to a significant extent our personality and life expectancy. *Environment* refers to everything around us, with a primary focus on the human-made environment. For example, exposure to toxic agents from environmental pollutants and occupational hazards can increase risk of ill health. *Social circumstance* refers to our level of income, housing, education, and employment (socioeconomic status). In general, people with a lower socioeconomic status have poorer health outcomes than those who are better off. *Medical care* refers to limited or inadequate services from the health care system. For those without health insurance, health problems are generally more serious because uninsured individuals use fewer screening and preventive services and delay seeking care when they are sick. As a result, when they enter the medical care system, they tend to be more ill and at more advanced disease stages than are insured persons. In the end, health is determined not by these factors acting alone, but by how they interact with one another (McGinnis, 2003).

An old military tactic is "know your enemy." Because we are in a war to increase our years of healthy life, it is important for us to know who that enemy is. At least half of this nation's premature deaths from the 10 leading causes of mortality are attributable to personal behavior and health habits such as tobacco use, lack of physical activity, alcohol and drug misuse, and risky sexual practices (Remington & Brownson, 2011). Lifestyle choices are also linked to higher ambulatory care and hospitalization costs, with preventable illness accounting for as much as 75 percent of all medical care spending (CDC, 2012b).

"We have met the enemy, and he is us" is the famous and most frequently quoted phrase of cartoonist Walt Kelly, and it is applicable here. As protectors of our own health, it is no secret that we are frequently our own worst enemy. We harm ourselves repeatedly in many ways. What is worse, we seldom realize it. We can be our own best friend, too, but more commonly we are our own worst enemy. After honest self-reflection, we are likely to see some ill-fated lifestyle choices we have made. Identifying these choices and evaluating their consequences is the first step toward being responsible for our own health.

Studies show that most Americans desperately want to have healthy lives, yet it's an elusive dream for so many because health is lost before it's valued and before its maintenance is understood. Choosing to participate in a healthy lifestyle requires self-responsibility and a self-change approach—you don't blame someone else, make excuses, or avoid personal accountability. Taking responsibility for your health is recognizing that your daily choices affect your total well-being. This includes being physically active, eating sensibly, maintaining a healthy weight, managing stress effectively, avoiding tobacco, following sensible drinking habits, and being safety conscious. Your challenge is to make smart decisions. Halbert Dunn (1967) states it simply: "We cannot take high-level wellness like a pill out of a bottle. It will come only to those who work at following its precepts."

A healthy lifestyle is a recurring pattern of health-promoting and disease-preventing behaviors undertaken to achieve wellness.

Healthy lifestyle A recurring pattern of health-promoting and disease-preventing behaviors undertaken to achieve wellness.

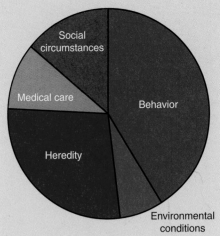

FIGURE 1.6 **Factors Influencing Premature Death or Longevity.**
Behavior is the single most important and modifiable factor influencing health and disease. SOURCE: McGinnis, J.M. (2003). A vision for health in our new century. *American Journal of Health Promotion* 18(2):146–150.

A self-change approach assumes that human beings can manage their lifestyle change and learn to control environmental factors that are detrimental to health.

No medicinal treatment in current or prospective use holds as much promise for sustained health as a regular program of physical activity.

Chronic diseases Illnesses that can develop early in life and last for many years.

Physical activity Any bodily movement produced by the contraction of skeletal muscle that increases energy expenditure above a basal (resting) level.

There is something truly remarkable in the fact that practically all of us want to better ourselves. Life continually presents opportunities for achieving what we desire. Most of us strive to be self-changers. A self-change approach puts you in control of your health and permits you to determine what to do, how, and when to do it. A self-change approach requires planning, time and effort, and, most important, the development of special lifestyle skills.

Physical Activity and Its Relationship to Health

Imagine picking up the daily newspaper and seeing the front-page headline: Miraculous New Health Pill Discovered. You read quickly through the article, which reports that this miracle drug can make you look younger, provide better weight control, give you more energy and a brighter mental outlook, relieve stress and anxiety, make you fit and flexible, and decrease your risk of serious diseases such as heart disease, cancer, diabetes, hypertension, depression, and osteoporosis. All of this with virtually no side effects. You would probably hurry to your physician to get a prescription for a supply of this remarkable new medication. Of course, this pill has not yet been discovered, and despite the miracles of modern medical research, it is not likely to happen any time soon. However, there is a prescription already available to everyone that can provide all of these benefits and many more. It is regular physical activity! In fact, no medicinal treatment in current or prospective use holds as much promise for sustained health as a regular program of physical activity (TABLE 1.1). This author believes that if physical activity could be packaged in a pill, it would be the most widely prescribed pill the world's ever seen.

Unfortunately, more than one in two U.S. adults (53 percent) are not getting enough leisure-time aerobic physical activity to benefit their health (CDC, 2012d). Furthermore, approximately one in four U.S. adults is completely inactive (sedentary) during their leisure time or is a genuine couch potato. Leading a sedentary lifestyle is common in the United States as well as in the rest of the world: 60 percent of the global population does not get the recommended amount of physical activity to promote health (WHO, 2012). This chapter explains later how we got this way. Right now, these enduring rates begin to show why some public health experts have declared that physical inactivity has become the biggest health problem in the twenty-first century (Blair, 2009). This declaration of crisis is based on decades of research by the finest scientists worldwide, who have revealed that sedentary living is a leading cause of **chronic diseases**—illnesses that can develop early in life and last for many years—poor quality of life, disability, and premature death in the United States, Canada, and many other developed countries (FIGURE 1.7). Such information shapes the case for current recommendations/ guidelines from many national health organizations and expert panels that advise that the first-line approach in preventing this unnecessary health crisis is encouraging physical activity. Simply put, their end purpose in recommending physical activity is the promotion of health and wellness.

This text emphasizes that regular physical activity is an essential lifestyle behavior for promoting health and preventing many major chronic diseases. It provides health benefits that cannot be obtained in any other way. Physical activity not only contributes directly to the physical health dimension but also contributes indirectly to the other six dimensions of health. It is important to establish what is meant by *physical activity* and the related term *exercise* when it comes to health.

Physical Activity, Exercise, and Physical Fitness

Physical activity refers to any bodily movement produced by the contraction of skeletal muscle that increases energy expenditure above a basal (resting) level (U.S. Department of Health and Human Services [USDHHS], 2008). The major

TABLE 1.1	The Health Benefits of Physical Activity

The table is based on a total physical activity program that includes activities and exercises to improve cardiorespiratory endurance, muscular strength and endurance, flexibility, neuromotor fitness, and body composition.

Physical Activity Benefit	Evidence	Physical Activity Benefit	Evidence
Physical Fitness		**Mental Health**	
Improves cardiorespiratory endurance	+++	Reduces stress symptoms	++
Improves muscular strength	+++	Reduces anxiety symptoms	++
Improves muscular endurance	+++	Reduces depression symptoms	++
Improves flexibility	+++	Enhances memory and learning	++
Decreases body fat percentage	+++	Enhances mood and self-esteem	++
Cardiovascular Disease		**Joint Health**	
Prevents coronary artery disease	+++	Prevents low-back pain	+
Prevents stroke	++	Prevents arthritis	+
Reduces atherosclerosis	+++	Treats arthritis	+
Treats heart disease	+++	Strengthens joint structure and functioning	+
High Blood Pressure		**Immune System**	
Prevents high blood pressure	+++	Improves overall immunity	++
Treats high blood pressure	+++	Prevents common cold	+
High Blood Lipids (Fats)		**Elderly**	
Lowers triglycerides	++	Increases years of healthy life	++
Lowers total cholesterol	++	Increases life expectancy	+
Lowers LDL cholesterol	++	Reduces risk of falling	+++
Raises HDL cholesterol	++	Reduces risk of Alzheimer's and dementia	+
Diabetes		**Bone Health**	
Prevents or delays type 2 diabetes	+++	Helps build bone density	+++
Treatment for type 2 diabetes	+++	Preserves bone mass and delays osteoporosis	++
Treatment for type 1 diabetes	+	Treats osteoporosis	++
Healthy Weight Management		**Occupational Health**	
Prevents fat gain	+++	Increases productivity	+
Maintains fat loss	++	Reduces short-term sick leave	+
Treats obesity	++	Reduces health insurance premiums	++
Cancer		**Pregnancy Benefits**	
Reduces risk of colon cancer	+++	Greater resistance to fatigue	+
Reduces risk of breast cancer	+++	Improved posture and stronger back muscles	+
Reduces risk of prostate cancer	++	May lead to easier labor and faster recovery	+
Reduces risk of endometrial cancer	++	Faster return to pre-pregnancy weight	+
Treats cancers	++	Reduces stress and elevates spirits	+
Medical Care Expenditures		**Morbidity and Mortality Rates**	
Lower annual direct medical care costs	+	Lower death rates for middle-age adults	++
Fewer hospital stays	+	Lower premature death rates	++
Fewer physician visits	+	Reduces and delays onset of illness	++
Reduced use of some medications	+	Reduces disease-related symtoms in many diseases	++

+++ Strong data support

++ Data supportive, but more research needed

+ Some data, but much more research needed

SOURCE: Kotecki, J.E. (2012). Updating the evidence that physical activity is good for health: An epidemiological review. A presentation delivered to the College of Pharmacy and Health Sciences, Butler University on October 8, 2012, in Indianapolis, Indiana.

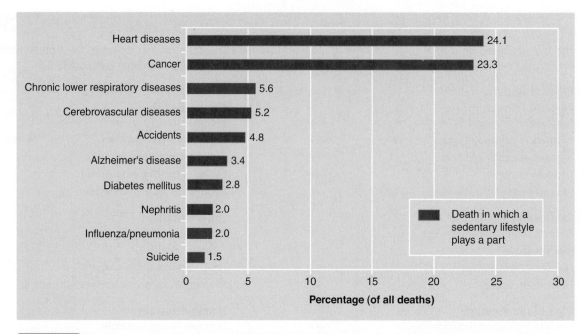

FIGURE 1.7 **The Ten Leading Causes of Death in the United States.** SOURCE: Data from Murphy, S.L., Jiaquan, X., & Kochanek, K.D. (2012). Deaths: Preliminary data for 2010. *National Vital Statistics Reports* 60(4):1–67.

Exercise A subset of physical activity that is a planned, structured, repetitive, and purposeful attempt to improve or maintain physical fitness, physical performance, or health.

Physical fitness A set of attributes a person has or achieves that relate to a person's ability or capacity to perform specific types of physical activity efficiently and effectively.

contributors to this form of energy expenditure usually are everyday light-intensity activities people undertake while performing other functions, such as standing and waiting in line, relaxed walking to class, riding a bike for transportation, climbing a couple of sets of stairs, lifting lightweight objects, or performing domestic duties such as shopping, sweeping floors, and dusting the furniture. Much physical activity occurs as an incidental part of your daily routines. Although these low levels of light-intensity activities of daily living are included under the broad definition of physical activity, they usually are insufficient for you to gain the more substantial health benefits provided by integrating medium levels of moderate-intensity physical activity into your daily routines.

Exercise, on the other hand, refers to a subset of physical activity that is a planned, structured, repetitive, and purposeful attempt to improve or maintain physical fitness, physical performance, or health. It usually includes more noticeable leisure-time activities such as distance running, swimming, aerobic dancing, mountain biking, weight lifting, yoga, and sporting activities such as basketball, racquetball, and tennis (FIGURE 1.8 and FIGURE 1.9). These activities generally require considerably more effort and energy expenditure than do the task-oriented activities of routine daily life.

Unlike physical activity and exercise, which are behavioral processes, **physical fitness** has been described as a set of attributes a person has or achieves. These attributes relate to a person's ability or capacity to perform specific types of physical activity efficiently and effectively. They are specific to the health-related components (cardiorespiratory endurance, muscular strength and endurance, flexibility, and body composition) and skill-related components (agility, coordination, balance, power, reaction time, and speed) of fitness required for the particular activity. For example, the fitness requirements for distance swimming, tennis, and yoga are very different in their physical demands and skills. Different fitness levels are mainly a result of the levels and types of physical activity you perform; therefore, exercise programs can be devised to produce a physiologic training effect to improve fitness attributes. You can attain these physical fitness attributes through individually tailored exercise programs using the FITT principle. The

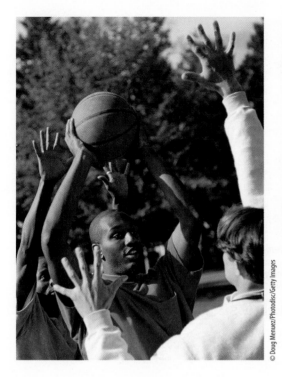

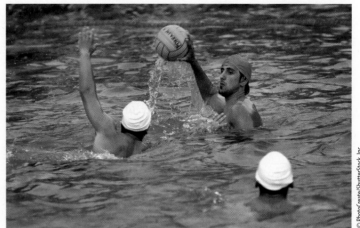

© Doug Menuez/Photodisc/Getty Images

© PhotoCreate/ShutterStock, Inc.

FIGURE 1.9 **Improving Physical Fitness.** Different fitness levels are the result of our levels of physical activity.

FIGURE 1.8 **Exercising for Health.** Recreational activities such as basketball can be an enjoyable way to exercise.

FITT principle includes specification of (F) frequency (days per week), (I) intensity (how hard, e.g., light, moderate, vigorous), (T) time (amount for each session or day), and (T) type of activity (e.g., running, weight training).

Physical Activity Recommendations for Health

Regular physical activity and exercise are critically important for the health and well-being of people of all ages. Recent research demonstrates that virtually all individuals can benefit from regular physical activity, whether they participate in vigorous exercise or some type of moderate health-enhancing physical activity. That's right—there is no need to think that only strenuous exercise training provides improved health benefits. In fact, individuals obtain the greatest proportional benefit to health when they change from inactivity or a low level of physical activity (activity beyond baseline but fewer than 150 minutes a week) to a regular pattern of medium moderate-intensity physical activity (150 minutes to 300 minutes a week) (**FIGURE 1.10**).

According to the recommendations in the *Physical Activity Guidelines for Americans* (USDHHS, 2008), for the broader population who have different and diverse health needs to attain the most benefits from physical activity:

Adults (ages 18–64)
- Adults should do 2 hours and 30 minutes a week of moderate-intensity, or 1 hour and 15 minutes a week of vigorous-intensity aerobic physical activity, or an equivalent combination of moderate- and vigorous-intensity aerobic physical activity. Aerobic activity should be performed in episodes of at least 10 minutes, preferably spread throughout the week.
- Additional health benefits are provided by increasing to 5 hours a week of moderate-intensity aerobic physical activity, or 2 hours and 30 minutes a week of vigorous-intensity physical activity, or an equivalent combination of both.
- Adults should also do muscle-strengthening activities that involve all major muscle groups on 2 or more days per week.

6

Current physical activity guidelines call attention to the health-related benefits of regular moderate physical activity that do not meet the traditional exercise/physical fitness guidelines.

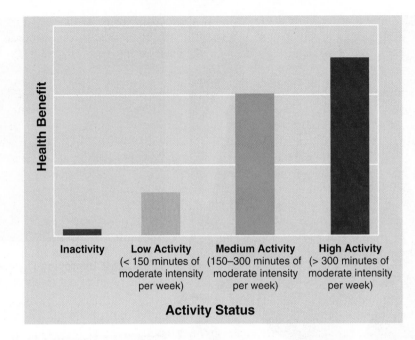

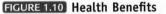 **Health Benefits and Activity Levels.** Individuals obtain the greatest proportional benefit to health when they change from inactivity or a low level of activity to a regular pattern of medium-intensity physical activity.

Older Adults (ages 65 or older)

- Older adults should follow the adult guidelines. If this is not possible due to limiting chronic conditions, older adults should be as physically active as their abilities allow. They should avoid inactivity. Older adults should do exercises that maintain or improve balance if they are at risk of falling.

Children and Adolescents (ages 6–17)

- Children and adolescents should do 1 hour or more of physical activity every day.
- Most of the 1 hour or more a day should be either moderate- or vigorous-intensity aerobic physical activity.
- As part of their daily physical activity, children and adolescents should do vigorous-intensity activity on at least 3 days per week. They also should do muscle-strengthening and bone-strengthening activity on at least 3 days per week.

Adults with Disabilities

- Follow the adult guidelines. If this is not possible, these persons should be as physically active as their abilities allow. They should avoid inactivity.

Children and Adolescents with Disabilities

- Work with the child's health care provider to identify the types and amounts of physical activity appropriate for them. When possible, these children should meet the guidelines for children and adolescents—or as much activity as their condition allows. Children and adolescents should avoid being inactive.

Pregnant and Postpartum Women

- Healthy women who are not already doing vigorous-intensity physical activity should get at least 2 hours and 30 minutes of moderate-intensity aerobic activity a week. Preferably, this activity should be spread throughout the week. Women who regularly engage in vigorous-intensity aerobic activity or high amounts of activity can continue their activity provided that their condition remains unchanged and they talk to their health care provider about their activity level throughout their pregnancy.

The primary intentions of these guidelines are to increase public awareness of the importance of moderate physical activity and provide a realistic goal as it relates to the achievement of health benefits that are attainable by all individuals. Despite the well-known benefits of physical activity, most teenagers and adults have relatively sedentary (inactive) lifestyles and are not active enough to achieve the health benefits that can result from following the *Guidelines*.

Levels and patterns of physical activity and inactivity are important indicators of the health of Americans. Physical activity is one of the leading health indicators established by *Healthy People 2020*, a set of health objectives for the nation to achieve over the second decade of the twenty-first century. *The Healthy People* project, currently in its fourth decade, provides a set of 10-year objectives that is a road map for improving the health of all people in the United States. *Healthy People 2020* builds on initiatives pursued by its predecessors *Healthy People*, *Healthy People 2000*, and *Healthy People 2010*. Each *Healthy People* document has brought together national, state, and local government agencies; nonprofit, voluntary, and professional organizations; businesses; communities; and individuals to identify the most significant preventable threats to health and to establish national goals to reduce these threats (USDHHS, 2010).

In addition to physical activity, other major indicators of health include overweight and obesity, tobacco use, substance use, sexual behavior, mental health, injury and violence, environmental quality, immunization, and access to health care. The fourth edition of *Healthy People* was published in 2010. The physical activity and fitness objectives for *Healthy People 2020* are provided in TABLE 1.2. Their overall goal is to improve the health, fitness, and quality of life of Americans through regular physical activity.

Why We Live Sedentary Lives

Over the last half century, a dramatic decrease in physical activity levels has occurred as a result of changes in society and in the economy. Among the major factors contributing to this decrease include technological changes in the workplace that led to a decline in physically active occupations, widespread use of the automobile as the major form of transportation, the introduction of labor-saving devices for the home, and increases in sedentary activities such as television watching, computer use, and video game playing during spare time. Your author finds the last factor notable because now people can find highly entertaining things to do in a sedentary position. It is hard to compete with 200+ stations on cable television, great video games, and other choices available on the computer. A recent study of Americans found that the average sedentary time was just over 8 hours a day (Clark et al., 2011). That equates to roughly half of our waking hours. The majority of this comes from chronic prolonged sitting related to screen time (time spent in front of the television, computer, or other screen-based device) on a daily basis.

In addition to the increases in low-activity occupations, conveniences that make people's lives easier, and the increase in sedentary activities during spare time, many personal variables, including individuals' underlying thoughts and feelings, make people resistant to being physically active. The most common reasons this instructor hears from students is that they lack time, they're too exhausted from other commitments, they don't like to sweat, and they don't like to go to the gym where they are afraid they may look inadequate.

TABLE 1.2	Healthy People 2020 Physical Activity and Fitness Objectives

1. Reduce the proportion of adults who engage in no leisure-time physical activity

2. Increase the proportion of adults who meet current Federal physical activity guidelines for aerobic physical activity and for muscle-strengthening activity

3. Increase the proportion of adolescents who meet current Federal physical activity guidelines for aerobic physical activity and for muscle-strengthening activity

4. Increase the proportion of the Nation's public and private schools that require daily physical education for all students

5. Increase the proportion of adolescents who participate in daily school physical education

6. Increase regularly scheduled elementary school recess in the United States

7. Increase the proportion of school districts that require or recommend elementary school recess for an appropriate period of time

8. Increase the proportion of children and adolescents who do not exceed recommended limits for screen time

9. Increase the number of States with licensing regulations for physical activity provided in child care

10. Increase the proportion of the Nation's public and private schools that provide access to their physical activity spaces and facilities for all persons outside of normal school hours (that is, before and after the school day, on weekends, and during summer and other vacations)

11. Increase the proportion of physician office visits that include counseling or education related to physical activity

12. Increase the proportion of employed adults who have access to and participate in employer-based exercise facilities and exercise programs

13. Increase the proportion of trips made by walking

14. Increase the proportion of trips made by bicycling

15. Increase legislative policies for the built environment that enhance access to and availability of physical activity opportunities

SOURCE: Reproduced from U.S. Department of Health and Human Services. (2010). Healthy People 2020 Topics & Objectives: Physical Activity and Fitness. Online: http://healthypeople.gov/2020/topicsobjectives2020/objectiveslist.aspx?topicId=33.

A Lifestyle Approach to Physical Activity

Most national goals address leisure time rather than occupational physical activity because people have more personal control over how they spend their leisure time and because most people do not have jobs that require regular physical activity. Furthermore, the use of labor-saving devices such as washing machines, dishwashers, garage door openers, and riding lawnmowers make tasks easier and leave people with more free time.

Earlier you read about the good news related to the scientific evidence that shows that physical activity done at a moderate intensity level can produce important health benefits. That's right—people really do not have to suffer. Furthermore, it's not necessary to carve out one 30-minute block of time from a busy schedule. The cumulative effect of physical activity throughout the day is what counts, and many types of activity can help (FIGURE 1.11).

College students usually have very busy schedules and often place exercise at the bottom of their list of priorities. It is easy to spend an entire day sitting in classes and meetings, studying in the library, and completing assignments using a computer. Some even have jobs and family commitments on top of their educational responsibilities. And, of course, they must allow for some social time with friends and classmates. What most of these pursuits have in common is that they are sedentary activities.

Even with all of the commitments you have as a college student, it is essential that you make time for moderate-intensity physical activity. For example, did you know that fitting regular moderate-intensity physical activity into your daily routine can help you better accomplish your educational goals for the day, such as studying and being attentive in class? Because regular moderate-intensity physical activity can increase your concentration, mental well-being, stamina, and energy, you are more likely to be more proficient when it comes to learning. Fitting moderate-intensity physical activity into your daily routine may be easier than you might think if you follow a lifestyle approach.

A lifestyle approach to physical activity includes accumulating at least 30 minutes of self-selected activities, which can include leisure, occupational, or domestic activities—either intentional or unintentional—that are at least moderate in their intensity and are part of everyday life. You may not even have to adjust your schedule. For instance, walk briskly to class, the library, or the campus dining hall. Include marching in place, jumping jacks, or walking around in your study breaks. These activities can be done in short duration intervals (lasting for at least 10 minutes at a time) several times a day, as long as they add up to at least a half hour each day. The health benefits will accumulate without you having to take a couple of hours to go to the gym or do some of the other things you may have a hard time fitting into your schedule.

Of course, you may intend to add an exercise program to your schedule and take advantage of the exercise facilities (e.g., weight room, track, tennis court) that your college offers. This is also a very good idea. Although participating in a regular exercise program can provide a higher intensity that can offer greater health benefits, it is imperative you remember that there are plenty of other ways to obtain the daily recommended amount of physical activity to accumulate the health benefits.

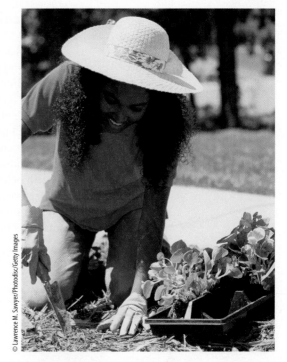

© Lawrence M. Sawyer/Photodisc/Getty Images

FIGURE 1.11 **Moderate-Intensity Physical Activity.** Gardening is enjoyable and expends energy.

Investing in Your Health

If good health came with a guarantee, the author bets most of you would pay any price asked. Obviously, that will never happen. However, you can invest in an insurance policy of sorts in the form of physical activity. Because physical activity is one of the most effective ways you can safeguard yourself from developing a number of major chronic degenerative diseases, it's really a major investment in minimizing the risks of developing debilitating conditions. You can also add years to your life and life to your years from this investment. As you have already learned, a little can go a long way, and it doesn't take as much of an investment to begin collecting quickly on the many benefits of physical activity.

If you are currently physically active, the author commends you for including this as part of your healthy lifestyle. You may already be aware of the many dividends you are reaping from this choice. It is important to remember that the benefits of physical activity last only as long as physical activity is accomplished. Large population studies show that currently the level of physical activity decreases throughout the entire human life span largely because of societal factors. No one is immune from becoming inactive. The most significant decline occurs in young people as they enter adolescence and young adulthood. This decrease generally continues throughout college and beyond.

Physical activity plays a role in your overall health and well-being. This *connection* between physical activity and health is one that is inseparable.

Physical Activity and Health Connection

Physical activity is an essential lifestyle behavior when it comes to promoting health and preventing many major chronic diseases. It provides health benefits that cannot be obtained in any other way. It can assist with every other aspect of a healthy lifestyle and is central to wellness.

One of the most important things you can do to promote well-being is to become knowledgeable enough to take responsibility for your own health. As a college student, you are beginning to develop a personal lifestyle, which, with slight modifications, you will likely follow for the rest of your life. Practicing positive health behaviors, with systematic reinforcement and follow-up throughout your college years, can provide you with the best opportunity for achieving wellness as well as preventing the development of dangerous and health-threatening behaviors that lead to serious diseases during the middle and later years of life.

concept connections

1 **Many of us are concerned about our present and future health.** We feel that we have some control over our health through our lifestyle or behaviors—things we can do or not do—that will promote health and prevent disease. However, the actions of far too many of us do not produce the good health we desire. As a college student, you face many health choices—choices that can affect you in the "here-and-now" and for the rest of your life. You are responsible for learning and implementing the best choices regarding your health. It is a responsibility only you can own.

2 **Wellness is conceptualized as a complex interaction and integration of the seven dimensions of health, each based on a dynamic level of functioning oriented toward maximizing our potential and based on self-responsibility.** When a person makes a conscious decision to work toward these enhanced aspects of health, well-being or wellness is identified. Halbert Dunn (1967) first wrote about the upper limits of health in his book *High Level Wellness*. Dunn saw wellness as a dynamic process of change and growth that was largely determined by the decisions we make about how to live our lives.

3 **A healthy lifestyle is a recurring pattern of health-promoting and disease-preventing behaviors undertaken to achieve wellness.** It is a way of life based on the idea that our chances of self-fulfillment are increased or decreased directly by our level of health. Further, it can decrease significantly the risk of disease and increase the chances of living a high quality of life into the later decades of life.

4 **A self-change approach assumes that human beings can manage their lifestyle change and learn to control environmental factors that are detrimental to health.** It puts you in control of your health and permits you to determine what to do, how, and when to do it. A self-help approach requires planning, time and effort, and, most important, the development of special lifestyle skills.

⑤ No medicinal treatment in current or prospective use holds as much promise for sustained health as a regular program of physical activity. Regular physical activity can make you look younger, provide better weight control, give you more energy and a brighter mental outlook, relieve stress and anxiety, make you fit and flexible, and decrease your risk of serious diseases such as heart disease, cancer, diabetes, hypertension, and osteoporosis.

⑥ Current physical activity guidelines call attention to the health-related benefits of regular moderate physical activity that do not meet the traditional exercise/physical fitness guidelines. Recent research demonstrates that virtually all individuals can benefit from regular physical activity, whether they participate in vigorous exercise or some type of moderate health-enhancing physical activity. Although both moderate- and vigorous-intensity activities have important health implications, you need to understand that physical activity does not have to be strenuous to provide health-promoting benefits. In fact, the greatest proportional benefit to health is obtained when individuals change from inactivity or a sedentary state to a regular pattern of moderate-intensity physical activity.

Terms

Chronic diseases, 10
Epidemiology, 8
Exercise, 12
Health, 5
Healthy lifestyle, 9

Pathogenesis, 7
Physical activity, 10
Physical fitness, 12
Protective factor, 8

Quality of life, 7
Risk factor, 8
Salutogenesis, 7
Wellness, 5

making the connection

Destiny realizes that she is in college to learn and do well academically. Her midterm grades are fine, but she doesn't like feeling tired all the time. After reading this chapter, Destiny realizes that she must take more responsibility for how she is feeling. She surmises that the lack of physical activity in her life may be contributing to her worn-out feeling and begins to think of ways she can find time to become more physically active while still maintaining other positive aspects of college life.

Critical Thinking

1. Are you feeling lethargic and tired, like Destiny? Could it be because of a lack of physical activity? If so, what physical activity are you currently doing? If none, what can you do to increase your physical activity? Develop a list of campus events or organizations that involve physical activity (e.g., hiking club, co-ed intramural volleyball, walking club, kick boxing). Investigate several of them to see which one best fits your needs and schedule. Begin adding this activity into your daily or weekly college routine.

2. Using the seven dimensions of health, identify two behaviors you do that would be an example of enhancing each dimension.

3. The morning newspaper headline is "Scientific Studies Indicate Physical Activity Is Important to Health and Quality of Life." The article mentions studies from the *Prestigious International Health and Medicine Journal*. Later that day, you hear a local radio report suggesting that too much physical activity can lead to an instant heart attack, maybe even death. We are bombarded with health messages daily. What is your major source of health information? Television? If so, which shows in particular? Magazines? School? Friends? How carefully do you analyze health information? Do you believe most of what you read about health, or does it depend on the source?

References
· · · · · · · · · · ·

Alpert, J.S. (2009). Failing grades in the adoption of healthy lifestyle choices. *American Journal of Medicine* 122(6):493–494.

American College of Sports Medicine. (2010). *ACSM's Guidelines for Exercise Testing and Prescription*, 8th ed. Baltimore: Lippincott Williams & Wilkins.

Blair, S. (2009). Physical inactivity: The biggest public health problem of the 21st century. *British Journal of Sports Medicine* 43(1):1–2.

Centers for Disease Control and Prevention, National Center for Chronic Disease Prevention and Health Promotion. (2012a). An introduction to epidemiology. Online: http://www.cdc.gov/EXCITE/classroom/intro_epi.htm.

Centers for Disease Control and Prevention, National Center for Chronic Disease Prevention and Health Promotion. (2012b). A national chronic disease crisis: The time to act is now. Online: http://www.cdc.gov/chronicdisease/resources/publications/aag/healthy_communities.htm#aag.

Centers for Disease Control and Prevention, National Center for Chronic Disease Prevention and Health Promotion. (2012c). Preventing chronic diseases and reducing health risk factors. Online: http://www.cdc.gov/healthycommunitiesprogram/overview/diseasesandrisks.htm.

Centers for Disease Control and Prevention, National Center for Chronic Disease Prevention and Health Promotion. (2012d). U.S. physical activity statistics 2012. Online: http://www.cdc.gov/nccdphp/dnpa/physical/stats/index.htm.

Clark, B.K., Healy, G.N., Winkler, E.A., Gardiner, P.A., Sugiyama, T., Dunstan, D.W., Matthews, C.E., & Owen, N. (2011). Relationship of television time with accelerometer-derived sedentary time: NHANES. *Medicine in Science & Sports Exercise* 43:(5):822–828.

Dunn, H. (1967). *High Level Wellness*. Arlington, VA: Charles B. Slack.

King, D.E., Mainous, A.G., Carnemolla, M., & Everett, C.J. (2009). Adherence to healthy lifestyle habits in US adults. *American Journal of Medicine* 122(6):528–534.

Kotecki, J.E., & Clayton, B.C. (2003). Educating pharmacy students about nutrition and physical activity counseling. *American Journal of Health Education* 34(1):28–34.

McGinnis, J.M. (2003). A vision for health in our new century. *American Journal of Health Promotion* 18(2):146–150.

Remington, P.L., & Brownson, R.C. (2011). Fifty years of progress in chronic disease epidemiology and control. *Morbidity and Mortality Weekly Report* 60(4):70–77.

U.S. Department of Health and Human Services. (2008). Physical activity guidelines for Americans. Online: http://www.health.gov/paguidelines/pdf/paguide.pdf.

U.S. Department of Health and Human Services. (2010). Healthy People 2020: The road ahead. Online: http://www.healthypeople.gov/hp2020.

World Health Organization. (1948). *Constitution of the World Health Organization*. Geneva, Switzerland: Author.

World Health Organization. (1986). *Ottawa Charter for Health Promotion, 1986*. Geneva, Switzerland: Author.

World Health Organization. (2012). Physical inactivity: A global public health problem. Online: http://www.who.int/dietphysicalactivity/factsheet_inactivity/en/index.html.

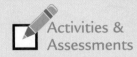

Activities & Assessments

Understanding and Enhancing Health Behaviors

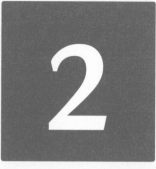

what's the connection?

Kevin is 20 years old, a college sophomore majoring in telecommunications and earning mostly As. Kevin is well liked by his classmates and is socially active in his fraternity. When he experienced low-back pain and visited the college health center, the attending physician noted that he was overweight with slightly elevated blood pressure. Questioned about physical activity, Kevin said he doesn't exercise at all. "Exercise involves a lot of discomfort and requires too much effort. The idea of participating in an activity whose mantra is 'No pain, no gain' just doesn't appeal to me," he explained. "Besides," he continued, "I'm way too busy, and don't have time to exercise. I'm here to receive treatment for low-back pain, not to start a physical activity program."

concepts

1. A self-change approach assumes that we can manage and control our own lives.

2. The transtheoretical model of health behavior change (TTM) is based on a time or temporal dimension, the stages of change, to integrate processes and principles of change using well-established psychological theories of behavioral change interventions.

3. The stages of change are a variable process that is organized on a continuum according to the decision-making process that is required to effect change.

4. Understanding or predicting when change occurs related to a specific behavior can largely be explained by decisional balance and self-efficacy.

5. The processes of change represent the mechanisms through which different techniques influence a change.

6. Successful behavior change requires careful assessment.

go.jblearning.com/kotecki4e
The website for this book is a great source for supplementary physical health information for both students and instructors. Visit **go.jblearning.com/kotecki4e** to find a variety of useful tools for learning, thinking, and teaching.

If it is to be, it is up to me.

Introduction

Lifestyle is the single most important and modifiable factor influencing health and disease today. A healthy lifestyle is described as a recurring pattern of health-promoting and disease-preventing behaviors undertaken to achieve wellness. Reducing risky behaviors is important in disease prevention. Risky behaviors eventually translate into disease, disability, and premature death. Today, the profile of diseases contributing most seriously to illness, extended pain, disability, and premature death is chronic diseases. Seven of the 10 leading causes of death each year are the result of degenerative chronic diseases (Centers for Disease Control and Prevention [CDC], 2012). The prolonged course of illness and disability from many chronic diseases is preventable. The underlying causes of these chronic diseases are common health habits that can be successfully modified years before they ultimately contribute to prolonged morbidity, needless suffering, and decreased quality of life (Cifuentes et al., 2005; Kotecki et al., 2004).

Pursuing healthy habits related to chronic disease prevention now may not seem important. Take the example of brushing your teeth, however: it prevents a lot of pain later from a dentist needing to use a high-speed drill to remove the decay (cavity) and prepare the tooth for a filling. Clean teeth look better too, and fresh breath is much more appealing. Similarly, healthy habits not only prevent or delay the onset of many chronic killers, but also add sparkle and vitality to our lives. You may be thinking that lifestyle-related chronic diseases are not likely to affect you at your age, and hopefully you are right. However, that does not mean that your current health habits are not contributing to the development of many asymptomatic disease processes. Preventing common chronic diseases and suffering later in life requires that you take action now, even though you have no symptoms of chronic disease. In fact, some health experts believe that today's youth and young adults are on their way to becoming the first generation in modern times who will have a shorter life expectancy than their parents as a result of their poor health habits (Olshansky et al., 2005). Therefore, it has become more important than ever to practice good health behaviors and eliminate detrimental ones as early in life as possible.

As a college student you are developing a personal health lifestyle, which, with slight modifications, you will likely follow for the rest your life (**FIGURE 2.1**). Every action you choose sets into motion a behavior that may become a health habit. A **health habit** is a health-related behavior that is firmly established and often performed automatically, without thought. Although the habit may have developed because it was reinforced by specific positive outcomes, eventually it becomes independent of the reinforcement process and is maintained by the environmental factors with which it is customarily associated (Hunt, Matarazzo, Weiss, & Gentry, 1979). As such, the habit can be highly resistant to change. The good news is that there are comprehensive self-change strategies available for modifying deeply rooted harmful behaviors.

> **Health habit** A health-related behavior that is firmly established and often performed automatically, without thought.

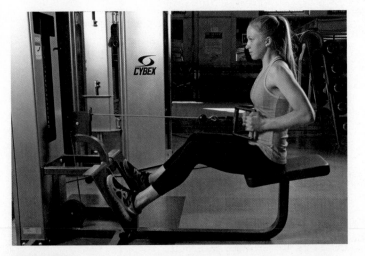

FIGURE 2.1 **Personal Health Lifestyle.** As a college student you are developing a personal health lifestyle that, with slight modifications, you will likely follow for the rest of your life.

Self-Change Approach

When you think about it, there is something truly remarkable in the fact that practically all of us want to be better than we are. Life continually presents us with opportunities for achieving what we desire (**FIGURE 2.2**). Most of us strive to be **self-changers**. Self-change means that our behavior is under our control—that when it is necessary to change, we can do it. We want to be able to control our behavior so that we can change in a desired way, increasing physical activity if we are sedentary and managing stress more effectively if we are feeling overwhelmed. Self-change means recognizing the changes you want and being able to actualize your own values. When it comes to an unhealthy lifestyle behavior, it can be a difficult task to change, however, because the thoughts that have fed our behavior for so long are deeply ingrained in our mind, and a habit of thought is hard to break. Many times our good intentions result in an unsuccessful attempt at behavior change. These failed attempts may occur because we pursue things the wrong way. Instead, we must learn to adequately prepare or ready ourselves for our eventual change.

Making important lifestyle changes—such as quitting smoking, becoming physically active, switching from junk food to nutritious food, or managing stress—requires that we go through a series of stages to adequately prepare or ready ourselves for that eventual change. Behavioral research suggests that you will more likely succeed if you think of change as a journey (**FIGURE 2.3**). It helps to have a map and to know where you are heading, the best ways to get there, and the ways to travel without getting lost or running into detours. There exists such a map, and it is discussed next. This map can keep you from getting lost and repeating errors that caused your previous good intentions to result in failures. It charts the path that successful self-changers have followed. The approach is simple to understand and makes a lot of sense when it comes to modifying problem behaviors and adding new, healthier behaviors. The approach or map is known as the transtheoretical model of behavior change, or the stages of change theory.

A self-change approach assumes that we can manage and control our own lives.

Self-changers Individuals who can manage and control their own lives.

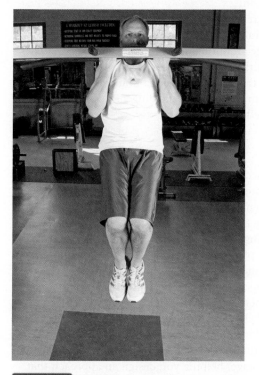

FIGURE 2.2 Self-Changers. Life continuously presents us with opportunities for achieving what we desire.

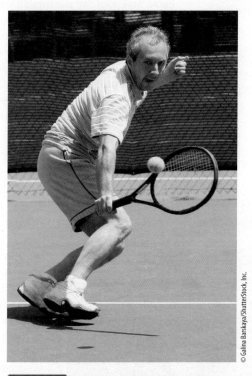

© Galina Barskaya/ShutterStock, Inc.

FIGURE 2.3 Lifestyle Changes. Behavioral research suggests that you will be more likely to succeed if you think of change as a journey.

The transtheoretical model of health behavior change (TTM) is based on a time or temporal dimension, the stages of change, to integrate processes and principles of change using well-established psychological theories of behavioral interventions.

Transtheoretical model of health behavior change (TTM) A change model that is based on a time or temporal dimension using well-established psychological theories of behavior change.

Stages of change A variable process that is organized on a continuum according to the decision-making process that is required to effect change.

Precontemplation Stage of change during which individuals are not intending to make a long-term lifestyle change in the foreseeable future (usually the next 6 months).

Transtheoretical Model of Behavior Change

The **transtheoretical model of health behavior change (TTM)** is based on a time or temporal dimension, the stages of change, to integrate processes and principles of change from other well-established psychological theories (this is the reason that it is called "transtheoretical") of behavioral interventions (Prochaska, Norcross, & DiClemente, 1994). Contrary to its long name, the TTM is a user-friendly model of change that is unique in four ways. First, it is evidence based—that means the conclusions have come out of many scientific studies of various individuals. By studying thousands of successful self-changers, scientists were able to describe how these individuals followed a commanding and controllable course to change a wide range of problem behaviors.

Second, the model conceptualizes change in stages, or as points on a motivational continuum that essentially begins with a firm conviction to maintain the status quo by never changing (precontemplation) and proceeds through the conditions of intending to change someday (contemplation), soon (preparation), now (action), and forever (maintenance/termination). The basic premise is that behavior change is a process and not an event, and that individuals are found at varying levels of motivation, or readiness, to change (**FIGURE 2.4**). They change their behavior incrementally or in a stepwise fashion.

Third, the model depicts change as a cycle as opposed to a linear progression. Typically, people move back and forth along the readiness continuum. It is not reasonable to expect everyone to be able to modify a habit perfectly without any slips. This cyclical nature of change is a normal part of the change process, indicating that it may take several trips through the various stages to make lasting change. More often, change evolves from a subtle, complex, and sometimes roundabout progression that involves thinking, hesitating, stepping forward, slipping back, and possibly starting all over again.

Fourth, each stage requires its own unique set of processes, or things people must think about or do, to be successful in moving through the stages. Identifying a person's stage of readiness for change and utilizing an intervention that matches readiness increases the likelihood that the individual will progress to at least the next stage of change. Research shows that getting someone to move just one stage forward can significantly increase his or her chances of being successful later down the road. Let's look at these distinctive features more closely.

Stages of Change or Motivational Readiness

The TTM describes change as progressing through six stages—precontemplation, contemplation, preparation, action, maintenance, and termination—that people go through along their way to eliminating problem behaviors or adopting new healthy habits. The **stages of change** are a variable process that is organized on a continuum according to the decision-making process that is required to effect change. Understanding each stage will help you determine where you are in relation to your different personal health behaviors. It is common to be at various stages of change for different behaviors. This will allow you to better match the specific behavioral-change processes with your current stage, helping you design an approach that promotes success and minimizes lapses.

Precontemplation is the stage during which individuals are not intending to make a long-term lifestyle change in the foreseeable future (usually the next 6 months); this

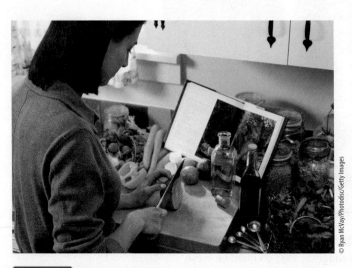

FIGURE 2.4 **Stages of Behavioral Change.** Successful self-changers recognize that behavioral change is a process.

is the "I won't" stage. Individuals in this stage are either unaware, unwilling, or too discouraged to change. They may be unaware of the risks associated with their behaviors. Or they may think, "It can't happen to me" or "It's not that serious." Or, they may want to change but do not intend to take action because they may have become discouraged as a result of being unsuccessful in previous attempts to change. A precontemplator may feel safe because he or she can't fail in this stage.

Hopefully you have discarded any lingering skepticism about the importance of regular physical activity. It should be perfectly clear that your regular participation in physical activity is vital for your health and well-being, especially as you move further through adulthood.

The **contemplation** stage begins when the individual starts to think seriously about intending to make a long-term change in the near future (within 6 months); this is the "I might" stage. In this stage, individuals are more open to information and want to learn more. They have become more aware of the problem behavior but have not yet made a commitment to act. Contemplators are not completely convinced that the effort to change is worth it and have indefinite plans to take action. It is easy to be stuck in this stage for a very long time.

Because you are reading this text, you are at least considering beginning a regular physical activity program even if it has been some time since you previously engaged in this important health behavior. You may now be thinking about getting in better shape, and specifically about how and where you might begin in the near future.

The **preparation** stage is when the individual intends to take action in the immediate future (usually in the next month); this is the "I will" stage. People in this stage realize that the behavior change is an important part of who they are. Preparers believe the effort to change is worth it and begin figuring out the best way to go about taking behavioral action. Although they have made a firm commitment to change, no consistent action has taken place.

In this stage, you feel certain that you will begin a regular exercise program soon. You might have already checked out various exercise facilities (e.g., weight room, track, basketball and tennis courts) that your college offers, signed up for an aerobics class, or talked to a friend about walking or running with you on a regular basis. As you continue to research you will have a better understanding of what types of activities are right for you.

In the **action** stage, the desired level of the new behavior has been reached, and it is consistently adhered to, although the individual has been doing it for less than 6 months; this is the "I am" stage. The individual has made significant effort to change and, more important, has achieved some degree of success with the change. Action takers need to be recognized and their new behaviors reinforced so that they continue their new behavior. Some encouragement and social support are essential because the risk for relapse in this stage is relatively high.

Have you started exercising with the intention of continuing on a regular basis? If so, you are in the action stage. In the past, you may have found it hard to adhere to an exercise program for more than a month or two. If this is the case, you will find many suggestions in this chapter to help sustain you.

The **maintenance** stage is when the behavioral practice is becoming habit; this is the "I still am" stage. People in this stage are strongly committed to their changed behavior and have maintained the desired level for more than 6 months (**FIGURE 2.5**).Maintainers have a much lower risk of relapse than action takers do. Generally, the maintenance stage lasts for up to about 5 years for many health behaviors. As the maintenance of the desired behavior becomes lengthened, heightened resistance to relapse develops over time;

The stages of change are a variable process that is organized on a continuum according to the decision-making process that is required to effect change.

Contemplation Stage of change that begins when the individual starts to think seriously about intending to make a long-term change in the near future (within 6 months).

Preparation Stage of change in which the individual intends to take action in the immediate future (usually in the next month).

Action Stage of change in which the desired level of the new behavior has been reached and is consistently adhered to, although the individual has been doing it for less than 6 months.

Maintenance Stage of change in which the behavioral practice is becoming habit.

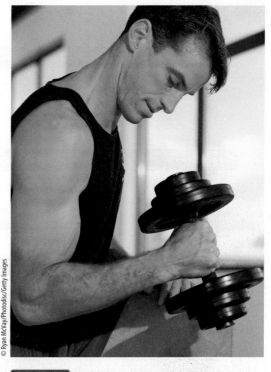

FIGURE 2.5 **Maintenance Stage.** People in this stage are strongly committed to their changed behavior and have maintained their desired level for more than 6 months.

individuals could theoretically exit the stages of change and find themselves in the termination stage.

The **termination** stage (sometimes referred to as "adoption") is when the individual no longer needs to attend to the task of maintaining the change; the behavior change is completely integrated into his or her lifestyle. This stage is usually after a positive behavior has been maintained for more than 5 years. In this stage it is no longer something you have to "do"—it's just who you are. The temptation to revert to the former behavior is completely gone and the new healthy behavior is almost an effortless part of who you are. People in this stage have complete confidence that they will cope without fear of relapse. They no longer are in the first five stages of willful change as they relate to a problem behavior and have exited the cycle of change. The whole point of mastering the skills of behavior change is to be in control of your behaviors and allow yourself to create a life of your highest choosing.

Look at the flowchart in FIGURE 2.6 . This is a useful visual aid for understanding the first five stages of change. By answering each question, you can identify your current stage or degree of intention for meeting the current recommendation for obtaining moderate-intensity physical activity. You can also substitute a number of other lifestyle questions in place of physical activity in the flowchart. It is common to be at various stages of change for different behaviors.

Understanding Relapse: The Spiral Model of Change

Linear progression through each of the five stages is a possible but relatively rare occurrence. Typically, individuals move back and forth along the change continuum a number of times before attaining their behavioral goal. Thus, the stages of change are better conceptualized as *spiraling* rather than linear (Prochaska et al., 1994) (FIGURE 2.7). In the **spiral model of change**, the good news is that all of your setbacks can be viewed positively because the path you are taking is always spiral-

> **Termination** Stage of change in which the individual's former problem behavior represents no threat or temptation; it denotes the concept of exiting the stages of change or the cycle of change.
>
> **Spiral model of change** A relapse model that demonstrates that individuals move back and forth along the change continuum a number of times before attaining their behavioral goal and therefore views setbacks as positive because changers are learning something new every time they change.

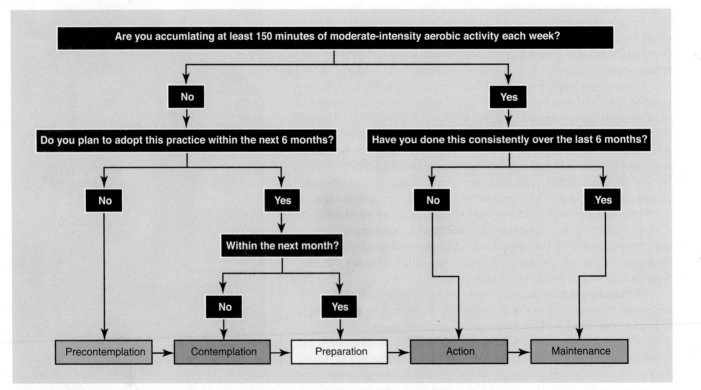

FIGURE 2.6 **Assessing Your Stage or Readiness to Change.**

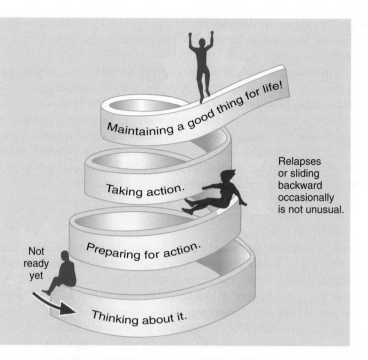

Maintaining a good thing for life!

Relapses
or sliding
backward
occasionally
is not unusual.

Taking action.

Preparing for action.

Not
ready
yet

Thinking about it.

FIGURE 2.7 **The Spiral Model of Change.** These stages represent a spiral path to adopting healthy behaviors. SOURCE: Centers for Disease Control and Prevention, National Center for Chronic Disease Prevention and Health Promotion. (2005). Physical activity for everyone: Getting started.

ing upward. Looking at relapse or a slip in this manner means that you are learning something new every time you change.

Despite our best efforts, relapses remain the rule rather than the exception when it comes to solving most of our health behavior problems. We make mistakes because we are human; we are imperfect. It is normal at the time of our relapse to be conscious of our incompetencies while lacking awareness of our abilities. The feelings and beliefs evoked by relapse are not pleasant. You may feel that you have completely failed, which may lead to guilt or embarrassment. You may begin to believe all of your efforts were wasted. A couple of setbacks in succession may trigger your wanting to give up completely on changing the problem behavior, so you slide from the action or maintenance stage back to contemplation or precontemplation and decide that you have gained nothing from your attempts. This is where you are dead wrong!

Changing unfavorable behavior patterns or adopting favorable health-enhancing ones usually requires a number of attempts. For example, even though you intend to remain an ex-smoker when you quit, you may slip up and smoke a cigarette. Slips often occur with any behavior change. Do not think about yourself as a failure; instead, think about a slip as a learning experience. Most people are not completely successful in their first couple of attempts of health behavior change. Mark Twain summed it up this way: "Quitting smoking is easy. I've done it a thousand times." Regression or relapse may occur at any part of the change sequence, but most often it happens in the action stage. For example, more than half of the individuals who begin an exercise program quit within the first 6 months, and most people need four attempts or more before they finally can quit smoking permanently.

With the stages of change, the good news is that all your setbacks are positive because you are learning new things every time you try. We can always rechart our steps and, armed with experience, make some corrections. Corrections triggered by our relapses lead to increased learning and can be responsible for improved outcomes. Never is a task completed without some modifications along the way. In fact, relapses may be thought of as necessary to focus on our health behavior change. We need to dwell not on the relapse but on the remedy. You have to have a relapse plan ready for just such a time. You need to have strategies in place that will help you get back on track, such as the support of family and friends, or a membership to a gym, or the presence of a store near you that carries fresh fruits and vegetables. You have to keep renewing your commitment to change even when it seems hardest.

One of the major reasons for relapse is that we rush through stages too quickly. When changing health habits, it is better to make one small change at a time rather than a series of sudden and dramatic changes. The latter are likely to be short-lived and you are likely to regress to your old habits very quickly. The likelihood of successfully changing problem behaviors improves when you make slow but sure changes, which give you time to unlearn negative patterns and substitute positive ones. Again, to quote Mark Twain: "Habit is habit and not to be flung out the window by man, but coaxed downstairs a step at a time."

When and Why We Change

Understanding or predicting when change occurs related to a specific behavior can largely be explained by two measures: decisional balance and self-efficacy (Prochaska & Velicer, 1997). **Decisional balance** reflects the individual's relative weighing of the pros and cons of changing (Janis & Mann, 1977). The *pros* represent the positive aspects of changing, or the benefits of change. In contrast, the *cons* are the negative aspects of changing, or the costs of change. During the precontemplation stage, the cons far outweigh the pros. In the contemplation stage, the pros and cons are balanced evenly. In the preparation stage, the balance has shifted and the pros outweigh the cons. In the advanced stages of action and maintenance, the pros continue to mount.

Listing the pros and cons as you contemplate a specific health behavior change is essential. However, many people do not correctly weigh the health and lifestyle pros and cons regarding participating or not participating in specific behaviors. For example, people who lead a sedentary lifestyle may want to spend their spare time relaxing after work by watching television or playing computer games. They may believe that exercising instead would take too much time away from their favorite activity. They are confusing what they want with what they need regarding their health. Our cultural environment further contributes to this confusion of what we want and what we need. For instance, advertisers send the messages that alcohol drinking and cigarette smoking are pleasurable and that fattening fast foods are good tasting, all of which promise immediate positive experiences. We pride ourselves on our intelligence and know that many of these products lead to harmful effects. In spite of this, we are not particularly good at weighing the short-term benefits against the long-term risks (Cloninger, 1987). This leads many of us to engage in a risky behavior and opt for short-term pleasure over long-term benefits.

So, slow down the decision-making process when you are listing your pros and cons and carefully consider the results of your specific behavior in both the short term and the long term. Become more familiar with the immediate short-term benefits associated with many health-promoting behaviors. In the previous example, people believed that participating in physical activity during their leisure time would cut into their relaxation time, as well as their television viewing time. Instead, they could relish the immediate reduction in mental and muscular tension that comes from taking a brisk 15-minute walk.

The other factor that greatly enhances motivation for change is self-efficacy. **Self-efficacy** is the confidence you have in your ability to perform specific behaviors in specific situations (Bandura, 1986). Self-efficacy assesses your belief that you can perform the behavior to achieve the desired outcome; it is your perceived confidence that you can change and maintain your behavior across a variety of difficult situations. Numerous research studies have substantiated what most people knew all along: people who strongly believe that they can initiate and adhere to a behavior change do. What's more, they exert an elevated level of effort to

Decisional balance An individual's relative weighing of the pros and cons of changing.

Self-efficacy The confidence one has in one's ability to perform specific behaviors in specific situations.

Understanding or predicting when change occurs related to a specific behavior can largely be explained by decisional balance and self-efficacy.

accomplish this goal, persisting in the face of the difficulties that inevitably rise. Similarly, people who believe they will fail usually do. In other words, there is truth to the adage "Whether you believe you can, or whether you believe you can't, you are probably right."

In studies that have measured the self-efficacy of people in different stages of change, self-efficacy has been found to increase steadily from precontemplation to contemplation to preparation, but rises significantly in the action and maintenance stages, when actual performance attainment is most evident and convincing. Highly self-efficacious persons invest more effort and persist longer to accomplish a specific behavior than those low in self-efficacy. Self-efficacy is specific to each behavior. A person who feels confident about exercising after work every day may have less belief in his or her ability to reduce saturated fat from his or her diet on a regular basis.

ENHANCING SELF-EFFICACY   According to Bandura (1986), you can enhance self-efficacy beliefs in four important ways: performance attainment, vicarious experience, verbal persuasion, and physiological states. *Performance attainments* are the most convincing because they are based on personal success experiences. Having swum on the high school swimming team will no doubt enhance your belief that you can choose swimming as part of your college physical activity program. Vicarious experience increases self-efficacy through observing the effective performances of others. If you are a nonswimmer, watching your friends swim may convince you that you can learn to swim. *Verbal persuasion*, or counseling, is thought to be less effective than vicarious experience, but it can be useful nevertheless to have a good friend talk you through the swim experience. The final source upon which self-efficacy beliefs are based are *physiological cues* that people experience when facing a challenge. These cues in turn affect performance (correctly or not). For example, you may feel a bit anxious about getting into the deep end of the pool, which leads to a racing heart rate or rapid breathing; this will adversely affect your performance in the water. You may question your ability to successfully complete the task. Conversely, if your friend reminds you that this is normal and that he is a certified lifeguard and will keep a close watch, you will be more relaxed and calm and more self-confident, enhancing your performance in the water. Physiological cues are the weakest influence of the four presented here.

How We Change

The stages of change call attention to particular shifts that occur in intention and behavior. This part of the TTM describes nine processes that we engage in when we attempt to modify our behaviors (Prochaska et al., 1994). The processes were identified by asking people how they changed, what helped, and what made change more difficult. The **processes of change** represent the mechanisms through which different techniques influence a change. The processes are divided into two categories: cognitive/emotional (involving thinking, attitudes, and feelings) and behavioral (involving actions). Cognitive/emotional processes include (1) increasing knowledge, (2) experiencing negative emotions, (3) caring about others, (4) comprehending personal benefits, and (5) committing yourself; behavioral processes include (1) rewarding yourself, (2) eliciting social support, (3) substituting alternatives, and (4) reminding yourself.

Furthermore, each stage requires its own unique set of processes, or things we must think about or do, to move to the next stage successfully (**FIGURE 2.8**). In summary, these processes are any activities you initiate to help modify your thinking, feelings, or behaviors to progress through the stages of change. Following is a brief description of the nine major processes of change, along with a single technique that may be used to mediate change. It is important to remember that for

The processes of change represent the mechanisms through which different techniques influence a change.

Processes of change The mechanisms through which different techniques influence a person's behavior change.

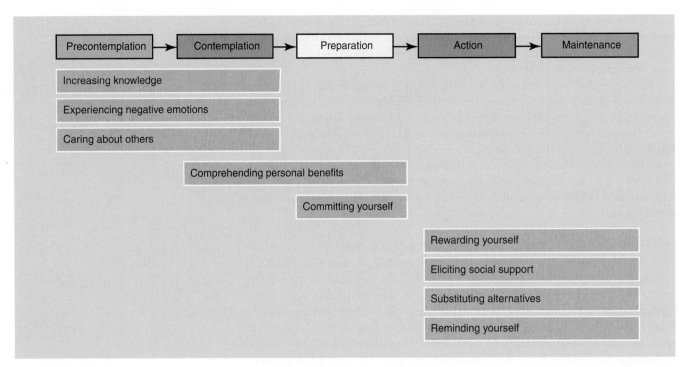

FIGURE 2.8 **The Process of Change, or How Change Occurs.** Applicable processes of change during each stage of change.

each process a myriad of techniques can be employed. Some of these techniques also can be used with more than one process.

INCREASING KNOWLEDGE   This process requires assimilating accurate and detailed information so that you can have an advanced understanding of the behavior. For example, not only do you know that a sedentary lifestyle and unhealthy eating habits are harmful to your health, but you know that they are linked to an increased risk of more than 20 physical ailments, as well as a number of psychological problems. One way to increase your knowledge or awareness related to your lifestyle is to measure what you are doing now.

EXPERIENCING NEGATIVE EMOTIONS   This process relates to a deeper way of increasing awareness by seeing when and how your problem behavior conflicts with your personal values. You begin to become afraid or fear the consequences of not participating in a particular health behavior. For example, how do you perceive yourself as a sedentary person? To express your emotions about it, try the following rational emotive technique recommended by Ellis and Harper (1971).
   Using a journal:
1. Record the events as they occurred at the time you felt emotionally uneasy about becoming physically active. Be objective and avoid judgments.
2. Next, write down your subjective assumptions, worries, and beliefs related to your emotions about becoming physically active.
3. Then, write down your emotions about physical activity, stating both appropriate and inappropriate emotions.
4. Finally, list your beliefs about why you had the right to be upset by the events and to respond the way you did. Is there support or truth for any of your beliefs? Explore appropriate alternative thoughts, emotions, and actions.

CARING FOR OTHERS   This process requires that you recognize the harmful effects of how participating in a problem behavior affects your family, friends, and others around you. A way to see if this is the case is to use a self-monitoring record-keeping technique (FIGURE 2.9). Record each of the times you practiced a problem behavior during the past 2 weeks. Next to each, write down whether you felt you were a poor role model for those around you or whether your problem behavior negatively affected others. For example, if you are a cigarette smoker, did children or young adults see you light up a cigarette or did others around you have to inhale the smoke from your cigarette?

COMPREHENDING PERSONAL BENEFITS   This process requires a thoughtful appraisal of what your self-concept or self-identity is like while continuing a problem behavior and what it would be after changing it. Several of the successes and failures that we experience in many areas of life are closely related to the ways that we have learned to view ourselves and our relationships with others. Some people tend to focus on their weaknesses rather than their strengths. For example, when it comes to exercise, they may see themselves as uncoordinated, too slow, or nonathletic. These are all self-limiting thoughts. Self-talk phrased in the negative regarding something positive is processed by the mind as a punishment and wastes valuable energy.

Instead, you could use positive affirmations or self-talk and thereby increase your self-concept regarding exercise. An *affirmation* is a statement that claims characteristics of the ideal self. Focus on your strengths rather than your weaknesses. Changing your statements to yourself to "I like to take brisk walks" or "I feel more confident when I exercise" or "I feel better about myself when I exercise" allows you to use energy as a positive search for ways that will eventually lead to your goal. Remember, your self-concept reflects years of experience and self-evaluation. It will take a few days to get to know and record the internal critic. Challenging or shutting up the critic may take weeks. Continually increase the number of positive affirmations you make about exercise. Self-talk, when positive, cultivates a healthy self-concept—one that offers security. Taking charge of the messages we send ourselves is an option that is always available to us (FIGURE 2.10).

COMMITTING YOURSELF   This process is related to the belief that you can change and the commitment to act on that belief. Making a self-contract is a very helpful technique in this process. Try making a physical activity contract with yourself. This interpersonal agreement to act should be consistent with your physically active self-image. You must understand what motivates you to be physically active and write it down. Research shows that goals are more likely to be accomplished when they are written down. Don't just think it, ink it. Be as specific as possible in detailing your goal of physical activity (FIGURE 2.11). When you commit in writing what you want to accomplish, you increase the likelihood that you will act accordingly within a certain period of time. Eliciting this type of personal commitment has been shown to be one of the most important aspects of health behavior change, especially when you share this self-contract with others close to you.

REWARDING YOURSELF   This process is based on the fact that a response followed promptly by an effective reward (reinforcement) is more likely to occur again. This is called the law of effect; it is the basis of operant conditioning and the major means of changing voluntary

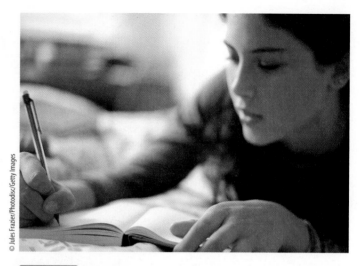

© Jules Frazier/Photodisc/Getty Images

FIGURE 2.9 **Self-Monitoring Technique.** A daily planner is a helpful behavior change tool.

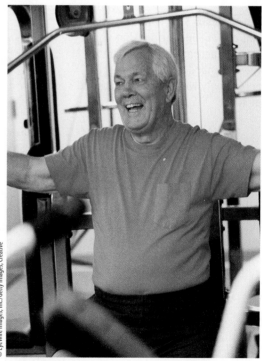

© EyeWire Images, Inc./Getty Images, Creative

FIGURE 2.10 **Positive Affirmations.** Repeated successful performances increase your confidence to perform the desired activity.

Start date: _____   Finish date: _____

Goal: _____

Motivation (benefits): _____

Identify your current stage of change: _____

Match your current stage of change and other stages you anticipate progressing through with the appropriate processes of change (refer to Figure 2.8):

_____   _____

_____   _____

What specific techniques will you use for each of the processes identified above?	
Processes	Specific Techniques
Stage of change on the finish date:	

Mini goals   Date   Reward

_____   _____   _____

_____   _____   _____

_____   _____   _____

I, _____, agree to work toward a healthier lifestyle and in doing so shall comply with the terms and dates of this contract.

Signature: _____   Date: _____

Witness: _____   Date: _____

FIGURE 2.11 Self-Contract. When you commit in writing what you want to accomplish, you increase the likelihood that you will act accordingly within a certain period of time.

behavior. Periodically check your goals and reward yourself for your progress toward specific goals. Internal reinforcement is generally better than external. However, this author recommends both. An internal reinforcement occurs when your own experience or perception of an event has value. For example, when you finish your run for the day, you feel a sense of enjoyment or accomplishment. Relive your positive experiences by stating aloud to yourself and others that you are proud of your recent accomplishments: "I feel good about myself after running 2 miles." Remember, positive self-talk allows a flow of positive energy that not only makes a goal obtainable, but also can significantly assist in maintaining it. An external reinforcement would be providing yourself with a special treat, such as buying a new outfit when a short-term weight goal has been reached.

ELICITING SOCIAL SUPPORT   One of the most important external resources is the availability of social support. This process is defined as information from others that one is loved, cared for, valued, and esteemed. It is much easier to maintain your habit of regular physical activity if you are encouraged by others. Share your goals with your friends and family. Obtaining encouragement and support from significant people in your life is a powerful reinforcement for keeping you on your physical activity program. Social support can be obtained by signing up for an exercise class at your college or university or organizing your own physical activity group that meets regularly.

SUBSTITUTING ALTERNATIVES   The basic idea with this process is that you substitute an alternate healthy behavior for those behavior traits that lead to the problem behavior. Because all of our behavior is conditional, it becomes important to anticipate the trigger situations and then counter the urges you know are coming by substituting a healthier alternative. For example, if you know that around 8:00 p.m. every evening you start craving sweets, eat a piece of fruit—a snack that's low-calorie, nutritious, and somewhat sweet. Alternatively, substitute a brisk walk in place of eating the sweets. Physical activity reduces cravings as effectively as sweets and expends calories rather than accumulating them. Furthermore, even something like a short, brisk walk can enhance your mood and relieve stress, as well as remove you physically from the temptation.

REMINDING YOURSELF   This process is similar to substituting alternatives in that it is action-oriented; however, cravings or temptations are eliminated by restructuring the environment to eliminate the stimulus. For example, try having cut-up fruit and vegetables ready to eat in the refrigerator rather than sweets such as soda and ice cream. If you are a smoker, remove the ashtrays from the house. Other techniques include using reminder systems. Place positive reminders throughout your environment to prompt you. These reminders can take the form of notes left in places where you will see them, such as your daily planner or the front of the refrigerator or television.

Making a Behavioral Change Plan

What one thing do you most want to change about your health this semester? Successful behavior change requires a careful assessment of exactly what it is that you want to change. Having a long laundry list of items only serves to discourage you, scatter your focus, and slow significant progress toward accomplishing even one goal. For instance, did you place becoming physically active at the top of the list and then follow that with four other items of equal importance? This may set the stage for failure. After assessing yourself, focus on one change; commit to it, and the rest may very well be addressed along the way. A resolution to achieve a healthy lifestyle, one goal at a time, opens the door to daily success.

If you are in the early cognitive stages of change—that is, thinking about whether the pros outweigh the cons of making the change (decisional balance) or making decisions about whether you have the skills and resources to make the necessary changes (self-efficacy)—you may not be ready for behavioral action. However, if you have committed to changing one specific behavior, your motivation is high enough to begin to set actual behavioral goals (preparation stage).

Setting SMART Goals

To properly set a goal, it is recommended that you follow a set of standard guidelines. An effective expression of these guidelines is that you should set SMART goals. SMART stands for specific, measurable, attainable, relevant, and trackable.

- *Specific.* A specific goal has a much greater chance of being accomplished than does a general goal. With a specific goal, you can clearly see what it is you want to achieve, and you have specific standards for that achievement. A general goal would be "get some physical activity." But a specific goal would be "I am going to make brisk walking part of my physical activity program."

Successful behavior change requires careful assessment.

- *Measurable.* A measurable goal establishes concrete criteria for quantifying progress. The goal needs to have a yardstick for measuring outcomes. It should take into account the principle of a specific goal as well. For example, "I am going to walk briskly for 30 minutes on Monday, Wednesday, and Friday."
- *Attainable.* A goal needs to stretch you slightly so that you feel you can do it, and it will need a real commitment from you. Although it is important to set goals just out of reach, it is imperative not to set goals that are so high that they are unattainable. If your goal is not attainable, chances are you will give up hope trying to reach it and quit. You may even want to break down your goal into different measured parts by setting short-term goals as well as long-term goals. Short-term goals are ones that you will achieve in the near future (e.g., in a day, within a week, within a few months). Long-term goals are ones that you will achieve over a longer period of time (e.g., 1 semester, 1 year, 5 years, 20 years).
- *Relevant.* Make sure the goal is consistent with other goals you have established for yourself and that it fits into your immediate and long-term plans. In other words, your goal should be important to you, rather than simply done as an assignment for class.
- *Trackable.* Trackable goals allow you to monitor your progress (**FIGURE 2.12**). By monitoring your progress, you will be able to see what you have achieved. Monitoring your progress is simply a case of writing down everything you did related to accomplishing your goal. For example, you may want to to record your physical activity sessions or use a food intake log to monitor your diet.

Using the flowchart in Figure 2.6, you can assess your level of readiness for a number of health behaviors. Depending on your stage of readiness, your goals will be different. You will learn to write SMART goals.

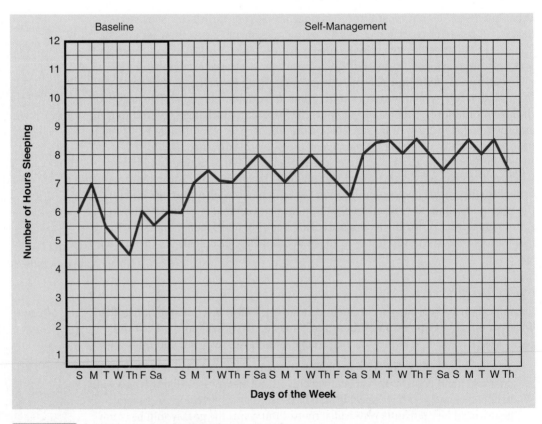

FIGURE 2.12 **Self-Managed Behavior Change Graph.**

Physical Activity and Health Connection

The path to obtaining a high quality of life, or a wellness lifestyle, lies in our behaviors. Our choices and subsequent actions make our lives what they are. They *do* make an enormous difference. With respect to overall health, no behaviors are more essential than performing regular stimulating physical activity and eating nutritious food. The human body is clearly designed for physical activity. If you want to remain healthy, regular physical activity should be part of your lifestyle.

In today's world, physical activity is a unique health behavior that encompasses a complex and dynamic range of behavioral demands. Planning for physical activity, its initial adoption, and your continued participation and maintenance involves different factors and justifies different self-change techniques. As a college instructor, I know that informing my students about the many benefits of physical activity is important but not necessarily enough to get my students to do it regularly. To become and stay physically active takes time, effort, and, most important, the development of special self-change skills. This chapter provides you with a state-of-the-art, step-by-step approach to behavior change that utilizes various skill-building strategies for including regular physical activity in your life. It concludes with ways to set a goal properly.

concept connections

1. **A self-change approach assumes that we can manage and control our own lives.** We want to be able to control our behavior so that we can change in a desired way, increasing physical activity if we are sedentary and managing stress more effectively if we are feeling overwhelmed. Self-change means recognizing the changes you want and being able to actualize your own values.

2. **The transtheoretical model of health behavior change (TTM) is based on a time or temporal dimension, the stages of change, to integrate processes and principles of change using well-established psychological theories of behavioral change interventions.** Behavioral research suggests that you will more likely succeed if you think of change as a journey. It helps to have a map and to know where you are heading, the best ways to get there, and the ways to travel without getting lost or running into detours. The transtheoretical model is such a map.

3. **The stages of change are a variable process that is organized on a continuum according to the decision-making process that is required to effect change.** This process begins with a firm conviction of maintaining the status quo by never changing (precontemplation) and proceeds through the conditions of intending to change someday (contemplation), soon (preparation), now (action), and forever (maintenance). The basic premise is that behavior change is a process and not an event, and that individuals are found at varying levels of motivation, or readiness to change.

④ **Understanding or predicting when change occurs related to a specific behavior can largely be explained by decisional balance and self-efficacy.** Decisional balance reflects your relative weighing of the pros and cons of changing. The *pros* represent the positive aspects of changing, or the benefits of change. In contrast, the *cons* are the negative aspects of changing, or the costs of change. Self-efficacy assesses your belief that you can perform the behavior to achieve the desired outcome; it is your perceived confidence that you can change and maintain your behavior across a variety of difficult situations.

⑤ **The processes of change represent the mechanisms through which different techniques influence a change.** The processes are divided into two categories: cognitive/emotional (involving thinking, attitudes, and feelings) and behavioral (involving actions). Cognitive/emotional processes include (1) increasing knowledge, (2) experiencing negative emotions, (3) caring about others, (4) comprehending personal benefits, and (5) committing yourself; behavioral processes include (1) rewarding yourself, (2) eliciting social support, (3) substituting alternatives, and (4) reminding yourself.

⑥ **Successful behavior change requires careful assessment.** To set a goal properly, you should follow a set of standard guidelines. An effective expression of these guidelines is that you should set SMART goals. SMART stands for specific, measurable, attainable, relevant, and trackable.

Terms
. . . .

making the connection

Based on what you have read in this chapter about the stages of change, Kevin would be considered to be in the precontemplation stage. Kevin is not ready to begin a physical activity program at this time. He may need to increase his knowledge about the benefits of participating in a regular physical activity program. In addition, Kevin may want to acknowledge his feelings related to participating in regular physical activity by using the rational emotive technique described in this chapter (see the section titled "How We Change").

Critical Thinking

1. Often, like Kevin, we are not ready to make a health behavior change, especially if we think our effort will be greater than the benefit of the behavior. List 10 reasons people begin a physical activity program (benefits) and 10 reasons people do not begin a physical activity program (barriers). Put an "L" next to the benefits that are long term and a "B" next to those that are short term. Turning to the barriers, indicate which you have control over and which you do not. Do the barriers seem to outweigh the benefits? Next, focus on short-term benefits and on barriers over which you have control. Does this change the picture?

2. As a friend, housemate, fraternity brother, or sorority sister, what role(s) can you play in supporting someone who is beginning a physical activity program? In analyzing your role, be aware of things you might do that would deter your friend from beginning or maintaining a physical activity program. Avoid those behaviors.

References

Bandura, A. (1986). *Social Foundations of Thought and Action: A Social Cognitive Theory*. Englewood Cliffs, NJ: Prentice Hall.

Centers for Disease Control and Prevention, National Center for Chronic Disease Prevention and Health Promotion. (2012). Chronic disease overview. Online: http://www.cdc.gov/NCCdphp/overview .htm.

Cifuentes, M., Fernald, D.H., Green, L.A., Niebauer, L.J., Stange, K.C., & Hassmiller, S.B. (2005). Prescription for health: Changing primary care practice to foster healthy behaviors. *Annuals of Family Medicine* 3(Suppl. 2):4–11.

Cloninger, C.R. (1987). A systematic method for clinical description and classification of personality variants. *Archives of General Psychiatry* 44:573–588.

Ellis, A., & Harper, R. (1971). *A Guide to Rational Living*. Hollywood, CA: Wilshire.

Hunt, W.A., Matarazzo, J.D., Weiss, S.M., & Gentry, W.D. (1979). Associative learning, habit, and health behavior. *Journal of Behavioral Medicine* 2:111–115.

Janis, I.L., & Mann, L. (1977). *Decision Making: A Psychological Analysis of Conflict, Choice and Commitment*. New York: Free Press.

Kotecki, J.E., McKenzie, J.F., Banter, A.E., Bird, J.C., Reece, J.S., & Brown, S.C. (2004). Indiana family physicians: Beliefs and practices regarding health promotion. *Journal of Eta Sigma Gamma* 36(1):13–22.

Olshansky, S.J., Passaro, D.J., Hershow, R.C., Layden, J., Carnes, B.A., Brody, J., Hayflick, L., Butler, R.N., Allison, D.B., & Ludwig, D.S. (2005). A potential decline in life expectancy in the United States in the 21st century. *New England Journal of Medicine* 352:1138–1145.

Prochaska, J.O., Norcross, J.C., & DiClemente, C.C. (1994). *Changing for Good*. New York: Avon.

Prochaska, J.O., & Velicer, W.F. (1997). The transtheoretical model of health behavior change. *American Journal of Health Promotion* 12(1):38–48.

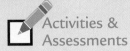

Activities &
Assessments

3.1   PAR-Q and You

3.2   Medical History
       Questionnaire

3.3   President's Challenge Adult
       Fitness Test

© Ryan McVay/Photodisc/Getty Images

Principles of Physical Fitness Development

3

what's the connection?

R on is planning to start a regular physical activity program soon. He has never participated in one before. Ron feels out of shape and has gained nearly 10 pounds over the last year. His schedule has been stressful, with university classes during the day and many hours of studying at night. After reading about how physical activity is an essential lifestyle behavior for promoting health and utilizing behavior change cognitive processes, Ron wants to learn more about how to get started and exactly which activities would be best for him to incorporate into his physical activity program.

concepts

1. The *Physical Activity Guidelines for Americans* published by the U.S. Department of Health and Human Services are designed to provide information and guidance on the types and amounts of physical activity that provide substantial health benefits for Americans age 6 years and older.

2. Health-related fitness contributes to developing optimum health, preventing the onset of chronic disease, or reversing an established chronic disease process associated with inactivity.

3. Several basic scientific fitness principles must be adhered to in order to develop an effective physical fitness program.

4. Before starting a physical activity program, it is important to complete a self-prescreening and self-assessment and to set specific goals.

5. Physical activity programs must be tailored to meet the needs of the individual.

go.jblearning.com/kotecki4e
The website for this book is a great source for supplementary physical health information for both students and instructors. Visit **go.jblearning.com/kotecki4e** to find a variety of useful tools for learning, thinking, and teaching.

Lack of activity destroys the good condition of every human being, while movement and methodical physical exercise save it and preserve it.

—Plato

Introduction

> **Physical activity** Any bodily movement produced by the contraction of skeletal muscle that increases energy expenditure above a basal (resting) level.

Physical activity is an essential lifestyle behavior when it comes to promoting health and preventing a myriad of disabling ailments and diseases. This statement is based on the conclusion of hundreds of scientists and health professionals who reviewed thousands of scientific studies showing that physically active people have higher levels of health-related fitness, a lower risk profile for developing a number of disabling medical conditions, and lower rates of various chronic degenerative diseases (U.S. Department of Health and Human Services [USDHHS], 2008).

This chapter provides an overview of the recommended amounts and types of physical activity for improved health and fitness. This includes both lifestyle physical activity and more formal exercise programs. It describes the components of physical fitness and outlines the systematic scientific principles that provide a framework to develop a personal conditioning program. Finally, fundamental elements on getting started and designing an exercise program that meets your own personal goals are explained.

The *Physical Activity Guidelines for Americans* published by the U.S. Department of Health and Human Services are designed to provide information and guidance on the types and amounts of physical activity that provide substantial health benefits for Americans age 6 years and older.

Physical Activity Guidelines for Americans

The main idea behind the *Physical Activity Guidelines for Americans*, which is published by the U.S. Department of Health and Human Services, is that regular physical activity over months and years can produce long-term health benefits (USDHHS, 2008). These *Guidelines* are necessary because of the importance of physical activity to the health of Americans, whose current inactivity puts them at unnecessary risk of developing many chronic degenerative diseases. The latest data show that inactivity among American adults and youth remains relatively high and insufficient progress has been made in increasing the level of physical activity in the population. Therefore, the guidelines' primary focus is on the strategy of physical activity for health rather than an exercise for fitness strategy.

According to the *Physical Activity Guidelines*, to attain the most benefit from physical activity by the broad population, who have different and diverse health needs:

> Adults need at least 150 minutes (2 hours and 30 minutes) of moderate-intensity aerobic activity or 75 minutes (1 hour and 15 minutes) of vigorous-intensity aerobic activity every week or an equivalent mix of moderate- and vigorous-intensity aerobic activity and muscle-strengthening activities on 2 or more days a week that work all major muscle groups (legs, hips, back, abdomen, chest, shoulders, and arms). (USDDHS, 2008)

TABLE 3.1 provides six different examples of how you can meet the *Guidelines* each week.

Note that there are differences in the duration and intensity of aerobic physical activity needed to obtain and maintain health in this recommendation. Time depends on intensity. The intensity of physical activity, or how hard your body is working, is usually categorized as light, moderate, or vigorous based on the amount of effort or energy you expend in performing physical activity. Light-intensity activities require more time than moderate-intensity activities, and moderate-intensity activities require more time than high-intensity activities. Light-intensity activities include walking slowly and easy gardening. Moderate-intensity activities are those that require you to exert some effort but not to push

TABLE 3.1	**There Are a Lot of Ways to Get the Physical Activity You Need!**

If you're thinking, "How can I meet the *Guidelines* each week?" don't worry. You'll be surprised by the variety of activities you have to choose from. Basically anything counts as long as it's at a moderate or vigorous intensity for at least 10 minutes at a time. If you're not sure where to start, here are some examples of weekly activity routines you may want to try.

Moderate Aerobic Activity Routines

	Monday	Tuesday	Wednesday	Thursday	Friday	Saturday	Sunday	Physical Activity TOTAL
Example 1	30 minutes of brisk walking	30 minutes of brisk walking	Resistance band exercises	30 minutes of brisk walking	30 minutes of brisk walking	Resistance band exercises	30 minutes of brisk walking	**150 minutes moderate-intensity aerobic activity AND 2 days muscle strengthening**
Example 2	30 minutes of brisk walking	60 minutes of playing softball	30 minutes of brisk walking	30 minutes of mowing the lawn		Heavy gardening	Heavy gardening	**150 minutes moderate-intensity aerobic activity AND 2 days muscle strengthening**

Vigorous Aerobic Activity Routines

	Monday	Tuesday	Wednesday	Thursday	Friday	Saturday	Sunday	Physical Activity TOTAL
Example 3	25 minutes of jogging	Weight lifting	25 minutes of jogging	Weight lifting	25 minutes of jogging			**75 minutes vigorous-intensity aerobic activity AND 2 days muscle strengthening**
Example 4	25 minutes of swimming laps		25 minutes of running	Weight training		25 minutes of singles tennis	Weight training	**75 minutes vigorous-intensity aerobic activity AND 2 days muscle strengthening**

Mix of Moderate and Vigorous Activity Routines

	Monday	Tuesday	Wednesday	Thursday	Friday	Saturday	Sunday	Physical Activity TOTAL
Example 5	30 minutes of water aerobics	30 minutes of jogging	30 minutes of brisk walking and yoga		30 minutes of brisk walking	Yoga		**90 minutes moderate-intensity aerobic activity AND 30 minutes vigorous-intensity aerobic activity AND 2 days muscle strengthening**
Example 6	45 minutes of doubles tennis and weight lifting		Rock climbing		30 minutes of vigorous hiking		45 minutes of doubles tennis	**90 minutes moderate-intensity aerobic activity AND 30 minutes vigorous-intensity aerobic activity AND 2 days muscle strengthening**

SOURCE: Centers for Disease Control and Prevention. (2009). Adding physical activity to your life. Online: http://www.cdc.gov/physicalactivity/downloads/pa_examples.

yourself as hard as more vigorous activities—for example, brisk walking (15 to 20 minutes per mile) as compared with running (8 to 12 minutes per mile).

Moderate-intensity activities can be distinguished from vigorous-intensity activities using the **talk test** (TABLE 3.2). As a general rule of thumb, if you are doing moderate-intensity aerobic activity, you can talk but not sing the words to your favorite song. When you perform vigorous-intensity aerobic activity you cannot say more than a few words without pausing for a breath (Centers for Disease Control and Prevention [CDC], 2009). To meet the guidelines for aerobic activity, basically anything counts, as long as it is done at a moderate or vigorous intensity for at least 10 minutes at a time.

Finally, the *Physical Activity Guidelines* state that adults should increase their aerobic activity time once initial levels are achieved to obtain additional health benefits. For even greater health benefits:

> adults should increase their activity to 300 minutes (5 hours) of moderate-intensity aerobic activity or 150 minutes (2 hours and 30 minutes) of vigorous-intensity aerobic activity every week or an equivalent mix of moderate- and vigorous-intensity aerobic activity and muscle-strengthening activities on 2 or more days a week that work all major muscle groups (legs, hips, back, abdomen, chest, shoulders, and arms). (USDDHS, 2008)

> **Talk test** A simply way to measure relative aerobic intensity.

TABLE 3.2   The Talk Test

How can I tell a moderate-level activity from a vigorous-level activity? Vigorous activities take more effort than moderate ones. Here are just a few moderate and vigorous aerobic physical activities. Do these for *10 minutes or more* at a time.

Moderate Activities *(I can talk while I do them, but I can't sing.)*
- Ballroom and line dancing
- Biking on level ground or with few hills
- Canoeing
- General gardening (e.g., raking, trimming shrubs)
- Sports where you catch and throw (e.g., baseball, softball, volleyball)
- Tennis (doubles)
- Using your manual wheelchair
- Using hand cyclers (also called ergometers)
- Walking briskly
- Water aerobics

Vigorous Activities *(I can only say a few words without stopping to catch my breath.)*
- Aerobic dance
- Biking faster than 10 miles per hour
- Fast dancing
- Heavy gardening (e.g., digging, hoeing)
- Hiking uphill
- Jumping rope
- Martial arts (e.g., karate)
- Race walking, jogging, or running
- Sports with a lot of running (e.g., basketball, hockey, soccer)
- Swimming fast or swimming laps
- Tennis (singles)

SOURCE: U.S. Department of Health and Human Services. (2008). *Physical Activity Guidelines for Americans.* Be active your way: A fact sheet for adults. Online: www.health.gov/paguidelines/pdf/fs_adult.pdf.

TABLE 3.3 provides a classification of the total weekly amounts of moderate-intensity aerobic physical activity and the accompanying health benefits based on four categories: inactive, low, medium, and high. Although the data are limited, the current research literature suggests that for health benefits, the frequency of aerobic activity is much less important than the amount or intensity. Besides aerobic activity, the *Guidelines* recommend that you do things to strengthen your major muscle groups at least 2 days a week (see Table 3.1). After you include the physical activity for health guidelines as part of your lifestyle, you can consider a variety of additional fitness and performance goals based on personal interests.

Exercise Guidelines for Obtaining Optimal Health and Fitness

The American College of Sports Medicine (ACSM) is the largest and foremost exercise science organization in the world and promotes fitness, physical performance, health, and quality of life. Consistent with the *Physical Activity Guidelines for Americans* that emphasize physical activity for health, the ACSM has also established exercise for fitness recommendations for individuals wishing to obtain optimal fitness and health benefits. According to the ACSM "a program of regular exercise that includes cardiorespiratory, resistance, flexibility, neuromotor exercise training *beyond* activities of daily living to improve and maintain physical fitness and health is *essential* for most adults" (ACSM, 2011). The ACSM recommendations on quantity and quality of exercise for adults fall into four categories (2011):

1. *Cardiorespiratory exercise.* Moderate-intensity cardiorespiratory exercise training for 30 minutes or more on at least 5 days a week for a total of 150 minutes a week, or vigorous-intensity cardiorespiratory exercise for 20 minutes or more on at least 3 days a week for a total of 75 minutes a week, or a combination of moderate- and vigorous-intensity exercise to achieve cardiorespiratory benefits.
2. *Resistance exercise.* Strength training or weight lifting should be performed on 2–3 days a week for each of the major muscle groups using a variety of exercises and equipment.

TABLE 3.3   Classification of Total Weekly Amounts of Aerobic Physical Activity Into Four Categories

Levels of Physical Activity	Range of Moderate-Intensity Minutes a Week	Summary of Overall Health Benefits	Comments
Inactive	No activity beyond baseline	None	Being inactive is unhealthy.
Low	Activity beyond baseline but fewer than 150 minutes a week	Some	Low levels of activity are clearly preferable to an inactive lifestyle.
Medium	150 minutes to 300 minutes a week	Substantial	Activity at the high end of this range has additional and more extensive health benefits than activity at the low end.
High	More than 300 minutes a week	Additional	Current science does not allow researchers to identify an upper limit of activity above which there are no additional health benefits.

SOURCE: U.S. Department of Health and Human Services. (2008). *Physical Activity Guidelines for Americans*. Online: http://www.health.gov/paguidelines/pdf/fs_adults.pdf.

3. *Flexibility exercise.* Stretching exercises for each of the major muscle–tendon groups on at least 2 or 3 days a week is recommended to improve and maintain joint range of movement.

4. *Neuromotor exercise.* Sometimes called "functional fitness training," this is recommended 2 to 3 days a week. Exercises should include activities that improve balance, stability, agility, and coordination.

The ACSM exercise recommendations are designed for the middle to higher end of the physical activity continuum.

My Physical Activity and Exercise Pyramid

The My Physical Activity and Exercise Pyramid is a great visual tool to help you integrate the *Physical Activity Guidelines for Americans* and the ACSM exercise guidelines for obtaining optimal health and fitness (FIGURE 3.1). The pyramid graphics and text convey the different types of activities, each with its own unique benefit, that help adults combine regular lifestyle physical activity with a comprehensive exercise program to improve and maintain physical fitness and health. By providing a visual, the pyramid not only shows you where you are starting but also lets you see where you want to go in terms of increasing physical activity and exercise levels throughout the day and week.

The four levels represent the incremental or progressive nature of physical activity and personal fitness conditioning. Additionally, each level expresses frequency by proportionality; as one moves up the levels of the pyramid, the frequency of participation decreases. Level 1 activities should be performed every day, but levels 2 and 3, because they are more intense, structured, and repetitive activities, can be performed less often. Level 4, sustained sitting or sedentary behavior, should be closely monitored because it has been shown to be a health risk on its own. It is a distinct form of human behavior and should not be regarded as the endpoint of the physical activity continuum (Katzmarzyk et al., 2009). A deeper understanding of each level will allow you to participate in all types of physical activity in the pyramid, and that should be the ultimate goal because it will produce optimal health and fitness benefits.

If you are not active at all, any amount of physical activity is a step in the right direction, and level 1 or the base is where you want to begin. Some physical activity is better than none. Labor-saving devices, cars, televisions, and other machines and gadgets can undermine the need for bodily movement. Even for those with hectic work schedules, being physically active can be achieved at home, at work, during a commute, or during leisure time. The goal is to engage in intermittent light- or moderate-intensity physical activity anytime, anywhere. Examples of lifestyle activities at this level include task-oriented physical activities like walking to class instead of driving, taking the stairs instead of the elevator, and doing household tasks. Regard this type of movement as an opportunity, not an inconvenience. Active leisure-time intermittent activities like playing golf, going bowling, and getting up to dance count as well. Pick an activity you like and one that fits your lifestyle. Health scientists have noted that regular lifestyle activities provide health and chronic disease risk reduction benefits for those who have been inactive (refer to Table 3.3). Because they are light- or moderate-intensity activities, they should be performed as often as possible. Begin by aiming for at least 30 minutes of lifestyle physical activity a day. It is not essential that you complete the 30 minutes at one time; any activities that last for 10 minutes can be added up over the course of the day to begin to accumulate health benefits. Aim to accumulate 150 minutes a week with the understanding that more minutes equals more health benefits.

Once you have built regular physical activity into your everyday life, your goal may be to challenge yourself by working up the pyramid by implementing a

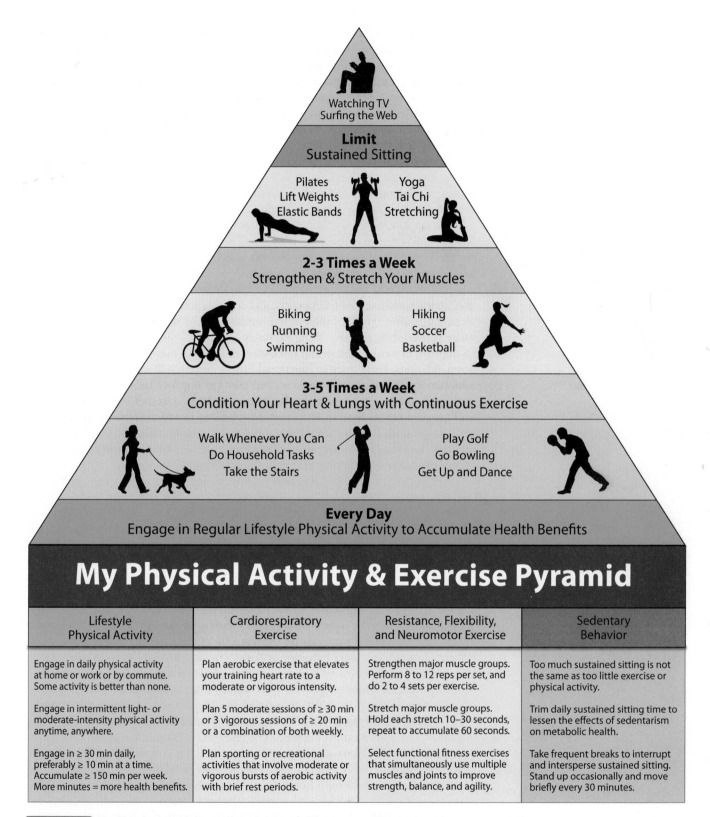

FIGURE 3.1 **My Physical Activity & Exercise Pyramid.** The graphics and text convey the different types of activities, each with its own unique benefit, that help adults link activities of daily living with a comprehensive exercise program to improve and maintain physical fitness and health. The levels further express frequency by proportionality of activity group and progressivity by encouraging individuals to start at the base and increase as their fitness grows.

SOURCE: Dr. Jerome E. Kotecki, Ball State University. Reprinted with permission of Ball State University © 2012.

systematic and structured exercise program to gain added health and fitness benefits beyond what can be achieved at level 1. The middle two levels illustrate the parts of a formal exercise program; they include more intense exercises and are the starting point for the irregular exerciser. To become consistent with activities in the middle levels of the pyramid, find exercises that you enjoy and plan them into your day. Always remember to start slowly, increase gradually, and set realistic goals. If continuous exercise is difficult for you, intermix several bouts of exercise with lifestyle activities from level 1.

Level 2 illustrates more structured and continuous aerobic exercises that condition your heart and lungs, such as brisk walking, running, biking, or swimming, as well as sporting or recreational activities like hiking, soccer, and basketball. Intensity matters. These exercises should elevate your training heart rate to a moderate or vigorous intensity. Because these activities are performed more intensely than the lifestyle activities at the base, they can be performed less frequently during the week. Plan five moderate sessions of at least 30 minutes, or three vigorous sessions of at least 20 minutes, or an equivalent combination of both.

The third level of the pyramid is occupied with muscular strength, stretching, and neuromotor exercises. Between 2 and 3 days a week adults need to participate in strengthening exercises such as free weights and/or weight machines, resistance bands/tubes, and stretching exercises for each of the major muscle groups to improve muscular fitness and flexibility. In order to meet the neuromotor recommendations, participate in functional fitness exercises like yoga or tai chi that simultaneously use multiple muscles and joints to improve balance, coordination, and agility. Many exercises at this level are multifaceted in that they provide several forms of fitness benefit. For example, yoga and tai chi exercises improve not only motor skills but also strength and flexibility; functional resistance exercises can involve a significant degree of stability and balance, fulfilling the recommendations for increasing flexibility and neuromotor exercise.

The pinnacle of the pyramid or level 4 is labeled "sustained sitting," and includes sedentary behaviors individuals should keep to a minimum during waking hours. The phrase *sedentary behavior* is derived from the Latin word *sedere*, meaning sitting, so it usually incorporates almost all sitting-based activity. Sedentary behavior is typically defined as any behavior with exceedingly low energy expenditure that causes muscular disuse, resulting in a cascade of harmful metabolic effects after a short period of time. These toxic metabolic effects lead to a considerable number of health disorders, such as obesity or cardiovascular and metabolic diseases (high blood pressure, an altered blood lipid profile, metabolic syndrome, diabetes, or inflammation) and a variety of cancers. In fact, adults and children in the United States spend the majority of their nonexercising waking day in some form of sedentary behavior or "couch potato activity," such as working or studying at a desk, riding in a car, eating a meal at a table, watching television, working on a computer, or playing video games (Katzmarzyk et al., 2009).

Patel and colleagues (2010) found that the amount of leisure time spent sitting is linked to increased risk of death, even if you exercise. Of course, they found it's much worse if you don't exercise. The researchers found that sitting 6 or more hours a day outside of work, compared to less than 3 hours, was significantly associated with a greater risk of death. Furthermore, compared to those who were most active, but still sat for 6 hours a day, those who got the least physical activity were more likely to die. Those who spent 6 hours or more sitting, but got physical activity every day, lowered their chances of dying. The goal is to limit the overall quantity of daily sustained sitting as well as to take frequent breaks to interrupt and intersperse sustained sitting by standing up occasionally and moving about briefly every 30 minutes.

In summary, you can meet your physical activity and fitness goals through different amounts and types of activity. Remember, this is your health and fitness program. There are no activities or exercises you must perform and there is no magic order in which exercises should be done. There are, however, systematic scientific principles that you need to understand to develop and maintain physical fitness. The following sections explain the components of physical fitness and outline the principles of their development that can provide you with a framework to develop a complete personal conditioning program.

Components of Health-Related Physical Fitness

Being physically fit provides an important foundation for overall health and well-being. Physical fitness is a set of attributes you have or achieve that relates to your ability or capacity to perform specific types of physical activity efficiently and effectively. The components of physical fitness may be categorized into health-related and skill-related fitness. **Health-related fitness** is how well the systems of your body work whereas skill-related fitness is generally associated more with your ability to perform a particular sport or athletic activity.

Health-related fitness is divided into five components: cardiorespiratory endurance, muscular strength and endurance, flexibility, and body composition. These five health-related components of physical fitness are largely independent of each other but overlap in complex ways. Because these components of fitness are independent of one another, it is possible to be well developed in one or more while being below average in others. Each component is influenced by a different part of the body or body systems. Understanding each of these components of physical fitness can help you better understand the importance of a regular physical activity program when it comes to achieving better health as well as assisting you in determining what the objective of your exercise program should be.

Cardiorespiratory endurance refers to the ability of the circulatory and respiratory systems to supply oxygen and fuel to the body during sustained physical activity. To do this the circulatory and respiratory systems must work together efficiently to provide the working muscles with enough oxygen and energy to sustain submaximal levels of physical activity. **Aerobic** (which means "using oxygen") **physical activity**, in which the body's larger muscles move in a rhythmic manner for a sustained period of time and increase the body's need for oxygen, are the best exercises to enhance cardiorespiratory endurance. When you participate in aerobic exercise that "gets your blood pumping," such as brisk walking, jogging, dancing, bicycling, and swimming, your heart and lungs have to work harder to supply your body with more oxygen for fuel (**FIGURE 3.2**). Over a given number of sessions the heart and lungs build up endurance and therefore are able to deliver oxygen more efficiently to the working muscles. This type of fitness has huge benefits to your daily lifestyle because it allows you more easily to meet the daily activity demands of life such as walking, climbing stairs, or running to catch the bus as well as allows you to get involved in recreational leisure-time activities and sports.

Practicing regular aerobic physical activity exercises that improve your ability to transport and use oxygen provides you with several benefits that go beyond performing daily activities and leisure-time activities with less fatigue. Aerobic physical activity assists in maintaining a healthy weight and lowering high blood pressure, lowering the "bad" cholesterol in your body (low-density lipoprotein [LDL]) while at the same time increasing the level of "good" cholesterol (high-density lipoprotein [HDL]). Over the long run, this helps prevent heart disease and stroke, two leading causes of death in the United States. Additionally higher levels of cardiorespiratory fitness can protect against type 2

Health-related fitness How well the systems of your body work; contributes to developing optimum health, preventing the onset of chronic disease, or reversing an established chronic disease process associated with inactivity.

Skill-related fitness Ability to perform a particular sport or athletic activity.

Cardiorespiratory endurance The ability of the circulatory and respiratory systems to supply oxygen and fuel to the body during sustained physical activity.

Aerobic physical activity Any activity that uses the body's larger muscles in a rhythmic manner for a sustained period of time and increases the body's need for oxygen.

Health-related fitness contributes to developing optimum health, preventing the onset of chronic disease, or reversing an established chronic disease process associated with inactivity.

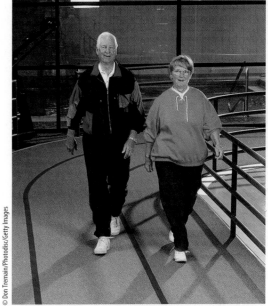

© Don Tremain/Photodisc/Getty Images

FIGURE 3.2 **Get Your Blood Pumping.** Brisk walking is an aerobic activity that enhances cardiorespiratory endurance.

Muscular strength The amount of force a muscle or muscle group can exert with a single maximum effort.

Muscular endurance The ability of a muscle or muscle group to exert repeated force against a resistance or to sustain muscular contraction for a given period of time.

Resistance training Any exercise that causes the muscles to contract against an external resistance with the expectation of increases in strength, endurance, tone, and/or mass.

Flexibility The ability to move a joint or group of joints through their complete range of motion.

Body composition The ratio of fat to fat-free mass (muscle, bone, organs, water) in the body.

diabetes and certain types of cancer and can decrease levels of stress, anxiety, and depression.

Muscular strength is the amount of force a muscle or muscle group can exert with a single maximum effort. This is in contrast to **muscular endurance**, which is the ability of a muscle or muscle group to exert repeated force against a resistance or to sustain muscular contraction for a given period of time. There are many different ways to develop muscular strength and endurance, but all plans include a form of physical activity referred to as resistance training. **Resistance training** (also called *anaerobic training*, a term that means "without oxygen") is any exercise that causes the muscles to contract against an external resistance with the expectation of increases in strength, endurance, tone, and/or mass. The external resistance can be free weights (e.g., dumbbells, barbells) or weight machines, your own body weight (e.g., pushups, chin-ups, sit-ups, leg lunges), or any other object that causes your muscles to contract (e.g., elastic exercise rubber tubing, jugs of water) (**FIGURE 3.3**).

The benefits of resistance exercise are well documented, and ongoing research continues to prove that it is an important activity for Americans to be engaged in when it comes to overall health. These benefits include improving or maintaining the integrity of the muscles and tendons, which is related to the risk of injury; being able to do more strenuous work and for a longer period of time as well as being less susceptible to muscular fatigue; improved appearance and improved athletic performance; building bone density, which is related to the risk of osteoporosis; increasing fat-free body mass and resting metabolic rate, which are related to weight gain and risk of obesity; and slowing down or even reversing the loss of muscle from aging (humans lose 5 pounds of muscle every decade after age 30).

Flexibility is the ability to move a joint or a group of joints through their complete range of motion. Several factors affect flexibility, including muscle elasticity, adequate warm-up, muscle temperature, and tightness of various other tissues such as ligaments and tendons. In physical activity programs, flexibility is enhanced through stretching exercises (**FIGURE 3.4**). Through stretching you attempt to improve muscle elasticity and compliance. Flexibility is necessary for normal activities that require bending, twisting, and reaching. Maintaining a range of motion allows us to do everyday tasks pain-free. In addition to making normal activities possible and pain-free, flexible muscles relieve stress, promote good posture, reduce the risk of pain and injury, and allow ease of movement through life.

Body composition refers to the ratio of fat to fat-free mass (muscle, bone, organs, water) in the body. Many health experts use the percentage of body fat in assessing health risk. Although there are no perfect criterion standards for ideal body fat percentage, most health professionals agree that fat percentages that range from 10 percent to 25 percent for men and 20 percent to 30 percent for women are considered to be below average or average risk. *Obesity* is the term used to define excessive accumulation of body fat that places individuals at greatest health risk. This is usually designated by a body fat percentage that exceeds 25 percent in males and 30 percent in females. A high proportion of body fat has serious health implications including increased risk of heart disease, stroke, high blood pressure, diabetes, high blood fats, some forms of cancer, back and joint problems, and gallbladder problems.

The best way to achieve and maintain a healthy body composition is to focus on regular physical activity (both aerobic and resistance training) and eat a healthy nutritious diet. By focusing on these two

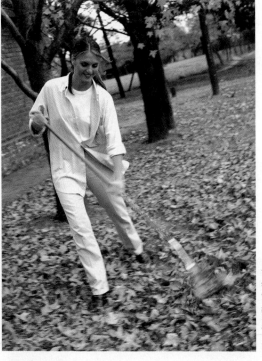

© Javier Pierini/Photodisc/Getty Images

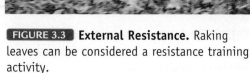

FIGURE 3.3 **External Resistance.** Raking leaves can be considered a resistance training activity.

major components, you can avoid the effects of creeping obesity and the negative consequences of repeated weight gains and losses.

Although you can improve your health by focusing on any one of these five components of health-related physical fitness, the best way to boost your well-being is to develop all five because a powerful synergy exists between these different components. For example, cardiovascular disease is the number one killer in the United States today, and many of its risk factors can be eliminated through both cardiorespiratory and muscular fitness training. Both aerobic and resistance training reduce cardiovascular disease by lowering blood pressure and cholesterol levels and improving body composition.

Skill-Related Components of Fitness

As mentioned previously, skill-related fitness is generally associated more with our ability to perform a particular sport or athletic activity than with our health. Skill-related fitness components include the following:

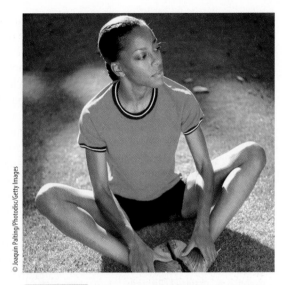

© Joaquin Palting/Photodisc/Getty Images

FIGURE 3.4 **Enhancing Flexibility.** Stretching exercises help to improve flexibility.

- *Agility*. The ability to quickly and accurately change the direction of the movement of the entire body in space. In games such as tennis, agility is important to reach the ball in time.
- *Balance*. The ability to maintain equilibrium while moving or stationary. Activities such as gymnastics, ballet, and skiing require balance.
- *Coordination*. The ability to combine the senses with different body parts to perform activities smoothly and accurately. Activities such as catching a baseball or kicking a football require the hands and eyes or foot and eyes to work together.
- *Power*. The ability to transfer energy into force at a fast rate or apply speed and strength to produce a muscular movement. Almost all sports require power to perform well.
- *Reaction time*. The amount of time it takes to respond and react to a stimulus. Activities such as returning a serve in tennis or badminton require fast reaction times.
- *Speed*. The ability to move quickly from one point to another. Activities such as the 100- or 200-meter sprint in track or running the bases in baseball require speed.

Health-related fitness is the primary focus of this text; however, components of skill-related and health-related fitness interlace with the importance of neuromotor exercise. Many skill-related fitness abilities can fade as we age. According to the ACSM, neuromotor exercise can be especially beneficial for older people to improve balance, coordination, and stability, thus reducing the risk of falls and other injury (ACSM, 2011). Additionally, in athletic events and recreational activities, many athletes develop high levels of cardiorespiratory and muscular fitness in combination with skill-related components to be competitive (for example, hockey and basketball players). As recreational athletes, many of us can get much satisfaction and enjoyment from being able to perform well in our favorite sporting activity.

Response and Adaptation to Physical Activity

The human body is remarkably adaptable. The greater the health-related fitness component demands made on the various physiological systems, the more the changes occur. Physical activity acts as a stimulus to the human body. Applied in appropriate doses, it can bring about positive changes in the way your body

Response A short-term change in an organ system.

Adaptation A long-term change in an organ system.

Principle of overload States that a greater than normal load or intensity on the body system is required for training adaptation or improved function to take place.

Principle of progression States that, to ensure safety and effectiveness, the overload must be applied in a systematic and logical fashion over an extended period of time.

FITT formula A basic set of rules about what is necessary to gain a training effect from an exercise program. FITT stands for frequency, intensity, time, and type.

Several basic scientific fitness principles must be adhered to in order to develop an effective physical fitness program.

functions. A short-term change in an organ system is termed a **response**. A long-term change is termed an **adaptation**. With respect to physical activity, organ system response and adaptation typically determine the fitness level of the body. For example, when you first start to move, there is almost an immediate change in your heart rate. With increasing workloads, the heart rate increases rapidly. Such a change is an example of a response of the cardiovascular system to the body's increasing demand for greater blood flow. If the body is regularly exposed to a stimulus that brings about this response, an adaptation occurs. For example, regular exposure to physical activity results in a lowering of the resting heart rate. The change in resting heart rate is the result of an adaptation in the cardiac muscle. This adaptation takes place in reaction to being regularly stimulated by progressive physical activity. The heart muscle becomes capable of contracting with greater force, thereby increasing the stroke volume, or the amount of blood forced out of the heart with each contraction. If more blood can be ejected with each contraction, the heart does not have to beat as often to circulate the same amount of blood.

All systems of the body that are regularly exposed to the stimulus of physical activity can undergo response and adaptation. Note that these responses and adaptations are not always positive. For instance, if a joint is exposed to a range of motion far beyond its normal functional capacity, the response may be swelling and pain to prevent further activity from potentially damaging the joint. With this in mind, the need to apply the correct amount of physical activity to the organ systems of the body becomes evident. Too much can cause damage, whereas just the right amount results in positive adaptation. Finally, many of the beneficial effects of physical activity diminish within a couple of weeks if physical activity is substantially reduced, and benefits completely disappear within 2 to 8 months if physical activity is not resumed.

The Principles of Training

Basic scientific fitness principles apply to everyone at all fitness levels, from the weekend jogger to the Olympic-caliber athlete. These principles govern how your body responds to the stimulus of physical activity and include overload, progression, specificity, reversibility, recovery, and individual differences. By following these principles, you can be sure to design a safe and effective activity program.

The **principle of overload** states that a greater than normal load or intensity on the body system is required for training adaptation or improved function to take place. In other words, you ask your body to do more than you usually require it to do in a normal day. Our bodies respond to this overload by increasing fitness to better handle the same load in the future. If the load is less than normal on a regular basis, your fitness level decreases.

The **principle of progression** states that, to ensure safety and effectiveness, the overload must be applied in a systematic and logical fashion over an extended period of time. If too much overload is applied too soon, the system does not have time to adapt properly and benefits may be delayed or injury may occur. You need to overload your body gradually so that it has time to respond and adapt. This does not mean you increase the overload every time you exercise or participate in physical activity. Rather, you attempt to achieve a new level of performance measured best by months rather than days or weeks.

You can use the FITT formula to help you determine how much exercise is enough for you to build fitness safely and effectively. The **FITT formula** is a basic set of rules about what is necessary to gain a training effect from an exercise program. FITT stands for frequency, intensity, time, and type. It is important to keep in mind that you can manipulate the FITT formula based on your fitness goals. For example, you may see fitness as a quality of life issue; in other words, being fit means being active and healthy to get the most out of life. Or you may see fitness as a way to enhance your ability to participate in various competitive sporting activities such as marathons and triathlons.

Frequency refers to how often you exercise and is most often expressed in the number of days per week. This number can vary based on the fitness component being developed as well as the fitness goal. For example, for important health benefits, cardiorespiratory endurance activities are recommended on most days of the week whereas muscular fitness and flexibility activities are recommended two to three times a week for adults to gain the most health benefits.

Intensity refers to how hard you exercise. Fitness develops when a greater than normal load or stimulus is placed on the body system. Intensity is measured differently for each fitness component because each is influenced by a different part of the body or body systems. Cardiorespiratory endurance is best increased by increasing the heart rate above resting; muscular strength and endurance are best increased by increasing the resistance a muscle or muscle group must contract against compared to at rest; and flexibility is best increased by stretching the muscles to a point of slight tension or mild discomfort.

Time is how long you exercise. Like intensity, time or duration varies by fitness component. To achieve health-related benefits from cardiorespiratory endurance activities, it is recommended that adults perform 20–60 minutes daily. Time in resistance training is most often measured by number of repetitions and sets you complete and how much time you rest between sets. A *repetition* is one complete movement of an activity, such as lifting a weight or doing a sit-up. Initially, it is recommended that you rest 2–3 minutes in between each set (a *set* is usually a group of 8 to 12 successive repetitions performed without resting) of exercise. As you become more conditioned, you may decrease the time between each set. For flexibility, it is recommended that you stretch at least 5 to 10 minutes in a way that involves the major muscle groups of the body after an aerobic or resistance training workout (ACSM, 2010).

Type dictates what kind of exercise you should choose to achieve the appropriate training response for the type of fitness you are trying to improve (refer to Figure 3.1). For example, if you are trying to improve cardiorespiratory fitness, you need to do an exercise that increases the need for oxygen consumption. This could be brisk walking, jogging, or swimming. If you are trying to increase your muscular strength and endurance, you can perform a resistance training exercise such as doing pull-ups, pushups, or sit-ups. If you are trying to increase flexibility, you can participate in stretching exercises.

The **principle of specificity** states that to develop a particular fitness component, activities must be performed to develop the various body parts or body systems for that fitness component. In other words, to improve muscular fitness, it is important to participate in resistance-type activities. Likewise, to improve cardiorespiratory endurance, you must participate in aerobic-type activities. This principle also implies that to become better at a particular activity or skill, you must perform that activity or skill. A marathon runner should train by running, a swimmer by swimming, and a tennis player by playing tennis.

The **principle of reversibility** states that changes occurring from physical activity are reversible and that if you stop being active for an extended period of time, your body deconditions and reverts back to its pretraining condition. Thus the maxim "use it or lose it," which is closely related to the biological principle of *use and disuse*. The **use and disuse** principle dictates that although rest periods are necessary for recovery after workouts, extensive rest intervals (more than a week or two) lead to a gradual loss of fitness. In fact, up to half of fitness improvements can be lost within 2 months if you completely stop exercising. If you must decrease activity, you can maintain many fitness benefits by reducing frequency and duration while maintaining intensity. This is why it is important to continue

---

Frequency How often you exercise, which is most often expressed as the number of days per week.

Intensity How hard you exercise.

Time How long you exercise.

Type Dictates what kind of exercise you should choose to achieve the appropriate training response for the type of fitness you are trying to improve.

Principle of specificity States that to develop a particular fitness component, activities must be performed to develop the various body part or body systems for that fitness component.

Principle of reversibility States that changes occurring from physical activity are reversible and that if a person stops being active for an extended period of time, the body deconditions and reverts back to its pretraining condition.

Use and disuse Dictates that, although rest periods are necessary for recovery after workouts, extensive rest intervals (more than a week or two) lead to a gradual loss of fitness.

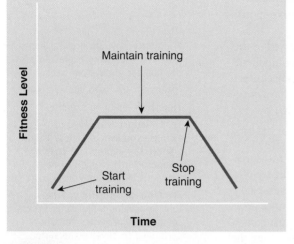

FIGURE 3.5 **Principle of Reversibility.** Avoiding extensive rest periods (more than a week or two) is important in limiting deconditioning of the body.

Principle of recovery States that physical activity, no matter how structured, requires a period of rest to permit the body to be restored to a state in which it can exercise once more.

Principle of individual differences States that we all vary in our ability to develop fitness in each of the fitness components.

Variability The differences among people.

Before starting a physical activity program, it is important to complete a self-prescreening and self-assessment and to set specific goals.

a modified activity program even if you become extremely busy for a period of time (**FIGURE 3.5**).

The **principle of recovery** states that physical activity, no matter how structured, requires a period of rest to permit the body to be restored to a state in which it can exercise once more. Adequate time is required for recovery of the large-scale systems that power the body during exercise and the restoration of the energy stores depleted by exercise. Both allow for adaptation to take place. The length of the recovery period in relation to the active exercise period is a function of the duration of the exercise as well as the intensity level at which the body performed the exercise. It is generally recommended that you rest 48 to 72 hours between exhaustive activity sessions that are similar in nature. This doesn't mean that you shouldn't be active at all for this period of time. It does mean that you should vary your activities so that one system is allowed time to recover before it is overloaded again.

The **principle of individual differences** states that we all vary in our ability to develop fitness in each of the fitness components. These differences have to do with genetics, age, body size and shape, chronic conditions, injuries, and gender. For example, the best estimates inform us that genetics accounts for approximately 10 to 25 percent of the variability in cardiorespiratory fitness, approximately 20 to 40 percent of the **variability** in muscular fitness, and about 25 percent of the variability in body fat levels (Beunen & Thomis, 2004; Lakka & Bouchard, 2004).

Not only do we differ in fitness based on heredity, but people of different genetic backgrounds respond differently to exercise. In other words, two people of different genetic backgrounds could do the same exercise program and get quite different benefits. Some people may get as much as 10 times the benefit from activity as others who do the same program (Lakka & Bouchard, 2004).

The genetic influence on how we respond to being physically active makes recognizing individual differences even more important. Assumptions about a person's fitness are not always good indicators of that person's current activity levels. Different people respond differently to each component of fitness. For example, whereas some people respond well to strength training, they may not respond as well to cardiorespiratory training. Typically, there is a 3- to 10-fold difference between low responders (people who don't show much change) and high responders (people who show a good deal of change) on the same standardized physical activity regimen if performed for a period of 15 to 20 weeks (Lakka & Bouchard, 2004). The magnitude of the difference is somewhat dependent on the component of fitness considered.

In summary, there is no question that some individuals have a higher natural capacity to develop the various components of physical fitness. Scientific evidence, however, suggests that it is regular participation in physical activity rather than our inherited component of fitness that is related to health. Those who feel they cannot benefit from physical activity because they have not been dealt genetic cards that allow them to obtain elite fitness levels are mistaken. Physical activity is required to make use of the genetic makeup of any individual. Sedentary individuals differ in their health-related fitness levels because of physical inactivity and not genetic capabilities. Although we cannot choose our parents, we can choose how we live our lives.

Designing Your Exercise Program

Although your enthusiasm and eagerness to begin an exercise program may be increasing, you should consider a few things before starting your program.

Prescreening

It is very important to make sure that your body is ready for physical activity before starting any activity program, and prescreening is the first step in ensuring safety and effectiveness. Several parts of the prescreening process can be completed on your own. Others may require that you consult with your health care provider.

The Physical Activity Readiness Questionnaire (PAR-Q) is a self-screening tool that anyone who is planning to start an exercise program can use. It is often used by certified fitness trainers to determine the safety or possible risk of exercising for an individual based on the individual's answers to specific health history questions.

Although physical activity is perfectly safe for most healthy people, sometimes it's important to get your health care provider's approval, particularly when contemplating vigorous-intensity activity, because the risks of this type of activity are higher than the risks for moderate-intensity activity (FIGURE 3.6). Certain chronic clinical conditions (e.g., arthritis, diabetes, hypertension, obesity, osteoporosis, peripheral arterial disease, pulmonary disease) may require adaptations in exercise programming (ACSM, 2010). It is very important to discuss your options with your health care provider before starting any exercise program to ensure safety.

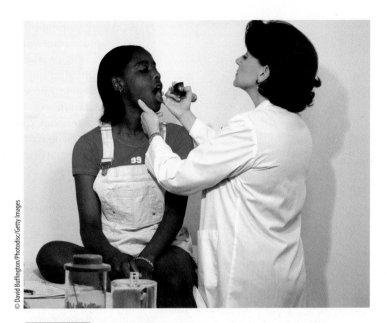

FIGURE 3.6 **Prescreening.** Although physical activity is perfectly safe for most people, sometimes it is important to get your health care provider's approval.

Self-Assessment

Whether you are beginning an exercise program for the first time or are a regular exerciser, consider assessing your current level of fitness for each of the five health-related components of physical fitness. The results of the assessment provide valuable information on your current fitness level and can help you set specific goals when planning or modifying your fitness program.

Goal Setting

If you are trying to get healthy and fit, you need specific goals. When you don't have a specific goal, it's difficult to keep exercising and to track your progress to see how far you have come. Before you begin your training, take time to consider goals and objectives regarding what you want to accomplish with an exercise program. People are active for a variety of reasons. To optimize the benefits associated with being regularly active, you must have a clear idea of what you wish to obtain from your activity program. Some people start activity programs to obtain health benefits; others are interested in improving their overall fitness levels; still others are simply interested in looking and feeling better.

In contemplating your reasons for becoming active, remember to be realistic when you define your goals and objectives. Goals and objectives should be attainable, adjustable, and allow for individual need. Remember that the overriding factors that must be incorporated into any physical activity program are safety and effectiveness. You want to make sure that you don't injure yourself, and you want to make sure that your goals are achieved. Planning a safe and effective program should influence your goal setting by encouraging you to think in terms of both short-term and long-term goals.

We are all born with different genetic blueprints. In terms of our responses and adaptations to physical activity, these genetic differences mean that we all respond and adapt at different physiological rates and magnitudes. Some people will see rapid changes in response to exercise, whereas others will see measurable change only over an extended period of time. Certain individuals will see their body function improve to an extent not achievable by other individuals, who might be working just as hard or harder. Taking the variation in improvement rate into consideration, you must individualize your program to bring about optimal benefit based on your particular needs and responses. Not everyone should be performing the same activities at the same intensities for the same period of time. You need to find the activities that are best suited to meet your individual needs.

Build Slowly

When beginning an activity program it is wise to start gradually, build slowly, and maintain consistency. A common mistake made by beginners is to try to do too much, too soon. Relying on what others are doing to determine how much you should do is not wise. Remember that fitness is individual in nature. What may appear to be a low-intensity warm-up for one person may be an exhaustive workout for another. It is far better to delay the acquisition of benefits to some degree rather than to do too much, become sore or injured, and set your program back significantly—or, worse, stop completely.

Selecting Activities

When creating your physical activity program, choose activities that are fun for you and that you think you would like to continue for some time. Be aware that by alternating activities or cross training, you are less likely to become bored and more likely to make physical activity a regular part of your lifestyle.

    FIGURE 3.7 shows several combinations of activities that you can choose. Cross training serves the purpose of adding variety to an activity program and making sure that various body systems and muscle groups are included. By using cross training effectively, you also allow one system (e.g., aerobic) to recover on a recovery day while developing another system (e.g., anaerobic).

Components of an Activity Session

All exercise and physical activity sessions should follow a similar format (**FIGURE 3.8**). This design allows you to optimize fitness gains while minimizing the risk of injury.

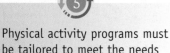

Physical activity programs must be tailored to meet the needs of the individual.

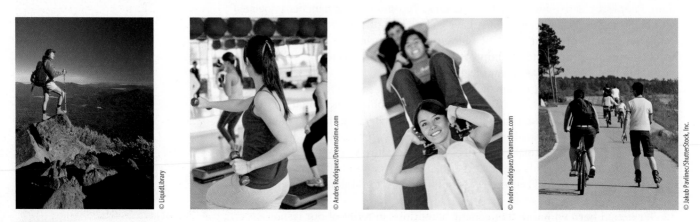

FIGURE 3.7 **Cross Training Combinations.** It is best to vary your activity program by combining different types of activities.

PREPARATION   The first stage is to prepare the body for physical activity. Make sure you are in appropriate attire that is designed for the activity to follow. For example, if you are preparing for a walking program, make sure you are in comfortable clothes and have proper walking shoes. Next, you must prepare your body to shift gradually from an inactive state to an active state or warm up. Low-intensity aerobic activity (slow walking) and light calisthenics (jumping jacks) movements usually characterize this portion of an exercise session. These light activities increase blood flow to the muscles and increase the temperature of the muscles. Though you may be performing an activity that is not traditionally "exercise," you still need to warm up. Muscle strains and low-back injuries can occur when you perform a sudden movement for which the body is not prepared.

TRANSITION   The second phase is one of transition in which you move gradually into the specific activity you will be performing. It is necessary to move gradually during this phase, increasing intensity as the body continually adjusts to the increased physiological demands of the activity.

ACTIVITY   The third phase is when you focus on the specific activity in which you are participating for its health benefit or for improvement of fitness (**FIGURE 3.9** and **FIGURE 3.10**). The intensity and duration of activity will be determined by your goals and fitness level and allotted time.

COOL-DOWN   The fourth and final phase is a combination cool-down phase. During this portion of an activity routine, you gradually bring the intensity down toward resting values. Reducing the intensity is important in keeping blood from pooling in the legs and in aiding the flow of blood back to the heart for recirculation. Breathing rate, heart rate, and temperature are all brought back to baseline levels. Stretching exercises are recommended during the cool-down because of the increased muscle temperature. Warm muscles are more pliable muscles, so performing stretching exercises at this time allows you to achieve improved range of motion around a joint.

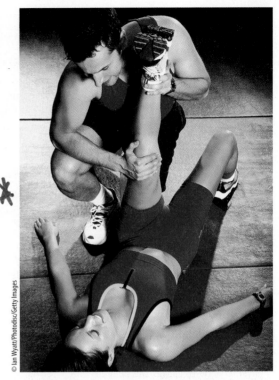

FIGURE 3.8 **Formatting Your Exercise Session.** Qualified instruction can enhance your physical activity experience.

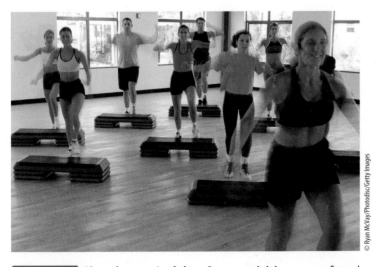

FIGURE 3.9 **Choosing an Activity.** Group activities are preferred by some people.

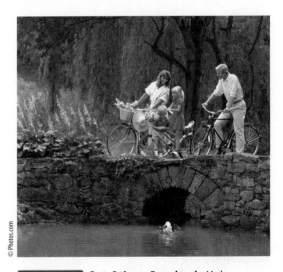

FIGURE 3.10 **Get Others Involved.** Make physical activity a family affair.

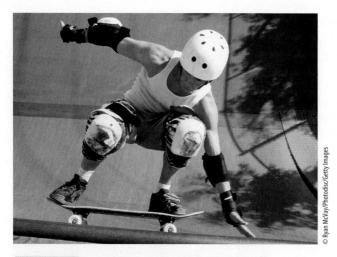

FIGURE 3.11 **Cornerstone of a Physical Activity Program.** Safety is an important factor to consider when participating in physical activity.

> **Overuse syndrome** Condition in which too much exercise or physical activity causes the body to start to break down (symptoms: increased risk of injury, lethargy, loss of appetite, irritability, decreased motivation).

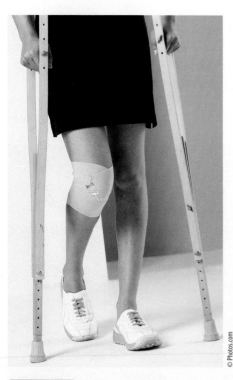

FIGURE 3.12 **Overuse Syndrome.** Too much activity for your level of fitness can lead to injury.

Monitoring Your Progress

It is important to check regularly to see whether your program is working and whether adjustments need to be made. Monitoring is accomplished by performing self-assessments on a regular basis. Another important aspect of monitoring your progress is that it can provide positive motivation as you see that what you are doing is actually producing benefits and moving you closer to the attainment of your goals. It also allows you to update your goals so that you can set new ones after you have achieved the initial ones.

Safety and Effectiveness

The cornerstones of any physical activity program are safety and effectiveness (**FIGURE 3.11**). According to the *Physical Activity Guidelines*, to perform physical activity safely and reduce risk of injuries and other adverse events, people should adhere to the following guidelines (USDHHS, 2008):

- Understand the risks and yet be confident that physical activity is safe for almost everyone.
- Choose to do types of physical activity that are appropriate for their current fitness level and health goals because some activities are safer than others are.
- Increase physical activity gradually over time whenever more activity is necessary to meet guidelines or health goals. Inactive people should "start low and go slow" by gradually increasing how often and how long activities are done.
  - Protect themselves by using appropriate gear and sports equipment, looking for safe environments, following rules and policies, and making sensible choices about when, where, and how to be active.
  - Be under the care of a health care provider if they have chronic conditions or symptoms. People with chronic conditions and symptoms should consult their health care provider about the types and amounts of activity appropriate for them.

Overuse Syndrome

Physical activity can provide wonderful benefits to those who participate regularly. However, too much physical activity can be harmful (**FIGURE 3.12**). If you exercise at a level well beyond your current state of fitness (overtrain), you may develop a condition called **overuse syndrome**. Overuse syndrome can involve symptoms of fatigue, lethargy, depression, more frequent colds and illnesses, muscular strain, joint soreness, and feelings of being overwhelmed. Overuse syndrome can be caused by a variety of factors, including an inadequate warm-up, poor conditioning, ill-fitting or worn-out shoes, biomechanical abnormalities, rushing results, or differences in activity surfaces. The best way to prevent overuse syndrome is to plan carefully, follow the plan, progress gradually, and listen to your body. If you start to feel that your body is not responding the way it should be, you need to reassess what you are doing.

Injuries

A common rule to follow in beginning an activity program is that it is better to progress slowly than to rush into activities for which your body is not prepared

TABLE 3.4	The Continuum of Injury Risk Associated with Different Types of Activity

Injury Risk Level	Activity Type	Examples
Lower risk	Commuting	Walking, bicycling
	Lifestyle	Home repair, gardening/yard work
	Recreation/sports (no contact)	Walking for exercise, golf, dancing, swimming, running, tennis
	Recreation/sports (limited contact)	Bicycling, aerobics, skiing, volleyball, baseball, softball
Higher risk	Recreation/sports (collison/contact)	Football, hockey, soccer, basketball

Note: The same activity done for different purposes and with different frequency, intensity, and duration leads to different injury rates. Competitive activities tend to have higher injury rates than noncompetitive activities, likely due to different degrees of intensity of participation.

SOURCE: U.S. Department of Health and Human Services. (2008). *Physical Activity Guidelines for Americans*. Online: http://www.health.gov/paguidelines/guidelines/default.aspx.

and risk injury. You can reduce your risk of injury by choosing appropriate types and amounts of activity. As TABLE 3.4 shows, the safest activities begin with every-day routine activities and noncontact recreational sports.

Physical Activity and Health Connection

Being physically fit provides an important foundation for overall health and well-being. Health-related fitness is how well the systems of your body work and contributes to developing optimum health, preventing the onset of chronic disease, or reversing an established chronic disease process associated with inactivity. Becoming more physically fit is something that everyone can achieve. As with other components of wellness, the transition to becoming physically fit requires lifestyle changes. To reap the benefits of regular physical activity you must be able to make a lifelong commitment to your program. It isn't necessary that you have any special equipment or join a health club or a gym. It requires only that you participate consistently in some type of moderate-intensity physical activity on most days of the week. Think of this movement as an opportunity, not an inconvenience. Finally, if you can, also enjoy some regular vigorous exercise for extra health and fitness benefits.

concept connections

(1) The *Physical Activity Guidelines for Americans* published by the U.S. Department of Health and Human Services are designed to provide information and guidance on the types and amounts of physical activity that provide substantial health benefits for Americans age 6 years and older. According to the *Guidelines*, for the broad population—who have different and diverse health needs—to attain the most benefits from physical activity,

Adults need at least 150 minutes (2 hours and 30 minutes) of moderate-intensity aerobic activity or 75 minutes (1 hour and 15 minutes) of vigorous-intensity aerobic activity every week or an equivalent mix of moderate- and vigorous-intensity aerobic activity and muscle-strengthening activities on 2 or more days a week that work all major muscle groups (legs, hips, back, abdomen, chest, shoulders, and arms).

2. **Health-related fitness contributes to developing optimum health, preventing the onset of chronic disease, or reversing an established chronic disease process associated with inactivity.** Health-related fitness is divided into five components: cardiorespiratory endurance, muscular strength and endurance, flexibility, and body composition. These five health-related components of physical fitness are largely independent of each other but overlap in complex ways. Because these components of fitness are independent of one another, it is possible to be well developed in one or more while being below average in others. Each component is influenced by a different part of the body or body systems.

3. **Several basic scientific fitness principles must be adhered to in order to develop an effective physical fitness program.** These principles apply to everyone at all fitness levels, from the weekend jogger to the Olympic-caliber athlete. These principles govern how your body responds to the physical stress of physical activity and include overload, progression, specificity, reversibility, recovery, and individual differences. Following these principles ensures that you design a safe and effective activity program.

4. **Before starting a physical activity program, it is important to complete a self-prescreening and self-assessment and to set specific goals.** The Physical Activity Readiness Questionnaire (PAR-Q) is a self-screening tool that anyone who is planning to start an exercise program can use. It is often used to determine the safety or possible risk of exercising for an individual based upon that person's answers to specific health history questions. Second, whether you are beginning an exercise program for the first time or are a regular exerciser, consider assessing your current level of fitness. The results of the assessment provide valuable information on your current fitness level and can help you set specific goals when planning or modifying your fitness program. Finally, before you begin your training, take time to consider goals and objectives regarding what you want to accomplish with an exercise program. When you don't have a specific goal, it's difficult to keep exercising and to track your progress to see how far you have come.

5. **Physical activity programs must be tailored to meet the needs of the individual.** Choose activities that are fun for you and that you think you would like to continue for some time. Be aware that by alternating activities or cross training, you are less likely to become bored and more likely to make physical activity a regular part of your lifestyle. Cross training serves the purpose of adding variety to an activity program and making sure that various body systems and muscle groups are included. By using cross training effectively, you also allow one system (e.g., aerobic) to recover while developing another system (e.g., anaerobic).

Terms

Adaptation, 52
Aerobic physical activity, 49
Body composition, 50
Cardiorespiratory endurance, 49
FITT formula, 52
Flexibility, 50
Frequency, 53
Health-related fitness, 49
Intensity, 53
Muscular endurance, 50

Muscular strength, 50
Overuse syndrome, 58
Physical activity, 42
Principle of individual
  differences, 54
Principle of overload, 52
Principle of progression, 52
Principle of recovery, 54
Principle of reversibility, 53
Principle of specificity, 53

Resistance training, 50
Response, 52
Skill-related fitness, 49
Talk test, 44
Time, 53
Type, 53
Use and disuse, 53
Variability, 54

Ron has learned that by following the *Physical Activity Guidelines for Americans*, which provide different amounts and types of activity, he can meet his personal goal of improving his health. Furthermore, he better understands how implementing specific systematic scientific principles (e.g., overload, progression, specificity, reversibility, recovery, individual differences) allows him to develop and maintain his physical fitness. Ron thinks of his physical activity program as an opportunity to improve his health, not an inconvenience. For example, he is now making a habit of speed walking or cycling instead of driving or getting a ride to class.

Critical Thinking

1. Explain the differences between health-related fitness and skill-related fitness.

2. Several scientific fitness principles (overload, progression, specificity, reversibility, recovery, individual differences) must be adhered to in order to develop an effective physical activity program. Select three different principles and explain them.

3. You can use the FITT formula to help you determine how much exercise is enough for you to build fitness safely and effectively. What does FITT stand for?

References

American College of Sports Medicine. (2011). Position stand: Quantity and quality of exercise for developing and maintaining cardiorespiratory, musculoskeletal, and neuromotor fitness in apparently healthy adults: Guidance for prescribing exercise. *Medicine and Science in Sports and Exercise* 43(7):1334–1359.

American College of Sports Medicine. (2010). *ACSM's Guidelines for Exercise Testing and Prescription*, 8th ed. Baltimore, MD: Lippincott Williams & Wilkins.

Beunen, G., & Thomis, M. (2004). Gene powered? Where to go from heritability (h2) in muscle strength and power. *Exercise and Sport Science Reviews* 32(4):148–154.

Centers for Disease Control and Prevention, National Center for Chronic Disease Prevention and Health Promotion. (2009). Physical activity for everyone: Measuring physical activity intensity. Online: http://www.cdc.gov/physicalactivity/everyone/measuring/index.html.

Katzmarzyk, P.T., Church, T.S., Craig, C.L., & Bouchard, C. (2009). Sitting time and mortality from all causes, cardiovascular disease, and cancer. *Medicine & Science in Sports & Exercise* 41(5):1486–1496.

Lakka, T.A., & Bouchard, C. (2004). Genetics, physical activity, fitness, and health: What does the future hold? *Journal of the Royal Society for the Promotion of Health* 124(1):14–15.

Patel, A.V., Bernstein, L., Deka, A., Feigelson, H.S., Campbell, P.T., Gapstur, S.M., Colditz, G.A., & Thun, M.J. (2010). Leisure time spent sitting in relation to total mortality in a prospective cohort of US adults. *American Journal of Epidemiology* 172:419–429.

U.S. Department of Health and Human Services. (2008). Physical Activity Guidelines for Americans. Online: http://www.health.gov/PAGuidelines/pdf/paguide.pdf.

© Andres Rodriguez/Dreamstime.com

The Heart of Physical Fitness: Cardiorespiratory Endurance

4

Like most of us, when Maria thinks about health and fitness, she thinks first of aerobic fitness or "cardio." Although Maria knows it is true that aerobic fitness is essential for an active, healthy life, she has uncertainty: what types of exercise options are best for aerobic fitness? How much aerobic activity does she need? How does she know whether she is working out hard enough? How often does she have to exercise?

concepts

1. Cardiorespiratory endurance is a crucial health-related component of fitness because it improves the quality of life and quantity of life and reduces the onset and symptoms of aging and illness.

2. The circulatory system consists of the heart and blood vessels—veins, arteries, and capillaries.

3. Cardiorespiratory endurance is the ability of the circulatory and respiratory systems to supply oxygen and fuel to the body during sustained physical activity.

4. A cardiorespiratory endurance session of 20–60 minutes is recommended to gain significant aerobic benefits.

go.jblearning.com/kotecki4e
The website for this book is a great source for supplementary physical health information for both students and instructors. Visit **go.jblearning.com/kotecki4e** to find a variety of useful tools for learning, thinking, and teaching.

Cardiorespiratory endurance is a crucial health-related component of fitness because it improves the quality of life and quantity of life and reduces the onset and symptoms of aging and illness.

Cardiorespiratory endurance
The ability of the circulatory and respiratory systems to supply oxygen and fuel to the body during sustained physical activity.

The circulatory system consists of the heart and blood vessels—veins, arteries, and capillaries.

We do not want in the United States a nation of spectators. We want a nation of participants in the vigorous life.
—President John F. Kennedy

Introduction

Cardiorespiratory endurance—the ability of the circulatory and respiratory systems to supply oxygen and fuel to the body during sustained physical activity—is a crucial health-related component of fitness because it improves the quality of life and quantity of life and reduces the onset and symptoms of aging and illness. The benefits of aerobic physical activity in which the body's larger muscles move in a rhythmic manner for a sustained period of time are many. Aerobic activities strengthen the heart and lungs, making them more efficient and resilient and allowing us to meet the daily activity demands of life, as well as to participate in recreational leisure-time activities and sports (**FIGURE 4.1**). Aerobic exercise improves the strength of your bones, ligaments, and tendons and enhances muscular endurance. Important systemic changes include reduced blood pressure and low-density lipoprotein (LDL) cholesterol, more efficient use of fats and sugars, the burning of lots of calories, and a healthier body composition. Aerobic exercise reduces your risk of cardiovascular disease and type 2 diabetes and has been shown to reduce stress and depression.

This chapter provides guidelines for designing your own cardiorespiratory endurance program. To help you design a more effective and safer cardiorespiratory endurance fitness program, it helps to have a basic understanding of how the cardiorspiratory system functions.

The Heart

The circulatory system consists of the heart (the pump) and a network of blood vessels that transport the blood throughout the body (**FIGURE 4.2**). The heart's primary function is to pump blood containing oxygen and nutrients throughout the body. The heart also receives blood filled with waste products (such as carbon dioxide) that need to be eliminated from the body. The heart is a highly specialized muscle about the size of an adult fist and is located under the rib cage to the left of the breast bone (sternum) and between the lungs. The heart pumps slightly more than a gallon of blood per minute through the approximately 60,000 miles of blood

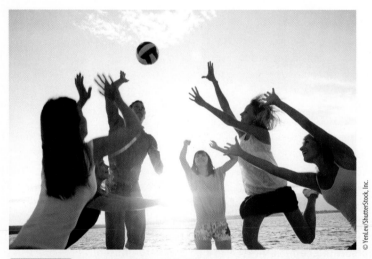

FIGURE 4.1 **Benefits of Aerobic Fitness.** A fit cardiorespiratory system allows us to participate in recreational sporting activities more easily.

© YenLev/ShutterStock, Inc.

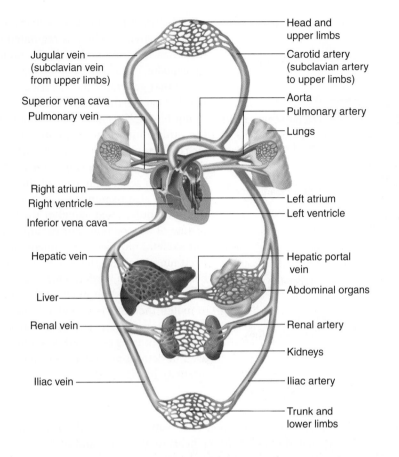

Jugular vein
(subclavian vein
from upper limbs)

Superior vena cava
Pulmonary vein

Head and
upper limbs

Carotid artery
(subclavian artery
to upper limbs)

Aorta
Pulmonary artery

Lungs

Right atrium
Right ventricle
Inferior vena cava

Left atrium
Left ventricle

Hepatic vein

Liver

Renal vein

Iliac vein

Hepatic portal
vein

Abdominal organs

Renal artery

Kidneys

Iliac artery

Trunk and
lower limbs

FIGURE 4.2 **The Circulatory System.** The circulatory system includes the heart, arteries, and veins. The heart receives oxygenated blood from the lungs and pumps it to all tissues in the body.

vessels in the body. Each day the heart expands and contracts 100,000 times, pumping about 2000 gallons of blood. In a 70-year lifetime, an average human heart beats more than 2.5 billion times. Maintaining a healthy heart and blood vessels is essential for survival. The walls of the heart are composed of three layers: the pericardium, the myocardium, and the endocardium. The **pericardium** is a thin, closed sac that surrounds the heart. The middle layer is the thickest, consists of muscle cells, and is called the **myocardium**. The **endocardium** is the inner layer that lines the heart chambers.

The heart contains four separate chambers: the upper two chambers are the left and right atria; the lower two chambers are the right and left ventricles (**FIGURE 4.3**). The heart also has four valves: the tricuspid valve (located between the right atrium and right ventricle), the pulmonary valve (between the right ventricle and pulmonary artery), the mitral valve (between the left atrium and left ventricle), and the aortic valve (between the left ventricle and aorta). To maintain uniform blood flow in one direction through arteries and veins, the cardiovascular system is equipped with one-way valves, both in the chambers of the heart and in blood vessels. With every heartbeat, the valves in the heart open and close to allow blood to circulate in just one direction.

Blood that is depleted of oxygen returns to the heart via the right atrium and then flows to the right ventricle. From there blood is pumped to the lungs, where it is reoxygenated and returned via the pulmonary artery to the left atrium. Finally, the fresh blood is pumped throughout the body's tissues from the left ventricle through the large artery called the **aorta**. The atria receive blood entering the heart: the right atrium receives **deoxygenated blood** returning from the various cells and muscles of the body, and the left atrium receives **oxygenated blood** from the lungs. The right ventricle pumps deoxygenated blood out to the lungs, and the left ventricle pumps oxygenated blood out to the cells and muscles of the body.

Pericardium Thin, closed outer sac that surrounds the heart.

Myocardium Muscular middle layer that surrounds the heart.

Endocardium Thin, inner layer that lines the heart.

Aorta Large artery that receives blood from the heart's left ventricle and distributes it to the body.

Deoxygenated blood Blood returned to the heart, to be replenished with oxygen in the lungs.

Oxygenated blood Blood leaving the heart that is oxygen-rich.

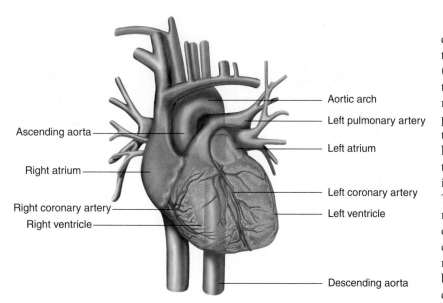

Ascending aorta

Right atrium

Right coronary artery

Right ventricle

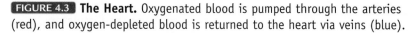

Aortic arch

Left pulmonary artery

Left atrium

Left coronary artery

Left ventricle

Descending aorta

FIGURE 4.3 **The Heart.** Oxygenated blood is pumped through the arteries (red), and oxygen-depleted blood is returned to the heart via veins (blue).

The heart has its own electrical conduction network, which is regulated by the sinoatrial (SA) node. The SA node (pacemaker) is a collection of specialized tissue that generates the electrical signal that causes the heart to contract and pump blood. This **autoregulation** allows the cardiac muscle to maintain a regular rhythm, or rate of beating, without the brain having to become consciously involved in setting the pace of the heart. The heart also responds to chemical and neural impulses that can alter the force or rate of contraction. For example, when our skeletal muscles send signals that they need more oxygen, the heart responds by beating faster or harder. This increases the quantity of blood pumped by the heart to match the increased skeletal muscle demand for oxygen. This is why heart rate (HR) monitoring is a method commonly used to determine and assess exercise intensity levels.

Autoregulation Self-regulation.

Arteries Blood vessels that carry oxygenated blood from the heart to the body.

Arterioles Small, muscular branches of arteries; when they contract, they increase resistance to blood flow, and blood pressure increases.

Capillaries Tiny blood vessels that circulate blood to all the body's cells.

Veins Blood vessels that return deoxygenated blood to the heart.

Venous return Blood returning through the veins to the heart.

The Blood Vessels

There are many different types of blood vessels that carry blood through the body. **Arteries** carry oxygenated blood from the heart to all organs and tissues in the body. The arteries closest to the heart are large; as they move farther from the heart they divide into smaller vessels called **arterioles**. Arterioles lead to **capillaries**, tiny blood vessels that branch out from arteries and veins and circulate blood to all the cells in the body. **Veins** return blood to the heart after oxygen and nutrients have been exchanged for carbon dioxide and waste products. Blood vessels can be damaged by injury or by disease; this damage may obstruct the flow of blood carrying oxygen and nutrients. The blood in the arterial system moves from the heart, which generates a great deal of pressure, into smaller and smaller vessels, which help to maintain a high-pressure outflow. This pressure is referred to as *blood pressure*. Maintaining adequate blood flow is important in the delivery of oxygen and the removal of carbon dioxide. If the blood pressure drops rapidly (for example, if you stand up too quickly), you feel dizzy. This dizziness is caused by diminished blood flow to the brain. Veins and arteries for the most part run side by side throughout the body.

The Circulation of Blood

When returning to the heart, blood moves from one-cell-thick capillaries into larger venules and then even larger veins. This movement from small vessels into larger vessels accounts for the low-pressure return system of our vascular network. One of the benefits of moving during the cooldown phase of a workout is that muscle contraction aids in **venous return**, making it easier for blood to return to the heart and helping you recover from exercise more rapidly. It also prevents you from fainting and keeling over from rapid blood pressure fluctuations.

The Function of Blood

The heart (a muscle) is responsible for circulating the blood that nourishes our cells and maintains life. Blood (the fluid circulated by the heart) plays an important role in removing waste products, assisting in *thermoregulation* (temperature control), and delivering hormones. A fluid portion of the blood, called *plasma*, consists primarily of water and thus makes circulation possible. The blood also contains **hemoglobin**, which is responsible for the transportation of oxygen. Oxygen binds to the hemoglobin found in red blood cells. Carbon dioxide is also carried in the blood, primarily in the form of **bicarbonate ions (HCO₃)**. The circulatory system functions to deliver oxygen to working muscles and remove carbon dioxide.

This closed system maintains blood pressure and flow. When you start to move, your heart must respond by beating more forcefully and rapidly to deliver the blood that the muscles need. The more fit you are, the easier your heart adjusts to the stimulus of physical activity.

Respiratory System

Your respiratory system is made up of the organs in your body that help you to breathe. The goal of breathing is to deliver oxygen to the body and to take away carbon dioxide. The lungs are the main organs of the respiratory system. Your lungs contain almost 1500 miles of airways and over 300 million alveoli (tiny sacs in the lungs that perform gas exchange). Every minute you inhale roughly 6 quarts of air.

In the lungs, oxygen is taken into the body and carbon dioxide is breathed out. The red blood cells are responsible for picking up the oxygen in the lungs and carrying the oxygen to all the body cells that need it. The red blood cells deliver oxygen to the body cells and then pick up carbon dioxide, which is a waste gas product produced by our cells. The red blood cells transport carbon dioxide back to the lungs, and we breathe it out when we exhale.

Cardiac Output, Stroke Volume, and Heart Rate

As stated previously, the heart is a special type of muscle (cardiac muscle). Like the other muscles in your body, the heart responds to the stimulus of physical activity by becoming stronger. One of the best measures of your heart's ability to function is its **cardiac output**. Cardiac output refers to the heart's ability to pump out blood every minute. When analyzing cardiac output, the amount of blood squeezed out of the heart with each contraction (**stroke volume**) is important, but so is the rate at which the blood is squeezed out (**heart rate**). With improved fitness, the force with which the heart can contract increases. Another adaptation to regular exercise is the improved ability of the heart to expand and allow more blood to flow into it. This increased contractile force and greater elasticity allow more blood to be squeezed out with each contraction. If you can squeeze more blood out with each contraction (greater stroke volume) the heart doesn't have to beat as often. Therefore, one way to monitor improvement in cardiovascular fitness is to measure your heart rate. The lower your resting heart rate, the higher your stroke volume and the stronger your heart.

With increasing amounts of work, a fit person's heart rate will be lower than an unfit person's heart rate at any workload. The lower heart rate is due to the fit person's heart being stronger (greater stroke volume), so it doesn't have to beat as often. As the workload continues to increase, the unfit person will fatigue before the fit person does. The fit person will be able to continue to be active at higher intensities and for a longer time than the unfit person can. The unfit person's weaker heart will reach its maximal rate and will not be able to maintain cardiac output. If cardiac output cannot be maintained, the unfit person fatigues. The fit person will be able to be active longer before reaching maximal heart rate because the stroke volume is greater. Therefore, the fit person will be able to postpone fatigue for a longer time.

Hemoglobin The oxygen-carrying pigment of the red blood cells.

Bicarbonate ions (HCO₃) As a buffer, they prevent a change in blood pH.

Cardiac output The amount of blood ejected from the heart each minute; calculated by multiplying heart rate by stroke volume.

Stroke volume The amount of blood ejected with each contraction of the heart.

Heart rate The frequency at which the heart beats (contracts).

Cardiorespiratory endurance is the ability of the circulatory and respiratory systems to supply oxygen and fuel to the body during sustained physical activity.

Assessing Cardiorespiratory Endurance

Cardiorespiratory endurance is defined as the ability of the circulatory and respiratory systems to supply oxygen and fuel to the body during sustained physical activity. To assess cardiorespiratory endurance, a measure that quantifies how effectively your body is using oxygen is required.

The best quantitative measure of cardiorespiratory endurance is maximum oxygen consumption or VO_2max (derived from V, volume per time; O_2, oxygen; max, maximum). VO_2max (also called maximal oxygen consumption, maximal oxygen uptake, or aerobic capacity) is the maximum capacity of your body to transport and utilize oxygen during maximum exercise. Tests measuring VO_2max can be time-consuming, require expensive equipment, and require highly trained professionals to conduct. Hence, many protocols for estimating VO_2max have been developed. These are similar to a VO_2max test but do not reach the maximum of the cardiovascular and respiratory systems and are called submaximal tests or field tests. Field tests are less expensive, require little to no equipment, are safer, can be conducted on your own, and therefore, are much more practical than a VO_2max test is.

A field test to estimate VO_2max is the Rockport Fitness Walking Test (**FIGURE 4.4**). The goal of the Rockport Fitness Walking Test is for you to walk as fast as possible for 1 mile. After you have completed the mile, immediately take your pulse rate. If you do not have a heart rate monitor, you can manually take your pulse and count the number of beats for 10 seconds and then multiple that number by 6 to get your minute heart rate. Another field test to estimate VO_2max is the Compiled Modified Canadian Aerobic Fitness Test (mCAFT). The mCAFT measures the rate at which the pulse returns to normal after completing a 3-minute step test (**FIGURE 4.5**).

Improvement in aerobic fitness level is measured by assessing changes in VO_2max. Increases in VO_2max may range from 5 to 30 percent when starting an aerobic physical activity program. Individuals with low initial levels of aerobic fitness will see the greatest percentage increase in VO_2max through aerobic activity. This happens because less fit individuals have more room for improvement.

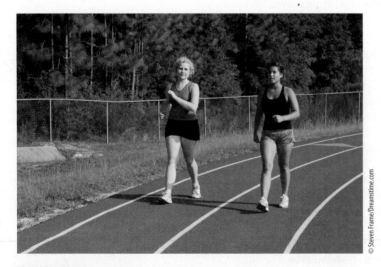

FIGURE 4.4 **Field Test.** A submaximal or field test such as the Rockport Fitness Walking Test can be used to assess cardiorespiratory fitness.

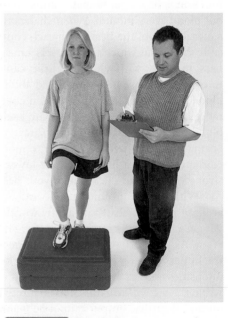

FIGURE 4.5 **Step Test.** A step test is another way to assess your cardiorespiratory fitness.

Designing Your Cardiorespiratory Fitness Program

Cardiorespiratory fitness should be the mainstay of any exercise program. You can use the FITT formula to help you determine how much exercise is enough for you to build aerobic fitness safely and effectively (TABLE 4.1). FITT stands for frequency, intensity, time, and type of activity.

Frequency

The American College of Sports Medicine recommends exercising 3 to 5 days a week (based on meeting certain intensity guidelines) to build cardiorespiratory fitness (ACSM, 2010). More frequent aerobic training provides few additional benefits and can increase the likelihood of injury. For general health, exercise classified as moderate-intensity aerobic activity or at the base of the My Activity and Exercise Pyramid, such as brisk walking, is recommended on a daily basis.

Intensity or How Hard

The recommended intensity (I) for developing optimal cardiorespiratory fitness is between 64 and 76 percent, up to 95 percent of your maximum heart rate (determined by using the equation $208 - 0.7$ [age]) (ACSM, 2010). An alternative way of setting your intensity is to use from between 40 and 59 percent up to 89 percent of your **heart rate reserve** (HRR) (ACSM, 2010). Both of these methods may be used to determine your aerobic capacity. Reserve methods utilize a percentage of the difference between your maximal score and your resting score. Reserve methods are preferred over the heart rate maximum (HR_{max}) method because they include an indirect measure of fitness (the resting score). Exercising at intensities beyond the recommended level shifts you from aerobic exercise into anaerobic exercise. Although this may increase your power, aerobic exercise is best for improvements in cardiorespiratory fitness.

Similar increases in cardiorespiratory endurance may be achieved by a moderate-intensity, longer-duration activity as opposed to a vigorous-intensity, shorter-duration activity. The moderate-intensity values—that is, 40 to 59 percent of HRR, and 64 to 76 percent of HR_{max}—are most applicable to individuals who are less fit (ACSM, 2010). Vigorous-intensity, shorter-duration activity is preferred by some people because they can be active for shorter periods of time. The drawback to this type of activity is that you are at greater risk of injury, and it can feel

Heart rate reserve The difference between maximum heart rate and resting heart rate.

TABLE 4.1	Cardiorespiratory Exercise FITT Guidelines
Frequency	5 days per week for moderate-intensity aerobic activity
	3 days per week for vigorous-intensity aerobic activity
Intensity	Based on heart rate reserve: 40–89%
	Based on maximum heart rate: 64–95%
	Based on rating of perceived exertion: 5–8
Time	Accumulate 30 or more minutes for moderate-intensity aerobic activity.
	Accumulate 20 or more minutes for vigorous-intensity aerobic activity.
Type	Choose an activity that uses repetitive, rhythmic, large-muscle movements performed continuously over an extended time.
	Start-and-stop sports such as basketball, tennis, and racquetball also are aerobic, if skill levels allow for continuous play and are intense enough to raise heart rate to target levels.

SOURCE: Adapted from the American College of Sports Medicine. (2010). *ACSM's Guidelines for Exercise Testing and Prescription*, 8th ed. Philadelphia: Lippincott Williams & Wilkins.

very strenuous mentally and physically. Moderate-intensity, longer-duration activity can provide the same benefits with a lower risk of injury and less mental and physical strain. The only drawback is that it takes longer to perform.

To reduce the risk of injury and to enhance adherence to your activity program, moderate-intensity, longer-duration activity is typically recommended for beginners. It is also recommended for those with previous injury and those who have no desire for physically challenging activities. However, athletes in training, those of higher fitness levels, and those who enjoy a physical challenge usually perform vigorous-intensity activities. Additionally, the more fit the person, the higher the intensity needs to be to bring about further improvement. For the majority of the healthy adult population, vigorous intensities within the range of 77 to 95 percent HR_{max} or 60 to 89 percent of HRR are sufficient to achieve improvements in cardiorespiratory fitness, when combined with an appropriate frequency and duration of training (ACSM, 2010).

You should consider several factors when determining exercise intensity. These include your level of fitness, any medications you might be taking, your risk for cardiovascular or orthopedic injury, your preference for different types of exercises, and your program objectives (ACSM, 2010). You will learn to modify the intensity of the activity you select to get the best response from your training program.

Monitoring Your Intensity

HEART RATE   You can monitor your cardiovascular response to aerobic physical activity in several ways (TABLE 4.2). The most common way is by measuring your heart rate response (FIGURE 4.6) This is most accurate when performing exercise of low to moderate intensities. During this type of exercise there is a linear relationship between heart rate and oxygen consumption. This means that as heart rate increases, oxygen consumption increases at the same rate and magnitude. When exercise intensities go beyond the moderate range, heart rate is not a good indicator of cardiovascular response. This is because as muscles go beyond 60 percent of their force-generating capacity, the muscles spend a longer time compressing the arteries and veins, and blood flow is reduced. Your body tries to compensate for this by having your heart beat more frequently. However, blood flow is still restricted, so heart rate increases at a much faster rate than oxygen delivery does. The rise in heart rate is therefore not a good indicator of oxygen consumption at higher intensities of activity.

TABLE 4.2	Classification of Aerobic Exercise Intensity Measurements		
Intensity	Heart Rate Reserve %	Maximal Heart Rate %	Rating of Perceived Exertion
Very light	< 30	< 57	1–2
Light	30–39	57–63	3–4
Moderate	40–59	64–76	5–6
Vigorous	60–89	77–95	7–8
Near-maximum to maximum	≥ 90	≥ 96	9–10

SOURCE: Adapted from the American College of Sports Medicine. (2010). *ACSM's Guidelines for Exercise Testing and Prescription*, 8th ed. Philadelphia: Lippincott Williams & Wilkins.

To monitor your exercise response using heart rate, you must first learn how to locate and measure your pulse (**FIGURE 4.7**). The next step involves calculating your target heart rate. Your *target heart rate* represents the zone that your heart rate needs to reach in order to receive optimal results from your activity session (**FIGURE 4.8**).

The American College of Sports Medicine (2010) reminds us that some people prefer to exercise at the low end of the target heart rate range and focus on long-duration activities to achieve their program goals. This may help adherence in certain populations. It is important to understand that different activities bring about different heart rate responses (ACSM, 2010). For example, the target heart rate you might choose while cycling would be different from the target heart rate when swimming. This reinforces the importance of selecting a prescreening test that is similar to the type of activity you plan on performing.

RATING OF PERCEIVED EXERTION (RPE) RPE is a subjective measure used to monitor your response to aerobic exercise. On a 0 to 10 scale, where 0 is the level of effort of sitting and 10 is maximal effort, you are asked to subjectively rate your exertion level based on physical sensations during aerobic activities, including increased heart rate, increased respiration or breathing rate, increased sweating, and muscle fatigue. A rating of 5 to 8 is recommended for cardiorespiratory training. Moderate intensity is a level of effort of 5 or 6 and vigorous intensity is a level of effort of 7 or 8 (see Table 4.2). Although this is a subjective measure, RPE values correlate highly with exercise heart rate percentages and provide an indication of the relative exercise intensity. As with heart rate, RPE scores are specific to the type of activity you perform.

TALK TEST The **talk test** is another relative method used for measuring exercise intensity. By judging your ability to talk during your aerobic workout, you can determine how hard you're working. A person who is active at a moderate intensity (around a level of 5 or 6 on the RPE scale) can talk or carry on a conversation during the activity, but cannot sing. If the person is not able to say more than a few words without pausing to take a breath (around a level of 7 or 8 on the RPE scale), they are doing vigorous-intensity activity (refer to Table 4.2).

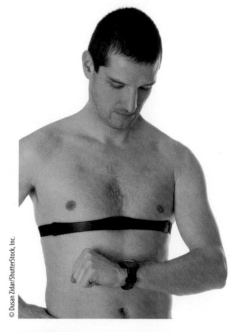

© Dusan Zidar/ShutterStock, Inc.

FIGURE 4.6 **Heart Rate Response.** A heart rate monitor can be used to track your heart rate and response to aerobic physical activity.

Talk test A simple way to measure relative aerobic intensity

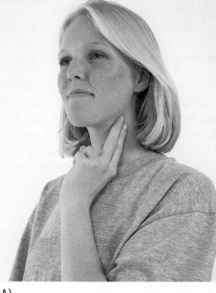

(A)

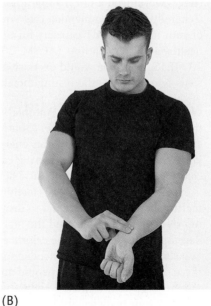

(B)

FIGURE 4.7 **How to Find Your Pulse.** The carotid artery (A) and radial artery (B) are frequently used to monitor heart rate response to aerobic physical activity.

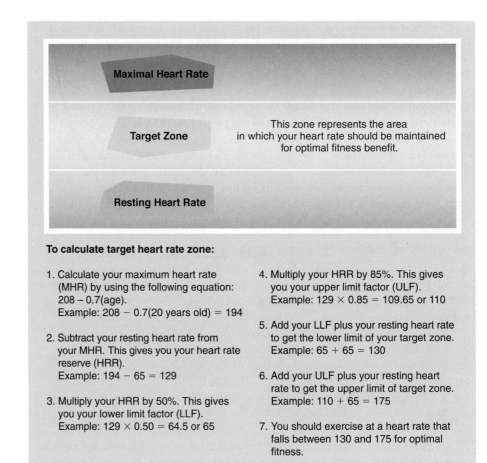

To calculate target heart rate zone:

1. Calculate your maximum heart rate (MHR) by using the following equation: 208 − 0.7(age).
Example: 208 − 0.7(20 years old) = 194

2. Subtract your resting heart rate from your MHR. This gives you your heart rate reserve (HRR).
Example: 194 − 65 = 129

3. Multiply your HRR by 50%. This gives you your lower limit factor (LLF).
Example: 129 × 0.50 = 64.5 or 65

4. Multiply your HRR by 85%. This gives you your upper limit factor (ULF).
Example: 129 × 0.85 = 109.65 or 110

5. Add your LLF plus your resting heart rate to get the lower limit of your target zone.
Example: 65 + 65 = 130

6. Add your ULF plus your resting heart rate to get the upper limit of target zone.
Example: 110 + 65 = 175

7. You should exercise at a heart rate that falls between 130 and 175 for optimal fitness.

FIGURE 4.8 **How to Calculate Your Target Heart Rate Using the Heart Rate Reserve Method.**

METS   You may also use *multiples of your resting metabolism*, or METS, to monitor exercise intensity. One MET is equal to your metabolic rate at rest. Its equivalent in VO_2 is $3.5 \text{ mL} \times \text{kg}^{-1} \times \text{min}^{-1}$. Exercising at 10 METS means that your metabolism is working at a rate 10 times its resting level, or at $35 \text{ mL} \times \text{kg}^{-1} \times \text{min}^{-1}$. Generally it is recommended that you use MET levels between 50 and 85 percent of your maximal MET capacity for optimal cardiorespiratory fitness benefit in healthy adult populations (ACSM, 2010). Thus, if a person had a MET capacity of 10 METS, he or she would exercise at an intensity of 5 to 8.5 METS. This represents 5 to 8.5 times the resting metabolic rate.

CALORIC EXPENDITURE   Another way of monitoring exercise intensity is through the use of caloric expenditure. All human movement requires the expenditure of energy. In the human body, this energy takes the form of a molecule called **adenosine triphosphate** (ATP). Monitoring caloric expenditure involves estimating the caloric cost of performing physical activity. The unit of heat produced when energy is expended is called a *calorie* (technically it's called a *kilocalorie [kcal]*, but in our metric-phobic society we tend to drop the *kilo* part). The more work we do, the more energy we expend, and the more calories we use. Several charts have been developed for estimating the caloric expenditure of a number of activities.

Caloric expenditure is dependent on body size and sex. Large people expend more energy than do small people doing the same activity. Men usually expend more energy than women do when performing the same activity. Additionally, whether your body weight is supported when performing an activity will affect

Adenosine triphosphate A high-energy phosphate that is the only useable form of energy in the human body.

caloric expenditure. For example, running expends more energy per unit of distance traveled than cycling does.

Generally, it is recommended that we expend approximately 150 to 400 kcal per activity session (ACSM, 2010). This would be equivalent to walking 1.5 to 4 miles. A goal to shoot for is a weekly caloric expenditure between 1000 and 2000 kcal, which has been associated with providing protection against cardiovascular disease. You can achieve 2000 kcal by performing activities that expend 400 kcal per session 5 days per week, 500 kcal per session 4 days per week, or any other combination that adds up to 2000 kcal for the week. It is best to spread the 2000 kcal over several days. See TABLE 4.3 on caloric cost of various activities to select the activities that will allow you to achieve this recommendation.

Time or Duration

A cardiorespiratory endurance session of 20–60 minutes is recommended to gain significant aerobic benefits. This does not include the warm-up and cool-down phases of your program. The duration of exercise can take place in a single session or in multiple sessions as long as each session lasts for 10 minutes or more. The total duration of exercise depends on intensity. The lower the intensity, the longer you need to be active. For example, to achieve general health-related benefits from cardiorespiratory endurance activities, it is recommended that adults should do 2 hours and 30 minutes (150 minutes) a week of moderate-intensity or 1 hour 15 minutes (75 minutes) a week of vigorous-intensity aerobic physical activity or an equivalent mix of moderate- and vigorous-intensity aerobic activity (U.S. Department of Health and Human Services [USDHHS], 2008; ACSM, 2011).

Type of Activity

Recommended forms of activity for improvement of cardiorespiratory fitness and cardiovascular health are usually focused on the larger muscle masses of the body and include such activities as walking, jogging, hiking, cycling, and swimming (FIGURE 4.9). These activities not only involve the larger muscles of the body but also are rhythmic in nature. The cyclical pumping action of the muscles assists blood flow, keeps blood pressure in healthy zones, and allows for the adequate delivery of oxygen. Activities that involve smaller muscle masses (e.g., arm cranking, heavy-resistance weight lifting) may actually restrict blood flow, elevate blood pressure, and retard the delivery of oxygen.

Activities that require the cardiovascular system to perform at a level above its normal resting state for an extended period of time are best for improving cardiovascular function. Such exercises are frequently referred to as being aerobic in nature. Examples include traditional exercises such as walking, jogging, cycling, swimming, inline skating, and cross-country skiing. Other activities that would help you improve your cardiovascular health include house and yard work and physically active recreational pursuits. TABLE 4.4 provides a few choices of indoor and outdoor aerobic activities, and the pros and cons of why you may or may not choose these activities for your exercise. You may wish to engage in several different types of activities to reduce repetitive stress to your bones and joints and to involve a greater number of muscle groups.

Progression

It is very important that you progress gradually whenever you start, or make significant changes to, a physical activity program. You must give your body time to adjust to being physically active. If you do not, you run the risk of injury and dissatisfaction with your program.

> A cardiorespiratory endurance session of 20–60 minutes is recommended to gain significant aerobic benefits.

TABLE 4.3	Caloric Expenditures	
Activity	**Calories per Minute per Pound**	**Calories per Hour per 150 Pounds**
Archery	0.034	305
Badminton		
Moderate	0.039	350
Vigorous	0.065	585
Baseball	0.031	279
Basketball (moderate)	0.047	423
Bicycling		
Slow (5 mph)	0.025	225
Moderate (10 mph)	0.05	450
Fast (15 mph)	0.072	550
Dancing		
Moderate	0.045	405
Fast	0.064	575
Fishing	0.018	165
Gardening	0.024	220
Golf	0.029	260
Hill climbing	0.06	540
Jogging (4.5 mph)	0.063	565
Karate	0.087	785
Rowing		
Light (2.5 mph)	0.036	325
Vigorous	0.118	1062
Running		
6 mph (10-min mile)	0.079	710
10 mph (6-min mile)	0.1	900
12 mph (5-min mile)	0.13	1170
Soccer	0.06	540
Swimming		
25 yd/min	0.058	520
50 yd/min	0.071	640
Table tennis	0.025	225
Tennis		
Moderate	0.046	415
Vigorous	0.06	540
Volleyball		
Moderate	0.036	325
Vigorous	0.065	585
Walking		
2 mph	0.022	200
3 mph	0.03	270
4 mph	0.039	350
5 mph	0.064	576
Wrestling	0.091	820

TABLE 4.4	Types of Indoor and Outdoor Aerobic Activity

Activity	Pros	Cons
Walking 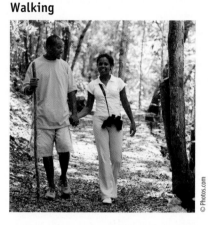	• Most popular of all activities • No age limit—a lifetime activity • Convenient • Easily incorporated into lifestyle • Little skill involved • No cost • Fewer injuries than jogging or running • You can take in seasonal changes or walk through city streets and people watch • This is a weight-bearing exercise • Uses most major lower-body muscle groups	• Not active enough for some • Takes three times longer to get the same aerobic benefit as from running • Injuries can occur, such as shin splints and blisters
Jogging/running 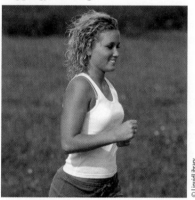	• Convenient • High levels of cardiorespiratory fitness benefits in short time periods • Few skills needed • Impact on hard surface builds stronger bones and offers protection against osteoporosis • Euphoric feeling or "runner's high" • In bad weather, you can run on an indoor track, if one is available • Low cost—just need a good pair of running shoes • Because it is often done outdoors, you get to view nature and a change of scenery	• Frequent, chronic injuries from impact to muscles, tendons, ligaments, and bones • Injuries such as shin splints and stress fractures due to: ◦ Improper warm-up ◦ Excessive distances ◦ Impact of feet and legs on ground ◦ Wearing inadequate shoes • Dangerous when done on roads with traffic • Poor outdoor conditions (e.g., snow, pollution) may prohibit
Bicycling (road or mountain) 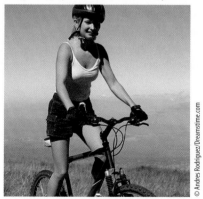	• No age limit—a lifetime activity • Fewer injuries than running because there is less impact on legs and feet • Because it is done outdoors, you get to view nature and a change of scenery	• May be difficult to locate a safe place to ride • Injuries include painful knees, feet, and back, and saddle soreness • Cost for the bike and other gear such as helmet, gloves, water bottle, sunscreen, and glasses

(continues)

TABLE 4.4 | **Types of Indoor and Outdoor Aerobic Activity** *(Continued)*

Activity

Inline skating/rollerblading

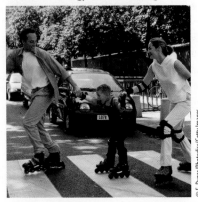

© E. Dygas/Photodisc/Getty Images

Pros

- Lots of fun—curving, turning, gliding, sprinting, and spinning
- Change of scenery
- Works thighs, hips, and buttocks muscles

Cons

- There is a learning curve, which could make the beginning stages a bit dangerous
- May be difficult to locate a safe place to skate
- Some people have difficulty stopping
- Injuries may result from collisions, falling, and blisters
- Requires skill and balance
- Coasting loses the aerobic effects
- Costs for skates, helmet, wrist guards, knee guards, elbow guards, and gloves

Swimming

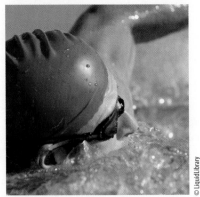

© LiquidLibrary

- Fewer injuries because there is no impact on legs and feet
- Good for people who are:
  - Injured and want to keep exercising
  - Pregnant
  - Overweight
- Works every part of the body, with an emphasis on the upper body
- Refreshing
- No age limit—lifetime activity

- You must locate a swimming pool and an available lane for swimming laps
- Requires skill
- Repetitive arm motions can result in pain and inflammation, leading to tendonitis and bursitis
- Swimming laps can be repetitive and seem boring
- Not a social activity
- Because this exercise doesn't involve impact, it does not help build bone density

Cross-country skiing

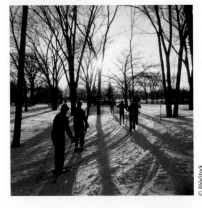

© AbleStock

- Involves both lower and upper body, including most major muscle groups when poles are used
- Rigorous workout obtained when at higher altitudes, in cold weather, and from added weight of clothing
- Scenery changes
- Low impact

- Risk of infections in the ears, eyes, and sinuses
- Exposure to cold conditions can lead to frostnip, frostbite, or hypothermia
- Requires accessibility to snow
- Skiing downhill decreases the aerobic effect

Treadmill

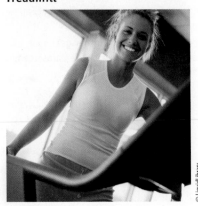

© LiquidLibrary

- Easily accessible no matter what the weather conditions
- Good for beginners, many levels
- Easy to use
- Easier on joints than walking or jogging on asphalt and concrete surfaces
- Can watch television while exercising
- Some machines have various personal high-tech computer programs that monitor heart rate

- Can get monotonous
- Can stumble and slide off
- Expensive to own; may require health club membership

TABLE 4.4 | **Types of Indoor and Outdoor Aerobic Activity** *(Continued)*

Activity	Pros	Cons
Stationary bicycle 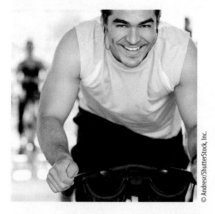	• Great thigh workout • Gives knees a rest • Can read or watch television while exercising • Easy to use • Convenient	• With stationary bikes you have added convenience, but lose the ability to ride outdoors • Expensive to own; may require health club membership
Rowing machine 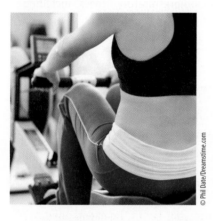	• Total body workout using most major muscle groups • Can watch television while exercising • Will prepare you for outdoor rowing or paddling on a canoe or kayak	• Can strain back if not performed correctly • Repetitive motion can become boring • Requires coordination
Aerobic dancing 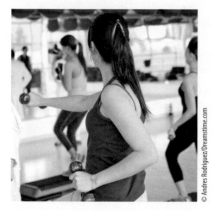	• Enjoyable • Can be done with a class or individually at home with a video or a televised class • Camaraderie can develop within a group of people working out together • Low injury rates • Different styles and variations of classes may be classified as follows: 　• High impact—more jumping and faster movement 　• Low impact—less jumping and slower movement 　• Aquatic—done in the water 　• Step aerobics using a 6- to 12-inch step—increases impact and weight-bearing movement 　• Kick boxing—uses movements of kick boxing for added variety and strength 　• Circuit—uses weights and aerobics to work out upper body as well as to increase aerobic endurance	• Possible injuries could occur, such as shin splints, tendonitis, muscle strain, back strain, and stress fracture • Cost of class or travel time to a gym

Physical Activity and Health Connection
. . . .

Practicing regular aerobic physical activity exercises that improve your ability to transport and use oxygen provides you with several benefits that go beyond performing daily activities and leisure-time activities with less fatigue. Aerobic physical activity assists in maintaining a healthy weight, lowering high blood pressure, lowering the "bad" cholesterol in your body (LDL), while at the same time increasing the level of "good" cholesterol (HDL). Over the long run, this helps prevent heart disease and stroke, two leading causes of death in the United States. Additionally, cardiorespiratory fitness can protect against type 2 diabetes and certain types of cancer and decrease levels of stress, anxiety, and depression.

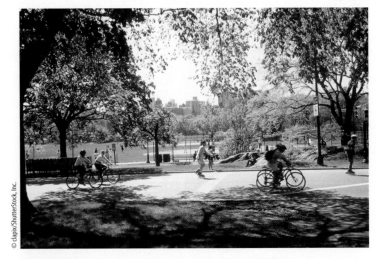

© dapix/Shutterstock, Inc.

FIGURE 4.9 **Choosing an Activity.** You can select from a variety of activities to improve your cardiorespiratory fitness, including walking, jogging, inline skating, and cycling.

concept connections

 1. **Cardiorespiratory endurance is a crucial health-related component of fitness because it improves the quality of life and quantity of life and reduces the onset and symptoms of aging and illness.** The benefits of aerobic physical activity in which the body's larger muscles move in a rhythmic manner for a sustained period of time are many. Aerobic activities strengthen the heart and lungs, making them more efficient and resilient and allowing you to meet the daily activity demands of life as well as participate in recreational leisure-time activities and sports. Aerobic exercise improves the strength of your bones, ligaments, and tendons and enhances muscular endurance. Important systemic changes include reduced blood pressure and LDL cholesterol, more efficient use of fats and sugars, the burning of lots of calories, and a healthier body composition. Aerobic exercise reduces your risk of cardiovascular disease and type 2 diabetes and has been shown to reduce stress and depression.

2. **The circulatory system consists of the heart and blood vessels—veins, arteries, and capillaries.** Arteries carry oxygenated blood from the heart to all organs and tissues, whereas veins return blood to the heart after oxygen and nutrients have been exchanged for carbon dioxide and waste products. Regular aerobic physical activity helps the circulatory system function properly.

3. **Cardiorespiratory endurance is the ability of the circulatory and respiratory systems to supply oxygen and fuel to the body during sustained physical activity.** Cardiorespiratory fitness should be the mainstay of any exercise program. You can use the FITT formula to help you determine how much exercise is enough for you to build aerobic fitness safely and effectively. FITT stands for frequency, intensity, time, and type of activity.

4. **A cardiorespiratory endurance session of 20–60 minutes is recommended to gain significant aerobic benefits.** This does not include the warm-up and cool-down phases of your program. The duration of exercise can take place in a single session or in multiple sessions as long each lasts for 10 minutes or more. The total duration of exercise depends on intensity. The lower the intensity, the longer you to need to be active.

Terms

Adenosine triphosphate, 72
Aorta, 65
Arteries, 66
Arterioles, 66
Autoregulation, 66
Bicarbonate ions (HCO$_3$), 67
Capillaries, 66
Cardiac output, 67

Cardiorespiratory endurance, 64
Deoxygenated blood, 65
Endocardium, 65
Heart rate, 67
Heart rate reserve, 69
Hemoglobin, 67
Myocardium, 65

Oxygenated blood, 65
Pericardium, 65
Stroke volume, 67
Talk test, 71
Veins, 66
Venous return, 66

making the connection

Maria learned from reading this chapter that to build her cardiorespiratory endurance she needs to exercise 3 to 5 days a week with each session lasting between 20 and 60 minutes and utilize activities that focus on the larger muscle masses of the body such as jogging, hiking, cycling, and swimming. After assessing her cardiorepiratory endurance via a the Rockport Fitness Walking Test, she decides to exercise at 65 to 75 percent of her heart rate reserve and will utilize a heart rate monitor.

Critical Thinking

1. In the vignette, Maria decides to use the heart rate reserve method to determine her aerobic exercise intensity. What other methods could she use to determine her exercise intensity?

2. Identify four activities in which you are likely to participate that will enhance your cardiovascular system. Describe how you will incorporate each activity into your daily and weekly routine.

3. You have been invited to speak at a local high school health class about how aerobic activity affects cardiorespiratory fitness. In 250 words, explain the impact that aerobic activity has on one's health.

References

American College of Sports Medicine. (2011). Position stand: Quantity and quality of exercise for developing and maintaining cardiorespiratory, musculoskeletal, and neuromotor fitness in apparently healthy adults: Guidance for prescribing exercise. *Medicine and Science in Sports and Exercise* 43(7):1334–1359.

American College of Sports Medicine. (2010). *ACSM's Guidelines for Exercise Testing and Prescription*, 8th ed. Baltimore, MD: Lippincott Williams & Wilkins.

U.S. Department of Health and Human Services. (2008). Physical Activity Guidelines for Americans. Online: http://health.gov/PAGuidelines/pdf/paguide.pdf.

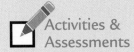

The Power of Resistance Training: Strengthening Your Health

5

what's the connection?

Kayleigh, a 19-year-old college sophomore, began taking aerobic dance classes during the fall semester to combat weight gain from her freshman year. She began with participating in two entry-level classes a week, gradually progressing up until she was completing three advanced classes a week by midsemester. Kayleigh dieted as well, but, despite "doing everything right," she was frustrated by her inability to lose weight fast enough. Her health instructor recommended that she include muscle-strengthening activities, or resistance exercises, along with her aerobic dance classes as a means to obtain a healthier body composition. Kayleigh was dumbfounded by her instructor's suggestion and thought to herself, "Oh yeah, right, I don't want to get bigger and bulkier!"

concepts

1. The health benefits of muscle-strengthening activities are well documented.

2. Skeletal muscles move and support the skeleton.

3. Skeletal muscle is made up of thousands of cylindrical muscle fibers.

4. Resistance training is essential for improving the health-related components of physical fitness—muscular strength and endurance.

5. Muscle-strengthening activities are recommended on 2 or more days a week for both adults and older adults.

6. A number of muscle-strengthening activities are available.

go.jblearning.com/kotecki4e
The website for this book is a great source for supplementary physical health information for both students and instructors. Visit **go.jblearning.com/kotecki4e** to find a variety of useful tools for learning, thinking, and teaching.

All parts of the body which have a function if used in moderation and exercised in labors in which each is accustomed, become thereby healthy, well developed and age more slowly, but if unused they become liable to disease, defective in growth and age quickly.

—Hippocrates

Introduction

The *Physical Activity Guidelines for Americans* recommend "muscle-strengthening activities on 2 or more days a week for all major muscle groups (legs, hips, back, chest, abdomen, shoulders, and arms)" for both adults and older adults (U.S. Department of Health and Human Services [USDHHS], 2008). This recommendation is consistent with that of the American College of Sports Medicine (ACSM, 2011), and recognizes the role of muscle-strengthening activities along with aerobic activity in obtaining substantial health benefits. The health benefits of muscle-strengthening activities—activities that cause skeletal muscles to contract against a resistance that leads to increases in strength and endurance—are well documented.

Muscle-strengthening activities or resistance training can increase lean body mass and lower body fat percentage, increase basal metabolism at rest, decrease the body's insulin response to changing glucose levels, lower the body's baseline insulin levels, and increase insulin sensitivity. Each of these factors is related to the body's ability to use sugars as fuel and aid in the prevention of type 2 diabetes. Participating in a regular resistance exercise program can maintain or improve your high-density lipoprotein (HDL) cholesterol levels and can decrease low-density lipoprotein (LDL) cholesterol levels, regulate diastolic blood pressure at rest, increase VO$_2$max, and improve cardiorespiratory endurance. All of these factors help to ensure a healthy cardiovascular system and protect against cardiovascular disease.

Fit muscles allow us to perform the tasks of daily living with less stress; help to protect our joints from injury; aid in sport and activity performance; assist in developing and maintaining strong bones, thereby reducing the risk of osteoporosis; and improve our body image and self-confidence. Older adults who perform resistance exercises regularly have shown improved ability to resist falls thanks to increased balance. These improvements are vital in maintaining independent living.

This chapter provides guidelines for designing your own resistance training program. To design an effective and safe resistance training program, it helps to have a basic understanding of muscle anatomy and physiology.

Muscle Anatomy and Physiology

Skeletal muscles move and support the skeleton. More than 600 individually named skeletal muscles make up 42 percent of an average adult male's and 36 percent of an average adult female's body mass (**FIGURE 5.1**). Skeletal muscles or "voluntary" muscles are joined to the bones by tendons. Tendons are bundles of tough fibers that differ in length and thickness. When a muscle contracts, the tendon exerts force on the bone, causing the bone to move (**FIGURE 5.2**). Most muscles work together in pairs. One muscle pulls while the other muscle relaxes. When you flex your arm, the biceps muscle pulls and the triceps muscle relaxes. When you extend your arm straight, the biceps muscle relaxes and the triceps muscle pulls.

Muscle Contraction and Relaxation

Skeletal muscle is not only highly organized to function at the macroscopic level, but the arrangement of muscle fibers at the microscopic level also demonstrates an

The health benefits of muscle-strengthening activities are well documented.

Skeletal muscles move and support the skeleton.

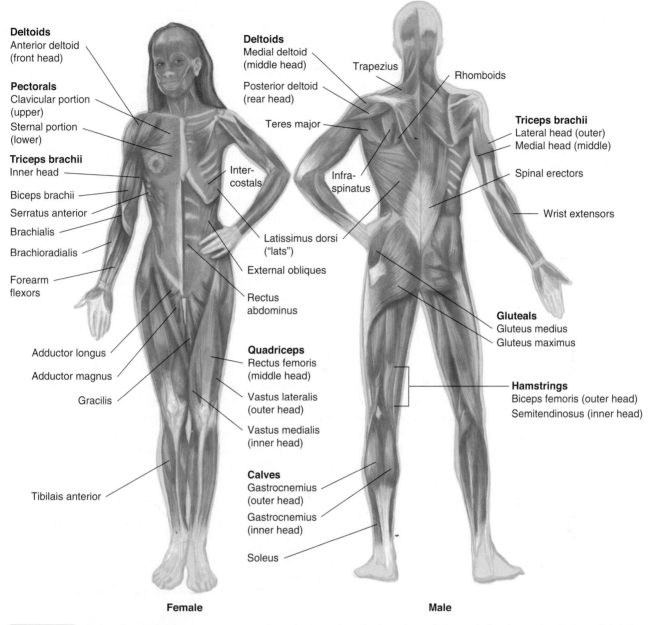

Deltoids
Anterior deltoid
(front head)

Pectorals
Clavicular portion
(upper)
Sternal portion
(lower)

Triceps brachii
Inner head

Biceps brachii

Serratus anterior

Brachialis

Brachioradialis

Forearm
flexors

Adductor longus

Adductor magnus

Gracilis

Tibilais anterior

Deltoids
Medial deltoid
(middle head)

Posterior deltoid
(rear head)

Teres major

Inter-
costals

Latissimus dorsi
("lats")

External obliques

Rectus
abdominus

Quadriceps
Rectus femoris
(middle head)

Vastus lateralis
(outer head)

Vastus medialis
(inner head)

Calves
Gastrocnemius
(outer head)

Gastrocnemius
(inner head)

Soleus

Trapezius

Rhomboids

Infra-
spinatus

Triceps brachii
Lateral head (outer)
Medial head (middle)

Spinal erectors

Wrist extensors

Gluteals
Gluteus medius
Gluteus maximus

Hamstrings
Biceps femoris (outer head)
Semitendinosus (inner head)

Female   **Male**

FIGURE 5.1 **Skeletal Muscle Groups, Front and Back.** Knowing the location of these skeletal muscles is beneficial for developing a resistance training program.

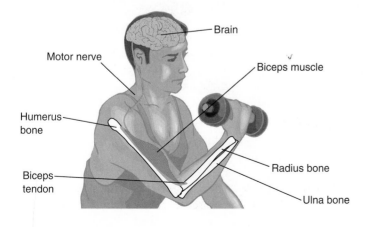

Brain

Motor nerve

Biceps muscle

Humerus
bone

Biceps
tendon

Radius bone

Ulna bone

FIGURE 5.2 **The Human Movement System.** This system consists of muscles, bones, tendons (which attach muscles to bones), and ligaments (which attach bones to bones). Movement occurs when the brain sends a signal via a specific nerve connecting it to a specific muscle. If the nerve signal directs a muscle to shorten, the two bones it connects move toward each other. If the nerve signal directs the muscle to lengthen, the two bones it connects move away from each other.

Skeletal muscle is made up of thousands of cylindrical muscle fibers.

Protein filaments Strands of protein (actin and myosin) that allow muscles to contract and relax.

Actin Filaments made of thin protein strands and located in the functional unit of the muscle cell.

Sarcomere The functional unit of the muscle cell.

Myosin Filaments made of thicker protein strands that must connect with the actin for muscle movement to occur.

amazing degree of organization (FIGURE 5.3). These muscle fibers are bound together by connective tissue through which run blood vessels and nerves. Between and within the muscle fibers is a complex structure of connective tissue, resembling struts and crossbeams, that helps to maintain the integrity of the muscle during contraction and relaxation (FIGURE 5.4). This connective tissue is composed of **protein filaments**, water, and minerals, which allow muscles to contract and relax. The protein filaments responsible for muscle contraction and relaxation are called *actin* and *myosin*. **Actin** filaments are made of thin protein strands and are located in the functional unit of a muscle cell, or **sarcomere**. **Myosin** filaments are thicker protein strands that must connect with the actin for movement to happen. Oarlike projections (myosin cross bridges) extend from the myosin and connect to active sites on the actin when the muscle is stimulated by a nerve impulse. As the muscle is innervated, energy is released, and the connected cross bridges swivel and rotate. This pulls the actin filaments over the myosin filaments, and the muscle shortens. The process of protein filaments sliding over the top of each other is referred to as the *sliding filament theory of muscle contraction*. As long as the muscle remains stimulated and energy is released, the muscle remains in this shortened state. When the stimulus is removed, the cross bridges detach and the filaments slide back over each other until they regain their elongated, resting state.

Slow-Twitch vs. Fast-Twitch Muscle Fibers

There are two broad types of skeletal muscle fibers: slow-twitch and fast-twitch. Each type influences how muscles respond to physical activity and training. Human muscles contain a genetically determined mixture of both slow and fast fiber types. On average, we have about 50 percent slow-twitch fibers and 50 percent fast-twitch fibers in most muscles used for movement.

Slow-twitch fibers are identified by a slow contraction time and a high resistance to fatigue, making them ideal for endurance activities. Slow-twitch muscles have a predominance of aerobic enzymes and therefore greater aerobic capacity,

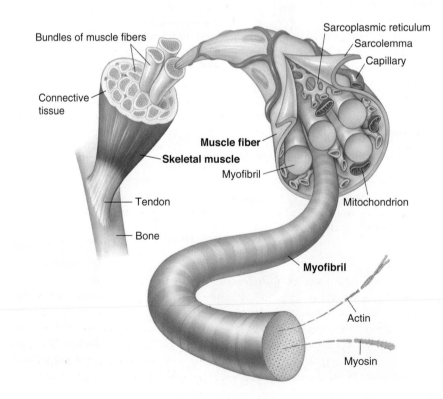

FIGURE 5.3 **The Structure of Skeletal Muscle.** Skeletal muscle is made up of thousands of cylindrical muscle fibers.

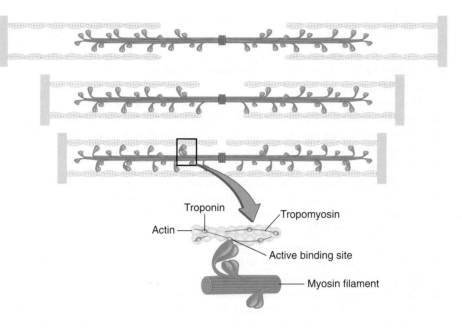

FIGURE 5.4 **Sliding Filament Theory of Muscle Contraction.** Your muscle filaments connect and slide to make your muscles move.

allowing them to generate more energy for continuous, extended muscle contractions over a long time. Aerobic activities and lower-intensity resistance training aimed at increasing muscular endurance better develop the functional capacity of our slow-twitch fibers.

Fast-twitch fibers are identified by a quick contraction time and a low resistance to fatigue, making them ideal for strength and power activities. Fast-twitch muscles do not use oxygen—they use glycogen. Reactions using glycogen require anaerobic enzymes to produce energy. Fast-twitch muscles allow us to perform rapid movements for shorter periods of time. Anaerobic activities such as sprinting and higher-intensity resistance training aimed at increasing muscular strength better develop the functional capacity of our fast-twitch fibers.

The contraction times of slow-twitch and fast-twitch muscle fibers are influenced by their number of motor units. A **motor unit** is a single nerve and all the corresponding muscle fibers it innervates. Muscles produce force by recruiting motor units. When you consciously flex your muscle, your brain informs the motor units in your muscle either to contract or to relax. Motor units that contain relatively few muscle fibers tend to be slow-twitch motor units. Motor units that contain large numbers of muscle fibers tend to be fast-twitch motor units. The more muscle fibers in a motor unit, the greater the force-generating capacity. This is why fast-twitch motor units are capable of generating more power than slow-twitch muscle fibers are. Fast-twitch motor units also have larger nerves than do slow-twitch motor units, which allows for greater speed of conduction of the nervous impulse that controls the muscle.

Functional Muscle Actions

There are four general types of muscle actions. The first is when unconscious nerve impulses maintain muscles in a partially contracted state that is passive and continuous. The presence of near-continuous innervations of muscle at a minimum is needed so that you can maintain normal posture. The second is when conscious nerve impulses actively increase voluntary muscle tension without moving the points of muscle origin and insertion because a counterforce equal to that of the contraction is being exerted. This is referred to as a static contraction.

Motor unit Single nerve cell and all of the corresponding muscle fibers it innervates.

The third is when the muscle's length shortens under tension against a counterforce less than that of the contraction, thus resulting in movement. This movement is called a concentric muscle action. For example, when you bend your arm at the elbow to lift a book, your biceps muscle undergoes concentric movement (FIGURE 5.5).

The fourth action is when a muscle contraction involving an external force lengthens the muscle. This is referred to as an eccentric muscle contraction. For example, when you are lowering the book and controlling how fast the book is moving by regulating how slowly you allow your arm to straighten, your biceps muscle is undergoing eccentric muscle action (refer to Figure 5.5).

The different functions muscles perform depend on the demands placed upon them. If a muscle is called upon to be responsible for the primary action of a desired movement, it is called the prime mover, or **agonist**. A muscle that resists the prime mover and helps to maintain joint integrity is called an **antagonist**. If you consider the example of lifting a book (refer to Figure 5.5), the biceps muscle of the upper arm that causes the arm to bend at the elbow is considered the agonist. The triceps muscle in the back of the upper arm resists the biceps and helps keep the elbow joint secure. In this example, the triceps is acting as an antagonist.

Muscles also can act as **synergists** if they assist the agonist but are not primarily responsible for carrying out the movement. In the previous example, the brachial radialis (a muscle that crosses the elbow and connects to the forearm) acts as a synergist. A **neutralizer**, or fixator, is a muscle whose action prevents unwanted activities of muscles not directly involved in the movement you wish to carry out. For example, the shoulder muscles frequently act as neutralizers to support the upper arm when it is bent at the elbow.

Muscle Strength and Size

Four main factors contribute to muscle strength and size. The first two factors are within your control (exercise and diet) whereas factors three and four are outside of your control (genetics and gender differences).

The first is the number of muscle-strengthening activities—activities that make the muscles do more work than they are accustomed to doing—that are included in your daily actions or as part of a resistance training program. For muscles to become stronger, they must regularly be exposed to more resistance than they are exposed to under normal resting conditions. Muscles that are regularly exposed to increased amounts of resistance also increase in size, or hypertrophy, as a result of their protein filaments increasing in size.

Agonist A muscle that acts as the prime mover; it is most responsible for the primary action of a desired movement.

Antagonist A muscle that resists the agonist; it helps to maintain joint integrity.

Synergists Muscles that assist the agonist.

Neutralizer A muscle that prevents unwanted activity in the muscles not directly involved in performing a movement.

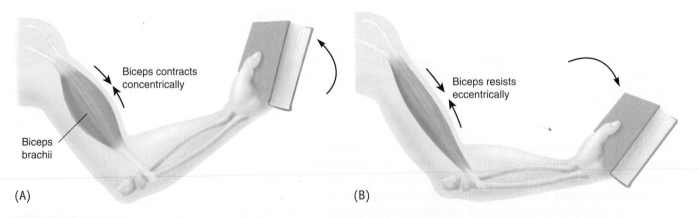

Biceps contracts concentrically

Biceps brachii

(A)

Biceps resists eccentrically

(B)

FIGURE 5.5 **Dynamic Muscle Contractions.** Your muscles shorten during concentric action (A) and lengthen during eccentric action (B).

It can take anywhere from a month or two for you to experience signs of structural changes in the size of protein filaments. However, most people show improvements in strength within a week or two of starting a resistance exercise program as a result of neuromuscular adaptations. The neuromuscular adaptations include the ability to selectively recruit the muscle fibers necessary to perform a given activity, the ability to synchronize the firing of these muscle fibers, and the ability to recruit more muscle fibers into action. In other words, as you experience increased coordination in performing a specific activity, this enables you to perform the activity with increasing levels of resistance.

The second factor contributing to muscle strength and size is making sure that you provide your muscles with enough energy from your diet by obtaining the recommended amounts of calories from carbohydrates, fats, and protein. Although you must consume the recommended daily allowance (RDA) of protein to build muscle, consuming protein in excessive amounts above the RDA to obtain greater muscle mass development is a mistake and can be harmful. Total dietary energy, specifically carbohydrate energy, is a very important nutritional factor affecting muscle gain and function (Fink, Burgoon, & Mikesky, 2012). Carbohydrates provide the main source of fuel for muscle contractions. Excessive intake of protein does not speed up the development of muscle mass or cause greater muscle mass to occur and can be harmful.

The third factor affecting muscle growth is genetics. Genetics, or your somatotype, contributes not only to the overall muscle-building process but also to the rate of muscle building. A somatotype is the kind of body type you have that is determined by your genes. There are three basic somatotypes: mesomorphs, ectomorphs, and endomorphs. **Mesomorphs** are naturally geared toward being muscular and therefore find it relatively easy to make gains in the muscle-building process. **Ectomorphs** are mainly those who are on the slender side and who typically have a genetic predisposition to being skinny. **Endomorphs** are people who are geared toward carrying around extra body fat and are typically known for having a rounder body shape.

The fourth factor is secretion of adequate amounts of the hormones responsible for causing muscle to grow (testosterone, androgens, human growth hormone). People who produce higher amounts of testosterone, androgens, and human growth hormone and combine this hormonal advantage with proper training and proper nutrition will generally have greater muscle mass development than those who have lower amounts. Men produce more of these hormones than women, so men tend to have the capacity for more muscle mass development than women. Women still have the capacity to show significant gains in muscle strength and muscle tone from regular resistance training, but they generally are not able to develop larger muscles.

Basics of Resistance Training

Types of Resistance Exercise

Knowing more about the types of resistance exercises available can help you make more informed decisions regarding the selection of muscle-strengthening activities for your fitness program. Resistance exercises are generally classified into static and dynamic.

Static, or isometric, resistance exercise involves muscular actions in which the length of the muscle does not change and there is no visible movement at the joint. An example of a static exercise is pushing against an immovable object such as a wall (FIGURE 5.6).

Mesomorphs Somatotype geared toward being muscular.

Ectomorphs Somatotype geared toward being slender.

Endomorphs Somatotype geared toward carrying more body fat.

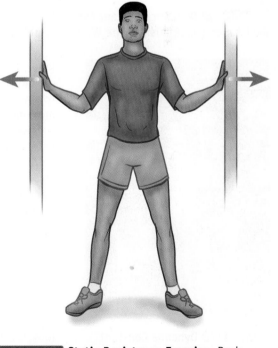

FIGURE 5.6 **Static Resistance Exercise.** Push against an inmovable object such as a wall.

Dynamic constant external resistance (DCER) Form of resistance training in which the external resistance or weight does not change and both a lifting (concentric) and lowering (eccentric) phase occur during each repetition; also known as isotonic resistance training.

Isokinetic resistance training Type of muscle contraction where the speed of movement is fixed and resistance varies with the force exerted.

Static exercises provide you with the opportunity to train anywhere because there is little or no equipment required. Static exercises increase strength at specific joint angles in which they are performed; however, they develop strength to a lesser extent at joint angles in which they are not performed. Dynamic resistance exercises are much better at increasing strength throughout a joint's full range of motion.

Dynamic resistance exercise involves muscular actions in which the length of the muscle does change and there is visible movement at the joint. Three examples of dynamic resistance exercise are **dynamic constant external resistance (DCER)**, also known as isotonic training, in which the prefix *iso* refers to constant and *tonic* refers to tension; isokinetic resistance exercise; and plyometrics.

DCER is a resistance training exercise in which the external resistance or weight does not change and both a lifting (concentric) and lowering (eccentric) phase occur during each repetition (Howley & Franks, 2007). This type of exercise is normally performed with free weights (dumbbells and barbells) (FIGURE 5.7) and various weight training machines (FIGURE 5.8).

A dilemma with training with free weights as a method of constant external resistance is the differences in the points of leverage. Because there are points in a joint's range of motion at which the muscle is stronger and points at which it is weaker, the amount of weight you can lift is limited by the weakest point. In other words, you experience various changes in resistance on the muscle at some points with the weight being easier to lift, and at other points being harder to lift because of the changing leverage points. Weight training machines/equipment have been designed to vary the resistance in an attempt to match the increases and decreases in strength throughout the range of motion of the exercise. These machines generally operate through a lever arm, cam, or pulley arrangement. These equipment designs attempt to create constant tension on the muscle under a constant load.

DCER exercises are the most well-liked type of resistance training for increasing muscular strength. Machines tend to be used more by beginners and by those who may have difficulty with balance (TABLE 5.1). Machines allow for an application of resistance in a guided or restricted manner. Free weights tend to be used by those who are more interested in developing control and balance when lifting as well as those who want to engage in more mechanical specificity or more lifelike or sporting movements (TABLE 5.2).

Isokinetic resistance training is a type of contraction where the speed of movement is fixed and resistance varies with the force exerted. In other words, the harder you push or pull, the more resistance you feel. This is referred to as *accommodating resistance* because the force generated is based on the person performing the activity. This method is mostly used for sports training or rehabilitation following an injury and requires special equipment (FIGURE 5.9). Isokinetic machines, such as the Cybex Orthotron, control the speed of motion and provide accommodating resistance through the use of hydraulics. For an example of how hydraulics can do this, consider a door with an automatic closer. If you allow the door to close at its preset rate, it takes little effort to move the door. However, if you try to speed the door up, the amount of resistance increases.

The major advantage to isokinetic training is that the resistance adjusts to the force you generate. This is important if you are rehabilitating injured or weak muscles. The disadvantages of isokinetic training include the high cost of the equipment, lack of access to this type of equipment (located mainly in rehabilitation clinics), and the inability to isolate individual muscle groups easily.

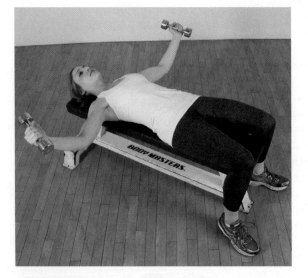

FIGURE 5.7 **Dynamic Constant External Resistance (DCER) Using Free Weight Dumbbells.**

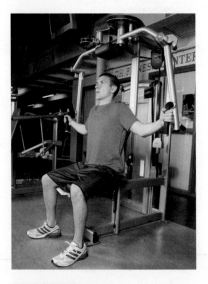

FIGURE 5.8 **Dynamic Constant External Resistance (DCER) Using a Weight Machine.**

TABLE 5.1	Advantages and Disadvantages of Weight Machines

Advantages
- Recommended for beginners
- Convenient
- Safe: weight cannot fall on you
- Less clutter: no weights scattered around
- No spotters needed
- No lifter needed to balance bar
- Offer variable resistance
- Ensure correct lifting movements, which prevents cheating when tired
- Easy to use: require less skill than free weights
- Easy to move from one exercise to the next
- Easier to adjust
- Easier to isolate specific muscle groups
- Back support (on most machines)
- Some offer high-tech options such as varying resistance during lifting motion

Disadvantages
- Limited availability: may need to go to a club
- Expensive
- Require a lot of space
- Do not allow natural movements
- Most machines have only one exercise
- Less motivation: only working against resistance on a machine

TABLE 5.2	Advantages and Disadvantages of Free Weights

Advantages
- Allow dynamic movements
- Allow a greater variety of exercises
- Widely available
- Require minimal space
- Strength transfers to daily activities
- Inexpensive
- Offer greater sense of accomplishment
- Most serious bodybuilders and lifters use free weights

Disadvantages
- Not as safe as exercise machines: weights can fall off the end of the bar or can pin or smash you when muscles tire
- Balancing is required, which can be difficult and dangerous (e.g., weights overhead, while doing squats)
- Require spotters for some exercises
- Allow cheating by swinging for momentum when muscles tire
- Require more time to change weights
- Can cause blisters and calluses
- Clutter creates hazard when weights are scattered

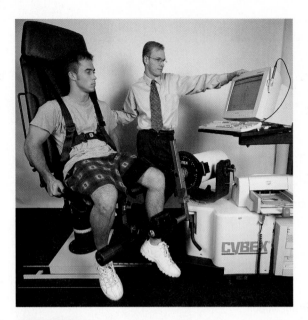

FIGURE 5.9 **Isokinetic Exercise.** Using a Cybex machine is a form of isokinetic resistance training.

Plyometrics Form of resistance training that uses rapid dynamic eccentric contraction and stretching of muscles followed by a rapid dynamic concentric contraction.

Valsalva maneuver Condition that occurs when you hold your breath and exert force (grunting action); causes elevated blood pressure that increases the risk for stroke, heart attack, or hemorrhage.

Plyometrics resistance training is a rapid dynamic eccentric contraction and stretching of muscles followed by a rapid dynamic concentric contraction. Plyometrics use bounding-type exercises to create these types of contractions. For example, depth jumping involves jumping off an elevated platform, landing on a surface, and then immediately performing a maximal vertical leap. Plyometrics are most often used by highly trained athletes because they can train at a normal speed of movement and overload the muscles in a way not possible with other training techniques. The disadvantage associated with plyometric training lies in the higher risk for injury resulting from the ballistic nature of the activity.

Proper Form and Technique

Any resistance exercise program should focus initially on proper form and technique. By doing so, you not only improve the safety of the activities you perform, but also increase the gains you receive. If you improperly perform a resistance exercise, you risk harming your joint ligaments and tendons as well as straining muscles.

Breathing

You should *never hold your breath when lifting*, particularly when you are exerting force. This may bring about a condition called the **Valsalva maneuver**. The Valsalva maneuver occurs when the windpipe is blocked off (as occurs when holding your breath). Pressure in your lungs begins to build up, which in turn causes an increase in blood pressure, which increases your risk of fainting or, even worse, suffering a heart attack or stroke. By breathing out when exerting force, you greatly reduce this risk. For example, when performing the bench press exercise, you breathe in when lowering the bar to your chest and breathe out when pressing the bar upward.

Proper Use of Equipment

For safe and effective training, it is important to understand how resistance strength equipment should be used. When it comes to the use of weight machines, typically several adjustments are required based on your body shape and size. It is important to understand the use of the equipment and how to adjust it properly to avoid injury. Ensure that you take the time to learn how equipment functions and how it adjusts.

Many individuals enjoy using free weight equipment such as dumbbells and barbells. Certain injuries can occur if proper technique and form are not followed. Injuries typically occur in training with free weights as a result of poor setup and lack of a spotter. *Setup* is doing the things possible to reduce the risk during exercise. Proper loading of the barbell in a balanced manner, using safety collars, and using a spotter are important. A *spotter* is a partner who provides hands-on assistance to you, most often during free weight training. The use of a spotter to assist you when potential muscle failure occurs is critical. If the lift becomes unattainable or unsafe because of improper technique, a spotter can assist.

Assessment

Assessment can be helpful in establishing beginning resistance workloads, monitoring progress, and enhancing safety. Several sample assessments are included in the activities and assessment manual.

Designing Your Resistance Training Program

Resistance training, along with cardiorespiratory endurance training, should serve as the foundation of any fitness program to improve muscular strength and endurance. **Muscular strength** is the amount of force a muscle or muscle group can exert with a single maximum effort. This is in contrast to **muscular endurance**, which is the ability of a muscle or muscle group to exert repeated force against a resistance or to sustain muscular contraction for a given period of time. You can use the FITT formula to help you determine how much exercise is enough for you to build muscle strength and endurance safely and effectively. FITT stands for frequency, intensity, time, and type of activity. There are many considerations and variations for frequency, intensity, time, and type when you consider muscle-strengthening activities to develop muscular endurance and strength. Your personal goals will influence how you apply the FITT principle to your resistance training program (ACSM, 2010).

Frequency of Exercise

For health-related fitness, the *Physical Activity Guidelines for Americans* recommend "muscle-strengthening activities on 2 or more days a week for all major muscle groups (legs, hips, back, chest, abdomen, shoulders, and arms) for both adults and older adults" (USDHHS, 2008). This recommendation is consistent with that of American College of Sports Medicine (2011). You can exercise these major muscle groups all on the same day or by utilizing a split routine, depending on your schedule.

Split routines are designed for the fitness participant who is unable to complete a full-body workout in a single day or who would like to work out more often. There are a number of ways to split your routine and there's no right or wrong way to do it. One of the most common ways of splitting up resistance exercises is dividing them into upper- and lower-body exercises. For example, you train your chest, back, abdomen, shoulders, and arms on Mondays and Thursdays and your legs and hips on Tuesdays and Fridays. Split routines are also designed to provide more advanced training for specific sports in which the resistance program has a greater volume demand and all training cannot be accomplished in a single full-body training session. For either health-related fitness or advanced training, recovery time is of vital importance.

Occasionally, people think that the more frequently you perform a resistance exercise, the more rapidly you will see improvement in fitness. If you do not allow adequate recovery time, your body does not have the chance to rebuild itself and make the structural changes necessary for muscular growth to occur. It is recommended that you allow 48 to 72 hours of recovery time between training sessions in which a muscle or group of muscles is exercised. This does not mean that you must remain inactive during this recovery time. You can perform muscle-strengthening activities that work other body parts or other aspects of health-related fitness (i.e., cardiorespiratory endurance activities) while you allow those muscles that were exercised time to recover. High-volume/intensity workouts may require extended rest intervals.

Intensity or Resistance of Exercise

The amount of resistance utilized to develop muscular endurance and strength is comparable to heart rate intensity in cardiorespiratory endurance training. To develop muscular endurance, choose resistances between 50 and 65 percent of your maximum capacity. To develop muscular strength, choose higher resistances between 70 and 85 percent of your maximum capacity. For a general health/fitness goal, which includes both endurance and strength, choose a resistance between 60

Resistance training is essential for improving the health-related components of physical fitness—muscular strength and endurance.

Muscle-strengthening activities are recommended on 2 or more days a week for both adults and older adults.

Muscular strength Amount of force a muscle or muscle group can exert with a single maximum effort.

Muscular endurance Ability of a muscle or muscle group to exert repeated force against a resistance or to sustain muscular contraction for a given period of time.

and 75 percent of your maximum capacity. [TABLE 5.3] provides guidelines for general resistance or intensity percentages based on one resistance exercise goal. As with any resistance exercise program, the amount of resistance applied also depends on your fitness level.

You can determine your resistances by using a one-repetition maximum (1-RM) measurement performed on a specific exercise. For example, if your maximum capacity for the bench press is 200 pounds, you would aim to lift between 100 and 130 pounds (between 50 and 65 percent) for endurance and aim to lift between 140 and 170 pounds for strength (between 70 and 85 percent). Because testing for a one-repetition maximum for each exercise can be time-consuming and requires special safety considerations, it is recommended that you select a resistance based on the number of repetitions you can perform on a given exercise based on your program goal (refer to Table 5.3).

Beginners or currently inactive individuals should focus on developing health/fitness and muscular endurance programs. Strength and power training are usually reserved for those individuals who have already developed a basic level of muscular fitness or training for sports. Training for strength requires including higher levels of resistance in your training. With increased resistance intensity, the number of repetitions performed is reduced. Training for power is very similar to training for strength, with the major difference that power training requires greater speed. By definition, power means that work is accomplished at a high rate of speed. Power is best developed through explosive training. Because of the dynamic nature of power training, there is a higher risk of injury.

The principle of progression is important in training for muscular strength, endurance, and power development. *Progressive resistance exercise* (PRE) refers to the logical and systematic application of the overload principle. Frequently misinformed or overeager people attempt to lift too much weight at the beginning stages of resistance training. This can lead to increased muscle soreness or injury risk. With any muscle-strengthening program, the body needs time to accommodate greater levels of resistance. Even the very basic new exercise regimens usually result in delayed onset of muscle soreness (DOMS), typically 48 hours post exercise.

The PRE model uses multiple sets in a training program that build upon each other to properly challenge the body toward overload. For example, in a three-set training model the first set is used as a warm-up with reduced load, the intensity is increased for the second set for greater challenge, and the intensity is increased again for the third set to provide the proper training stimulus for the training goals. This PRE approach has been shown to be an effective way to increase

TABLE 5.3	Resistance Exercise Guidelines				
Goal	Exercises	Sets	Repetitions	Resistance	Rest Between Sets*
Health/fitness	8–10	1–2	8–12	60–75% of 1-RM	45–90 seconds
Endurance	8–12	2–3	12–20	50–65% of 1-RM	≤30–60 seconds
Strength	6–10	3–6	4–8	70–85% of 1-RM	2–3 minutes
Power	3–5	3–5	2–4	80–90% of 1-RM	4–5 minutes

Note: These are basic guidelines. Additional combinations of sets and repetitions may elicit greater fitness gains based on individual differences.
*Rest requirements vary depending on training goals and the level of experiences of the lifter. You should always rest long enough to achieve the desired repetitions.

strength, size, and endurance. During resistance exercise the muscle is not the only area that is accommodating higher levels of resistance; adaptations to ligaments, tendons, and bone also occur.

Time or Repetitions and Sets of Exercise

Time in resistance training is most often measured by the number of reps and sets you complete and how much time you rest between sets. *Reps* is short for repetitions. A repetition is one complete movement through an exercise. A bicep curl is an example. You curl your arm up and then back down. A set is a group of repetitions. A typical set can range from 4 to 8 reps for strength training to 12 to 20 reps for endurance training and is based on your program goal (refer to Table 5.3). The objective behind a set is to use a resistance or weight that will fatigue the muscle or muscle group that you are exercising by the end of the set. It is important to utilize a rest period between sets. A typical rest period ranges from 1 to 2 minutes (refer to Table 5.3). There are a number of different types of set systems. They range from the most basic (e.g., multi-set) training to the advanced (e.g., pyramiding, compound and tri-sets, supersetting).

Research indicates that multi-set or simple-set training is the best approach to elicit advanced muscular strength, endurance, and power gains (ACSM, 2009; Fleck & Kraemer, 2004). Multi-set training includes completing more than one set of a particular exercise using the same resistance intensity. Multi-set training includes exercises for all the major muscle groups. As indicated in Table 5.3, most resistance training program goals are met through a multi-set approach.

Pyramid lifting is an advanced level resistance exercise technique. Pyramiding up is when the resistance is increased and the repetitions are reduced for each set. For example, you may start at 6 reps at 70 percent of 1-RM followed by 4 reps at 80 percent of 1-RM, followed by 2 reps at 90 percent of 1-RM, followed by 1 rep at 100 percent of 1-RM. Pyramiding down is when you decrease the resistance and increase the repetitions for each set (FIGURE 5.10).

Compound sets and tri-sets are advanced level resistance exercise techniques that involve performing two (compound) or three (tri) exercises in a row that work the same muscle groups with little or no rest between the sets. This ensures that the muscle group is optimally fatigued. The disadvantage of using compound and tri-sets is the increase in discomfort caused by the lack of rest between sets.

Supersetting is an advanced level resistance exercise technique in which you perform two different exercises targeting two different muscles with little or no rest between sets. For example, you work your biceps and then immediately work your triceps with no rest. Each set consists of both biceps and triceps instead of just one or the other. Supersetting is designed to ensure that both muscle groups are actively fatigued. If done correctly, supersetting has the potential to speed up the development of muscular strength. A disadvantage is the discomfort associated with the increased muscle fatigue.

Many advanced bodybuilders and athletes also use a periodization program in their resistance training program. Periodization refers to the planned manipulation of your resistance training program at regular time

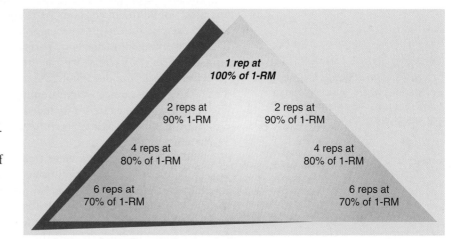

FIGURE 5.10 **Pyramid Lifting Chart by One-Repetition Maximum (1-RM) Percentages.** *Pyramiding up* is when the resistance is increased and the repetitions are decreased for each set. *Pyramiding down* is when the resistance is decreased and the repetitions are increased for each set.

intervals to bring about optimal gains in strength, muscle hypertrophy, power, and motor performance (Fleck & Kraemer, 2004). A periodization program is divided into a number of distinct cycles. The longest cycle is called a macrocycle and usually spans a period of one year, although shorter macrocycles are generally used. For example, you can subdivide the year into four macrocycles. During the first cycle, you focus on the development of muscular strength; during the second cycle, you focus on the development of muscular power. During the third cycle, you focus on the development of muscular endurance, and during the fourth cycle you focus on cross training to allow adequate recovery from the three preceding resistance training cycles. In the case of a competitive athlete, a goal may be to bring peak physical performance for a major competition (Fleck & Kramer, 2004).

For those interested in overall health-related muscular fitness, periodization can provide for a greater variety in their training while allowing for enhanced fitness levels. Periodization applies the principles of progressive training—by varying the repetitions, sets, weight, and intensity during each cycle—which allows for continual improvements in fitness throughout the year, thus avoiding reaching a plateau. If you follow the same workout for any length of time, the body soon adapts to the constant load and your gains diminish.

A number of muscle-strengthening activities are available.

Type of Resistance Exercise

There are a number of muscle-strengthening activities available, ranging from using your own body weight as resistance (e.g., pushups, chin-ups, sit-ups, leg lunges) to free weights (e.g., dumbbells, barbells) to weight machines to any other object that causes your muscles to contract (e.g., elastic exercise rubber tubing). Whatever form of resistance exercise you select, it is important to focus on all major groups of the body (legs, hips, back, chest, abdomen, shoulders, and arms).

Multi-joint exercises are recommended over single-joint exercises because they affect more than one muscle group. A multi-joint exercise is any movement in which your body must change the angles of more than one joint while performing the motion. Multi-joint exercises that work the major muscle groups include the bench press and pushups (chest, shoulders, and arms) and pulldowns or chin-ups (back and arms).

The sample program in TABLE 5.4 lists exercise recommendations in a systematic order for all the major body parts and corresponding muscle groups. This sample exercise routine provides a proper sequencing to achieving a balance between working all major body parts and corresponding muscle groups. Table 5.4 also references the exercise with figures in this text to provide visual familiarity.

Circuit weight training involves setting up a series of stations where you perform different resistance weight training (and/or aerobic) exercises. You can use any combination of exercises included in the basic lifts (refer to Table 5.4). By reducing the time between exercises/stations, you can develop muscular endurance and aerobic capacity.

For beginners, circuit weight training is a good place to start because it provides them with muscle system balance and both strength and endurance gains. In addition it provides safe exercises, is good for improving technique through the use of manageable loads, and aids in dissipating the soreness that typically accompanies new exercises. Circuit weight training is also a good approach for older adults because the repetition ranges are reasonable and the exercises are basic yet effective in keeping the body healthy. Finally, circuit training is an excellent way to meet the *Physical Activity Guidelines for Americans*, which recommends "muscle-strengthening activities on 2 or more days a week for all

Circuit weight training A series of stations where you can perform different resistance training (and/or aerobic) exercises.

TABLE 5.4	A Sample Circuit Weight Training Program		
Body Part	**Exercise**	**Muscles Trained**	**Figure**
1. Legs	Leg press	Gluteals, quadriceps	Figure 5.11
	Leg curls	Hamstrings	Figure 5.12
2. Chest	Bench press	Pectorals	Figure 5.13
3. Back	Lat pulldown	Latissimus dorsi	Figure 5.14
4. Shoulders	Seated press	Deltoids	Figure 5.15
5. Arms	Arm curl	Biceps	Figure 5.16
	Overhead arm extension	Triceps	Figure 5.17
6. Abdomen	Sit-up and curl-up	Rectus abdominis	Figure 5.18
7. Calves	Heel raises	Gastrocnemius, soleus	Figure 5.19

major muscle groups (legs, hips, back, abdomen, chest, shoulders, and arms)" (USDHHS, 2008).

It is recommended that you alternate between agonist and antagonists when setting the order of exercises to avoid muscle imbalances. It is also recommended that you start with large muscle groups and then move to the smaller assistive muscle groups. For example, you might want to perform leg extensions (refer to Figure 5.25) followed by leg curls (flexion) (refer to Figure 5.12), and then move to heel raises (refer to Figure 5.19). Another example is to perform bench presses (refer to Figure 5.13) followed by a back exercise (lat pulldown) (refer to Figure 5.14), and then move on to overhead arm extensions (refer to Figure 5.17). Table 5.4 illustrates a properly ordered circuit of exercise that incorporates the previously mentioned design parameters of alternating exercises and sequencing of large to small muscle groups.

In summary, you can choose to participate in a variety of exercises to enhance your muscular strength, endurance, and power. The figures that follow provide a sample of common resistance exercises. They are divided into basic (**FIGURE 5.11** to **FIGURE 5.29**) and advanced resistance exercises (**FIGURE 5.30** to **FIGURE 5.36**). The basic resistance exercises require little time to learn proper technique, work the major muscle groups, and are safe if you perform them properly. The advanced lifts are offered for those seeking optimal muscular fitness goals or those competing in sports. They require more time to learn proper technique (professional instruction is recommended), place a great deal of stress on the specific areas of the body, and are associated with a higher risk of injury if performed improperly.

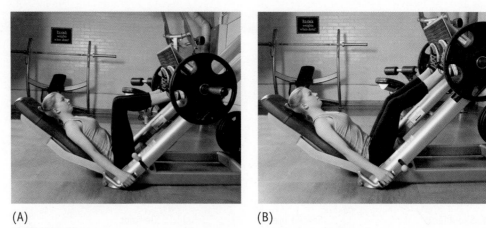

(A)   (B)

FIGURE 5.11 **Leg Exercise.** Double-leg press. (A) start (B) finish

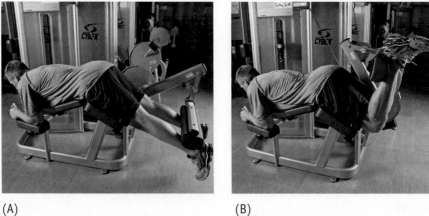

(A)   (B)

FIGURE 5.12 **Leg Exercise.** Lying leg curl. (A) start (B) finish

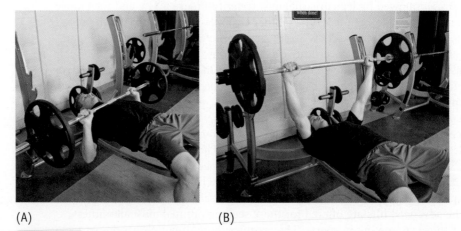

(A)   (B)

FIGURE 5.13 **Chest Exercise.** Flat bench press. (A) start (B) finish

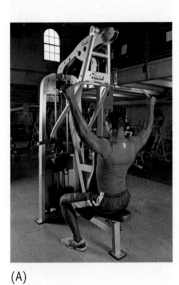
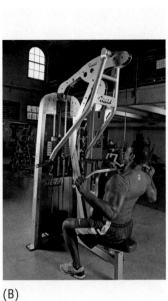

(A) (B)

FIGURE 5.14 **Back Exercise.** Lat pulldown press. (A) start (B) finish

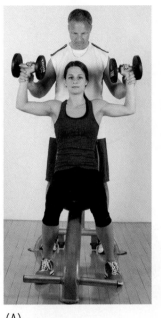
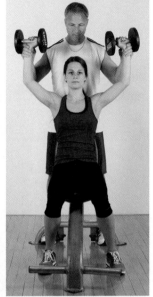

(A) (B)

FIGURE 5.15 **Shoulder Exercise.** Seated dumbbell press. (A) start (B) finish

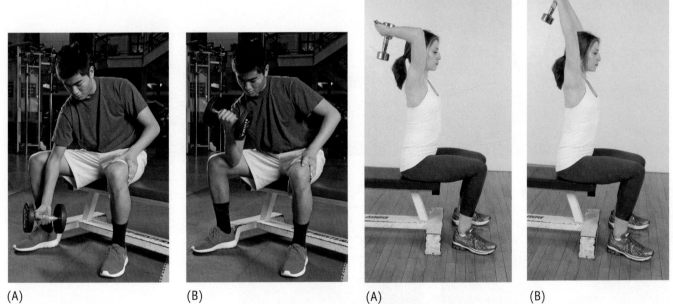

(A) (B)

FIGURE 5.16 **Arm Exercise.** One-arm bicep curl. (A) start (B) finish

(A) (B)

FIGURE 5.17 **Arm Exercise.** Overhead dumbbell tricep extension. (A) start (B) finish

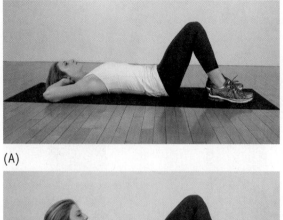

(A)

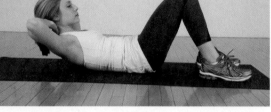

(B)

FIGURE 5.18 **Abdomen Exercise.** Lying on the floor curl-up. (A) start (B) finish

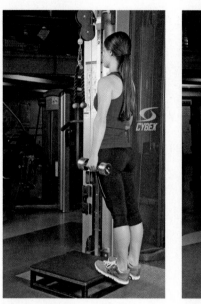
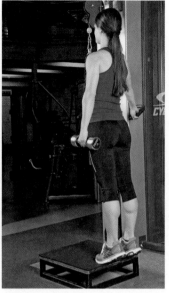

(A)   (B)

FIGURE 5.19 **Leg Exercise.** Standing heel raise for calve muscles. (A) start (B) finish

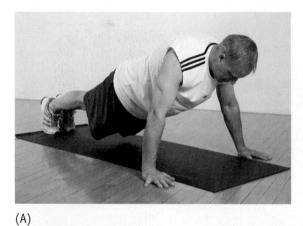

(A)

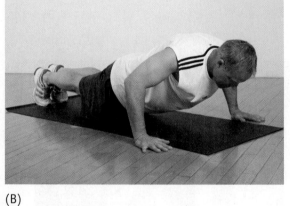

(B)

FIGURE 5.20 **Chest Exercise.** Pushup. (A) start (B) finish

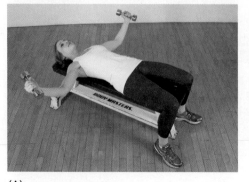

(A)

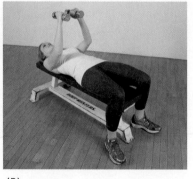

(B)

FIGURE 5.21 **Chest Exercise.** Dumbbell flys. (A) start (B) finish

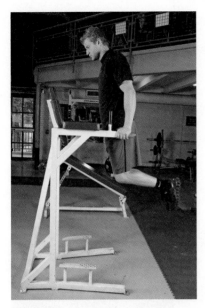

(A)

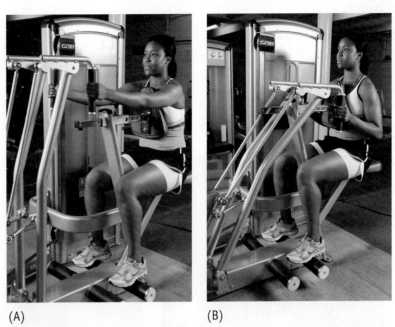

(A) (B)

FIGURE 5.23 **Back Exercise.** Upper back row. (A) start (B) finish

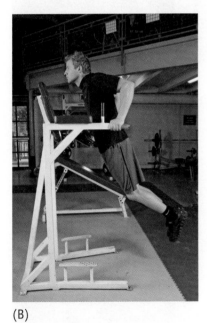

(B)

FIGURE 5.22 **Chest Exercise.** Dips.
(A) start (B) finish

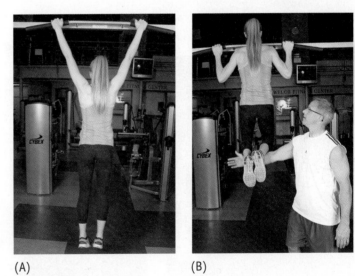

(A) (B)

FIGURE 5.24 **Back Exercise.** Pull-up. (A) start (B) finish

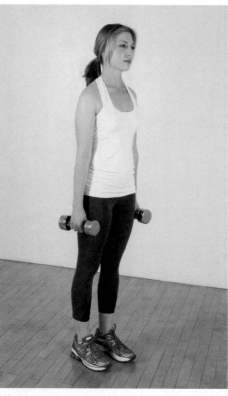

(A)

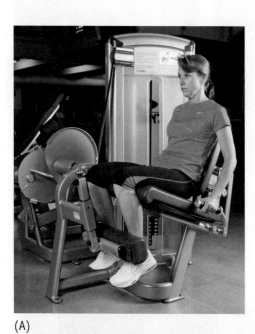

(A)

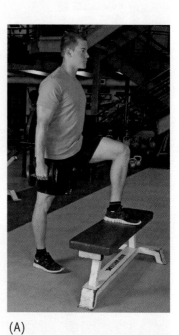

(A)

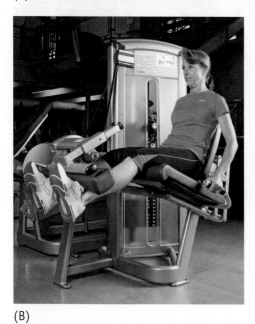

(B)

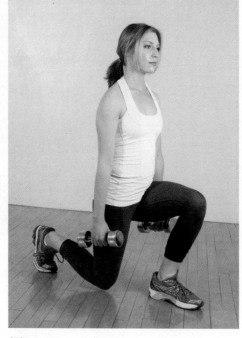

(B)

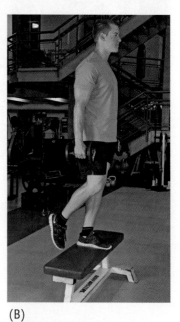

(B)

FIGURE 5.25 **Leg Exercise.** Quadricep extension. (A) start (B) finish

FIGURE 5.26 **Leg Exercise.** Lunges. (A) start (B) finish

FIGURE 5.27 **Leg Exercise.** Bench step-ups. (A) start (B) finish

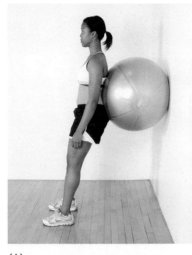

(A)

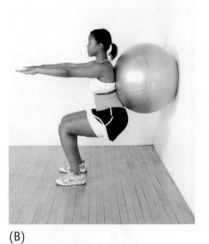

(B)

FIGURE 5.28 **Leg Exercise.**
Stability ball wall squat. (A) start
(B) finish

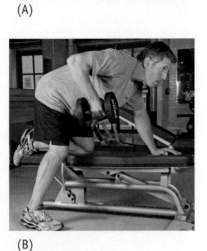

(A)

(B)

FIGURE 5.29 **Back Exercise.**
One-arm dumbbell row. (A) start
(B) finish

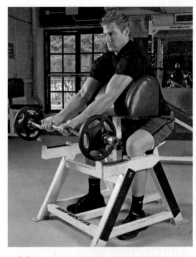

(A)

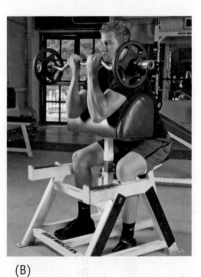

(B)

FIGURE 5.30 **Arm Exercise.**
Preacher curl. (A) start (B) finish

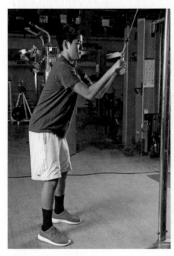

(A)   (B)

FIGURE 5.31 **Arm Exercise.** Tricep
pushdowns. (A) start (B) finish

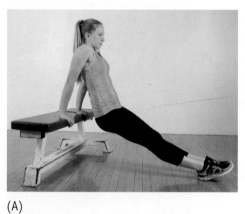

(A)

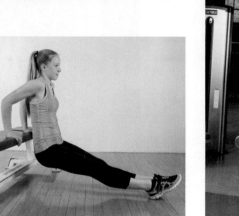

(B)

FIGURE 5.32 **Arm Exercise.** Bench dips. (A) start (B) finish

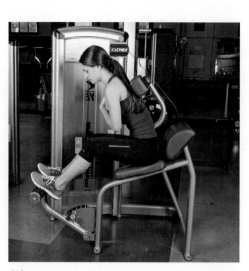

(A)

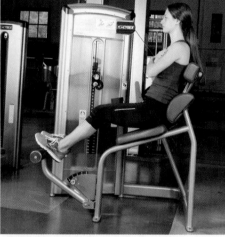

(B)

FIGURE 5.33 **Back Exercise.** Lower back extension. (A) start (B) finish

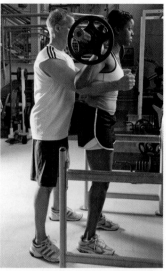

(A)

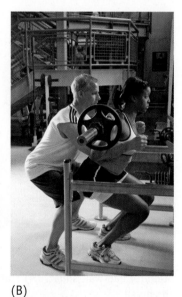

(B)

FIGURE 5.34 **Advanced Lifts: Leg Exercise.** Squat. (A) start (B) finish

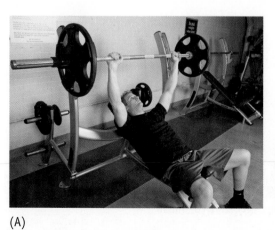

(A)

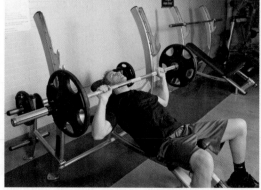

(B)

FIGURE 5.35 **Advanced Lifts: Chest Exercise.** Incline bench press. (A) start (B) finish

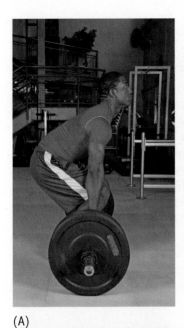
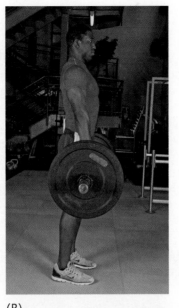

(A)   (B)

FIGURE 5.36 **Advanced Lifts: Back Exercise.** Deadlift. (A) start (B) finish

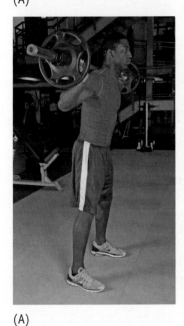
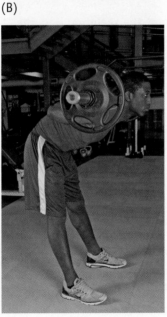

(A)   (B)

FIGURE 5.37 **Advanced Lifts: Back Exercise.** Good morning. (A) start (B) finish

Physical Activity and Health Connection

Resistance exercise boosts our health in a variety of ways. When you incorporate resistance exercise properly as part of your physical activity program you can expect to end up stronger and more energetic and with more muscle tone. This can have a positive impact on how you look and improve your body image and self-confidence. Fit muscles allow us to perform the tasks of daily living with less stress, help to protect our joints from injury, aid in sport and activity performance, and assist in developing and maintaining strong bones, thereby reducing the risk of osteoporosis. Resistance exercise can increase lean body mass and lower body fat percentage (improving body composition), thereby contributing to enhanced metabolic health (our ability to use sugars as fuel properly) and aiding in the prevention of cardiovascular disease, type 2 diabetes, and some cancers. Understanding the realm of possibilities afforded by resistance exercise and its relationship to good health is important in your overall wellness.

concept connections

1 **The health benefits of muscle-strengthening activities are well documented.** Muscle-strengthening activities, or resistance training, can increase lean body mass and lower body fat percentage, increase basal metabolism at rest, decrease the body's insulin response to changing glucose levels, lower the body's baseline insulin levels, and increase insulin sensitivity. Each of these factors is related to the body's ability to use sugars as fuel and aid in the prevention of type 2 diabetes. Participating in a regular resistance exercise program can maintain or improve your HDL cholesterol levels and decrease LDL cholesterol levels, regulate diastolic blood pressure at rest, increase VO$_2$max, and improve cardiorespiratory endurance. All of these factors help to ensure a healthy cardiovascular system and protect against cardiovascular disease.

Fit muscles allow us to perform the tasks of daily living with less stress, help to protect our joints from injury, aid in sport and activity performance, improve our body image and self-confidence, and assist in developing and maintaining strong bones, thereby reducing the risk of osteoporosis.

2 **Skeletal muscles move and support the skeleton.** More than 600 individually named skeletal muscles make up 42 percent of an average adult male's and 36 percent of an average adult female's body mass, respectively. Skeletal muscles or "voluntary" muscles are joined to the bones by tendons. Tendons are bundles of tough fibers that differ in length and thickness. When a muscle contracts, the tendon exerts force on the bone, causing the bone to move.

3 **Skeletal muscle is made up of thousands of cylindrical muscle fibers.** These muscle fibers are bound together by connective tissue through which run blood vessels and nerves. Between and within the muscle fibers is a complex structure of connective tissue, resembling struts and crossbeams, that helps to maintain the integrity of the muscle during contraction and relaxation. This connective tissue is composed of protein filaments, water, and minerals that allow muscles to contract and relax.

4 **Resistance training is essential for improving the health-related components of physical fitness—muscular strength and endurance.** Muscular strength is the amount of force a muscle or muscle group can exert with a single maximum effort. This is in contrast to muscular endurance, which is the ability of a muscle or muscle group to exert repeated force against a resistance or to sustain muscular contraction for a given period of time. You can use the FITT formula to help you determine how much exercise is enough for you to build muscle strength and endurance safely and effectively. FITT stands for frequency, intensity, time, and type of activity.

5 **Muscle-strengthening activities are recommended on 2 or more days a week for both adults and older adults.** The major muscle groups include the legs, hips, back, chest, abdomen, shoulders, and arms. These major muscle groups may be exercised all on the same day or by using a split routine, depending on your schedule.

6 **A number of muscle-strengthening activities are available.** Whatever form of resistance exercise you select, it is important that you focus on all major groups of the body (legs, hips, back, chest, abdomen, shoulders, and arms).

Terms

Actin, 84
Agonist, 86
Antagonist, 86
Circuit weight training, 94
Dynamic constant external
 resistance (DCER), 88
Ectomorphs, 87
Endomorphs, 87

Isokinetic resistance
 training, 88
Mesomorphs, 87
Motor unit, 85
Muscular endurance, 91
Muscular strength, 91
Myosin, 84
Neutralizer, 86

Plyometrics, 90
Protein filaments, 84
Sarcomere, 84
Synergists, 86
Valsalva maneuver, 90

making the connection

Kayleigh learned from reading this chapter that her skepticism about resistance exercise or weight training making her look bigger was based on a myth. Kayleigh learned that rather than causing women to get bigger, resistance exercise generally leads to a toned, "tighter" body. After instituting a weight training program, she found that she lost inches rather than weight. More important, resistance exercise helped Kayleigh achieve many of her other health goals, including having a positive effect on her mood and assisting in developing and maintaining strong bones, thereby reducing her risk for osteoporosis.

Critical Thinking

1. List five ways resistance training improves your health.
2. Explain the sliding filament theory of muscle contraction.
3. Explain two differences between slow-twitch and fast-twitch muscle fibers.
4. Explain the differences between static and dynamic resistance-type exercises.
5. Explain the FITT principle as it applies to a resistance training program.

References

American College of Sports Medicine. (2011). Position stand: Quantity and quality of exercise for developing and maintaining cardiorespiratory, musculoskeletal, and neuromotor fitness in apparently healthy adults: Guidance for prescribing exercise. *Medicine and Science in Sports and Exercise* 43(7):1334–1359.

American College of Sports Medicine. (2010). *ACSM's Guidelines for Exercise Testing and Prescription*, 8th ed. Baltimore: Lippincott Williams & Wilkins.

American College of Sports Medicine. (2009). Position stand: Progression models in resistance training for healthy adults. *Medicine and Science in Sports and Exercise* 41(3):687–708.

Fink, H., Burgoon, L.A., & Mikesky, A.E. (2012). *Practical Applications in Sports Nutrition*, 3rd ed. Burlington, MA: Jones & Bartlett Learning.

Fleck, S.J., & Kraemer, W.J. (2004). *Designing Resistance Training Programs*, 3rd ed. Champaign, IL: Human Kinetics.

Howley, E.T., & Franks, B.D. (2007). *Fitness Professionals Handbook*, 5th ed. Champaign, IL: Human Kinetics.

U.S. Department of Health and Human Services. (2008). Physical Activity Guidelines for Americans. Online: http://www.health.gov/PAGuidelines/pdf/paguide.pdf.

Activities & Assessments

Focus on Flexibility: Stretching for Better Health

6

Budd is currently meeting the recommended physical activity guidelines for health by participating in at least 150 minutes (2 hours and 30 minutes) of moderate-intensity aerobic activity every week along with incorporating muscle-strengthening activities on 2 or more days a week that work all major muscle groups. However, Budd remembers reading that stretching exercises to enhance flexibility are recommended as part of a comprehensive health-related fitness program. Budd is unsure of what types of stretching exercises to perform and what guidelines to follow to implement a safe and effective stretching program.

concepts

1. Significant health benefits are associated with being flexible.

2. Many factors can influence range of motion around a joint.

3. A regular stretching program is an important part of a comprehensive health-related fitness program.

4. Three common types of stretching exercises are static, ballistic, and PNF.

5. Select stretching exercises that stretch the major muscle groups of the body.

go.jblearning.com/kotecki4e
The website for this book is a great source for supplementary physical health information for both students and instructors. Visit **go.jblearning.com/kotecki4e** to find a variety of useful tools for learning, thinking, and teaching.

Every human being is the author of his own health or disease.

—Hindu Prince Siddhartha Gautama

Significant health benefits are associated with being flexible.

Introduction

The health benefits of being flexible—the ability to move a joint or a group of joints through their complete range of motion—are many. Flexibility is necessary for normal everyday activities that require bending, twisting, and reaching. Maintaining a "range of motion" enables us to do everyday tasks pain-free and experience greater ease of movement through life.

In addition to making typical activities possible and pain-free, a regular stretching program can relieve neuromuscular tension buildup from chronic stress, promote good posture, prevent lower-back pain, reduce the risk of pain and injury, and aid in providing better balance, making you less prone to falls and related injuries—especially as you age (American College of Sports Medicine [ACSM], 2011) (**FIGURE 6.1**). Stretching after either a cardiorespiratory endurance or resistance training workout can help relax and increase circulation and speed up recovery time in muscles that have just been exercised. In summary, a regular stretching program contributes to both physical fitness and preventive health care.

This chapter provides guidelines for designing your own stretching program. To help you design a more effective and safer stretching program, it is helpful to have a basic understanding of the factors that determine flexibility and range of motion around a joint.

Factors Influencing Flexibility

Many factors can influence range of motion around a joint.

Many factors can influence range of motion around a joint, including joint structure (shape and alignment of bones), muscle elasticity and compliance, nervous system activity, activity status, age, and sex.

Joint structure varies from joint to joint in your own body and among individuals. The achievable range of motion around a joint is highly specific to the type of joint because various types of joints allow our bodies to perform more than one kind of motion. A **hinge joint** allows for movement in only one plane so that the body parts bend and straighten. Some examples of hinge joints are the elbow, knee, ankle, and joints in the fingers. A **ball and socket joint** allows one part to rotate at almost any angle with respect to another. The shoulder and hip are examples. The shoulder joint is the most flexible joint in the body; good hip joint flexibility plays a major role in the prevention of lower-back pain.

There are other types of movable joints in the body. **Gliding joints** allow two flat bones to slide over each other such as in the bones of the wrist and foot. A **condyloid joint** allows the head to nod and the fingers to bend. The thumbs have a **saddle joint** that allows enough flexibility for the thumb to touch any other finger.

Soft tissues, including muscles, tendons, ligaments, joint cartilage, fat, and skin, also influence the range of motion around a joint. Of these, muscle tissue is central to improving range of motion of a joint because of its elasticity and compliance properties. **Elasticity** is the degree to which a material resists deformation and quickly returns to its normal shape. **Compliance** is the ease with which a material is elongated or stretched.

Our muscles are held together by a series of elastic connective tissues that both surround each muscle and are found throughout each muscle. These connective tissues come together at the ends of the muscles into tendons. Tendons connect muscle to bone. When we move a muscle, we stretch these connec-

Hinge joint A joint that allows for movement in only one plane so that the body parts can bend and straighten.

Ball and socket joint A joint that allows one body part to rotate at almost any angle with respect to another.

Gliding joint A joint that allows two flat bones to slide over each other.

Condyloid joint A joint that allows the head to nod and the fingers to bend.

Saddle joint A joint that allows for the thumb to touch any other finger.

Soft tissues Include muscles, tendons, ligaments, joint cartilage, fat, and skin.

Elasticity The degree to which a material resists deformation and quickly returns to its normal shape.

Compliance The ease with which a material is elongated or stretched.

tive tissues. When the muscle relaxes, the connective tissue recoil helps the muscle return to its original resting length. Slow, sustained stretching exercises have the greatest impact on the elastic and compliant properties of the tissues, resulting in a short-term increase in muscle and tendon length. Regularly stretching these connective tissues through a proper exercise program enhances the elongation of the connective tissues of the muscle and tendon and produces a lasting increase through alteration in the surrounding connective tissue matrix. Similarly, loss of muscle elasticity and compliance is caused by chronic disuse. This is why a sedentary lifestyle is a major contributing factor to reduced flexibility.

Muscle temperature also affects elasticity and compliance and therefore has a direct impact on flexibility. Warmer muscles have increased elastic and compliant properties, whereas cooler muscle temperatures have the opposite effect. This is why individuals who warm up are able to have better flexibility than when they do not warm up.

In addition to the elasticity and compliance properties of muscles, nervous system activity plays a role in flexibility. Throughout our body we have **proprioceptors**, or sense receptors, that provide feedback to the central nervous system. The primary proprioceptors in the muscles are called **stretch receptors** (or muscle spindles) and are located within the thick center portion (belly) of the muscles. Stretch receptors detect stretching in a muscle and are essential for coordinated muscle activity, passing information about the state of muscles to the central nervous system. The stretch receptors are sensitive to rapid forceful stretching, responding with a reflexive contraction of the muscle called the **stretch reflex**. This dynamic component of the stretch reflex (which can be very powerful) lasts for only a moment and is in response to the initial sudden increase in muscle length. If you happen to stretch a muscle abruptly when performing a stretching exercise, you are more likely to elicit an enhanced stretch reflex and increase the potential to cause muscle injury.

Our tendons also have sense receptors imbedded in them that are called Golgi tendon organs. **Golgi tendon organs** are also sensitive to rapid forceful contractions and cause a reflexive relaxation to occur within the muscle. As the tension increases in the muscle and tendon, these sense receptors detect the rate of force change and regulate further muscle action. Muscle action might be inhibited to induce relaxation. This reflex inhibition can prevent injury from excessive strain and may account for short-term increases in flexibility immediately after stretching.

Last, age and sex affect flexibility. As we age, the elastic and compliant properties of muscles and tendons diminish for both sexes. The rate and degree at which the natural aging process limits flexibility and functional ability can be significantly delayed by a regular stretching program (ACSM, 2010). On average, women are more flexible than men are, particularly when it comes to hip joint flexibility.

Assessing Flexibility

Assessment can be helpful in establishing which of your body joints would benefit most from stretching exercises. The most commonly employed flexibility assessment is the sit-and-reach test (**FIGURE 6.2**). This test is used to measure hamstring and

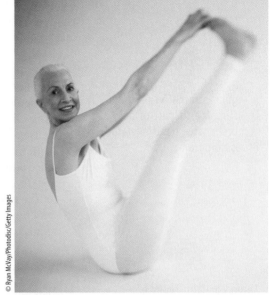

© Ryan McVay/Photodisc/Getty Images

FIGURE 6.1 **Regular Stretching Program.** Maintaining flexibility is important throughout your life span.

Proprioceptors Sense receptors that provide feedback to the central nervous system.

Stretch receptors Primary proprioceptors located within the thick center portion (belly) of the muscle that detect stretching in the muscle.

Stretch reflex Reflexive response to rapid forceful stretching that causes a muscle to contract.

Golgi tendon organs Sense receptors that are sensitive to rapid forceful contractions and cause a reflexive relaxation to occur within the muscle.

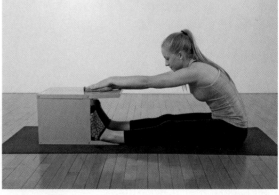

FIGURE 6.2 **Sit-and-Reach Test.** This test can be used to assess hamstring flexibility and trunk/hip flexion.

lower-back flexibility, which allow the hip to rotate forward, and upper-back flexibility, which allows the arms to reach forward.

Designing Your Stretching Program

A regular stretching program is all too often overlooked when a fitness program is being planned. Inflexible joints and muscles can limit movement efficiency and cause an individual to have problems such as those related to lower-back pain. As with fitness programs designed to maintain or improve cardiorespiratory endurance and muscular strength and endurance, the FITT principle provides guidelines for developing a safe and effective stretching program. This includes consideration of the types of stretching exercises, how often (frequency), how hard (intensity), and how long (time or duration) so that you can design a stretching exercise program based on your individual needs.

Types of Stretching Exercises

The three most common types of stretching methods are static stretching, ballistic stretching, and proprioceptive neuromuscular facilitation (PNF) stretching. Each type has advantages and disadvantages and can be performed actively or passively. In **active stretching** you apply the force for a stretch; for example, the seated hamstring and lower back stretch in **FIGURE 6.3** requires the woman to lean her upper torso to her lower torso and hold for a period of time. **Passive stretching** requires the assistance of a device or a trained partner to apply the force to the stretch.

Static Stretching

Static stretching is slowly elongating a muscle to the point of slight tension or mild discomfort (not to a point of pain) and then holding it at that position (Figure 6.3). A slow and smooth stretch prompts a reduced response from stretch receptors, thereby decreasing the stretch reflex response (reflexive contraction) and allowing the muscle to stretch farther. You then hold the stretch in this position for 15 to 60 seconds. One of the reasons for holding a stretch for a prolonged period of time is that as you hold the muscle in a stretched position, the stretch receptors in the muscle habituate (become accustomed to the new length) and reduce its signaling. Gradually, you can train your stretch receptors to allow great-

A regular stretching program is an important part of a comprehensive health-related fitness program.

Three common types of stretching exercises are static, ballistic, and PNF.

Active stretching Requires you to apply the force for a stretch.

Passive stretching Requires the assistance of a device or a trained partner to apply the force to the stretch.

Static stretching Elongating a muscle and holding that position.

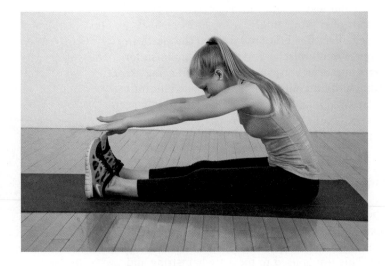

FIGURE 6.3 **Static Stretching.** This entails slowly elongating a muscle to the point of slight tension or mild discomfort and then holding it at that position.

er lengthening of the muscles. The nonmoving state of the elongated muscle gives static stretching its name.

Static stretching activities are best practiced after the body is sufficiently warmed up or after an aerobic or resistance training workout. Static stretching is the type most often recommended and used because it is effective and safe (ACSM, 2010). Additionally, static stretching exercises take a lesser degree of training to perform compared to either ballistic or PNF stretching. The use of static stretching technique is recommended for the common stretching exercises illustrated later in this chapter.

A potential disadvantage of static stretching is that it may take a good deal of time to stretch out all of your muscles. For this reason, multiple-joint stretching is recommended over single-joint stretching so that you can stretch more than one muscle group at a time. Figure 6.3 is an example of a multijoint static stretching involving the upper trunk and the hips.

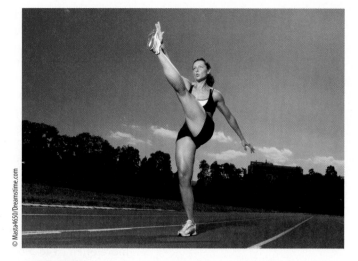

FIGURE 6.4 **Ballistic Stretching.** Dynamic movement, such as high leg kicks, are an example of ballistic hamstring stretching.

Ballistic Stretching

Ballistic stretching is a form of dynamic stretching that utilizes a bouncing motion to move a muscle beyond its normal range of motion (**FIGURE 6.4**). Dynamic or ballistic stretching performed in a nonfatiguing manner is an effective means of warming up the body for advanced explosive athletic activity (National Strength and Conditioning Association [NSCA], 2009). Another advantage to this type of stretching is that you can stretch rather rapidly and use specific dynamic movement patterns. However, ballistic stretching activities have the potential to cause injury to the muscle if the body is not properly warmed up or if the bouncing is too forceful and rapid. Forceful and rapid stretching of the muscle stimulates the stretch receptors to activate the stretch reflex, which causes a reflexive contraction. Ballistic stretching is therefore not recommended unless you have proper supervision or advanced training experience.

> **Ballistic stretching** Fast, momentum-assisted, pulsing movements used to stretch muscles.
>
> **Proprioceptive neuromuscular facilitation (PNF) stretching** Utilization and integration of the nervous and muscular systems to enhance flexibility.

Proprioceptive Neuromuscular Facilitation Stretching

Proprioceptive neuromuscular facilitation (PNF) stretching utilizes and integrates the nervous and muscular systems to enhance flexibility. As mentioned earlier, Golgi tendon organs are located in the tendons that connect muscle to bone. They are sensitive to rapid forceful contraction and respond by causing the muscle to relax. In PNF stretching, you take advantage of the way Golgi tendon organs work and use them to enhance flexibility (Holcomb, 2000). You do this by causing a muscle to contract and then relaxing the muscle. The forced contraction aids in getting the muscle to relax.

One example of PNF stretching is the hold–relax method (**FIGURE 6.5**). In this stretching method you first start out with passively stretching the muscle, for example, the hamstring, to the point of mild discomfort for 10 seconds; this is followed by a maximal isometric contracting of the hamstring against a fixed resistance for 6 seconds. You then relax the hamstring muscle and stretch it passively to a greater range

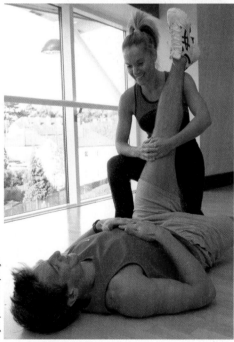

FIGURE 6.5 **PNF Stretching.** This utilizes a hold–relax method to stretch the hamstring muscle.

for 30 seconds. The final stretch should be a greater range because of the Golgi tendon organ feedback. The relaxation phase and subsequent contraction of the hamstring muscle further enhance the degree of relaxation felt in the muscle. There are several variations on PNF stretching involving hold–relax and contracting combinations.

There is some evidence that PNF may bring superior results compared with the other types of exercises done to increase flexibility (Holcomb, 2000). However, it usually takes a greater degree of training to perform PNF safely and effectively. It is therefore recommended that professionals familiar with PNF stretching either directly assist or supervise this type of stretching activity.

Frequency, Intensity, and Time

Exercises that stretch the major muscle groups should be performed a minimum of 2 to 3 days per week (ACSM, 2010). You can perform stretching exercises more often (3 to 5 days a week) for even greater progress and benefits. The best time to stretch is when your muscles are warmed up because warmer muscles are elastic and compliant. This is usually after completing your cardiorespiratory or resistance exercises. This is why the most improvements in flexibility occur during the cooldown phase. If your muscles are not already warm before you wish to stretch, then you need to warm them up yourself, usually by performing some type of brief general warm-up (e.g., joint rotations, aerobic activity) for 5 to 10 minutes. If the weather is very cold, or if you are feeling very stiff, then you need to take extra care to warm up before you stretch to reduce the risk of injuring yourself.

In terms of intensity, slowly apply each stretch to your muscles to the point of slight tension or mild discomfort (ACSM, 2010). Applying the stretch slowly allows for greater reflexive relaxation in both the muscle spindles and the Golgi tendon organs. All the way through the stretch it is important that you continue to breathe easily and rhythmically and try to remain relaxed. Do not hold your breath at any time during the stretch. If the feeling of slight tension subsides as you hold your stretch, feel free to try to stretch slightly farther.

It is recommended that static stretches be held for 15 to 60 seconds whereas PNF stretches be performed utilizing a 6-second contraction followed by a 10- to 30-second assisted stretch (ACSM, 2010). Each stretch should be completed four times, allowing 30 to 60 seconds between each stretch (ACSM, 2010).

Common Stretching Exercises

When selecting the stretching exercises that are right for you, remember to choose those that stretch the major muscle groups of the body and make the best use of your time. The major muscle groups that should be stretched include the neck, arms, shoulders, upper and lower trunk, hips, and legs (ACSM, 2010). Multiple-joint stretches or exercises that stretch multiple muscle groups are typically suggested because they allow you to stretch more muscles, more thoroughly, and in a shorter period of time. These include the hamstring (back of thigh) muscles, the quadriceps (front of thigh) muscles, and the calf muscles.

A complete full-body stretching workout usually takes between 10 and 20 minutes. TABLE 6.1 provides a sample stretching program. Static stretching is recommended because it is easy to learn, safe, and effective in improving flexibility. FIGURE 6.6 through FIGURE 6.26 illustrate suggested static stretching exercises.

Select stretching exercises that stretch the major muscle groups of the body.

TABLE 6.1   Sample Stretching Program

Upper Body/Torso Stretching

	Stretch	Figure	Area of Proposed Stretch	Secondary Stretch Location
1	Ear to shoulder left and right	6.6	Neck lateral flexion	
2	Chin to chest and chin raised	6.7	Neck flexion and extension	
3	Look right and left	6.8	Neck stretch	

Note: Perform these neck stretching exercises in circuit format. Neck rotations are not advised.

	Stretch	Figure	Area of Proposed Stretch	Secondary Stretch Location
4	Arm across chest	6.9	Rear shoulder and arm	
5	Shoulder girdle stretch	6.10	Front shoulder and chest	
6	Handcuff stretch	6.11	Shoulders, chest, and upper back	
7	Overhead triceps	6.12	Upper arms and shoulders	
8	Seated side reach	6.13	Back and shoulders	
9	Bent over lat stretch	6.14	Back and shoulders	
10	Prone torso extension	6.15	Lower back and shoulders	

Lower Body/Torso Stretching

	Stretch	Figure	Area of Proposed Stretch	Secondary Stretch Location
1	Elbow to knee	6.16	Gluteal and lower trunk	
2	Modified hurdler	6.17	Hamstring, lower back, and groin	
3	Lying iliotibial stretch	6.18	Quadricep and hip	
4	Side-lying infraspinatus stretch	6.19	Quadricep and hip	
5	Kneeling stretch	6.20	Lower back and hip flexor	
6	Standing heel to buttocks	6.21	Quadricep	
7	Lunging hip flexor stretch	6.22	Quadricep and hip flexor	
8	Prone glute stretch	6.23	Glute and lower back	
9	Hip abductors stretch	6.24	Hip abductors	
10	Wall lean	6.25	Calf	
11	Seated shin stretch	6.26	Shin	

All stretching activities should be preceded by a 5–10 minute warm-up period consisting of large muscle group activity. It is recommended that all static stretches be held for 15 to 60 seconds. Do not hold your breath at any time during a stretch. Exercises that stretch the major muscle groups should be performed a minimum of 2 to 3 days a week.

Note: It is suitable to stretch the upper body one day and the lower body the next.

Note: It is advisable to take note of where the stretching exercise is felt. Even though the primary function of the muscle stretch may be felt, pay close attention to secondary stretch locations in other areas. Chart these areas because this is a sign of tightness in other areas, which should be addressed for balance.

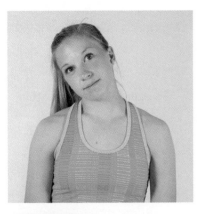

FIGURE 6.6 **Ear to Shoulder, Left to Right.** Neck stretch.

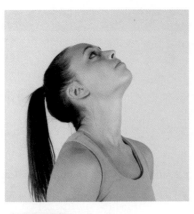

FIGURE 6.7 **Chin to Chest and Chin Raised.** Neck stretch.

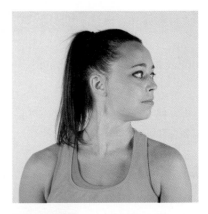

FIGURE 6.8 **Look Right and Left.** Neck stretch.

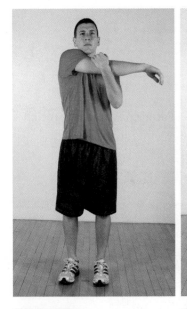

FIGURE 6.9 **Arm Across Chest.** Rear shoulder and arm stretch.

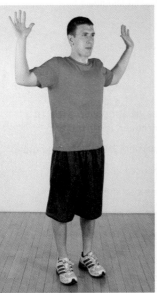

FIGURE 6.10 **Outstretched Arms.** Rear shoulder girdle stretch.

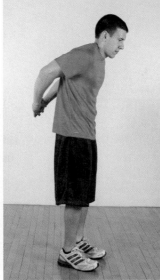

FIGURE 6.11 **Handcuff Stretch.** Shoulders, chest, and upper back stretch.

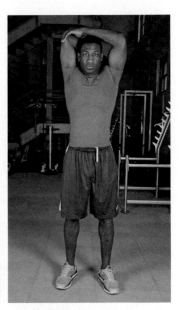

FIGURE 6.12 **Overhead Triceps Stretch.** Upper arms and shoulders stretch.

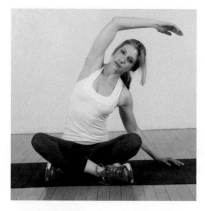

FIGURE 6.13 **Seated Side Reach.** Side lat stretch.

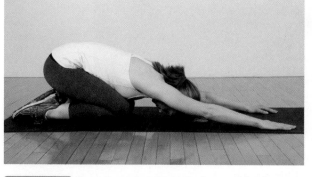

FIGURE 6.14 **Bent Over Lat Stretch.** Lat and back stretch.

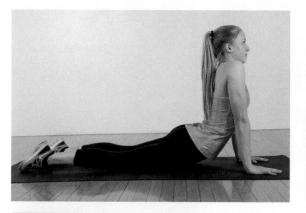

FIGURE 6.15 **Prone Torso Extension.** Lower back and shoulders stretch.

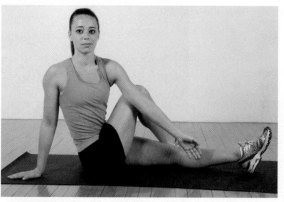

FIGURE 6.16 **Elbow to Knee.** Gluteal and lower trunk stretch.

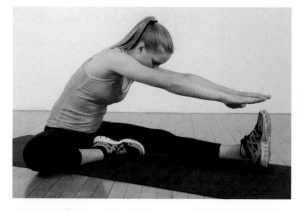

FIGURE 6.17 **Modified Hurdler.** Hamstrings, lower back, and groin stretch.

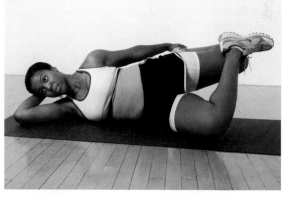

FIGURE 6.18 **Lying Iliotibial Stretch.** Quadricep and hip stretch.

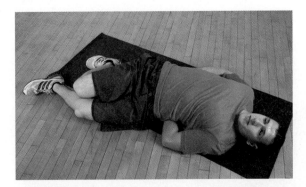

FIGURE 6.19 **Side-Lying Infraspinatus Stretch.** Quadricep and hip stretch.

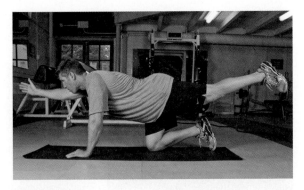

FIGURE 6.20 **Kneeling Stretch.** Lower back and hip flexors stretch.

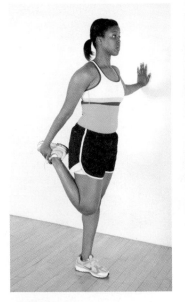

FIGURE 6.21 **Standing Heel to Buttock Stretch.** Quadricep stretch.

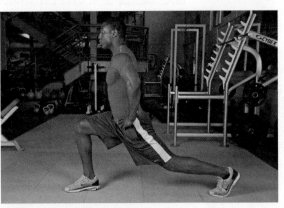

FIGURE 6.22 **Lunging Hip Flexor Stretch.** Quadriceps and hip flexors stretch.

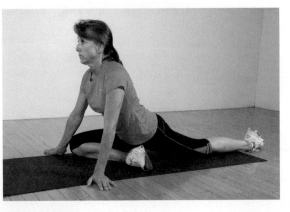

FIGURE 6.23 **Prone Glute Stretch.** Glute and lower back stretch.

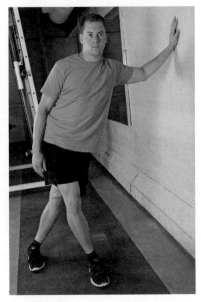

FIGURE 6.24 **Arm on Wall.** Hip abductors stretch.

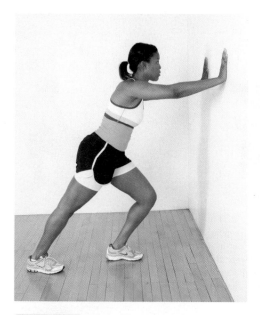

FIGURE 6.25 **Wall Lean.** Calf stretch.

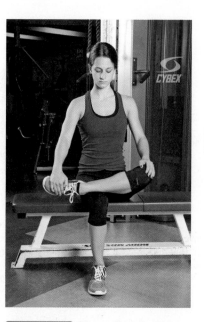

FIGURE 6.26 **Sit on Bench.** Shin stretch.

Yoga and Tai Chi

The movements found within the practices of both yoga and tai chi contain many effective stretching poses, or postures. The word *yoga* means "union" in Sanskrit, the language of ancient India where yoga originated. Think of the union occurring between the mind, body, and spirit. Although stretching is certainly involved, yoga is really about creating balance in the body through developing both strength and flexibility. This is done through the performance of poses or postures, each of which has specific physical benefits that rely on mental concentration for balance, flexibility, and strength enhancements. Of the several kinds of yoga, the most common is Hatha yoga. **FIGURE 6.27** illustrates a combination of postures called the Sun Salute. This Hatha yoga exercise is a series of 12 postures intended to be done in one flowing routine. Each posture should be held for a full breath (inhale and exhale), and some are held for up to five breaths.

Tai chi originated in China, and many of its movements are derived from the martial arts. Tai chi, as it is practiced in the West today, can perhaps best be thought of as a moving form of yoga and meditation combined. There are a number of so-called forms (also called sets) that consist of a sequence of movements. These movements are performed slowly, softly, and gracefully with smooth and even transitions between them (**FIGURE 6.28**). As with the different forms of yoga, tai chi includes both basic and more challenging exercise series depending on the practice selected. The principal physical fitness benefits of yoga and tai chi are enhancing flexibility, muscular fitness, and neuromotor fitness. Although most forms of yoga and tai chi are suitable for everyone regardless of age or physical ability, it is recommended you learn the correct posture forms from a class taught by an experienced and certified instructor.

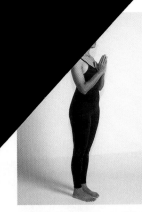

Position 1. Stand erect with your feet hip-width apart and palms together in front of your chest. Inhale and exhale slowly and calmly.

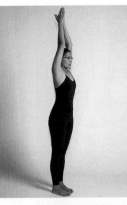

Position 2. Inhaling, raise your arms above your head, palms facing in. Lengthen through the spine, but do not arch your back.

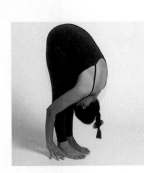

Position 3. Exhaling, bend forward from the hips, keeping your arms extended and your head hanging loosely between them. Keep your legs slightly bent and relax your neck and shoulders.

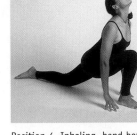

Position 4. Inhaling, bend both knees and place your palms flat on the floor by the outside of your feet. Extend your left leg back. Stretch your chin toward the ceiling.

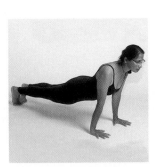

Position 5. Continue while holding the breath if you can—do not strain. Reach your forward leg back next to the other leg. Hold your body straight, supported by your hands and toes, with ankles, hips, and shoulders in a straight place.

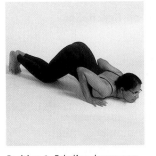

Position 6. Exhaling, lower your knees, chest, and chin or forehead to the floor, keeping your hips up and toes curled under.

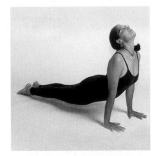

Position 7. Inhaling, bring the tops of your feet to the floor, straighten your legs, and come up to straight arms, opening the chest and stretching your chin toward the ceiling. Be careful not to overarch your lower back.

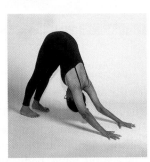

Position 8. Exhaling, curl your toes under and raise your hips into an inverted V. Push back with your hands and lengthen your spine by reaching your hips outward. Keep your head hanging loosely.

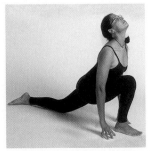

Position 9. Inhaling, lift your head and bring your left leg between your hands, keeping the right leg back. Raise your chin toward the ceiling.

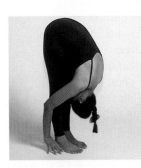

Position 10. Exhaling, bring your left foot forward so your feet are together. Bend forward from the hips, keeping your legs slightly bent and your upper body relaxed. If you can, touch your head to your knees and place your palms beside your feet.

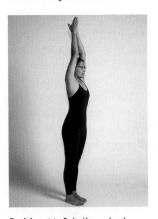

Position 11. Inhaling, slowly straighten up with your arms extended above your head. If you have any lower back pain, be sure to bend your knees.

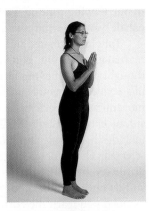

Position 12. Exhaling, bring your hands together in front of you. Close your eyes for a moment and feel the sensations in your body.

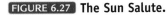

FIGURE 6.27 **The Sun Salute.**

Low-Back Pain Prevention and Rehabilitation

Low-back pain is a complaint common to many individuals. It is estimated that 80 percent of all Americans will experience some degree of low-back pain over the course of their lifetime. A combination of weak core muscles (muscles that run the length of the trunk and torso of the body) and limited hip flexibility are main contributors to the development of low-back pain.

With the approval of your health care provider, or as a preventive measure, you may wish to try the following exercises to improve lower-back health. The major core muscle lacking sufficient strength is the abdominal muscle. Exercises such as the curl-up are recommended to strengthen the abdominal muscles (FIGURE 6.29).

To improve hip flexibility you also should implement exercises that stretch the hamstring muscles, hip flexors, and back extensors. Exercises such as the knee to chest stretch (FIGURE 6.30) or the seated toe stretch (FIGURE 6.31) are recommended. To stretch the hip flexors a lunge stretch is recommended (FIGURE 6.32). To stretch the back extensors a cat and camel stretch is recommended (FIGURE 6.33).

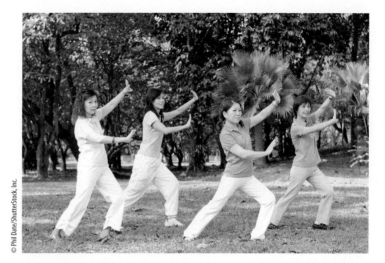

© Phil Date/ShutterStock, Inc.

FIGURE 6.28 **Tai Chi.** Tai chi exercises help maintain flexibility and mind–body harmony.

Physical Activity and Health Connection

Good flexibility contributes to overall physical fitness and preventive health care. Maintaining a range of motion allows us to do everyday tasks pain-free and experience a greater ease of movement through life. In addition to making typical activities possible and pain-free, a regular stretching program can relieve neuromuscular tension buildup from chronic stress, promote good posture, prevent lower-back pain, reduce the risk of pain and injury, and aid in providing better balance, making you less prone to falls and related injuries—especially as you age.

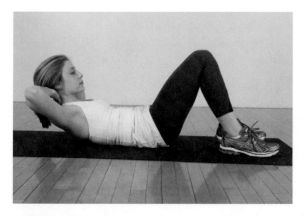

FIGURE 6.29 **Curl-Up.** Abdominal strengthening exercise to support lower back.

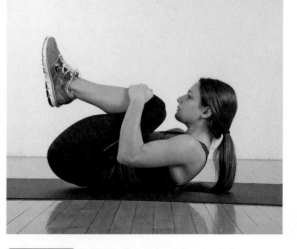

FIGURE 6.30 **Roll-Up Stretch.** Bring both knees to the chest and hold.

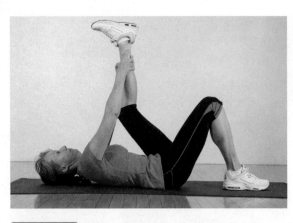

FIGURE 6.31 **Lying Glute Stretch.** Bring leg to chest.

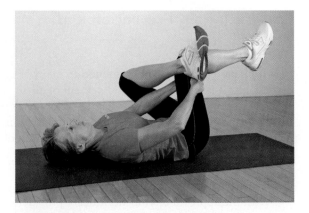

FIGURE 6.32 **Lying Hamstring Stretch.** Bring leg to chest.

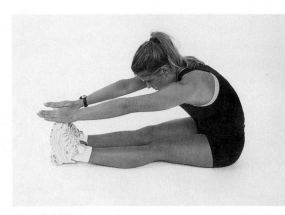

FIGURE 6.33 **Lower-Back Exercise.** Seated toe touch to stretch the hamstrings.

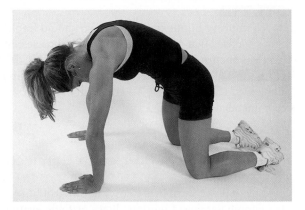

FIGURE 6.34 **Lower-Back Exercise.** Cat and camel to stretch the lower back.

concept connections

1   **Significant health benefits are associated with being flexible.** Flexibility is necessary for normal everyday activities that require bending, twisting, and reaching. Maintaining a range of motion allows us to do everyday tasks pain-free and experience a greater ease of movement through life. In addition to making typical activities possible and pain-free, a regular stretching program can relieve neuromuscular tension buildup from chronic stress, promote good posture, prevent lower-back pain, reduce the risk of pain and injury, and aid in providing better balance, making you less prone to falls and related injuries—especially as you age.

2   **Many factors can influence range of motion around a joint.** Joint structure (shape and alignment of bones), muscle elasticity and compliance, nervous system activity, activity status, age, and sex can all influence range of motion around a joint.

3   **A regular stretching program is an important part of a comprehensive health-related fitness program.** Inflexible joints and muscles can limit movement efficiency and cause an individual to have problems such as those related to lower-back pain. As with fitness programs designed to maintain or improve cardiorespiratory endurance and muscular strength and endurance, the FITT principle provides guidelines for developing a safe and effective exercise stretching program. This includes consideration of the types of stretching exercises, how often (frequency), how hard (intensity), and how long (time or duration) so that you can design a stretching exercise program based on your individual needs.

4   **Three common types of stretching exercises are static, ballistic, and PNF.** Static stretching is slowly elongating a muscle to the point of slight tension or mild discomfort (not to a point of pain), and then holding it at that position. Ballistic stretching, a form of dynamic stretching, utilizes a bouncing motion to move a muscle beyond its normal range of motion. PNF stretching, or proprioceptive neuromuscular facilitation, utilizes and integrates the nervous and muscular systems to enhance flexibility.

5   **Select stretching exercises that stretch the major muscle groups of the body.** The major muscle groups that you should stretch include the neck, arms, shoulders, upper and lower trunk, hips, and legs. Multiple-joint stretches or exercises that stretch multiple muscle groups are typically suggested because they allow you to stretch more muscles, more thoroughly, and in shorter period of time. These include the hamstring (back of thigh) muscles, the quadriceps (front of thigh) muscles, and the calf muscles.

Terms

Active stretching, 110
Ball and socket joint, 108
Ballistic stretching, 111
Compliance, 108
Condyloid joint, 108
Elasticity, 108
Gliding joint, 108

Golgi tendon organs, 109
Hinge joint, 108
Passive stretching, 110
Proprioceptive neuromuscular facilitation (PNF) stretching, 111
Proprioceptors, 109

Saddle joint, 108
Soft tissues, 108
Static stretching, 110
Stretch receptors, 109
Stretch reflex, 109

making the connection

Budd has learned that there are many health benefits to flexibility. Budd has decided to incorporate static stretching exercises into his exercise program at least twice a week, immediately following his resistance training exercises. Budd includes stretching exercises that involve all major muscle groups of the body.

Critical Thinking

1. The health benefits of being flexible—the ability to move a joint through its complete range of motion—are many. List three health benefits and how each could enhance your quality of life.

2. Based on your current flexibility program and time commitments, identify three different types of stretching exercises and briefly explain which type you would prefer and why.

3. Many factors influence the amount of flexibility you have at a joint. List two factors over which you have control and whether or not you have taken action on these factors.

References

American College of Sports Medicine. (2011). Position stand: Quantity and quality of exercise for developing and maintaining cardiorespiratory, musculoskeletal, and neuromotor fitness in apparently healthy adults: Guidance for prescribing exercise. *Medicine and Science in Sports and Exercise* 43(7):1334–1359.

American College of Sports Medicine. (2010). *ACSM's Guidelines for Exercise Testing and Prescription*, 8th ed. Baltimore: Lippincott Williams & Wilkins.

Holcomb, W.R. (2000). Improved stretching with proprioceptive neuromuscular facilitation. *Strength and Conditioning Journal* 22(1):59–61.

National Strength and Conditioning Association. (2009). *Essentials of Strength Training and Conditioning*, 3rd ed. Champaign, IL: Human Kinetics.

Activities & Assessments

Optimal Nutrition for an Active Lifestyle

what's the connection?

Mare is a junior in college and is extremely attentive to her physical health. She began her weekly running program as a freshman and is now very fit. She runs approximately 20 miles a week and lifts weights twice a week. Mare adheres strictly to the MyPlate food guidance system when selecting foods for her daily diet. In addition, she closely follows the recommended number of servings from each food group, selecting the most nutrient-dense foods from each group. Recently, a number of friends with whom Mare exercises have recommended that she take special vitamin and mineral supplements because she is physically active. Mare is uncertain about whether she needs to supplement her diet. Besides, dietary supplements can be expensive and she is on a tight budget. Mare schedules a meeting with the nutritionist at the university health center. The nutritionist asks Mare to record her food intake for a week so they can analyze Mare's diet.

concepts

1. Nutrition plays a major role in our overall health.

2. Nutrients provide energy, regulate body processes, and nourish tissues.

3. Food can be divided into six classes, and each class plays a different role.

4. The *Dietary Guidelines for Americans* provides general recommendations that focus attention on the association between diet and chronic diseases.

5. The MyPlate food guidance system provides information to help implement the recommendations of the *Dietary Guidelines* and make better food choices.

6. The diet recommended for a person who participates in physical exercise differs little in nutrient composition from the diet advised for any healthy individual.

go.jblearning.com/kotecki4e
The website for this book is a great source for supplementary physical health information for both students and instructors. Visit **go.jblearning.com/kotecki4e** to find a variety of useful tools for learning, thinking, and teaching.

To eat is a necessity, but to eat intelligently is an art.

—François de la Rochefoucauld

Introduction

Good nutrition is vital to your good health—both in the present and in the distant future. Hippocrates, an ancient Greek physician, commonly regarded as one of the most outstanding figures in medicine of all time and known as the "father of medicine," recognized the value of diet and nutrition to enhance health and declared, "Let food be your medicine and medicine be your food." Hippocrates said this more than two thousand years ago, and it is still meaningful today, as the preventive and therapeutic health values of food relative to the development of chronic diseases are unraveled. Today, scientific studies indicate that diet and nutrition often play a crucial role in the development and progression of chronic diseases that are the major killers of adults: cardiovascular disease, stroke, high blood pressure, diabetes, and some types of cancer. Obesity and osteoporosis also have been associated with faulty nutrition. Consequently, sensible lifelong eating habits play an important role in maintaining good health and preventing chronic disease (**FIGURE 7.1**).

Healthy eating is defined as the practice of making choices about what you eat with the intention of improving or maintaining good health. Typically this means following the recommendations of "experts" regarding a nutritional diet. Regrettably, there are many misconceptions and misunderstandings as to what constitutes a good, nutritional diet. This is seen by the many different diets available, the articles written in popular magazines and books, and the eating patterns of people. What is needed are very clear science-based dietary guidelines that you can follow in selecting your nutritional plan. As you increase your knowledge about nutrition and gain a better understanding of your eating habits, you improve your chances of enjoying good health now and later in life.

This chapter highlights the nutrients, their major food sources and roles in the body, and their recommended dietary allowances. It introduces you to science-based guidelines that you can use to design a healthy diet plan as well as several practical tools designed to help guide you in making healthy food selections. The information in this chapter, along with the accompanying activities and assessments, will assist you in evaluating the nutritional adequacy of your diet and

---

1

Nutrition plays a major role in our overall health.

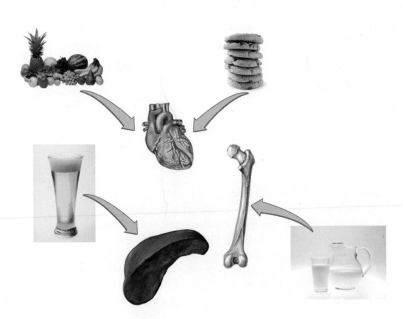

FIGURE 7.1 **Nutrition and Your Health.** Many health conditions are related to diet. For example, consuming fruits and vegetables can be helpful to your heart, whereas eating too much saturated fat can be harmful to your heart; drinking too much alcohol can lead to cirrhosis of the liver; and an adequate amount of calcium is important for strong bones.

(fruits) © Photodisc/Getty Images (cookies) © Samantha Grandy/ShutterStock, Inc. (milk) © LiquidLibrary (beer) © AbleStock

planning nutritious menus. Finally, information about nutrition should always be linked to information about physical activity because the health benefits of each support those of the other.

Nutrition Basics

Nutrition is all about the study of food and how our bodies use food as fuel for growth and daily activities. The Council on Food and Nutrition of the American Medical Association (AMA) defines *nutrition* as "the science of food, the nutrients and the substances therein, their action, interaction, and balance in relation to health and disease, and the process by which the organism ingests, digests, absorbs, transports, utilizes, and excretes food substances" (International Food Information Council Foundation [IFICF], 2011). This definition stresses the biochemical or physiological functions of food we eat, but public health experts note that nutrition may be interpreted in a broader sense and be affected by our behavior and environment as it relates to these functions (Johnson-Askew, Fisher, & Yaroch, 2009).

Most people know that nutrients in food nourish the body and are essential for promoting health. Nevertheless, most people choose foods for reasons other than their nutrient content. Instead, people's food choices tend to be influenced by a variety of personal factors, including pleasure or preference, emotional comfort, values, attitudes, social pressure, image, habit, ethnic and cultural background, availability, convenience, and cost (Johnson-Askew, Fisher, & Yaroch, 2009). In principle, eating well is not difficult. Yet to master that principle and put it into practice can be challenging because of the powerful preferences just noted. Simply put, even though we may know about nutritious foods, that doesn't mean we actually eat such foods all the time. Although our food selection and nutritional status are greatly influenced by these personal factors, it is in every person's best interest to understand optimal nourishment first; therefore, this chapter begins with the primary purpose of why we must eat food—for the nutrients themselves.

Nutrient Needs

The principal purpose of eating is to provide our body with **nutrients**. Nutrients perform three major functions in the body that are essential for life: (1) provide energy, (2) help regulate body processes, and (3) build and repair tissues.

Nutrients provide energy, regulate body processes, and nourish tissues.

ENERGY All biological and physiological body functions require energy. The human body must be supplied continuously with its own form of energy to perform its many complex functions. The nutrients contained in food provide the energy necessary to maintain bodily functions both at rest and during various forms of physical activity. The most obvious example of our body's need for energy is the mechanical work generated by muscle contraction. Our muscles must be provided with chemical energy from food to accomplish this mechanical work. Your physical functioning related to jogging, swimming, aerobic dancing, and weight lifting is considerably influenced by your capacity to extract energy from food nutrients and deliver it to the skeletal muscles.

In addition to the energy required for physical activity, the body requires considerable energy for absorption and assimilation of food nutrients during **digestion**, a series of complex mechanical and chemical reactions. **FIGURE 7.2** depicts the digestive system and its major organs. The raw fuel for both biological and mechanical energy requirements comes in the form of three **macronutrients**: carbohydrates, fats, and proteins. These energy-yielding nutrients continuously replenish the energy you expend daily from biological and mechanical work.

There are a variety of ways to express the energy value of food. The term used and understood by most people is *calorie*. A **calorie** is the amount of heat it takes to raise the temperature of 1 gram of water 1 degree Celsius. Calories are such

Nutrients Elements in foods that are required for energy, growth, and repair of tissues and regulation of body processes.

Digestion Metabolizing of food through a series of complex mechanical and chemical reactions.

Macronutrients Raw fuel, in the form of protein, carbohydrates, and fats, for biological and mechanical energy requirements.

Calorie Amount of heat it takes to raise the temperature of 1 gram of water 1 degree Celsius.

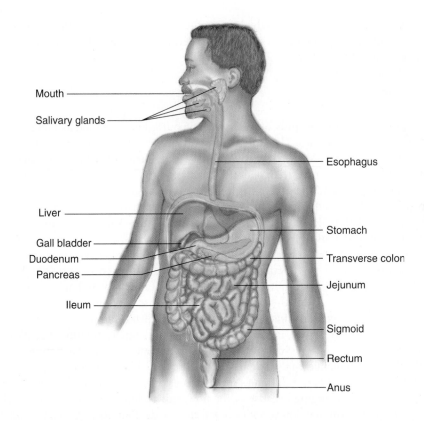

FIGURE 7.2 **The Human Digestive System.** Teeth and glandular secretions in the mouth help break up food, which the esophagus transports to the stomach. The stomach breaks down some of the food molecules and passes the food to the rest of the digestive tube: the duodenum, jejunum, ileum, colon, and rectum. The pancreas secretes enzymes and fluid into the duodenum to help the digestive process while the liver controls the release of absorbed nutrients into the body. Undigested material is eliminated from the body at the anus.

small units of measurement that nutrition scientists find it easier to express food energy in 1000-calorie units called *kilocalories* (abbreviated kcalories, or kcal). When you see the term *calorie* on a food label, or when you calculate your energy expenditure in calories, you are actually using kilocalories, but because the term *calorie* is commonly used in everyday life, we use it here.

The energy in a particular food depends on how much carbohydrate, protein, and fat the food contains. Carbohydrate and protein yield 4 calories of energy from each gram, and fat yields 9 calories per gram (TABLE 7.1). Once you know the

TABLE 7.1	Classes of Nutrients	
Nutrient	**Function**	**Major Sources**
Proteins (4 kcal/g)	Form important parts of muscles, bone, blood, enzymes, some hormones, and cell membranes; repair tissue; regulate water and acid–base balance; help in growth; supply energy	Meat, fish, poultry, eggs, milk products, legumes, nuts, soybeans
Carbohydrates (4 kcal/g)	Supply energy to cells in brain, nervous system, and blood; supply energy to muscles during exercise	Grains (breads and cereals), fruits, vegetables, milk
Fats (9 kcal/g)	Supply energy; insulate, support, and cushion organs; provide medium for absorption of fat-soluble vitamins	Saturated fats primarily from animal sources, palm and coconut oils, and hydrogenated vegetable fats; unsaturated fats from grains, nuts, seeds, fish
Vitamins	Promote (initiate or speed up) specific chemical reactions within cells	Abundant in fruits, vegetables, and grains; also found in meat and dairy products
Minerals	Help regulate body functions; aid in the growth and maintenance of body tissues; act as catalysts for the release of energy	Found in most food groups
Water	Makes up 50–70% of body weight; provides a medium for chemical reactions; transports chemicals; regulates temperature; removes waste products	Fruits, vegetables, and other liquids

number of grams of each of these substances contained in a certain food, you can derive the number of calories available in that food. Simply multiply the carbohydrate grams times 4, the protein grams times 4, and the fat grams times 9, and add all three together.

Calories are a highly desirable feature of food because they are used to do the body's physiological work or to exercise the muscles. Without calories, we would not survive. A constant flow of energy is so vital to life that other functions are sacrificed to maintain it. The average adult requires about 2000 calories per day to meet energy needs. The "evil" reputation of calories relates to energy storage in the body and is not deserved. If your body doesn't use all the energy-yielding nutrients to fuel its requirements, it rearranges them into storage compounds, primarily body fat, and puts them away for later use. This connection with excess body weight is the way many people think about calories, but it is a distortion of the true value of calories.

REGULATE BODY PROCESSES   The second function of food is to regulate body processes. Although the raw fuel for biological and mechanical work comes from calories in the form of carbohydrates, fats, and proteins (or *macronutrients*), the systematic removal and utilization of energy from these nutrients requires an assortment of additional **micronutrients**. Vitamins, minerals, and water play crucial roles in regulating the body's processes related to activating energy release. The regulating of energy processes and tissue maintenance is referred to as human metabolism. *Human metabolism* is the sum total of all chemical and physical reactions that go on in living cells. Metabolic processes allow for the release and use of energy from food compounds, the making of new compounds, and the transporting of compounds from place to place. For example, certain vitamins are essential for facilitating the release of the energy found in food and for controlling growth of body tissues. Like vitamins, minerals also play a regulatory role in metabolism and are essential for the synthesis of nutrients.

MAINTENANCE, REPAIR, AND GROWTH   The third function of food is to supply the required nutrients for body tissue maintenance, repair, and growth. Nearly all body cells are constantly being replaced. For example, red blood cells are useful for about a month and then must be replaced, and the cells that line the intestinal tract live less than a week. Various nutrients must be available to build the new cells for the body tissues: protein is a major material for red blood cells, muscle cells, and various enzymes; certain minerals such as calcium and phosphorus make up the cells that form the skeletal system.

Classes of Nutrients

Six classes of nutrients are considered necessary in human nutrition: proteins, carbohydrates, fats, vitamins, minerals, and water (refer to Table 7.1). Some nutritional scientists further distinguish nutrients into **essential nutrients** and **nonessential nutrients**. The term *essential nutrients* describes nutrients the body cannot make for itself and that must be obtained from foods we eat. TABLE 7.2 lists the specific nutrients currently known to be essential. Essential nutrients are necessary for human life. Inadequate intake of essential nutrients can lead to certain disease states and, eventually, death.

Other nutrients either come from the foods we eat or can be made by the body. For example, the body can convert protein or fats into a carbohydrate, if needed. Because it is not crucial that we obtain them from food, we refer to these nutrients as *nonessential nutrients*. This is not to say that nonessential nutrients are unimportant, just that they can be made by the body. As noted earlier, there are six classes of nutrients that your body needs for normal functioning and

Micronutrients Nutrients required in small amounts; includes vitamins and minerals.

Essential nutrients Nutrients the body cannot make for itself; must be obtained from food.

Nonessential nutrients Nutrients made by the body from the foods we eat.

Food can be divided into six classes, and each class plays a different role.

TABLE 7.2	The Essential Nutrients*			
Amino Acids	**Vitamins**	**Minerals**	**Fats**	**Water**
Isoleucine	Ascorbic acid	Calcium	Linoleic acid	
Leucine	(vitamin C)	Chlorine	Linolenic acid	
Lysine	Biotin	Chromium		
Methionine	Cobalamin	Cobalt		
Phenylalanine	(vitamin B_{12})	Copper		
Threonine	Folic acid	Iodine		
Tryptophan	Niacin (vitamin B_3)	Iron		
Valine	Pantothenic acid	Magnesium		
	Pyridoxine	Manganese		
	(vitamin B_6)	Molybdenum		
	Riboflavin	Phosphorous		
	(vitamin B_2)	Potassium		
	Thiamine	Selenium		
	(vitamin B_1)	Sodium		
	Vitamin A	Sulfur		
	Vitamin D	Zinc		
	Vitamin E			
	Vitamin K			

*Must be obtained from food.

good health. These six classes—proteins, carbohydrates, fats, vitamins, minerals, and water—provide energy, regulate body processes, and contribute to the maintenance, repair, and growth of body structures. Each class can be further described by their composition, functions in the body, and dietary recommendations. The following sections examine these key differences.

Proteins

Protein is one of our most essential nutrients. The body uses it in more ways than any other nutrient. Protein was named after the Greek word *proteios*, meaning "of prime importance." The prime importance of protein is reflected by its uses in the body. The body uses proteins for new growth and to build such body proteins as hemoglobin, enzymes, hormones, and antibodies. Proteins constantly help to replace worn-out cells in the body. Protein has a number of physiological functions that are essential to optimal physical performance. People think of proteins as body-building nutrients, the material of strong muscles, and rightly so. Protein forms the structural basis for muscle tissue and is a major component of most enzymes in the muscle.

To appreciate the many vital functions of protein, we need to understand its structure. Protein is a complex chemical containing atoms of carbon, hydrogen, oxygen, and nitrogen that are combined in a structure called an **amino acid**. There are 20 different amino acids that are important to human nutrition. Humans can synthesize some amino acids in the body but cannot synthesize others. The eight amino acids that the body cannot make are referred to as **essential amino acids** (refer to Table 7.2). Two of the essential amino acids, *lysine* and *tryptophan*, are poorly represented in most plant proteins. Thus, strict vegetarians should make special plans to ensure that their diet contains sufficient amounts of these two amino acids. It should be noted that all 20 amino acids are necessary for protein

Protein An essential nutrient that the body uses in more ways than any other nutrient.

Amino acid Complex chemical structure of protein, containing atoms of carbon, hydrogen, oxygen, and nitrogen.

Essential amino acids The eight amino acids that the body cannot make.

(synthesis) in the body and must be present simultaneously for optimal maintenance of body growth and function. Protein foods that contain all of the essential amino acids in adequate amount, and in the correct ratio to maintain nitrogen balance and allow for tissue growth and repair, are known as *complete proteins*. Excellent sources of complete protein are eggs, milk, meat, fish, poultry, and soybeans (FIGURE 7.3).

DIETARY RECOMMENDATION FOR PROTEIN   According to the Food and Nutrition Board, the Recommended Dietary Allowance (RDA) for both adult men and women is 0.8 grams of good quality protein per kilogram (2.2 lb) of ideal weight (Institute of Medicine [IOM], 2005). Ideal weight is used rather than actual weight because protein is needed for lean body tissues, not for fat tissue. Thus, a reference 150-lb person (68 kilograms) needs approximately 55 grams of protein a day.

A second way to estimate protein needs is the **Acceptable Macronutrient Distribution Range** (AMDR). The AMDR is expressed as the percentage of total daily calorie intake for all three macronutrients that provide calories: protein, carbohydrates, and fat. The adult AMDR for protein is 10–35 percent of daily calories (IOM, 2005). This recommendation may be slightly higher than the RDA, depending on actual calorie intake. The RDA assumes that the protein in your diet is from a variety of sources and that enough carbohydrate and fat calories are consumed so that protein is not used for energy. The AMDRs are set to provide essential nutrients like vitamins and minerals as well as reduce the risk from chronic diseases. The ranges are quite wide, which allows individuals to have a lot of flexibility in their eating patterns.

Does the highly physically active individual or athlete need more protein in the diet? A position paper from the American Dietetic Association (ADA), the Dietitians of Canada, and the American College of Sports Medicine states that all athletes, as well as those who train like athletes, have higher protein needs than do sedentary people (ADA, 2009a). Recommendations exist for different categories of athletes. They recommend 1.2 to 1.4 grams of protein per kilogram each day for endurance athletes. Strength athletes should consume slightly more or between 1.5 and 1.7 grams of protein per kilogram each day. Although adequate protein consumption is of great importance to athletes, more is not always better. The overconsumption of protein, in excess of 2 grams per kilogram per day, could potentially be harmful to the body. Based on the AMDR for protein, individuals should not exceed 35 percent of total daily calories from protein. It is important to realize that additional calories from protein are used for energy or stored as fat; protein is not an efficient source of energy compared to carbohydrates and fats.

> **Acceptable Macronutrient Distribution Range** (AMDR) A range of intakes for a particular energy source that is associated with reduced risk of chronic disease while providing adequate intakes of essential nutrients. An AMDR is expressed as a percentage of total daily calorie intake for protein, carbohydrates, and fat.

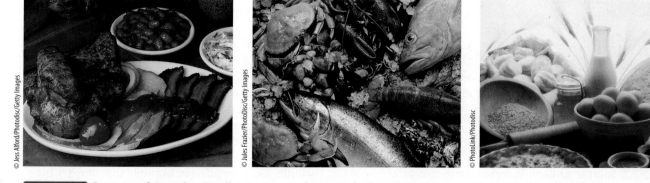

FIGURE 7.3 **Sources of Protein.** Excellent sources of protein include fish, meat, poultry, milk, and soybeans.

Carbohydrates

Carbohydrates are the preferred energy source for most of the body's functions. Carbohydrates are found in all foods, but are especially plentiful in grains, fruits, and vegetables (FIGURE 7.4). Carbohydrates are organic compounds that contain carbon, hydrogen, and oxygen. A wide variety exists in nature and in the body. Carbohydrates are generally divided into two categories: simple and complex.

SIMPLE CARBOHYDRATES

Simple carbohydrates are divided into one-sugar or two-sugar molecules. A one-sugar molecule is referred to as a **monosaccharide** (saccharide means "sugar" or "sweet"). More than 200 monosaccharides are found in nature, with the most common types being glucose, fructose, and galactose (FIGURE 7.5). Almost all of the body's cells use glucose as their chief energy source. Fructose is one of the sweetest sugars and is found in fruits and honey. Galactose is produced from milk sugar. Both must be converted to glucose to be used for energy by the cells.

The combination of two monosaccharides yields a **disaccharide**, which sucrose, maltose, and lactose are. All three have glucose as one of their single sugars. Glucose occurs naturally in many fruits and vegetables. The most familiar source of sucrose is table sugar. Table sugar is a concentrated sweetener that is derived by refining the juice from sugar cane. Monosaccharides and disaccharides are known as simple carbohydrates, or simple sugars, because there is only one bond in each that must be broken down by the digestive enzymes before they can be absorbed by the blood.

COMPLEX CARBOHYDRATES

Complex carbohydrates are known as polysaccharides. The term polysaccharide is used when three or more sugar molecules are linked. In fact, from 300 to 26,000 monosaccharides can be linked together to form a complex carbohydrate. The three most common forms of complex carbohydrates are starch, glycogen, and dietary fiber.

Starches are the storage form of carbohydrates for plants. Grains such as wheat, rice, and corn are the richest food sources of starch. Other important sources include the foods from the legume family (e.g., peanuts, kidney beans, chickpeas, soybeans) and root vegetables (e.g., potatoes, yams).

As starch stores energy for plants, glycogen stores energy for humans and animals. If the blood delivers more glucose than the cells need, the liver and muscles take up a certain amount and build the polysaccharide **glycogen**. Glycogen plays an important role in the body as a readily available source of glucose, especially during physical activity. The well-nourished human body can store approximately 400 to 500 grams or 1600 to 2000 calories of energy (Wilmore, Costill, & Kenney, 2008). Excess glucose beyond what the body is able to use immediately, or deposit as glycogen, is stored as fat.

DIETARY RECOMMENDATION FOR ENERGY-YIELDING CARBOHYDRATES

Carbohydrates are the body's main source of energy. The adult AMDR for carbohydrates is 45–65 percent of daily calories (U.S. Department of Health and Human Services [USDHHS] & U.S. Department of Agriculture [USDA], 2010; IOM, 2005). To calculate how many carbohydrate calories that means for you, start with the number of calories you normally eat. Multiply that number by the recommended percentages to get the range of car-

Carbohydrates Organic compounds that contain carbon, hydrogen, and oxygen.

Simple carbohydrates Either one-sugar or two-sugar molecules.

Monosaccharide One-sugar molecule.

Disaccharide Two-sugar molecule.

Complex carbohydrates Called polysaccharides, these link three or more sugar molecules.

Starches Storage form of carbohydrates for plants.

Glycogen Storage form of sugar energy for humans and animals.

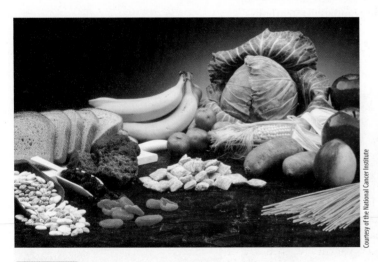

Courtesy of the National Cancer Institute

FIGURE 7.4 **Sources of Carbohydrates.** Good sources of carbohydrates include fruit, vegetables, and grains.

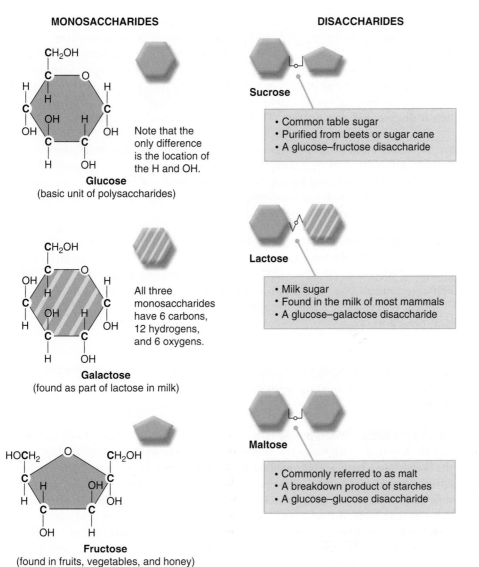

MONOSACCHARIDES

Glucose
(basic unit of polysaccharides)

Note that the only difference is the location of the H and OH.

Galactose
(found as part of lactose in milk)

All three monosaccharides have 6 carbons, 12 hydrogens, and 6 oxygens.

Fructose
(found in fruits, vegetables, and honey)

DISACCHARIDES

Sucrose

- Common table sugar
- Purified from beets or sugar cane
- A glucose–fructose disaccharide

Lactose

- Milk sugar
- Found in the milk of most mammals
- A glucose–galactose disaccharide

Maltose

- Commonly referred to as malt
- A breakdown product of starches
- A glucose–glucose disaccharide

FIGURE 7.5 **Some Common Sugars.** Sucrose and fructose are the most common sugars in our diets.

bohydrate calories. For example, based on a 2200-calorie-a-day diet, the range of carbohydrate calories would be 990 (45 percent) to 1430 (65 percent). To determine how many grams of carbohydrate that is, divide the total carbohydrate calories by 4 (calories in a gram of carbohydrate). This translates to approximately 248 to 358 grams of carbohydrates a day.

The type of carbohydrates is vital. Some provide health benefits whereas others should be limited. Added sugar should account for 10 percent or less of total calories because it supplies relatively few nutrients (USDA, 2012). Added sugar is the sugar added to processed food and drinks while they are being made, as well as sugar you may add to your food at home. Food manufacturers may add both natural sugars (such as fructose) and processed sugars (such as high-fructose corn syrup) to processed food and drinks. Similarly, limit refined grains because they are missing the key nutrients that their whole-grain counterparts retain. Refined grains include white rice, white bread, regular white pasta, and other foods that have been made with enriched flour or all-purpose flour, including many cookies, cakes, breakfast cereals, crackers, and snack foods. Rather, you should consume whole grains, vegetables, fruits, and beans because they promote good health by providing vitamins, minerals, fiber, and a mass of significant phytonutrients.

Dietary fiber Diverse carbohydrate polysaccharides of plants that cannot be digested by the human stomach or small intestine.

Insoluble fibers Dietary fibers not soluble in water or metabolized by the intestines; make feces bulkier and softer, promoting decreased passage time.

Soluble fibers Dietary fibers soluble in water, metabolized in the large intestine; assist in removing cholesterol from the body.

Fats Members of a family of compounds called lipids.

Triglycerides Fatty acids that provide the body's largest energy store, act as insulation, transport fat-soluble vitamins, and contribute to satiety.

Dietary fiber is a general term for diverse carbohydrate polysaccharides of plants that cannot be digested by the human stomach or small intestine. Technically, dietary fiber is not an essential nutrient, but it has demonstrated benefits of health maintenance and disease prevention, making it a highly recommended functional food. Long praised as part of a healthy diet, fiber appears to reduce the risk of developing various conditions, including heart disease, diabetes, diverticular disease, and constipation (Park, Subar, Hollenbeck, & Schatzkin, 2011).

Dietary fiber exists in two basic forms: insoluble and soluble. **Insoluble fibers** are not dissolved in water or metabolized by the intestines; they make the feces bulkier and softer, thus decreasing passage time. They are made up mostly of cellulose, hemicelluloses, and lignins. **Soluble fibers** are dissolved in water and are metabolized in the large intestine; they assist in draining cholesterol from the body. They include pectins, gums, and mucilages.

DIETARY RECOMMENDATIONS FOR FIBER The Institute of Medicine's Food and Nutrition Board (FNB) recommends 20 to 35 grams of fiber per day, or 10 to 13 grams per 1000 calories (IOM, 2005). To achieve adequate dietary fiber intake, the FNB recommends you include at least two to three servings of whole grains as part of the daily servings of grains, five servings of fruits and vegetables, and legumes at least twice a week.

Fats

Fats (also known as lipids) are found in foods and in the body (FIGURE 7.6). Fats can be categorized into three main groups: triglycerides, cholesterol, and phospholipids.

TRIGLYCERIDES When people talk about body fat, or fat in their food, they are usually referring to triglycerides. **Triglycerides** perform many important functions in the body. These fatty acids constitute the body's largest energy store, provide insulation, transport fat-soluble vitamins, and contribute to satiety (satisfaction). More than 95 percent of our body fat is in the form of triglycerides. The chemical name helps explain itself. A triglyceride molecule consists of three fatty acid atoms attached to a glycerol molecule. Fatty acids are chains of carbon, oxygen, and hydrogen atoms (FIGURE 7.7). Fatty acids chains may differ from one another in two ways: chain length and saturation. The chain length affects the way fat is absorbed and its solubility in water (shorter chains are more soluble). Saturation refers to the chemical structure—specifically, to the number of hydrogens the fatty acid chain is holding. The basic structures of fatty acid molecules are *saturated* and *unsaturated*.

If every available bond from the carbons is holding a hydrogen atom, the fatty acid is saturated. In some fatty acid chains there is a place where hydrogens are missing; this is the point of unsaturation, and the fatty acid is unsaturated. If there is one point of unsaturation the chain is *monounsaturated*; if there is more than one point of unsaturation the chain is *polyunsaturated*.

Both plants and animals provide ready sources of fat. All dietary fats contain a mixture of saturated and unsaturated fatty acids (FIGURE 7.8). The type of fatty acid that predominates determines whether the fat is solid or liquid and whether it is characterized as saturated or unsaturated. Coconut and palm oil, for example, contain high levels of saturated fatty acids and are relatively hard at room temperature. Oils such as soybean, canola, cottonseed, corn, and

© Mark Adams/SuperStock, Inc.

FIGURE 7.6 **Sources of Fats.** Sources of fats in foods include oil, ice cream, cheese, and margarine.

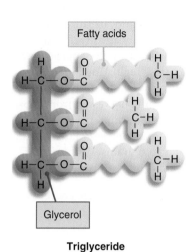

Fatty acids

Glycerol

Triglyceride

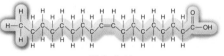

Stearic Acid

Saturated Fatty Acid
(no double bonds between carbon atoms)

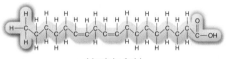

Oleic Acid

Monounsaturated Fatty Acid
(one double bond between carbon atoms)

Linoleic Acid

Polyunsaturated Fatty Acid
(two or more double bonds between carbon atoms)

FIGURE 7.7 **Chemical Structure of Saturated and Unsaturated Fats.** Triglyceride consists of a molecule of glycerol with three fatty acids attached. Fatty acids can differ in the lengths of their carbon chains and degree of saturation.

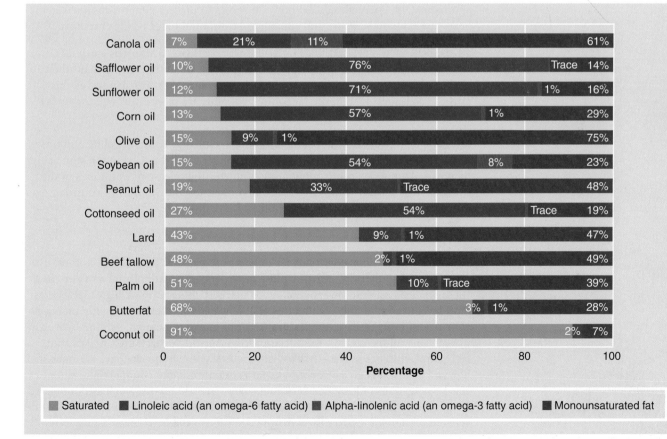

Oil/Fat	Saturated	Linoleic acid (an omega-6 fatty acid)	Alpha-linolenic acid (an omega-3 fatty acid)	Monounsaturated fat
Canola oil	7%	21%	11%	61%
Safflower oil	10%	76%	Trace	14%
Sunflower oil	12%	71%	1%	16%
Corn oil	13%	57%	1%	29%
Olive oil	15%	9%	1%	75%
Soybean oil	15%	54%	8%	23%
Peanut oil	19%	33%	Trace	48%
Cottonseed oil	27%	54%	Trace	19%
Lard	43%	9%	1%	47%
Beef tallow	48%	2%	1%	49%
Palm oil	51%	10%	Trace	39%
Butterfat	68%	3%	1%	28%
Coconut oil	91%		2%	7%

Percentage

■ Saturated ■ Linoleic acid (an omega-6 fatty acid) ■ Alpha-linolenic acid (an omega-3 fatty acid) ■ Monounsaturated fat

FIGURE 7.8 **Comparison of Dietary Fats.**

other vegetable oils contain higher levels of unsaturated fatty acids and are liquid at room temperature.

ESSENTIAL FATTY ACIDS   The body can synthesize all the fatty acids it needs from carbohydrate, fat, or protein except for linoleic acid (omega-6) and alpha-linolenic acid (omega-3). Both are unsaturated fatty acids and, because they must be obtained from food, are referred to as **essential fatty acids** (refer to Table 7.2). These fatty acids are essential for the body because they participate in triggering immune responses, forming cell structures, regulating blood pressure, determining blood lipid concentration, and supporting clot formation. Linoleic acid is found in the seeds of plants and in the oils harvested from those seeds. Alpha-linolenic acid is found in fish such as salmon, tuna, trout, and sardines. Canola or soybean oil and nuts also supply these omega-3 fatty acids. The FNB recommends a minimum daily amount of 3 to 6 grams, or 1 to 2 percent of your total calories from the essential fatty acids (IOM, 2005).

ENERGY SOURCE AND RESERVE   One gram of fat contains twice the energy (9 calories) of an equal gram of carbohydrate or protein. The utilization of fat provides energy at rest and during specific types of physical activity. We store most of our energy in the form of triglycerides, or body fat. Ideally, approximately 15 percent of body weight for males and 25 percent for females is fat. Each pound of body fat provides 3500 calories of energy; therefore, for an average male the energy stored in fat is about 100,000 calories. Compare this with the 2000 calories of stored energy from carbohydrate.

INSULATION AND PROTECTION   The layer of fat just beneath our skin is made up of triglycerides and insulates the body against extreme cold. Furthermore, approximately 4 percent of total body fat serves to protect vital organs such as the heart, liver, kidneys, brain, and spinal cord from injury as a result of trauma.

TRANSPORTING VITAMINS   Triglycerides and other fats in foods carry fat-soluble vitamins—vitamins A, D, E, and K—to the small intestine and aid their absorption. The ingestion of approximately 20 grams of fat per day serves this purpose. Without this fat, the fat-soluble vitamins are passed through the body and eliminated in the feces.

SATIETY   Triglycerides in foods help give us a full and content feeling and offset hunger feelings. The fat we eat takes much longer to be digested in the stomach than carbohydrate or protein. Fat also stimulates the release of hormones in the stomach that decrease hunger feelings. If you cut too much fat from your diet, you lose satiety value and may become hungry more quickly.

Trans Fat

Health researchers consider **trans fat** to be a very harmful type of fat (Hunter, Zhang, & Kris-Etherton, 2010). Unlike other fats, trans fat both raises your "bad" (LDL) cholesterol and lowers your "good" (HDL) cholesterol. A high LDL cholesterol level in combination with a low HDL cholesterol level significantly increases your risk of heart disease, the leading killer of men and women. Adding hydrogen to vegetable oil through an industrial process called hydrogenation makes trans fat. Manufacturers use trans fats to help foods stay fresh longer, have a longer shelf life, and have a less greasy feel. Trans fat is found in many commercially baked snack goods like cookies, crackers, and cakes, and fried foods, such as donuts and french fries. Most of the trans fat Americans consume comes from partially hydrogenated oil. Look for partially hydrogenated oils on the ingredient list on food packages. According to the U.S. Dietary Guidelines, Americans should eat less than 2 grams of trans fat per day (USDA, 2012).

Essential fatty acids Support immune responses, form cell structures, regulate blood pressure, affect blood lipid concentration, and promote clot formation; must be obtained from food.

Trans fats Unsaturated fatty acids formed when vegetable oils are processed (hydrogenation) and made more solid.

Phospholipids and Cholesterol

Phospholipids and cholesterol make up the remaining 5 percent of lipids in the diet. **Phospholipids** are a component of all cells, and many types exist in the body; they are made by the body and therefore are not considered essential nutrients. Among these, the lecithins are of particular interest. *Lecithin* functions as a fat emulsifier in the small intestine, breaking fat into small globules that are suspended in water. This separation of fat in water helps create more fat surface area for the fat-digesting enzymes to work on. There is no need to supplement lecithin in your diet because the body makes its own lecithin and because it is so readily available in the diet through a variety of foods, including soybeans, nuts, egg yolks, beef, oatmeal, and wheat germ.

Cholesterol is vital to the body in a variety of ways. Cholesterol forms part of many important hormones and is an essential structural component of cells. However, like the lecithins, cholesterol can be manufactured by the body and therefore is not an essential nutrient. In addition to the cholesterol made by the body from fats, carbohydrates, or proteins, it can be obtained through eating foods of animal origin, such as eggs, red meat, and fish. Eating saturated fats raises your blood cholesterol level more than anything else in your diet. Elevated blood cholesterol levels have been shown to be related to an increased incidence of coronary heart disease (Expert Panel, 2001). The goal is to encourage people to eat less than 300 mg of cholesterol a day. In addition, less than 10 percent of their fat calories should come from saturated fat.

DIETARY RECOMMENDATION FOR FAT   Dietary fat is essential for the body because it provides us with a source of essential fatty acids, provides a means to transport fat-soluble vitamins, and supplies a concentrated and efficient energy source. Although no specific RDA has been established for the total amount of fat, the adult AMDR for fat is 20–35 percent of daily calories (IOM, 2005). To figure out how many fat calories that means for you, start with the number of calories you normally eat or want to eat a day. Multiply that number by the recommended percentages to get the range of fat calories. For example, based on a 2200-calorie-a-day diet, the range of fat calories would be 440 (20 percent) to 770 (35 percent). To determine how many grams of fat that is, divide the total fat calories by 9 (calories in a gram of fat). This translates to approximately 49 to 86 fat grams a day.

In terms of influencing disease risk, the total amount of fat you consume in a day is less important than the type of fat you consume (USDA, 2012). You should consume less than 10 percent of calories from saturated fatty acids and replace them with monounsaturated and polyunsaturated fatty acids. These unsaturated fatty acids, or "good fats," have been shown to protect against cardiovascular disease and diabetes (Gillingham, Harris-Janz, & Jones, 2011). One should also keep trans fatty acid consumption as low as possible (less than 1 percent of total calories), especially by limiting foods that contain synthetic sources of trans fats, such as partially hydrogenated oils, and by limiting other solid fats. Finally, dietary cholesterol should be limited to less than 300 mg per day.

Vitamins

Vitamins are essential organic substances needed by the body to perform highly specific metabolic processes in the cells. They are indispensable nutrients because they can't be synthesized by the body and must be obtained from food. Additionally, for a substance to be classified as a vitamin, its absence from the diet over a period of time must lead to deficiency symptoms. For example, vitamin A deficiency over an extended period of time can cause blindness, and a lack of niacin can cause mental illness.

> **Phospholipids** Lipids made by the body and therefore not considered essential fatty acids.
>
> **Vitamins** Essential organic substances needed by the body to perform highly specific metabolic processes in the cells.

Vitamins contribute no energy to the body; instead they assist the enzymes that release energy from carbohydrate, fat, and protein. Thirteen different vitamins have been isolated, analyzed, and synthesized, and their recommended dietary intakes established (TABLE 7.3). They are needed in small amounts in the diet for normal function, growth, and maintenance of the body. In fact, the body requires only about 350 grams of vitamins from the nearly 1900 pounds of food consumed by the average adult during the year. Vitamins fall into two classes, fat-soluble and water-soluble. The solubility of a vitamin refers to how it is absorbed and transported, whether it can be stored, and how easily it is lost from the body.

The four **fat-soluble vitamins** (A, D, E, K) are absorbed into the body with fats. These vitamins travel with dietary fats through the bloodstream to reach the cells.

> **Fat-soluble vitamins** Vitamins A, D, E, K; must travel with dietary fats in the bloodstream to reach the cells.

| TABLE 7.3 | Water-Soluble and Fat-Soluble Vitamins |

Water-Soluble Vitamins	Why Needed?	Primary Sources	Deficiency Results in
Ascorbic acid (vitamin C)	Tooth and bone formation; production of connective tissue; promotion of wound healing; may enhance immunity	Citrus fruits, tomatoes, peppers, cabbage, potatoes, melons	Scurvy (degeneration of bones, teeth, and gums)
Biotin	Involved in fat and amino acid synthesis and breakdown	Yeast, liver, milk, most vegetables, bananas, grapefruit	Skin problems; fatigue; muscle pains; nausea
Cobalamin (vitamin B_{12})	Involved in single carbon atom transfers; essential for DNA synthesis	Muscle meats, eggs, milk, and dairy products (not in vegetables)	Pernicious anemia; nervous system malfunctions
Folacin (folic acid)	Essential for synthesis of DNA and other molecules	Green leafy vegetables, organ meats, whole-wheat products	Anemia; diarrhea and other gastrointestinal problems
Niacin	Involved in energy production and synthesis of cell molecules	Grains, meats, legumes	Pellagra (skin, gastrointestinal, and mental disorders)
Pantothenic acid	Involved in energy production and synthesis and breakdown of many biological molecules	Yeast, meats, and fish, nearly all vegetables and fruits	Vomiting; abdominal cramps; malaise; insomnia
Pyridoxine (vitamin B_6)	Essential fat synthesis, breakdown of amino acids, manufacture of unsaturated fats from saturated fats	Meats, whole grains, most vegetables	Weakness; irritability; trouble sleeping and walking; skin problems
Riboflavin (vitamin B_2)	Involved in energy production; important for health of the eyes	Milk and dairy foods, meats, eggs, vegetables, grains	Eye and skin problems
Thiamine (vitamin B_1)	Essential for breakdown of food molecules and production of energy	Meats, legumes, grains, some vegetables	Beri-beri (nerve damage, weakness, heart failure)
Fat-Soluble Vitamins	**Why Needed?**	**Primary Sources**	**Deficiency or Excess Results in**
Vitamin A (retinol)	Essential for maintenance of eyes and skin; influences bone and tooth formation	Liver, kidney, yellow and green leafy vegetables, apricots	*Deficiency:* night blindness; eye damage; skin dryness. *Excess:* loss of appetite; skin problems; swelling of ankles and feet
Vitamin D (calciferol)	Regulates calcium metabolism; important for growth of bones and teeth	Cod-liver oil, dairy products, eggs	*Deficiency:* rickets (bone deformities) in children; bone destruction in adults. *Excess:* thirst; nausea; weight loss; kidney damage
Vitamin E (tocopherol)	Prevents damage to cells from oxidation; prevents red blood cell destruction	Wheat germ, vegetable oils, vegetables, egg yolk, nuts	*Deficiency:* anemia; possibly nerve cell destruction
Vitamin K (phylloquinone)	Helps with blood clotting	Liver, vegetable oils, green leafy vegetables, tomatoes	*Deficiency:* severe bleeding

They are not readily excreted by the body. Once absorbed, excessive amounts of fat-soluble vitamins are stored in the liver and fat cells until the body needs them. The ability to store fat-soluble vitamins makes daily ingestion of the fat-soluble vitamins unnecessary.

Nine vitamins are classified as water-soluble because they are transported throughout the watery medium of the body. **Water-soluble vitamins** are more readily excreted than are fat-soluble vitamins and are not stored in tissues. Excess water-soluble vitamins are excreted through the urine.

Minerals

Minerals are inorganic substances that are vital to many body functions. Minerals help build strong bones and teeth, aid in accurate muscle function, help nervous systems transmit messages, help balance the amount of water in the body, and work closely with vitamins to perform our body's chemical and hormonal activities. Like vitamins, minerals do not provide any energy for the body. In the body, minerals are classified as **major minerals** if their requirement exceeds 100 milligrams per day and **trace minerals** if their requirement is less than 100 milligrams per day. (TABLE 7.4) lists the minerals, their major functions, and their food sources.

> **Water-soluble vitamins** Vitamins that can be transported throughout the body by a watery medium.
> **Minerals** Inorganic substances vital to many body functions.
> **Major minerals** Mineral requirements that exceed 100 mg per day.
> **Trace minerals** Mineral requirements of less than 100 mg per day.

TABLE 7.4	**Essential Minerals**		
Mineral	**Why Needed?**	**Primary Sources**	**Deficiency Results in**
Calcium	Bone and tooth formation; blood clotting; nerve transmission	Milk, cheese, dark-green vegetables, dried legumes	Stunted growth; rickets; osteoporosis; convulsions
Chlorine	Formation of gastric juice; acid–base balance	Common salt	Muscle cramps; mental apathy; reduced appetite
Chromium	Glucose and energy metabolism	Fats, vegetable oils, meats	Impaired ability to metabolize glucose
Cobalt	Constituent of vitamin B_{12}	Organ and muscle meats	Not reported in humans
Copper	Constituent of enzymes of iron metabolism	Meats, drinking water	Anemia (rare)
Iodine	Constituent of thyroid hormones	Marine fish and shellfish, dairy products, many vegetables	Goiter (enlarged thyroid)
Iron	Constituent of hemoglobin and enzymes of energy metabolism	Eggs, lean meats, legumes, whole grains, green leafy vegetables	Iron-deficiency anemia (weakness, reduced resistance to infection)
Magnesium	Activates enzymes; involved in protein synthesis	Whole grains, green leafy vegetables	Growth failure; behavioral disturbances; weakness, spasms
Manganese	Constituent of enzymes involved in fat synthesis	Widely distributed in foods	In animals: disturbances of nervous system, reproductive abnormalities
Molybdenum	Constituent of some enzymes	Legumes, cereals, organ meats	Not reported in humans
Phosphorus	Bone and tooth formation; acid–base balance	Milk, cheese, meat, poultry, grains	Weakness, demineralization of bone
Potassium	Acid–base balance; body water balance; nerve function	Meats, milk, many fruits	Muscular weakness; paralysis
Selenium	Functions in close association with vitamin E	Seafood, meat, grains	Anemia (rare)
Sodium	Acid–base balance; body water balance; nerve function	Common salt	Muscle cramps; mental apathy; reduced appetite
Sulfur	Constituent of active tissue compounds, cartilage, and tendon	Sulfur amino acids (methionine and cysteine) in dietary proteins	Related to intake and deficiency of sulfur amino acids
Zinc	Constituent of enzymes involved in digestion	Widely distributed in foods	Growth failure

Minerals can be found in most food items that we eat daily. For example, if you were to consume dark-green leafy vegetables, grain products, and meat and dairy products every day, you would get plenty of the minerals listed in Table 7.4.

In general, the human body maintains a proper balance of many minerals through a number of precise control mechanisms, but deficiencies and excesses of any mineral may disturb this balance. Some minerals interact and compete with each other, and consuming excesses of some minerals can affect the absorption of others; this is referred to as a mineral–mineral interaction. For example, iron and magnesium absorption is hindered if too much calcium is taken in.

Another interaction that is important is the vitamin–mineral interaction. This refers to the importance of certain vitamins and minerals being available at the same time. Iron absorption is improved when it is consumed with vitamin C, and the presence of vitamin D improves the absorption of calcium. Because of mineral–mineral and vitamin–mineral interactions, people should avoid taking individual supplements for minerals unless they have a specific condition that warrants it.

DIETARY RECOMMENDATIONS FOR VITAMINS AND MINERALS A well-balanced diet will satisfy all the vitamin and mineral requirements of most individuals, including those who are physically active. Select a wide variety of foods from all food groups. *For those receiving the RDA of vitamins and minerals, there is no research evidence that supplementation enhances exercise performance.* It is important to remember that excess vitamin and mineral intake does not improve health or exercise performance, but it can be toxic. For example, excessive amounts of vitamin A can lead to weakness, headache, nausea, pain in the joints, and liver damage. Too much vitamin D may lead to vomiting, diarrhea, loss of weight, loss of muscle tone, and soft-tissue damage. Vitamin and mineral excesses generally occur as a result of supplementation.

SPECIAL NEEDS FOR IRON AND CALCIUM Two minerals of special interest, especially for adolescents, adults older than 50, and physically active individuals, are iron and calcium. Women need more of both nutrients than men do. In all cases, individuals need to be particularly aware of obtaining good sources of nutrients in their diet.

The mineral *iron* has many diverse biological functions, but none more important than its role in the transport of oxygen in blood. Iron forms a major part of the hemogloblin in red blood cells. Red blood cells play a major role in aerobic capacity. Nearly 75 percent of the body's iron is found in hemogloblin. If neither diet nor body stores supply the iron needed, hemogloblin concentration levels eventually fall, leading to iron depletion and anemia. **Anemia** is a deficiency in red blood cells and is generally recognized to be the most common single nutritional deficiency, not just in developing countries but around the world.

Several factors are responsible for iron deficiency, including inadequate dietary iron, absorption disturbances, illness, and exercise. Treatment of iron deficiency includes prudent use of MyPlate (**FIGURE 7.9**) and possibly iron supplements. High-iron foods are meat, poultry, fish, dry beans, eggs, and nuts found in the Protein group from MyPlate and from fortified foods such as breakfast cereals. Women between the ages of 19 and 50 require 18 milligrams per day. Women older than 50 and men older than the age of 18 need 8 milligrams of iron daily. The higher RDA for young and middle-aged women is chiefly to counteract menstrual blood loss.

The body contains more *calcium* than any other mineral. Calcium's primary role in the body is that of forming and maintaining bones. Osteoporosis, a major health concern for women, is related to calcium deficiency. Calcium is also important for muscle contraction, nerve transmission, and cellular metabolism. Muscles cannot relax after contraction if blood calcium levels fall below a crucial point.

Anemia Deficiency in red blood cells.

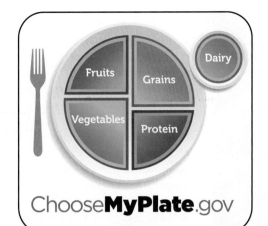

Vegetables	Fruits	Grains	Dairy	Protein Foods
Vary your veggies	*Focus on fruits*	*Make half your grains whole*	*Get your calcium-rich foods*	*Go lean with protein*
Eat more red, orange, and dark-green veggies like tomatoes, sweet potatoes, and broccoli in main dishes. Add beans or peas to salads (kidney or chickpeas), soups (split peas or lentils), and side dishes (pinto or baked beans), or serve as a main dish. Fresh, frozen, and canned vegetables all count. Choose "reduced sodium" or "no-salt-added" canned veggies.	Use fruits as snacks, salads, and desserts. At breakfast, top your cereal with bananas or strawberries; add blueberries to pancakes. Buy fruits that are dried, frozen, and canned (in water or 100% juice), as well as fresh fruits. Select 100% fruit juice when choosing juices.	Substitute whole-grain choices for refined-grain breads, bagels, rolls, breakfast cereals, crackers, rice, and pasta. Check the ingredients list on product labels for the words "whole" or "whole grain" before the grain ingredient name. Choose products that name a whole grain first on the ingredients list.	Choose skim (fat-free) or 1% (low-fat) milk. They have the same amount of calcium and other essential nutrients as whole milk, but less fat and calories. Top fruit salads and baked potatoes with low-fat yogurt. If you are lactose intolerant, try lactose-free milk or fortified soymilk (soy beverage).	Eat a variety of foods from the protein food group each week, such as seafood, beans and peas, and nuts as well as lean meats, poultry, and eggs. Twice a week, make seafood the protein on your plate. Choose lean meats and ground beef that are at least 90% lean. Trim or drain fat from meat and remove skin from poultry to cut fat and calories.

Be physically active your way
Children and adolescents: get 60 minutes or more a day.
Adults: get 2 hours and 30 minutes or more a week of activity that requires moderate effort, such as brisk walking.

Cut back on sodium and empty calories from solid fats and added sugars
Look out for salt (sodium) in foods you buy. Drink water instead of sugary drinks.
Eat sugary desserts less often. Make foods that are high in solid fats occasional choices, not everyday foods.

FIGURE 7.9 **The MyPlate Food Guidance System Icon.** MyPlate illustrates the five food groups that are the building blocks for a healthy diet using a familiar image—a place setting for a meal. Each colored section of the plate represents a food group; an interactive tool on www.choosemyplate.gov provides personalized amounts for users. SOURCE: Reproduced from U.S. Department of Agriculture. Online: http://www.ChooseMyPlate.gov.

Daily calcium intake allows good muscle contractions and relaxations during physical activity.

The dairy group of MyPlate and calcium-fortified foods (orange juice, breakfast cereals) provide the best sources of calcium. Adults need between 1000 and 1500 milligrams of calcium daily. Surveys indicate that Americans consume only half of this requirement. If you are having difficulty maintaining a well-balanced diet, consider supplementing your diet with calcium.

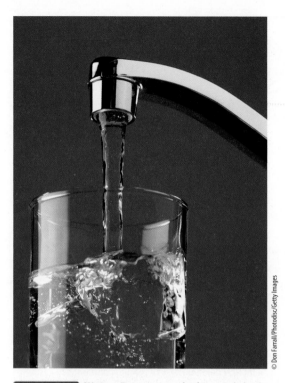

FIGURE 7.10 **Water Recommendation.** Drink six to eight glasses of water a day.

Water

Water makes up about 60 percent of the body's weight and is involved in virtually every body process. Water could be considered the most essential nutrient. Our bodies can survive deficiency of all the other nutrients for a few weeks or more but can survive only a few days without water. Water serves as the body's transport solvent, distributing nutrients throughout the body and conducting waste products to be excreted through the water in urine and feces. Water serves as the body's reactive medium, participating in every chemical reaction in the body. Water plays a major role in regulating the maintenance of body temperature because it is able to absorb a significant amount of body heat with only a small change in its temperature. Because water is vital to these and other functions, it is essential to maintain a healthy level in the body.

Proper fluid replacement is important for both health and physical activity. The sedentary body loses about 2 to 3 liters of water each day through urination, perspiration, breathing, and defecation. To replace this water, the RDA recommendation is that, under normal dietary and environmental conditions, the average adult who expends 2000 calories a day should consume 2 to 3 liters, or about six to eight glasses, of water each day (**FIGURE 7.10**). In addition to the water we drink, nearly all foods provide water (IOM, 2004). Fruits and vegetables are generally high in water content, whereas many meats and fatty foods are low.

Water is a crucial nutrient for those engaged in physical activity, especially if the activity is strenuous and performed in extreme environmental temperatures and humidity. To find out how much water you need to replenish from losses occurring during exercise, weigh yourself before and after exercise; the difference is all water. One pound equals approximately two glasses of water. Plain cool water is the best choice for drinking because it leaves the digestive system rapidly, is quickly absorbed by tissues, and cools the body.

Functional Foods

We now know that the minimum diet for human growth, energy, and regulating body processes requires six classes of essential nutrients. Within the emerging area of food and nutrition science, however, is the expanding knowledge of the role of other physiologically active components in foods that provide health benefits beyond those supplied by the traditional nutrients. Examples include carotenoids, dietary fiber, flavonoids, and phenols, all of which can be found in fruits and vegetables (TABLE 7.5). The International Food Information Council (IFIC) defines **functional foods** as those that contain significant levels of biologically active components that provide health benefits beyond basic nutrition (IFIC, 2012). The increasing comprehension of the role of physiologically active food components, both from plant (*phytochemicals*) and animal (*zoochemicals*) sources, has notably changed the role of diet in health. Interest in functional foods continues to evolve as food and nutrition science has advanced beyond studying nutritional deficiencies to studying foods for biologically active components that impart health benefits or desirable physiological effects beyond basic nutrition. To obtain the many potentially beneficial components from functional foods, the best advice is to include foods from all of the food groups represented in MyPlate.

Functional foods Foods that contain significant levels of biologically active components that provide health benefits beyond basic nutrition.

TABLE 7.5	Examples of Functional Components

Class/Components	Source*	Potential Benefit(s)
Carotenoids		
Beta-carotene	Carrots, pumpkin, sweet potato, cantaloupe	Neutralizes free radicals, which may damage cells; bolsters cellular antioxidant defenses; can be made into vitamin A in the body
Lutein, zeaxanthin	Kale, collards, spinach, corn, eggs, citrus	May contribute to maintenance of healthy vision
Lycopene	Tomatoes and processed tomato products, watermelon, red/pink grapefruit	May contribute to maintenance of prostate health
Dietary (Functional and Total) Fiber		
Insoluble fiber	Wheat bran, corn bran, fruit skins	May contribute to maintenance of a healthy digestive tract; may reduce the risk of some types of cancer
Beta glucan††	Oat bran, oatmeal, oat flour, barley, rye	May reduce risk of coronary heart disease (CHD)
Soluble fiber††	Psyllium seed husk, peas, beans, apples, citrus fruit	May reduce risk of CHD and some types of cancer
Whole grains††	Cereal grains, whole wheat bread, oatmeal, brown rice	May reduce risk of CHD and some types of cancer; may contribute to maintenance of healthy blood glucose levels
Fatty Acids		
Monounsaturated fatty acids (MUFAs)††	Tree nuts, olive oil, canola oil	May reduce risk of CHD
Polyunsaturated fatty acids (PUFAs)—omega-3 fatty acids—ALA	Walnuts, flax	May contribute to maintenance of heart health; may contribute to maintenance of mental and visual function
PUFAs—omega-3 fatty acids—DHA/EPA	Salmon, tuna, marine, other fish oils	May reduce risk of CHD; may contribute to maintenance of mental and visual function
Conjugated linoleic acid (CLA)	Beef and lamb; some cheese	May contribute to maintenance of desirable body composition and healthy immune function
Flavonoids		
Anthocyanins (cyanidin, delphinidin, malvidin)	Berries, cherries, red grapes	Bolsters cellular antioxidant defenses; may contribute to maintenance of brain function
Flavanols (catechins, epigallocatechin, procyanidins, epicatechins)	Tea, cocoa, chocolate, apples, grapes	May contribute to maintenance of heart health
Flavanones (hesperetin, naringenin)	Citrus fruits	Neutralize free radicals, which may damage cells; bolster cellular antioxidant defenses
Flavonols (quercetin, kaempferol, isorhamnetin, myricetin)	Onions, apples, tea, broccoli	Neutralize free radicals, which may damage cells; bolster cellular antioxidant defenses
Proanthocyanidins	Cranberries, cocoa, apples, strawberries, grapes, wine, peanuts, cinnamon	May contribute to maintenance of urinary tract health and heart health
Isothiocyanates		
Sulforaphane	Cauliflower, broccoli, broccoli sprouts, cabbage, kale, horseradish	May enhance detoxification of undesirable compounds; bolsters cellular antioxidant defenses
Phenolic Acids		
Caffeic acid, ferulic acid	Apples, pears, citrus fruits, some vegetables, coffee	May bolster cellular antioxidant defenses; may contribute to maintenance of healthy vision and heart health
Plant Stanols/Sterols		
Free stanols/sterols††	Corn, soy, wheat, wood oils, fortified foods and beverages	May reduce risk of CHD
Stanol/sterol esters††	Stanol ester dietary supplements, fortified foods and beverages, including table spreads	May reduce risk of CHD

(continues)

TABLE 7.5	Examples of Functional Components *(Continued)*	
Class/Components	**Source***	**Potential Benefit(s)**
Polyols		
Sugar alcohols[††] (xylitol, sorbitol, mannitol, lactitol)	Some chewing gums, other food applications	May reduce risk of dental caries
Prebiotics/Probiotics		
Inulin, fructo-oligosaccharides (FOS), polydextrose	Whole grains, onions, some fruits, garlic, honey, leeks, fortified foods and beverages	May improve gastrointestinal health; may improve calcium absorption
Yeast, *Lactobacilli, Bifidobacteria*, and other specific strains of beneficial bacteria	Certain yogurts, other cultured dairy and nondairy applications	May improve gastrointestinal health and systemic immunity; benefits are strain-specific
Phytoestrogens		
Isoflavones (daidzein, genistein)	Soybeans and soy-based foods	May contribute to maintenance of bone health, healthy brain and immune function; for women, may contribute to maintenance of menopausal health
Lignans	Flax, rye, some vegetables	May contribute to maintenance of heart health and healthy immune function
Soy Protein		
Soy protein[††]	Soybeans and soy-based foods	May reduce risk of CHD
Sulfides/Thiols		
Diallyl sulfide, allyl methyl trisulfide	Garlic, onions, leeks, scallions	May enhance detoxification of undesirable compounds; may contribute to maintenance of heart health and healthy immune function
Dithiolthiones	Cruciferous vegetables	May enhance detoxification of undesirable compounds; may contribute to maintenance of healthy immune function

*Examples are not an all-inclusive list. [††]FDA-approved health claim established for component.

SOURCE: International Food Information Council. (2009). Foundation Functional Foods Backgrounder. Online: http://www.ific.org/nutrition/functional/index.cfm.

Planning a Nutritious Diet

One of the most important features of a nutritious diet is to obtain all required nutrients through a reasonable calorie or energy intake approach. In other words, you should not only nourish your body with the proper amounts of nutrients, but also understand that how much you eat contributes to your weight, which plays a major role in your long-term health. Basically, you must meet your nutrient requirements within the constraints of your energy demands. Nutrient–calorie benefit ratio, or nutrient density, is a simple way to connect nutrients with calories.

Nutrient Density and Why It Is Important

The American diet is said to be increasingly energy rich but nutrient poor. To help improve the nutrient-to-energy ratio, the 2010 *Dietary Guidelines for Americans* recommends that consumers replace some foods in their diets with more nutrient-dense options. **Nutrient-dense foods** are those foods and beverages that provide substantial amounts of vitamins, minerals, and other substances that provide many positive health effects with relatively few calories. In essence, a food with a high nutrient density possesses a significant amount of a specific nutrient or nutrients per serving compared with its calorie content. For example, a candy bar contains many calories in the form of added simple sugars but has few vitamins and minerals, so it has a low nutrient density. A serving of soybeans, on the other hand,

Nutrient-dense foods Foods and beverages that provide substantial amounts of vitamins, nutrients, and other substances that have many positive health effects with relatively few calories.

has a moderate amount of calories but is rich in high-quality protein, healthy fats, complex carbohydrates, vitamins and minerals, and sterols (a functional food component), and therefore has a high nutrient density.

Nutrient-rich, low-calorie foods can enhance your wellness and support healthy, long-term weight management, whereas nutrient-poor, high-calorie foods—sometimes called empty calorie foods—do not. The greater the consumption of foods or beverages that are low in nutrient density or provide empty calories, the more difficult it is to consume enough nutrients without gaining weight, especially for sedentary individuals. The consumption of added sugars, saturated and trans fats, and alcohol provides calories while providing little, if any, of the essential nutrients.

Dietary Reference Intakes

Ever wonder how much of the nutrients listed in Table 7.2 you really need to eat every day to be healthy? The first set of recommendations, Recommended Dietary Allowances (RDAs), was published by the Institute of Medicine's Food and Nutrition Board of the National Academy of Sciences in 1941 and revised periodically over the years. The RDAs were originally designed to prevent nutritional deficiencies in large groups of people such as the armed forces and children in school lunch programs. From a statistical standpoint, this means that the RDAs were set to prevent nutritional deficiencies in 97 percent of the population. In other words, the RDAs are intentionally set somewhat higher than the body's actual physiological needs.

Times have changed. In 1993, the Food and Nutrition Board (FNB), working with Health Canada, began a major overhaul of the RDAs that continues today. With increased understanding of the relationship between nutrition and chronic diseases, the FNB is redefining nutrient requirements and developing new RDAs based on three overriding principles. The first two principles supporting the current revision are: (1) incorporating the concept of risk reduction for chronic diseases, not just prevention of nutrient deficiencies, and (2) recommending nutrient intakes that are thought to help people achieve good health by providing multiple reference points for nutrient intake instead of one number for each nutrient. The reference points are collectively referred to as the **Dietary Reference Intakes (DRIs)**. DRI serves as an umbrella term that includes the following values.

Dietary Reference Intakes (DRIs) Umbrella term that includes Estimated Average Requirement, Recommended Dietary Allowance, Adequate Intake, and Tolerable Upper Intake Level.

ESTIMATED AVERAGE REQUIREMENT (EAR)   The Estimated Average Requirement (EAR) is estimated to meet the requirement of half the healthy individuals for a specific age–gender group. For example, the iron EAR for women of childbearing age will likely be different than that for adult males. The EAR is used to assess nutritional adequacy of intakes of population groups. In addition, EARs are used to calculate RDAs.

RECOMMENDED DIETARY ALLOWANCE (RDA)   The Recommended Dietary Allowance (RDA) is a goal for individuals and is based on the EAR. Unlike earlier RDAs, these are designed to *reduce disease risk*, not just prevent deficiency. It is the daily dietary intake level that is sufficient to meet the requirements of 97 percent of all healthy individuals in a group and is meant for use by individuals. If an EAR cannot be set, no RDA value can be proposed.

ADEQUATE INTAKE (AI)   Adequate Intake (AI) is used when an RDA cannot be determined. In other words, scientific data are not strong enough to come up with a final number, yet there is enough evidence to give a general guideline. Like the RDA, individuals can use this number to set their personal dietary goals.

TOLERABLE UPPER INTAKE LEVEL (UL) The Tolerable Upper Intake Level (UL) is the highest level of daily nutrient intake that is likely to pose no risks of adverse health effects to almost all individuals in the general population. Anything above the UL might result in toxic reactions. The higher the intake, the higher the risk.

The third principle behind the nutrient revisions is that both essential nutrients and food components—deemed valuable even if not essential nutrients—will be considered. This principle allows the Food and Nutrition Board to consider components such as fiber and carotenoids.

The *Dietary Guidelines for Americans* provides general recommendations that focus attention on the association between diet and chronic diseases.

Dietary Guidelines for Americans

In recognition of the role that dietary factors play in promoting health and causing many major chronic diseases, the U.S. Departments of Agriculture (USDA) and Health and Human Services (USDHHS) periodically issue the *Dietary Guidelines for Americans*. The recommendations contained within the *Dietary Guidelines* provide authoritative advice for people 2 years and older about how proper dietary habits can promote health and reduce risk for major chronic diseases (USDHHS & USDA, 2010). The *Dietary Guidelines*, first published in 1980, are reviewed every 5 years by a committee of nutrition and health scientists who recommend changes based on current knowledge of the influence of diet on health and disease. The seventh edition of the *Dietary Guidelines*, published in 2010, includes 23 key recommendations for all Americans, and 6 additional recommendations for specific population groups. The four interrelated themes and the key recommendations from the 2010 *Dietary Guidelines* report are as follows (USDA, 2012):

1. **Balancing Calories to Manage Weight**
- Prevent and/or reduce overweight and obesity through improved eating and physical activity behaviors.
- Control total calorie intake to manage body weight. For people who are overweight or obese, this will mean consuming fewer calories from foods and beverages.
- Increase physical activity and reduce time spent in sedentary behaviors.
- Maintain appropriate calorie balance during each stage of life–childhood, adolescence, adulthood, pregnancy and breastfeeding, and older age.

2. **Reduce the Following Foods and Food Components**
- Reduce daily sodium intake to less than 2300 milligrams (mg) and further reduce intake to 1500 mg among persons who are 51 and older and those of any age who are African American or have hypertension, diabetes, or chronic kidney disease. The 1500 mg recommendation applies to about half of the U.S. population, including children and the majority of adults.
- Consume less than 10 percent of calories from saturated fatty acids by replacing them with monounsaturated and polyunsaturated fatty acids.
- Consume less than 300 mg per day of dietary cholesterol.
- Keep trans fatty acid consumption as low as possible by limiting foods that contain synthetic sources of trans fats, such as partially hydrogenated oils, and by limiting other solid fats.
- Reduce the intake of calories from solid fats and added sugars.
- Limit the consumption of foods that contain refined grains, especially refined grain foods that contain solid fats, added sugars, and sodium.
- If alcohol is consumed, it should be consumed in moderation—up to one drink per day for women and two drinks per day for men—and only by adults of legal drinking age.

3. Increase Intake of the Following Foods and Nutrients

Individuals should meet the following recommendations as part of a healthy eating pattern and while staying within their calorie needs:

- Increase vegetable and fruit intake.
- Eat a variety of vegetables, especially dark-green and red and orange vegetables and beans and peas.
- Consume at least half of all grains as whole grains. Increase whole-grain intake by replacing refined grains with whole grains.
- Increase intake of fat-free or low-fat milk and milk products, such as milk, yogurt, cheese, or fortified soy beverages.
- Choose a variety of protein foods, which include seafood, lean meat and poultry, eggs, beans and peas, soy products, and unsalted nuts and seeds.
- Increase the amount and variety of seafood consumed by choosing seafood in place of some meat and poultry.
- Replace protein foods that are higher in solid fats with choices that are lower in solid fats and calories and/or are sources of oils.
- Use oils to replace solid fats where possible.
- Choose foods that provide more potassium, dietary fiber, calcium, and vitamin D, which are nutrients of concern in American diets. These foods include vegetables, fruits, whole grains, and milk and milk products.

Recommendations for specific population groups:

- *Women capable of becoming pregnant*
  a. Choose foods that supply heme iron, which is more readily absorbed by the body; additional iron sources; and enhancers of iron absorption such as vitamin C–rich foods.
  b. Consume 400 micrograms (mcg) per day of synthetic folic acid (from fortified foods and/or supplements) in addition to food forms of folate from a varied diet.
- *Women who are pregnant or breastfeeding*
  a. Consume 8 to 12 ounces of seafood per week from a variety of seafood types.
  b. Due to their methyl mercury content, limit white (albacore) tuna to 6 ounces per week and do not eat the following four types of fish: tilefish, shark, swordfish, and king mackerel.
  c. If pregnant, take an iron supplement as recommended by an obstetrician or other health care provider.
- *Individuals age 50 years or older*
  a. Consume foods fortified with vitamin B_{12}, such as fortified cereals, or dietary supplements.

4. Build Healthy Eating Patterns

- Select an eating pattern that meets nutrient needs over time at an appropriate calorie level.
- Account for all foods and beverages consumed and assess how they fit within a total healthy eating pattern.
- Follow food safety recommendations when preparing and eating foods to reduce the risk of foodborne illnesses.

In summary, the *Dietary Guidelines* are designed to help Americans choose diets that will meet nutritional requirements, promote health, support active lives, and reduce chronic disease risks. To obtain the most benefit, individuals should carry out the *Dietary Guidelines* recommendations in their totality as part of an overall healthy eating pattern. The MyPlate food guidance system can be used to further plan your daily food intake by practically applying the information in the *Dietary Guidelines*.

The MyPlate food guidance system provides information to help implement the recommendations of the *Dietary Guidelines* and make better food choices.

The MyPlate Food Guidance System

The MyPlate food guidance system provides information to help implement the recommendations of the *Dietary Guidelines* and make better food choices. The MyPlate icon illustrates the five food groups that are the building blocks for a healthy diet using a familiar image, a place setting for a meal (refer to Figure 7.9). The icon is a plate split into four sections, each representing a different type of food (protein, whole grains, fruits, and vegetables). The sections vary in size depending on the recommended portion of each food a person should eat. The MyPlate graphic shows that half of your plate should be fruits and vegetables; less than one-quarter should be protein foods, such as meat, beans, or eggs; and more than one-quarter of your plate should be grain products. A circle shape next to the plate represents dairy products, especially milk. Visiting MyPlate.gov online allows consumers to learn more about each food group and examples of healthy food choices. The key messages and concepts in each food category from MyPlate.gov are described in the following paragraphs (USDA, 2012).

VEGETABLES   The key message in the vegetable group is "vary your veggies." Any vegetable or 100% vegetable juice counts as a member of the vegetable group. Vegetables may be raw or cooked; fresh, frozen, canned, or dried/dehydrated; and may be whole, cut up, or mashed. The vegetables are organized into five subgroups based on their nutrient content: dark green, starchy, red and orange, beans and peas, and other vegetables, based on their nutrient content TABLE 7.6 .

FRUITS   The key message in the fruit group is to "focus on fruits." Any fruit or 100% fruit juice counts as part of the fruit group. Fruits may be fresh, canned, frozen, or dried, and may be whole, cut up, or pureed. Commonly eaten fruits are provided in Table 7.6.

GRAINS   The key message in the grain group is to "make half your grains whole." Any food made from wheat, rice, oats, cornmeal, barley, or another cereal grain is a grain product. Bread, pasta, oatmeal, breakfast cereals, tortillas, and grits are examples of grain products. Grains are divided into two subgroups, whole grains and refined grains. Whole grains contain the entire grain kernel—the bran, germ, and endosperm. Examples include whole-wheat flour, bulgur (cracked wheat), oatmeal, whole cornmeal, and brown rice. Consumers can check the food label for the words "whole" or "whole grain" before the grain ingredient.

Refined grains have been milled, a process that removes the bran and germ. This is done to give grains a finer texture and improve their shelf life, but it also removes dietary fiber, iron, and many B vitamins. Examples of refined grain products are white flour, de-germed cornmeal, white bread, and white rice. Most refined grains are *enriched*. This means certain B vitamins (thiamin, riboflavin, niacin, folic acid) and iron are added back after processing. Fiber is not added back to enriched grains. Check the ingredient list on refined grain products to make sure that the word "enriched" is included in the grain name. Some food products are made from mixtures of whole grains and refined grains. Commonly eaten grain products are provided in Table 7.6.

DAIRY   The key message in the dairy group is to "get your calcium-rich foods." All fluid milk products and many foods made from milk are considered part of this food group. Most dairy group choices should be fat-free or low-fat. Foods made

| TABLE 7.6 | **Commonly Eaten Food from the Food Groups** |

Grain Products

Whole Grains

- Amaranth
- Brown rice
- Buckwheat
- Bulgur (cracked wheat)
- Millet
- Oatmeal
- Popcorn
- Rolled oats
- Quinoa
- Sorghum
- Triticale
- Whole grain barley
- Whole grain cornmeal
- Whole rye
- Whole wheat bread
- Whole wheat crackers
- Whole wheat pasta
- Whole wheat sandwich buns and rolls
- Whole wheat tortillas
- Wild rice

Ready-to-eat breakfast cereals:

- Whole wheat cereal flakes
- Muesli

Refined Grains

- Cornbread
- Corn tortillas
- Couscous
- Crackers
- Flour tortillas
- Grits
- Noodles
- Pitas
- Pretzels
- White bread
- White sandwich buns and rolls
- White rice

Pastas

- Spaghetti
- Macaroni

Ready-to-eat breakfast cereals:

- Corn flakes

Vegetables

Dark Green Vegetables

- Bok choy
- Broccoli
- Collard greens
- Dark green leafy lettuce
- Kale
- Mesclun
- Mustard greens
- Romaine lettuce
- Spinach
- Turnip greens
- Watercress

Starchy Vegetables

- Cassava
- Corn
- Fresh cowpeas, field peas, or black-eyed peas (not dry)
- Green bananas
- Green lima beans
- Green peas
- Plantains
- Potatoes
- Taro
- Water chestnuts

Red and Orange Vegetables

- Acorn squash
- Butternut squash
- Carrots
- Hubbard squash
- Pumpkin
- Red peppers
- Sweet potatoes
- Tomatoes
- Tomato juice

Beans and Peas

- Black beans
- Black-eyed peas (mature, dry)
- Garbanzo beans (chickpeas)
- Kidney beans
- Lentils
- Navy beans
- Pinto beans
- Soy beans
- Split peas
- White beans

Other Vegetables

- Artichokes
- Asparagus
- Avocado
- Bean sprouts
- Beets
- Brussels sprouts
- Cabbage
- Cauliflower
- Celery
- Cucumbers
- Eggplant
- Green beans
- Green peppers
- Iceberg (head) lettuce
- Mushrooms
- Okra
- Onions
- Parsnips
- Turnips
- Wax beans
- Zucchini

(continues)

TABLE 7.6	Commonly Eaten Food from the Food Groups *(Continued)*

Fruits

- Apples
- Apricots
- Bananas
- Grapefruit
- Grapes
- Kiwi fruit
- Lemons
- Limes
- Mangoes
- Nectarines
- Oranges
- Papaya
- Peaches
- Pears
- Pineapple
- Plums
- Prunes
- Raisins
- Tangerines

Berries

- Blueberries
- Cherries
- Raspberries
- Strawberries

Melons

- Cantaloupe
- Honeydew
- Watermelon

Mixed Fruits

- Fruit cocktail

100% Fruit Juice

- Apple
- Grape
- Grapefruit
- Orange

Protein Foods

Meats
Lean cut of

- Beef
- Ham
- Lamb
- Pork
- Veal

Game Meats

- Bison
- Rabbit
- Venison

Lean Ground Meats

- Beef
- Lamb
- Pork

Organ Meats

- Giblets
- Liver

Nuts and Seeds

- Almonds
- Cashews
- Hazelnuts (filberts)
- Mixed nuts
- Peanuts
- Peanut butter
- Pecans
- Pistachios
- Pumpkin seeds
- Sesame seeds
- Sunflower seeds
- Walnuts

Processed Soy Products

- Tempeh
- Texturized vegetable protein
- Tofu (bean curd made from soy beans)
- Veggie burgers

Seafood
Finfish such as:

- Catfish
- Cod
- Flounder
- Haddock
- Halibut
- Herring
- Mackerel
- Pollock

Shellfish such as:

- Clams
- Crab
- Crayfish
- Lobster
- Mussels
- Octopus
- Oyters
- Scallops
- Shrimp
- Squid (calamari)

Canned fish such as:

- Anchovies
- Clams
- Tuna
- Sardines

Poultry

- Chicken
- Duck
- Goose
- Ground chicken and turkey
- Turkey

Eggs

- Chicken eggs
- Duck eggs

TABLE 7.6	Commonly Eaten Food from the Food Groups *(Continued)*

Daily Products

Milk

All fluid milk:
- Fat-free (skim)
- Low fat (1%)
- Reduced fat (2%)
- Whole milk
- Chocolate (flavored)
- Strawberry (flavored)
- Lactose-reduced milks
- Lactose-free milks

Milk-based Desserts
- Frozen yogurt
- Ice cream
- Ice milk
- Puddings

Calcium-fortified soymilk (soy beverage)

Cheese

(hard natural cheese)
- Cheddar
- Mozzarella
- Parmesan
- Swiss

(soft cheese)
- Cottage cheese
- Ricotta

(processed cheese)
- American

Yogurt
- Fat-free
- Low fat
- Reduced fat
- Whole milk

Commonly Eaten Oils

- Canola
- Corn
- Cottonseed
- Olive
- Safflower
- Soybean
- Sunflower

Some oils are used mainly as flavorings, such as walnut oil and sesame oil. A number of foods are naturally high in oils like:
- Nuts
- Olives
- Some fish
- Avocados

SOURCE: Modified from ChooseMyPlate.gov. Food Groups Overview. Online: http://www.choosemyplate.gov/food-groups.

from milk that retain their calcium content are part of the group. Foods made from milk that have little to no calcium, such as cream cheese, cream, and butter, are not. Calcium-fortified soymilk (soy beverage) also is part of the dairy group. Commonly eaten dairy products are provided in Table 7.6.

Choose fat-free or low-fat milk, yogurt, and cheese. If you choose milk or yogurt that is not fat-free, or cheese that is not low-fat, the fat in the product counts against your maximum limit for "empty calories" (calories from solid fats and added sugars). If sweetened milk products are chosen (flavored milk, yogurt, drinkable yogurt, desserts), the added sugars also count against your maximum limit for empty calories. Finally, for those who are lactose intolerant, smaller portions (such as 4 fluid ounces of milk) may be well tolerated. Lactose-free and lower-lactose products are available. These include lactose-reduced or lactose-free milk, yogurt, and cheese, and calcium-fortified soymilk (soy beverage). Also, enzyme preparations can be added to milk to lower the lactose content. Calcium-fortified foods and beverages such as cereals, orange juice, or rice or almond beverages may provide calcium, but may not provide the other nutrients found in dairy products.

PROTEIN   The key message in the protein group is to "go lean with protein." All foods made from meat, poultry, seafood, beans and peas, eggs, processed soy products, nuts, and seeds are considered part of the protein foods group. Beans and peas are also part of the vegetable group. Select a variety of protein foods to improve nutrient intake and health benefits, including at least 8 ounces of cooked seafood per week. Young children need less, depending on their age and calorie needs. The advice to consume seafood does not apply to vegetarians. Vegetarian options in the protein foods group include beans and peas, processed soy products, and nuts and seeds. Meat and poultry choices should be lean or low-fat. Commonly eaten protein products are provided in Table 7.6.

A related topic at MyPlate.gov is empty calories. Currently, many of the foods and beverages Americans eat and drink contain **empty calories**—calories from solid fats and/or added sugars. Solid fats and added sugars add calories to the food but few or no nutrients. For this reason, the calories from solid fats and added sugars in a food are often called empty calories. Learning more about solid fats and added sugars can help you make better food and drink choices. **Solid fats** are fats that are solid at room temperature, like butter, beef fat, and shortening. Some solid fats are found naturally in foods. They can also be added when foods are processed by food companies or when they are prepared. **Added sugars** are sugars and syrups that are added when foods or beverages are processed or prepared. Solid fats and added sugars can make a food or beverage more appealing, but they also can add a lot of calories. The foods and beverages that provide the most empty calories for Americans are:

- Cakes, cookies, pastries, and donuts (contain both solid fat and added sugars)
- Sodas, energy drinks, sports drinks, and fruit drinks (contain added sugars)
- Cheese (contains solid fat)
- Pizza (contains solid fat)
- Ice cream (contains both solid fat and added sugars)
- Sausages, hot dogs, bacon, and ribs (contain solid fat)

A small amount of empty calories is okay, but most people eat far more than is healthy. It is important to limit empty calories to the amount that fits your calorie and nutrient needs. You can lower your intake by eating and drinking foods and beverages containing empty calories *less often* or by decreasing the *amount* you eat or drink.

Your Personal Nutrition Plan

To personalize a nutrition plan, you can go to www.ChooseMyPlate.gov to obtain information that is specific to what and how much to eat within your calorie allowance based on your physical activity level. Select Daily Food Plans from the menu. You will be asked to enter your age, sex, weight, height, and the amount of moderate or vigorous activity (such as brisk walking, jogging, biking, aerobics, or yard work) you do in addition to your normal daily routine, on most days of the week. For example, a 20-year-old female who is 5 feet 6 inches and weighs 125 pounds and jogs between 30 and 40 minutes on most days of the week would enter her age, sex, height, weight, and the 30- to 60-minute level of daily physical activity into the online Daily Food Plan program. The Daily Food Plan program will then calculate the recommended servings in each of the five major food groups and provide information on the amount of oils and discretionary calories per day based on these five characteristics. **FIGURE 7.11** shows the results of the calculations for this 20-year-old female jogger. Following the recommendations from these calculations will help this woman maintain a healthy weight and meet nutrient requirements. If this jogger decides to increase her physical activity level to 60 minutes or more daily, she would need to enter the new information using the 60-minute or more physical activity level. A new calorie amount and recommended servings would be calculated. This individualization is helpful because not all individuals of the same age, sex, height, and weight have the same physical activity level and energy needs.

Empty calories Measurement of the digestible energy present in high-energy foods with poor nutritional profiles, with most of the energy typically coming from processed carbohydrates, fats, or alcohol.

Solid fats Fats that are solid at room temperature, like beef fat, butter, and shortening.

Added sugars Sugars and syrups added when foods or beverages are processed or prepared.

My Daily Food Plan

Based on the information you provided, this is your daily recommended amount for each food group.

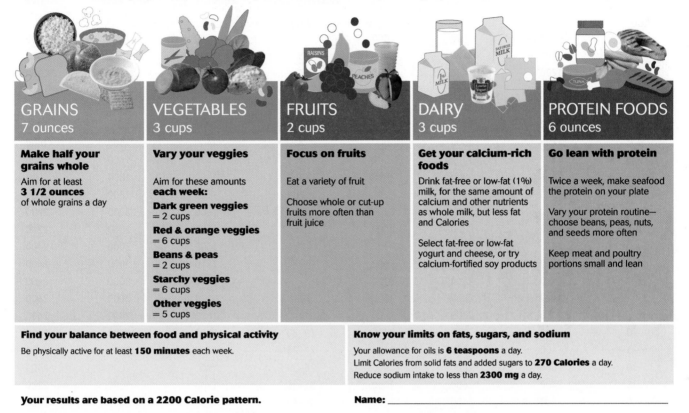

GRAINS 7 ounces	VEGETABLES 3 cups	FRUITS 2 cups	DAIRY 3 cups	PROTEIN FOODS 6 ounces
Make half your grains whole Aim for at least **3 1/2 ounces** of whole grains a day	**Vary your veggies** Aim for these amounts **each week:** **Dark green veggies** = 2 cups **Red & orange veggies** = 6 cups **Beans & peas** = 2 cups **Starchy veggies** = 6 cups **Other veggies** = 5 cups	**Focus on fruits** Eat a variety of fruit Choose whole or cut-up fruits more often than fruit juice	**Get your calcium-rich foods** Drink fat-free or low-fat (1%) milk, for the same amount of calcium and other nutrients as whole milk, but less fat and Calories Select fat-free or low-fat yogurt and cheese, or try calcium-fortified soy products	**Go lean with protein** Twice a week, make seafood the protein on your plate Vary your protein routine— choose beans, peas, nuts, and seeds more often Keep meat and poultry portions small and lean

Find your balance between food and physical activity Be physically active for at least **150 minutes** each week.	**Know your limits on fats, sugars, and sodium** Your allowance for oils is **6 teaspoons** a day. Limit Calories from solid fats and added sugars to **270 Calories** a day. Reduce sodium intake to less than **2300 mg** a day.

Your results are based on a 2200 Calorie pattern.   **Name:** _____

This Calorie level is only an estimate of your needs. Monitor your body weight to see if you need to adjust your Calorie intake.

FIGURE 7.11 Personalized MyPlate Plan. This plan is personalized for a 20-year female who is 5 feet 6 inches and weighs 125 pounds and jogs between 30 and 60 minutes on most days of the week. SOURCE: Reproduced from U.S. Department of Agriculture. Online: www.ChooseMyPlate.gov.

TABLE 7.7 provides the individual differences the MyPlate food guidance system uses to calculate calorie needs based on age, sex, and physical activity level. It is flexible enough to help you make simple, small improvements in your food and lifestyle decisions and to match these steps with your own calorie needs, lifestyle, and food preferences. The suggested amounts of food from the basic food groups to meet the recommended nutrient intakes at 12 different calorie levels are shown in TABLE 7.8.

The MyPlate food guidance system provides a wealth of information for you to apply in developing your nutritious eating and physical activity lifestyle. In summary, MyPlate provides detailed guidelines for improving overall health through proper nutrition and physical activity.

Food Labeling

As a health-conscious consumer, you know how important it is to choose foods that offer high nutritional value. But how can you be sure you are making the wisest selections of foods as you roll your grocery cart down the supermarket aisles? Considering that the average supermarket stocks over 40,000 different products

TABLE 7.7	MyPlate Food Intake Pattern Calorie Levels

		Males				Females		
Activity Level	Sedentary*	Mod. Active*	Active*	**Activity Level**	Sedentary*	Mod. Active*	Active*
Age				**Age**			
2	1000	1000	1000	2	1000	1000	1000
3	1000	1400	1400	3	1000	1200	1400
4	1200	1400	1600	4	1200	1400	1400
5	1200	1400	1600	5	1200	1400	1600
6	1400	1600	1800	6	1200	1400	1600
7	1400	1600	1800	7	1200	1600	1800
8	1400	1600	2000	8	1400	1600	1800
9	1600	1800	2000	9	1400	1600	1800
10	1600	1800	2200	10	1400	1800	2000
11	1800	2000	2200	11	1600	1800	2000
12	1800	2200	2400	12	1600	2000	2200
13	2000	2200	2600	13	1600	2000	2200
14	2000	2400	2800	14	1800	2000	2400
15	2200	2600	3000	15	1800	2000	2400
16	2400	2800	3200	16	1800	2000	2400
17	2400	2800	3200	17	1800	2000	2400
18	2400	2800	3200	18	1800	2000	2400
19–20	2600	2800	3000	19–20	2000	2200	2400
21–25	2400	2800	3000	21–25	2000	2200	2400
26–30	2400	2600	3000	26–30	1800	2000	2400
31–35	2400	2600	3000	31–35	1800	2000	2200
36–40	2400	2600	2800	36–40	1800	2000	2200
41–45	2200	2600	2800	41–45	1800	2000	2200
46–50	2200	2400	2800	46–50	1800	2000	2200
51–55	2200	2400	2800	51–55	1600	1800	2200
56–60	2200	2400	2600	56–60	1600	1800	2200
61–65	2000	2400	2600	61–65	1600	1800	2000
66–70	2000	2200	2600	66–70	1600	1800	2000
71–75	2000	2200	2600	71–75	1600	1800	2000
76 and up	2000	2200	2400	76 and up	1600	1800	2000

*Calorie levels are based on the Estimated Energy Requirements (EER) and activity levels from the Institute of Medicine Dietary Reference Intakes Macronutrients Report, 2002.

Sedentary = less than 30 minutes a day of moderate physical activity in addition to daily activities.

Mod. active = at least 30 minutes up to 60 minutes a day of moderate physical activity in addition to daily activities.

Active = 60 or more minutes a day of moderate physical activity in addition to daily activities.

SOURCE: Reproduced from U.S. Department of Agriculture, Center for Nutrition Policy and Promotion. (2012). MyPlate food intake pattern calorie levels. Online: http://www.choosemyplate.gov.

TABLE 7.8	MyPlate Food Intake Patterns											

Daily Amount of Food from Each Group

Calorie Level[1]	1000	1200	1400	1600	1800	2000	2200	2400	2600	2800	3000	3200
Fruits[2]	1 cup	1 cup	1.5 cups	1.5 cups	1.5 cups	2 cups	2 cups	2 cups	2 cups	2.5 cups	2.5 cups	2.5 cups
Vegetables[3]	1 cup	1.5 cups	1.5 cups	2 cups	2.5 cups	2.5 cups	3 cups	3 cups	3.5 cups	3.5 cups	4 cups	4 cups
Grains[4]	3 oz-eq	4 oz-eq	5 oz-eq	5 oz-eq	6 oz-eq	6 oz-eq	7 oz-eq	8 oz-eq	9 oz-eq	10 oz-eq	10 oz-eq	10 oz-eq
Protein foods[5]	2 oz-eq	3 oz-eq	4 oz-eq	5 oz-eq	5 oz-eq	5.5 oz-eq	6 oz-eq	6.5 oz-eq	6.5 oz-eq	7 oz-eq	7 oz-eq	7 oz-eq
Dairy[6]	2 cups	2 cups	2 cups	3 cups	3 cups	3 cups	3 cups	3 cups	3 cups	3 cups	3 cups	3 cups

[1]**Calorie Levels** are set across a wide range to accommodate the needs of different individuals. The table "Estimated Daily Calorie Needs" can be used to help assign individuals to the food intake pattern at a particular calorie level.

[2]**Fruit Group** includes all fresh, frozen, canned, and dried fruits and may be whole, cut-up, or pureed. Any 100% fruit juice created as a form of fruit. In general, 1 cup of fruit, or 100% fruit juice, or ½ cup of dried fruit can be considered as 1 cup from the fruit group.

[3]**Vegetable Group** includes all fresh, frozen, canned, and dried vegetables and vegetable juices. In general, 1 cup of raw or cooked vegetables or vegetable juice or 2 cups of raw leafy greens can be considered as 1 cup from the vegetable group.

[4]**Grains Group** includes all foods made from wheat, rice, oats, cornmeal, and barley, such as bread, pasta, oatmeal, breakfast cereals, tortillas, and grits. In general, 1 slice of bread, 1 cup of ready–to-eat cereal, or ½ cup of cooked rice, pasta, or cooked cereal can be considered as 1 ounce equivalent from the grains group. At least half of all grains consumed should be whole grains.

[5]**Protein Foods Group** in general, 1 ounce of lean meat, poultry, or fish, 1 egg, 1 tablespoon peanut butter, ¼ cup cooked dry beans, or ½ ounce of nuts or seeds can be considered as 1 ounce equivalent from the meat and beans group.

[6]**Dairy Group** includes all fluid milk products and foods made from milk that retain their calcium content, such as yogurt and cheese. Foods made from milk that have little to no calcium, such as cream cheese, cream, and butter, are not part of the group. Most dairy group choices should be fat-free or low-fat. In general, 1 cup of milk or yogurt, 1½ ounces of natural cheese, or 2 ounces of processed cheese can be considered as 1 cup from the dairy group.

Although MyPlate does not include "oils" group, some fat is essential for good health. Oils include fats from many different plants and from fish that are liquid at room temperature, such as canola, corn, olive, soybean, and sunflower oil. Some foods are naturally high in oils, like nuts, olives, some fish, and avocados. Foods that are mainly oil include mayonnaise, certain salad dressings, and soft margarine.

SOURCE: Reproduced from the U.S. Department of Agriculture, Center for Nutrition Policy and Promotion. (2011, April).

and that many food manufacturers use health advertising claims to get you to purchase their products, you have to make many decisions in a short shopping trip.

Fortunately for you, the U.S. government requires by law that all manufactured foods must be labeled with the name of the food, name and address of the manufacturer, and quantity of the contents. The food label must also include the Nutrition Facts label, sometime called the Nutrition Facts panel, and the list of ingredients. The food label also may include FDA-approved health claims or nutrient content claims. Each is discussed in the following sections.

NUTRITION FACTS LABEL   The Nutrition Facts label **FIGURE 7.12** is a simple, graphical nutrition tool that can serve as a key to planning a healthful diet. The label provides comprehensive information on the nutritional composition of food products that facilitates comparison of food products and assists in the selection of foods for a diet that will meet the *Dietary Guidelines for Americans*.

Most of the information needed to adhere to the MyPlate food guidance system is provided on the Nutrition Facts label. The following 15 nutrients must be listed: total calories, calories from fat, total fat, saturated fat, trans fat, cholesterol, sodium, total carbohydrate, dietary fiber, sugars, protein, vitamin A, vitamin C, calcium, and iron. The 15 mandatory nutrients were selected because they are most relevant to our national health problems. If optional nutrients are listed by the manufacturer to make a health claim—for example, naming other essential vitamins and minerals, or whether the food is fortified or enriched with any of them—nutrition figures for these optional nutrients become mandatory as well.

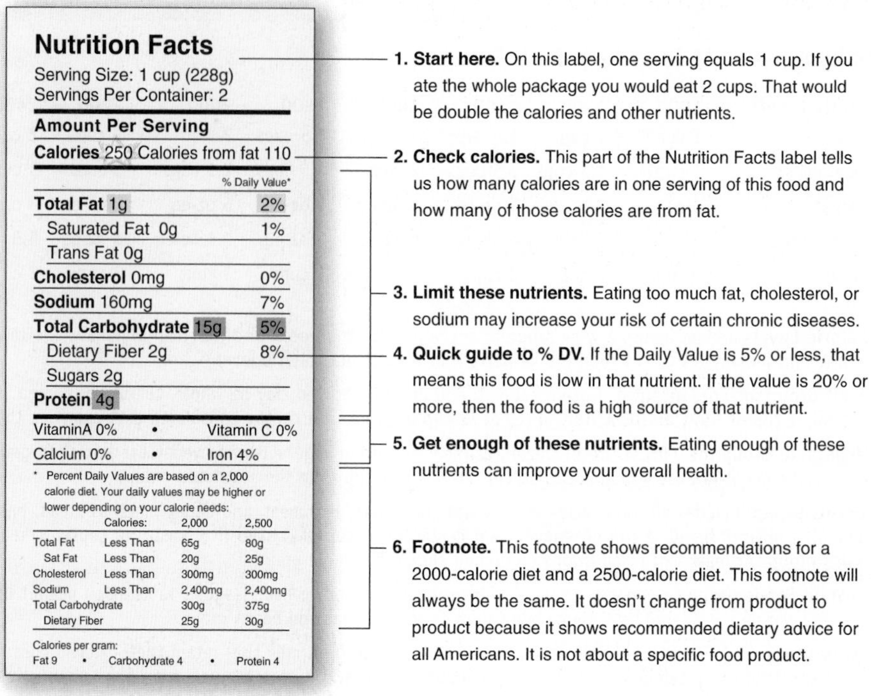

Nutrition Facts
Serving Size: 1 cup (228g)
Servings Per Container: 2

Amount Per Serving

Calories 250 Calories from fat 110

	% Daily Value*
Total Fat 1g	2%
Saturated Fat 0g	1%
Trans Fat 0g	
Cholesterol 0mg	0%
Sodium 160mg	7%
Total Carbohydrate 15g	5%
Dietary Fiber 2g	8%
Sugars 2g	
Protein 4g	

VitaminA 0%	•	Vitamin C 0%
Calcium 0%	•	Iron 4%

* Percent Daily Values are based on a 2,000 calorie diet. Your daily values may be higher or lower depending on your calorie needs:

	Calories:	2,000	2,500
Total Fat	Less Than	65g	80g
Sat Fat	Less Than	20g	25g
Cholesterol	Less Than	300mg	300mg
Sodium	Less Than	2,400mg	2,400mg
Total Carbohydrate		300g	375g
Dietary Fiber		25g	30g

Calories per gram:
Fat 9 • Carbohydrate 4 • Protein 4

1. **Start here.** On this label, one serving equals 1 cup. If you ate the whole package you would eat 2 cups. That would be double the calories and other nutrients.

2. **Check calories.** This part of the Nutrition Facts label tells us how many calories are in one serving of this food and how many of those calories are from fat.

3. **Limit these nutrients.** Eating too much fat, cholesterol, or sodium may increase your risk of certain chronic diseases.

4. **Quick guide to % DV.** If the Daily Value is 5% or less, that means this food is low in that nutrient. If the value is 20% or more, then the food is a high source of that nutrient.

5. **Get enough of these nutrients.** Eating enough of these nutrients can improve your overall health.

6. **Footnote.** This footnote shows recommendations for a 2000-calorie diet and a 2500-calorie diet. This footnote will always be the same. It doesn't change from product to product because it shows recommended dietary advice for all Americans. It is not about a specific food product.

FIGURE 7.12 **The Nutrition Facts Label.**

Another important way the Nutrition Facts label helps you meet the *Dietary Guidelines* is that the % daily value is given for each nutrient. The *% daily value* is a measure of the contribution of one serving of the food product to the recommended daily intake of the nutrient based on a daily intake of 2000 calories. This % daily value information permits comparison of food products without the need for calculations. Also, by scanning the % daily value column, you can see how a product's protein, carbohydrate, fiber, fat, and sodium fit within your total diet. Simple math calculations can help you keep track of how much of each of the various nutrients you have obtained for the day. All of this information can help you balance your food choices and develop improved eating habits.

INGREDIENT LIST   The ingredient list on food labels also provides very important information. The ingredients must be listed in order of their weight, with the ingredient present in the largest amount listed first. An ingredients list that contains "wheat flour, malted barley flour, and salt" informs you that wheat flour is proportionally the largest ingredient and that the second largest is barley flour. As a general rule of thumb, choose foods with as few ingredients as possible. If the list of ingredients is long, there are probably a lot of chemical additives in the product; if the list of ingredients is short, it may or may not have harmful additives in it, so read the ingredients carefully before you decide to purchase it.

The nutrition quality of a product can be evaluated by the presence of a specific ingredient as well as the order of the listed ingredients, which can help you identify "hidden" harmful ingredients, like added sugars, refined grains, and partially hydrogenated oils. For example, if you are choosing a breakfast cereal and the first ingredient is sugar, you may want to select another cereal. If you are looking for whole grains, which are healthier and are preferred to refined grains, it is important to remember that a food is not made with whole grains if it is labeled with the words multi-grain, 100% wheat, seven-grain, stone-ground, bran, or cracked wheat. Finally, partially hydrogenated oils are the primary source of trans fats, which have been shown to be potentially more harmful to arteries than saturated fat. Foods can call themselves "trans-fat free" even if they contain up to half a gram of trans fats per serving. Look on the ingredients list. If a food contains partially hydrogenated oils, it contains trans fats.

NUTRIENT CONTENT CLAIMS   Understanding the many nutrient content claims made by companies touting products that contain "low," "less," "free," or "reduced" ingredients can help you make informed decisions about what you purchase and put into your body. The FDA requires that a nutrient content claim on a food package be based on the amount of that food that most people usually eat or drink. This is called a reference amount. Usually the serving size and the reference amount are the same. This ensures that they mean the same thing on every product in which they appear, making it easier for you to compare similar products with the same nutrition claim. The FDA provides the types of descriptive words used to make health-related claims and their specific meanings that all food-manufacturing companies must adhere to TABLE 7.9 .

HEALTH CLAIMS ON FOOD PRODUCTS   The U.S. Food and Drug Administration (FDA) defines the health-related claims that manufacturers can use in labeling and advertising to help consumers identify foods that are rich in nutrients and that may help to prevent chronic disease conditions. Manufacturers are allowed to make health claims about certain nutrients that are found naturally in foods. Claims must be balanced and based on current, reliable scientific studies and must be approved by the FDA.

To date, the following health claims have been approved (FDA, 2011):

- *Calcium, vitamin D, and osteoporosis:* Adequate calcium and vitamin D along with regular exercise may reduce the risk of osteoporosis.
- *Dietary fat and cancer:* Low-fat diets may reduce the risk of some types of cancer.
- *Dietary fiber, such as that found in whole oats, barley, and psyllium seed husk, and coronary heart disease (CHD):* Diets low in fat and rich in these types of fiber can help reduce the risk of heart disease.
- *Dietary noncariogenic carbohydrate sweeteners and dental caries (tooth decay):* Foods sweetened with sugar alcohols do not promote tooth decay.
- *Dietary saturated fat, cholesterol, and trans fat and heart disease:* Diets low in saturated fat and cholesterol and as low as possible in trans fat may reduce the risk of heart disease.
- *Fiber-containing grain products, fruits, and vegetables and cancer:* Diets low in fat and rich in high-fiber foods may reduce the risk of certain cancers.
- *Fluoridated water and dental caries:* Drinking fluoridated water may reduce the risk of dental caries.
- *Folate and neural tube defects:* Adequate folate intake prior to and early in pregnancy may reduce the risk of neural tube defects (a birth defect).
- *Fruits and vegetables and cancer:* Diets low in fat and rich in fruits and vegetables may reduce the risk of certain cancers.
- *Fruits, vegetables, and grain products that contain fiber, particularly pectins, gums, and mucilages, and CHD:* Diets low in fat and rich in these types of fibers may reduce the risk of heart disease.
- *Plant sterol/stanol esters and CHD:* Diets low in saturated fat and cholesterol that contain significant amounts of these additives may reduce the risk of heart disease.
- *Potassium and high blood pressure/stroke:* Diets that contain good sources of potassium may reduce the risk of high blood pressure and stroke.

TABLE 7.9	Approved Nutrient Content Claims: What Words on Food Products Mean

Free   Food contains no amount (or trivial or "physiologically inconsequential" amounts). May be used with one or more of the following: fat, saturated fat, cholesterol, sodium, sugar, and calorie. Synonyms include *without, no,* and *zero.*

   Fat-free   Less than 0.5 mg of fat per serving.

   Saturated fat-free   Less than 0.5 mg of saturated fat per serving.

   Cholesterol-free   Less than 2 mg of cholesterol and 2 g or less of saturated fat and trans fat combined per serving.

   Sodium-free   Less than 5 mg of sodium per serving.

   Sugar-free   Less than 0.5 g of sugar per serving.

   Calorie-free   Fewer than 5 calories per serving.

Low   Food can be eaten frequently without exceeding dietary guidelines for one or more of these components: fat, saturated fat, cholesterol, sodium, and calories. Synonyms include *little, few,* and *low source of.*

   Low fat   3 g or less per serving.

   Low saturated fat   1 g or less of saturated fat; no more than 15% of calories from saturated fat and trans fat combined.

   Low cholesterol   20 mg or less and 2 g or less of saturated fat per serving.

   Low sodium   140 mg or less per serving.

   Low calorie   40 calories or less per serving.

High   Food contains 20% or more of the daily value for a particular nutrient in a serving.

Good source   Food contains 10% to 19% of the daily value for a particular nutrient in one serving.

Lean and extra lean   The fat content of meat and main dish products, seafood, and game products.

Lean   Less than 10 g fat, 4.5 g or less saturated fat, and less than 95 mg of cholesterol per serving and per 100 g.

Extra lean   Less than 5 g fat, less than 2 g saturated fat, and less than 95 mg of cholesterol per serving and per 100 g.

Reduced   Nutritionally altered product containing at least 25% less of a nutrient or of calories than the regular or reference product. (*Note:* A "reduced" claim can't be used if the reference product already meets the requirement for "low.")

Less   Food, whether altered or not, contains 25% less of a nutrient or of calories than the reference food. *Fewer* is an acceptable synonym.

Light   This descriptor can have two meanings:

1. A nutritionally altered product contains one-third fewer calories or half the fat of the reference food. If the reference food derives 50% or more of its calories from fat, the reduction must be 50% of the fat.

2. The sodium content of a low-calorie, low-fat food has been reduced by 50%. Also, *light in sodium* may be used on a food in which the sodium content has been reduced by at least 50%.

   Note: The term *light* can still be used to describe such properties as texture and color as long as the label explains its meaning (e.g., "light brown sugars" "light and fluffy").

More   A serving of food, whether altered or not, contains a nutrient that is at least 10% of the daily value more than the reference food. This also applies to fortified, enriched, and added claims, but in those cases, the food must be altered.

Healthy   A healthy food must be low in fat and saturated fat and contain limited amounts of cholesterol (less than 60 mg) and sodium (less than 360 mg for individual foods and less than 480 mg for meal-type products). In addition, a single-item food must provide at least 10% or more of one of the following: vitamins A or C, iron, calcium, protein, or fiber. A meal-type product, such as a frozen entrée or dinner, must provide 10% or two or more of these vitamins or minerals, or protein, or fiber, in addition to meeting the other criteria. Additional regulations allow the term *healthy* to be applied to raw, canned, or frozen fruits and vegetables and enriched grains even if the 10% nutrient content rule is not met. However, frozen or canned fruits or vegetables cannot contain ingredients that would change the nutrient profile.

Fresh   Food is raw, has never been frozen or heated, and contains no preservatives. *Fresh frozen, frozen fresh,* and *freshly frozen* can be used for foods that are quickly frozen while still fresh. Blanched foods also can be called fresh.

Percent fat-free   Food must be a low-fat or a fat-free product. In addition, the claim must reflect accurately the amount of nonfat ingredients in 100 g of food.

Implied claims   These are prohibited when they wrongfully imply that a food contains or does not contain a meaningful level of a nutrient. For example, a product cannot claim to be made with an ingredient known to be a source of fiber (such as "made with oat bran") unless the product contains enough of that ingredient (in this case, oat bran) to meet the definition for "good source" of fiber. As another example, a claim that a product contains "no tropical oils" is allowed, but only on foods that are "low" in saturated fat, because consumers have come to equate tropical oils with high levels of saturated fat.

SOURCE: U.S. Food and Drug Administration. (2011). Nutrient content claims. Online: http://www.fda.gov/Food/LabelingNutrition/LabelClaims/default.htm.

- *Sodium and hypertension (high blood pressure):* Low-sodium diets may help lower blood pressure.
- *Soy protein and CHD:* Foods rich in soy protein as part of a low-fat diet may help reduce the risk of heart disease.
- *Substitution of saturated fat with unsaturated fat and heart disease:* Replacing saturated fat with similar amounts of unsaturated fats may reduce the risk of heart disease.
- *Whole-grain foods and CHD or cancer:* Diets high in whole-grain foods and other plant foods and low in total fat, saturated fat, and cholesterol may help reduce the risk of heart disease and certain cancers.

A new health claim may be proposed at any time based on scientific evidence, and therefore this list may expand in the future.

SERVING SIZES   Knowing how much food is considered a serving is an important element of any nutrition plan. However, the serving size listed on the nutrition facts label may not be the same as the serving size for the food groups in MyPlate. The serving sizes on the food label and MyPlate serve different purposes. The serving size declared on the food label is to allow you to compare serving amounts from similar product categories. The serving sizes must be expressed in consumer-friendly units, such as ounces, cups, or gram weights. This means that all brands of tuna fish, for example, must use the same serving size (2 oz) on their labels. The serving sizes in the MyPlate system are specified for each food group, using simple, easy-to-remember household units that allow people to *estimate visually* the amount of food they are eating (TABLE 7.10). In most cases the serving sizes are similar on food labels and in the MyPlate system. It is important to remember that the "serving size" is a unit of measure and may not be the *portion* an individual actually eats.

If you are not accustomed to judging the amount, or portion, of food you eat, you will find it helpful to weigh and measure foods for a brief time, using a food scale or measuring spoons or cups. This will help you become familiar with visually estimating a recommended serving size. Using the same size and type of bowl, plate, or glass will assist even further in learning to eyeball approximate serving sizes.

Dietary Supplements

The best way to get the nutrients you need to promote health is through the food you eat, not any supplements you might take. Nutrients are generally absorbed better from food than from tablets or capsules. Additionally, foods contain an array of nutrients that facilitate each other's absorption, whereas individual supplements must go it alone. If you stick to a healthy diet (MyPlate and the *Dietary Guidelines*), you can obtain all the vitamins, minerals, fiber, calories, and other substances—presently known and yet to be discovered—that you need to maintain good health. However, if you do not consume a variety of foods as recommended by MyPlate and the *Dietary Guidelines*, some supplements may help ensure that you get the adequate amounts of essential nutrients you need.

For example, multiple vitamin-mineral supplements, sometimes known as multivitamin-mineral (MVM) supplements, contain a variable number of essential and nonessential nutrients. Their primary purpose is to provide a convenient way to take a variety of supplemental nutrients from a single product to prevent vitamin or mineral deficiencies as well as to achieve higher intakes of nutrients believed to be of benefit above typical dietary levels. Many MVMs contain at least 100 percent of the daily value or RDA of all vitamins and minerals that have been assigned RDAs. Taking one MVM daily can provide you with dietary insurance against any diet deficiencies and may help to protect against future disease.

TABLE 7.10 **Playing with MyPlate Portions**

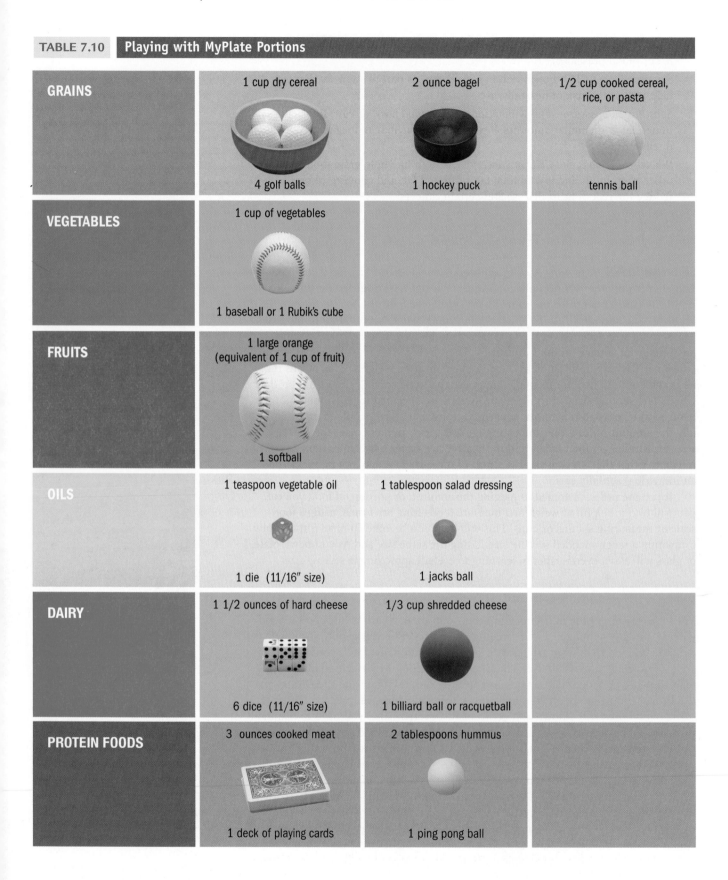

GRAINS	1 cup dry cereal 4 golf balls	2 ounce bagel 1 hockey puck	1/2 cup cooked cereal, rice, or pasta tennis ball
VEGETABLES	1 cup of vegetables 1 baseball or 1 Rubik's cube		
FRUITS	1 large orange (equivalent of 1 cup of fruit) 1 softball		
OILS	1 teaspoon vegetable oil 1 die (11/16″ size)	1 tablespoon salad dressing 1 jacks ball	
DAIRY	1 1/2 ounces of hard cheese 6 dice (11/16″ size)	1/3 cup shredded cheese 1 billiard ball or racquetball	
PROTEIN FOODS	3 ounces cooked meat 1 deck of playing cards	2 tablespoons hummus 1 ping pong ball	

However, you should always avoid megadoses (doses 10 times or more of the RDA) of vitamins and minerals.

Vegetarian Diets

Vegetarian diets depend largely or entirely on plant products and restrict intake of animal products. There is a variety of ways to be a vegetarian, ranging from being a strict vegetarian, eating no animal products of any kind, to being one who eats certain types of animal products.

Strict vegetarians are known as **vegans** because they eat no animal products. Most nutrients are obtained from breads, cereals, vegetables, fruits, legumes, seeds, and nuts. Less strict vegetarian diets include some foods derived from animals. **Ovovegetarians** include eggs (ovo) in their diet, and **lactovegetarians** include foods in the milk (lacto) group such as yogurt and cheese. An **ovolactovegetarian** eats both eggs and milk products. Finally, **semivegetarians** may eat fish and poultry, but do not eat red meat such as beef and pork.

The American Dietetic Association, in a position paper devoted to vegetarian diets, noted that such diets are healthful and nutritionally adequate, but deficiencies may occur if the diet is not planned appropriately (ADA, 2009b). If foods are not selected carefully, the vegetarian may suffer nutritional deficiencies involving calories, vitamins, minerals, and protein. Vegetarians can modify their consumption of foods according to the traditional vegetarian diet pyramid (**FIGURE 7.13**). The healthy vegetarian diet pyramid presents a helpful plan for people wishing to avoid meats. The recommended number of servings of grains, vegetables, fruits, and milk products is identical to the recommended amounts on MyPlate. The major difference is the exclusion of meat in favor of legumes, nuts, seeds, and eggs.

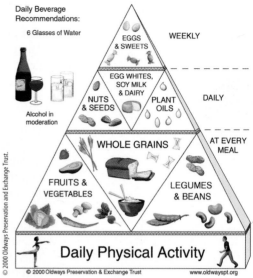

FIGURE 7.13 **The Traditional Healthy Vegetarian Diet Pyramid.** With careful planning, a diet that lacks animal products can be nutritionally complete.

Nutrition and Physical Activity

Good nutrition plays an important role in maximizing your capacity to maintain elevated levels of physical activity. In fact, most researchers feel that proper nutrition ranks right behind proper training principles and heredity in influencing exercise performance (Wilmore, Costill, & Kenney, 2008). This factor, however, may contribute to the widespread belief among those engaging in exercise that additional protein, vitamins, and minerals, sometimes in the form of energy bars or drinks, are necessary for optimal exercise performance. You will discover that the same diet principles that enhance health are advocated for exercise enthusiasts, along with a few commonsense guidelines for managing energy intake and fluid replacement. The following information will help you meet your nutrient needs when you participate in regular physical activity and is presented to dispel some myths related to exercise and food.

The ideal distribution of protein, carbohydrate, and fat for physically active individuals is comparable to the recommendations provided by the *Dietary Guidelines for Americans* and presented in MyPlate (refer to Figure 7.9). The main difference is in the quantity of calories consumed to produce the extra energy required by increased physical activity. As the amount of physical activity increases, so does the amount of energy required to maintain our energy reserves. Individuals who are highly active can expend high levels of daily energy, usually in a short period of time.

Similar to a healthy diet, a high-carbohydrate diet is probably the most important nutritional concern for regular exercisers. Carbohydrates are one of the main

The diet recommended for the person who participates in physical exercise differs little in nutrient composition from the diet advised for any healthy individual.

Vegan A strict vegetarian who eats no animal products.

Ovovegetarian A vegetarian who includes eggs in the diet.

Lactovegetarian A vegetarian who includes milk in the diet.

Ovolactovegetarian A vegetarian who eats both eggs and milk products.

Semivegetarian A vegetarian who may eat fish and poultry, but not eat red meat.

sources of energy for working muscles. Additionally, body carbohydrate stores (glycogen) are extremely important for maximizing the muscle glycogen stores that provide greater energy reserve for both aerobic and anaerobic activities. Therefore, heightened glycogen stores are important for increasing endurance and delay of fatigue. Because glycogen synthesis is directly related to dietary carbohydrate intake, it is recommended that 60 to 65 percent of the exerciser's total energy intake should come from carbohydrates.

Many exercisers, especially weight lifters and bodybuilders, feel that extra protein is needed to build muscle mass. Indeed, regular exercisers may require approximately 1.5 grams per kilogram of body weight compared to the Recommended Dietary Allowance of 0.8 gram per kilogram of body weight. This increased requirement is minor. More important to remember is that the body's protein need is driven more by body-tissue maintenance, repair, and growth (see protein section) than energy needs. During exercise there is relatively little protein loss through energy metabolism. In fact, the limiting factor in the use of protein for tissue growth and repair is energy intake, not protein intake. This means that you must first meet your energy requirements with an adequate intake of carbohydrates and then determine your protein requirements via the biologically driven protein-grams-per-kilogram ratio method. This has been referred to as the *protein-sparing* effect of protein.

Following the serving recommendations of the MyPlate system for dairy products and meat or meat substitutes will provide the necessary daily RDA protein requirements. Americans already eat more protein than they need and do not require protein supplements. Excess protein is used as energy and can be stored as body fat. Furthermore, too much protein can increase calcium loss (contributing to osteoporosis) and put an added burden on the kidneys and liver, which are required to filter out the nitrogen by-product (ketones) of the protein.

Probably the second most important dietary principle for regular exercisers is to consume the right amount of fluids before, during, and after exercise. Losing as little as 2 to 3 percent of body weight by dehydration can adversely affect exercise performance. Moreover, if exercisers are not careful about avoiding dehydration, they run the risk of heat exhaustion and even heat stroke. Water and fluids are essential to maintaining good hydration and body temperature.

Increased muscular activity from exercise leads to an increase in heat production in the body. The body's chief way to lose heat is evaporation from the skin. To keep the body cool, sweat losses can exceed a liter in a 1-hour period under normal conditions, and be even higher in extremely hot and humid conditions. Any lost body weight during exercise should be replaced with equal amounts of fluids immediately following the exercise. If exercise is longer than an hour or in extremely warm and humid conditions, or if body weight drops more than 3 percent, regular intervals of fluid replacements during exercise are imperative. Cool water (refrigerator cold) is the best choice. The addition of electrolytes (through "sport" drinks such as All Sport, Gatorade, and Powerade) is generally not justified. Sweat is about 99 percent water and only 1 percent electrolytes and other substances.

As you learned earlier, vitamins and minerals play an important role in the metabolism of carbohydrates, protein, and fats. Physical activity slightly increases the need for some vitamins and minerals (iron, calcium, and ascorbic acid, to name a few) because of the increased metabolism. However, these demands for vitamins and minerals can be easily met through the increased calories consumed from carbohydrate-rich foods. Remember, people who exercise are at an advantage because they need to eat more than sedentary people to account for their increased caloric expenditure, thereby providing their bodies with more vitamins and minerals. Vitamin and mineral supplements are generally not needed if you follow the MyPlate food guidance system.

Physical Activity and Health Connection

Sound nutritional advice for good health is also sound nutritional advice for physical activity. Although proper exercise and sound nutrition habits may confer health benefits separately, a reduction in risk factors can be maximized when both are part of a healthy lifestyle. A healthy diet may prevent disease in a variety of ways, but the health benefits multiply when healthful nutrition and proper exercise are combined. For example, dieting and aerobic exercise may combat obesity independently, but together sound eating practices and participation in a physical activity program are more effective.

Proper nutritional practices may complement physical activity as a means to enhance health status. Nutrition forms the foundation for physical activity; it provides both the fuel for mechanical work and the elements for extracting and using the potential energy contained within the fuel. Food also provides the essential elements for the synthesis of new tissue and the repair of existing cells. A nutrient-dense diet provides the minerals for strong bones and muscles. Adequate consumption of water helps keep you hydrated when you are active in warm climates. Expending energy through physical activity helps maintain healthy body composition. As you increase your level of physical activity, you will find that you are much more successful if you are also following sound nutritional practices.

concept connections

1. **Nutrition plays a major role in our overall health.** Today, scientific studies indicate that diet and nutrition often play a crucial role in the development and progression of chronic diseases that are the major killers of adults: cardiovascular disease, stroke, high blood pressure, diabetes, and some types of cancer. Obesity and osteoporosis also have been associated with faulty nutrition. Consequently, sensible lifelong eating habits play an important role in maintaining good health and preventing chronic disease.

2. **Nutrients provide energy, regulate body processes, and nourish tissues.** These major functions are essential for life.

3. **Food can be divided into six classes, and each class plays a different role.** Proteins, carbohydrates, and fats are macronutrients that provide the raw fuel for both biological and mechanical energy requirements. Vitamins, minerals, and water play crucial roles in regulating the body's processes related to activating energy release.

4. **The *Dietary Guidelines for Americans* provides general recommendations that focus attention on the association between diet and chronic diseases.** The recommendations contained within the *Dietary Guidelines* provide authoritative advice for people 2 years and older about how proper dietary habits can promote health and reduce risk for major chronic diseases. The *Dietary Guidelines*, first published in 1980, are reviewed every 5 years by a committee of nutrition and health scientists who recommend changes based on current knowledge of the influence of diet on health and disease. The seventh edition of the *Dietary Guidelines*, published in 2010, includes 23 key recommendations for all Americans, and 6 additional recommendations for specific population groups.

⑤ **The MyPlate food guidance system provides information to help implement the recommendations of the *Dietary Guidelines* and make better food choices.** The MyPlate icon illustrates the five food groups that are the building blocks for a healthy diet using a familiar image, a place setting for a meal (refer to Figure 7.9). The icon is a plate split into four sections, each representing a different type of food (protein, whole grains, fruits, and vegetables). The sections vary in size depending on the recommended portion of each food a person should eat. The MyPlate graphic shows that half of your plate should be fruits and vegetables; less than one-quarter should be protein foods, such as meat, beans, or eggs; and more than one-quarter of your plate should be grain products. A circle shape next to the plate represents dairy products, especially milk. Visiting MyPlate.gov allows consumers to learn more about each food group and examples of healthy food choices.

⑥ **The diet recommended for the person who participates in physical exercise differs little in nutrient composition from the diet advised for any healthy individual.** The most important dietary concerns for regular exercisers are meeting their increased caloric requirements with complex carbohydrates and drinking enough fluids before, during, and after exercise to ensure proper hydration.

Terms
. . . .

Acceptable Micronutrient Distribution Range (AMDR), 131
Added sugars, 152
Amino acid, 130
Anemia, 140
Calorie, 127
Carbohydrates, 132
Complex carbohydrates, 132
Dietary fiber, 134
Dietary Reference Intakes (DRIs), 145
Digestion, 127
Disaccharide, 132
Empty calories, 152
Essential amino acids, 130

Essential fatty acids, 136
Essential nutrients, 129
Fat-soluble vitamins, 138
Fats, 134
Functional foods, 142
Glycogen, 132
Insoluble fibers, 134
Lactovegetarian, 161
Macronutrients, 127
Major minerals, 139
Micronutrients, 129
Minerals, 139
Monosaccharide, 132
Nonessential nutrients, 129
Nutrients, 127
Nutrient-dense foods, 144

Ovolactovegetarian, 161
Ovovegetarian, 161
Phospholipids, 137
Protein, 130
Semivegetarian, 161
Simple carbohydrates, 132
Solid fats, 152
Soluble fibers, 134
Starches, 132
Trace minerals, 139
Trans fats, 136
Triglycerides, 134
Vegan, 161
Vitamins, 137
Water-soluble vitamins, 139

making the connection

Meeting with the nutritionist at the university health center, Mare learns that she is meeting all of her daily nutrient requirements for vitamins and minerals, including iron and calcium. Mare is relieved to discover that, by following the MyPlate food guidance system and its basic principles of variety, balance, and moderation, she is obtaining all the needed nutrient requirements to maintain her physically active lifestyle.

Critical Thinking

1. Like Mare, we sometimes rely on dietary supplements. What supplements are you currently taking or have you taken? For each supplement, list natural foods that you could have eaten that would have provided you the same nutritional value as the supplement.

2. Identify three barriers you face in trying to follow the *Dietary Guidelines for Americans*. For each barrier, identify a strategy and timeline to overcome each barrier.

3. You are 1 of 12 students at your university who is asked to assist the dietetics staff in developing healthy, nutritious, and appealing meals for college students. Using your nutrition knowledge, develop a well-balanced menu for breakfast, lunch, and dinner.

4. Go to a local health food store (these are often found in a shopping mall). Walk through the store, looking at the products and their health claims. Find two products, identify the claims made, and note any scientific research that supports the claim. Would you, based on the information provided, use this product? Why or why not?

References

American Dietetic Association. (2009a). Position of the American Dietetic Association, Dietitians of Canada, and the American College of Sports Medicine: Nutrition and athletic performance. *Journal of the American Dietetic Association* 109:509–527.

American Dietetic Association. (2009b). Position of the American Dietetic Association: Vegetarian diets. *Journal of the American Dietetic Association* 109:1266–1282.

Expert Panel on Detection, Evaluation, and Treatment of High Blood Cholesterol in Adults. (2001). Executive summary of the third report of the National Cholesterol Education Program (NCEP) Expert Panel on Detection, Evaluation, and Treatment of High Blood Cholesterol in Adults. *Journal of the American Medical Association* 285:2486–2497.

Food and Drug Administration. (2011). Summary of qualified health claims subject to enforcement discretion. Online: http://www.fda.gov/Food/LabelingNutrition/LabelClaims/QualifiedHealthClaims/ucm073992.htm.

Gillingham, L.G., Harris-Janz, S., & Jones, P.J. (2011). Dietary monounsaturated fatty acids are protective against metabolic syndrome and cardiovascular disease risk factors. *Lipids* 46(3):209–228.

Hunter, J.E., Zhang, J., & Kris-Etherton, P.M. (2010). Cardiovascular disease risk of dietary stearic acid compared with trans, other saturated, and unsaturated fatty acids: A systematic review. *American Journal of Clinical Nutrition* 9(1):46–63.

Institute of Medicine, Food and Nutrition Board. (2005). *Dietary Reference Intakes for Energy, Carbohydrate, Fiber, Fat, Fatty Acids, Cholesterol, Protein, and Amino Acids (Macronutrients)*. Washington, DC: National Academy Press.

Institute of Medicine, Food and Nutrition Board. (2004). *Dietary Reference Intakes for Water, Potassium, Chloride, and Sulfate*. Washington, DC: National Academy Press.

International Food Information Council Foundation. (2012). Functional foods. Online: http://www.foodinsight.org.

International Food Information Council Foundation. (2011). Food Science and Nutrition: A Journey Toward Health and Wellness. Online: http://www.foodinsight.org/Newsletter/Detail.aspx?topic=Food_Science_and_Nutrition_a_Journey_toward_Health_and_Wellness.

Johnson-Askew, W.L., Fisher, R.A., & Yaroch, A.L. (2009). Decision making in eating behavior: State of the science and recommendations for future research. *Annals of Behavioral Medicine* 38(Suppl. 1):s88–s92.

Park, Y., Subar, A.F., Hollenbeck, A., & Schatzkin, A. (2011). Dietary fiber intake and mortality in the NIH-AARP diet and health study. *Archives of Internal Medicine* 171(12):1061–1068.

U.S. Department of Agriculture. (2012). ChooseMyPlate. Online: http://choosemyplate.gov.

U.S. Department of Health and Human Services & U.S. Department of Agriculture. (2010). *Dietary Guidelines for Americans 2010*. Online: http://www.cnpp.usda.gov/dietaryguidelines.htm.

Wilmore, J., Costill, D., & Kenney, W. (2008). *Physiology of Sport and Exercise*, 4th ed. Champaign, IL: Human Kinetics.

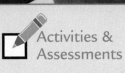
NOT LEGAL FOR TRADE

CAP-350 lb.   300   250   150   100   50   0

© Tim Ricks/age fotostock

Achieving and Maintaining a Healthy Weight

what's the connection?

Leah is a freshman in college; she is 5'6" tall and weighs about 130 pounds. Previously, when Leah was happy, she looked in the mirror and thought "Hey, I am not that bad!" However, if Leah was in a bad mood, she would think "I am so fat!" and get mad at herself. Recently, things are not going well in Leah's life and, when she looks in the mirror, she often sees herself as fat. It seems to her that the weight is piling on and she cannot stop it. To Leah, every part of her body looks bigger—her legs, her arms, her face—and she hates it. Leah thinks "I just want to be thin. I never really noticed how fat I was until yesterday when I looked in the mirror." Leah is not sure what to do. "I don't eat that much. Really I eat only a little, and I'm not sure why I even eat that." Leah is thinking about fasting as a means to deal with her image of being fat.

concepts

1. Achieving and maintaining a healthy body weight has long been identified as a major public health challenge in the United States, and remains one of the most challenging health crises the country has ever faced.

2. The body mass index (BMI) uses weight and height to produce a number that enables health professionals to gauge risk of weight-related illnesses.

3. Individuals with more abdominal body fat tend to have a more adverse metabolic profile and an increased risk for diabetes and cardiovascular disease.

4. A body composition analysis allows for the assessment of the percentage of fat tissue versus the percentage of fat-free tissue.

5. Obesity is a complex disorder with multiple contributing factors.

6. A lifestyle approach that includes regular physical activity and a nutritious diet is essential in achieving and maintaining a healthy weight.

7. A negative sign of dissatisfaction with body weight, when basing it on the "ideal" weight portrayed by the mass media, is the development of eating disorders.

To feel "fit as a fiddle," you must tone down your middle.
—Unknown

Introduction

Achieving and maintaining a healthy body weight has been identified as a major public health challenge in the United States.

Achieving and maintaining a healthy body weight has long been identified as a major public health challenge in the United States and remains one of most challenging health crises the country has ever faced. The U.S. prevalence data for overweight continues to be high, with two-thirds of adult Americans currently obese or overweight, double the rate from 30 years ago (Centers for Disease Control and Prevention [CDC], 2012c). Additionally, one-third of children and teenagers are currently obese or overweight, triple the rate from 30 years ago (CDC, 2012c). These enduring high prevalence rates raise fear because of their implications for Americans' health, putting obese and overweight individuals at increased risk for developing more than 20 major diseases, including heart disease, type 2 diabetes, and cancer (CDC, 2012b). **FIGURE 8.1** further outlines a number of other important health problems related to overweight and obesity that impact a person's health-related quality of life.

Individuals with excess body weight not only experience substantial harm to their physical function, vitality, and quality of life, but also have an increased mortality rate and a reduced life expectancy (Flegal, Graubard, Williamson, & Gail, 2010). Furthermore, obesity is now a bigger problem in the United States than smoking in terms of quality of life, shortening of healthy life, morbidity, and mortality (Jia & Lubetkin, 2010).

It's not just one's physical health that may suffer; being overweight or obese may result in *psychosocial morbidity*, where an individual suffers from psychological and social consequences due to depression, social stigma, and discrimination (Puhl, Heuer, & Brownell, 2010). Our modern culture idealizes thinness and disparages obesity (Markey, 2010). Because weight is an important aspect of appearance in our society, especially for women, it seems likely that basing one's self-esteem on appearance would be a particular risk factor for mental health (**FIGURE 8.2**). Indeed, those who are overweight and base their self-esteem on their appearance have lower self-esteem, more symptoms of depression, and more symptoms of eating disorders (Puhl, Heuer, & Brownell, 2010). Furthermore, overweight or obese individuals have suffered from weight bias and discrimination in various areas of society, including employment practices, salary and promotion decisions, education and housing opportunities, and the portrayal of obese persons in popular media as physically unattractive, lazy, and lacking in willpower (Puhl & Heuer, 2009). Not surprisingly, many overweight or obese individuals are dissatisfied and preoccupied with their weight and body image (Puhl, Heuer, & Brownell, 2010).

Overweight and obesity and their associated health problems have a significant economic impact on the U.S. health care system. Considerable health care dollars are spent each year on the treatment and management of obesity-related diseases, including high blood pressure;

Type 2 diabetes (noninsulin dependent)

Back pain

Heart disease (coronary and congestive)

Stroke

Asthma; shortness of breath

Cancer (endometrial, colon, prostate, kidney, gallbladder, and postmenopausal breast cancer)

Bladder control problems (stress incontinence—urine leakage caused by weak pelvic-floor muscles)

Hypertension (high blood pressure)

High blood cholesterol

Premature death

Complications of pregnancy

Gallbladder disease (gallstones)

Menstrual irregularities

Osteoarthritis (degeneration of cartilage and bone in joints)

Increased surgical risk

Sleep apnea (intermittent cessation of breathing while sleeping) and respiratory problems

Psychological disorders (e.g., depression, eating disorders, distorted body image, low self-esteem)

FIGURE 8.1 **Health Risks for Overweight and Obese People.** Overweight people have a great likelihood of developing certain health problems.

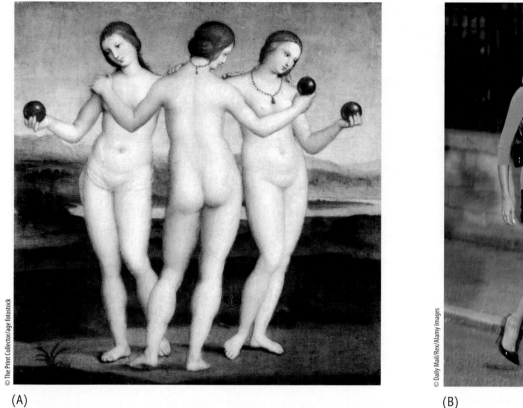

(A)   (B)

FIGURE 8.2 **Changing Standards.** (A) Voluptuous women were once considered the female ideal. (B) In today's society, Victoria Beckham embodies a popular standard.

type 2 diabetes; dyslipidemia (abnormalities in blood lipid and lipoprotein concentrations); heart disease and stroke; respiratory problems, including obstructive sleep apnea (interrupted breathing during sleep) and asthma; osteoarthritis (wearing away of the joints); gallstones; and certain cancers, including endometrial, breast, prostate, and colon cancer. Treating obesity-related illnesses costs about $117 billion annually, or approximately 10 percent of total health care expenditures (Finkelstein, Trogden, Cohen, & Dietz, 2009). Yet, obesity remains one of the most preventable health problems in the United States today.

Health experts use the terms *overweight* and *obesity* as nouns to reflect conditions characterized by excessive and unhealthy amounts of body fat that lead to an increase in disease risks. Therefore, the characterization of people as overweight and obese has to be evaluated within the context of their overall health. The current prevailing scientific consensus is that the increased health risks blamed on being overweight and obese are really the result of many overweight people being sedentary and having detrimental diets and other unhealthful habits. Therefore, one's weight is not just about the numbers on the scale and body image, but also about the lack of regular physical activity and poor eating habits. Engaging in regular physical activity and following proper eating habits have a positive impact on your health no matter what your current weight may be (**FIGURE 8.3** and **FIGURE 8.4**).

This chapter is divided into three basic sections. The first section provides an overview of the current research literature on the relationship between weight and health. This section provides a better understanding of how America's public health authorities determine whether you are medically at risk based on your current weight and related conditions. The second section provides an overview of your body's intricate mechanism for maintaining a healthy weight and how this mechanism can be altered. The third section provides information related to a

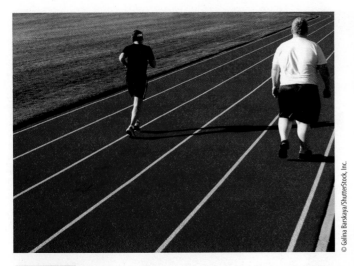

FIGURE 8.3 **Get Out and Move.** Regular physical activity is important at all weight levels.

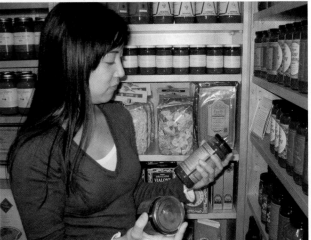

FIGURE 8.4 **Be an Informed Consumer.** Reading food labels to compare calorie content is important to understanding your overall caloric intake.

lifestyle approach to maintaining a healthy weight that focuses on developing a lifelong commitment to regular physical activity and suitable eating practices that are sustainable and enjoyable.

Overweight and Obesity and Health Risk

To understand both the statistics and the significance of health risk related to overweight and obesity, it is important to know how they are defined and measured. **Overweight** is generally defined as weight that exceeds the threshold of a health criterion standard. The health criterion standard is based on the relationship of weight to morbidity (disease) or mortality (death) outcomes. In quantifiable terms, it refers to a body weight that is at least 10 percent over an ideal weight for a specified height (National Heart, Lung, and Blood Institute [NHLBI], 2000). Many people who are classified as overweight are also overfat, and the health risks they face are a result of the latter condition. **Obesity**, like overweight, is a weight that exceeds the threshold of a health criterion standard but to a greater degree. The health criterion standard for obesity refers to a body weight that is at least 30 percent over an ideal weight for a specified height (NHLBI, 2000).

The excessive weight mentioned in these definitions generally refers to an excessive amount of body fat in relation to lean body mass. The proportion of lean tissue—bone, muscle, and water—to fat tissue and the distribution of fat tissue are important to health and are the basis of body composition. If a person's weight is disproportionally fat, he or she will have greater health risks than someone whose ratio of fat to lean tissue mass is better proportioned. Clinical or laboratory measures to determine fat weight and fat-free weight (body composition) are discussed following an explanation of the two most common measures to screen for whether a person is overweight: the body mass index (BMI) and waist circumference. BMI and waist circumference are simple, inexpensive, and reliable measurements known as *anthropometrics*—measures of body size and proportions that provide an initial screening for overfatness and potential health risk.

Body Mass Index

The BMI uses weight and height to produce a number that enables health professionals to gauge risk of weight-related illnesses. The BMI criterion standards recom-

Overweight A weight that exceeds the threshold of a health criterion standard.

Obesity A weight that exceeds the threshold of a health criterion standard to a greater degree than overweight.

The body mass index (BMI) uses weight and height to produce a number that enables health professionals to gauge risk of weight-related illnesses.

TABLE 8.1	Body Mass Index Classifications
BMI (kg/m²)	**Classification**
< 18.5	Underweight
18.5–24.99	Normal weight
25.0–29.99	Overweight
30.0–34.99	Obesity class 1
35.0–39.99	Obesity class 2
> 40	Obesity class 3 (extreme obesity)

mended by the National Heart, Lung, and Blood Institute (NHLBI) Expert Panel on the Identification, Evaluation, and Treatment of Overweight and Obesity in Adults are as follows: underweight, BMI less than 18.5; normal or healthy weight, BMI of 18.5 to 24.99; overweight or preobesity, BMI of 25.0 to 29.99; and class 1, 2, and 3 obesity, BMI of 30 to 34.99, 35 to 39.99, and 40.0 or greater, respectively (NHLBI, 2000) (TABLE 8.1). Therefore, an adult BMI under 18.5 or greater than 25.0 indicates a potential health risk. The link between being screened with a BMI classified as underweight or overweight/obese and the chance of becoming ill is not definite. The research is ongoing; however, when data from large groups of people from the general population are analyzed, a J-shaped association is found between BMI and mortality rate (FIGURE 8.5). For example, BMIs lower than 18.5 are associated with a slight increase in mortality; as weights increase past BMIs of 25 or greater, a successively larger association with mortality is represented. This successively larger association between increasing weight and risk of death is visually represented by the slight increase (20 to 30 percent) as BMI rises from 25 to 27 and the steeper increase (60 percent) as BMI rises above 27.

Although the greatest number of deaths is associated with the overweight categories, there is an increased risk of death for underweight as well. This primarily results from *unhealthy* underweight people, not *healthy* underweight people. Most deaths associated with a low BMI are usually among elderly people who have suffered from underlying chronic diseases that cause low body weight. Cancer, heart failure, chronic lung disease, alcoholism, depression, digestive disease, malnourishment, eating disorders, and osteoporosis (low bone density) are associated with low body weight as well as ill health. The key to knowing whether there is a link

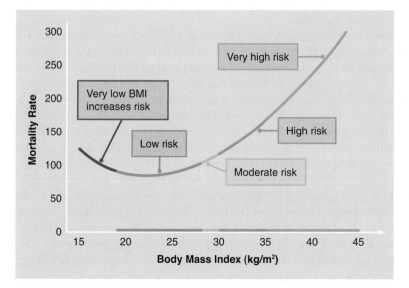

FIGURE 8.5 **BMI and Mortality.** People with a very low or high BMI have a higher relative mortality rate.

between underweight and disease is in determining whether low body weight is voluntary or involuntary, explained or unexplained. An underweight person in poor health should be medically evaluated to rule out an underlying disease or medical condition. For example, many college students are socialized to believe their worth and power come from rigid cultural definitions of beauty, including thinness. The emphasis on extreme thinness, to which women are subjected, may lead to the development of eating disorders—a severe medical condition that involves serious disturbances in eating behavior, such as the extreme and unhealthy reduction of food intake. Eating disorders are discussed at the end of this chapter.

Adult BMIs are calculated using a mathematical formula that takes into account both a person's height and weight. BMI equals a person's weight in kilograms divided by height in meters squared (BMI = kg/m^2). TABLE 8.2 has already calculated the math and metric conversions. To determine your BMI, find your height on the left side of the chart and go straight across from that point until you come to your weight in pounds. The number at the top of the column is your BMI for your height and weight. Compare your BMI with the recommended classifications in Table 8.1.

If you were classified as overweight or obese, you should try not to gain any additional weight. You may even begin thinking about a small decrease of 10 percent of your total body mass. But before you take action, it is important to look at other factors—namely, your waist circumference and conditions associated with being overweight or obese—when it comes to assessing your overall risk for developing a chronic health condition. Before discussing waist circumference and associated conditions, the advantages and limitations of BMI will be addressed.

The BMI is an easy and quick noninvasive method to assess weight-related health status. You only need to measure your height in inches (without shoes) and weight in pounds (obtained with minimal clothing—only undergarments). The BMI is not gender specific, and therefore is appropriate for all men and nonpregnant women older than 20 years of age. For children and teenagers, weight status is defined differently than it is for adults. Because children and teenagers are still growing, and boys and girls develop at different rates, BMIs for children 2 to 20 years old are determined by comparing their weight and height against growth charts that take their age and gender into account.

There is much evidence to support the predictive power of BMI in risk assessment because it provides a more accurate measure of total body fat compared with the assessment of body weight alone (NHLBI, 2000). Given that BMI correlates well with health risk, it is one of the many tools available to identify individuals who would benefit from weight loss, thus lowering their risk of developing a chronic disease condition.

Although a BMI measurement may be good for predicting health risks associated with excess weight due to fat, including high blood pressure, diabetes mellitus, and coronary heart disease, as the name suggests, it measures body mass, not body fat. Any measure of obesity that relies primarily on weight, an indirect estimate of body fat, has limitations. A high BMI may indicate obesity, but a high value may also occur in people who are not overfat. The BMI may overestimate fatness in lean, muscular athletes or people with high bone densities. Conversely, older individuals who have gained fat, lost muscle and bone mass as a result of a sedentary lifestyle, or lost weight to an underlying chronic illness may have a BMI in the normal healthy range but may actually be at greater risk for disease because of a higher percentage of body fat. Determining whether an individual is obese from simply being overweight or because of increased muscle mass, or is underweight because of a lack of muscle tissue, requires body composition techniques for quantifying fat mass and fat-free mass. Finally, the BMI provides no information about fat distribution (site of fat), which is a more important risk factor than overall body fat.

TABLE 8.2 Body Mass Index Table

Body Weight (pounds)

Height (inches)	Normal						Overweight					Obese										Extreme Obesity														
BMI	19	20	21	22	23	24	25	26	27	28	29	30	31	32	33	34	35	36	37	38	39	40	41	42	43	44	45	46	47	48	49	50	51	52	53	54
58	91	96	100	105	110	115	119	124	129	134	138	143	148	153	158	162	167	172	177	181	186	191	196	201	205	210	215	220	224	229	234	239	244	248	253	258
59	94	99	104	109	114	119	124	128	133	138	143	148	153	158	163	168	173	178	183	188	193	198	203	208	212	217	222	227	232	237	242	247	252	257	262	267
60	97	102	107	112	118	123	128	133	138	143	148	153	158	163	168	174	179	184	189	194	199	204	209	215	220	225	230	235	240	245	250	255	261	266	271	276
61	100	106	111	116	122	127	132	137	143	148	153	158	164	169	174	180	185	190	195	201	206	211	217	222	227	232	238	243	248	254	259	264	269	275	280	285
62	104	109	115	120	126	131	136	142	147	153	158	164	169	175	180	186	191	196	202	207	213	218	224	229	235	240	246	251	256	262	267	273	278	284	289	295
63	107	113	118	124	130	135	141	146	152	158	163	169	175	180	186	191	197	203	208	214	220	225	231	237	242	248	254	259	265	270	278	282	287	293	299	304
64	110	116	122	128	134	140	145	151	157	163	169	174	180	186	192	197	204	209	215	221	227	232	238	244	250	256	262	267	273	279	285	291	296	302	308	314
65	114	120	126	132	138	144	150	156	162	168	174	180	186	192	198	204	210	216	222	228	234	240	246	252	258	264	270	276	282	288	294	300	306	312	318	324
66	118	124	130	136	142	148	155	161	167	173	179	186	192	198	204	210	216	223	229	235	241	247	253	260	266	272	278	284	291	297	303	309	315	322	328	334
67	121	127	134	140	146	153	159	166	172	178	185	191	198	204	211	217	223	230	236	242	249	255	261	268	274	280	287	293	299	306	312	319	325	331	338	344
68	125	131	138	144	151	158	164	171	177	184	190	197	203	210	216	223	230	236	243	249	256	262	269	276	282	289	295	302	308	315	322	328	335	341	348	354
69	128	135	142	149	155	162	169	176	182	189	196	203	209	216	223	230	236	243	250	257	263	270	277	284	291	297	304	311	318	324	331	338	345	351	358	365
70	132	139	146	153	160	167	174	181	188	195	202	209	216	222	229	236	243	250	257	264	271	278	285	292	299	306	313	320	327	334	341	348	355	362	369	376
71	136	143	150	157	165	172	179	186	193	200	208	215	222	229	236	243	250	257	265	272	279	286	293	301	308	315	322	329	338	343	351	358	365	372	379	386
72	140	147	154	162	169	177	184	191	199	206	213	221	228	235	242	250	258	265	272	279	287	294	302	309	316	324	331	338	346	353	361	368	375	383	390	397
73	144	151	159	166	174	182	189	197	204	212	219	227	235	242	250	257	265	272	280	288	295	302	310	318	325	333	340	348	355	363	371	378	386	393	401	408
74	148	155	163	171	179	186	194	202	210	218	225	233	241	249	256	264	272	280	287	295	303	311	319	326	334	342	350	358	365	373	381	389	396	404	412	420
75	152	160	168	176	184	192	200	208	216	224	232	240	248	256	264	272	279	287	295	303	311	319	327	335	343	351	359	367	375	383	391	399	407	415	423	431
76	156	164	172	180	189	197	205	213	221	230	238	246	254	263	271	279	287	295	304	312	320	328	336	344	353	361	369	377	385	394	402	410	418	426	435	443

SOURCE: Adapted from National Heart, Lung, and Blood Institute. (1998). *Clinical Guidelines on the Identification, Evaluation, and Treatment of Overweight and Obesity in Adults: The Evidence Report.* Bethesda, MD: National Institutes of Health.

Individuals with more abdominal body fat have a more adverse metabolic profile and an increased risk for diabetes and cardiovascular disease.

Visceral fat Located inside the peritoneal cavity, packed in between internal organs.

Omentum A large fold of visceral peritoneum that hangs down from the stomach.

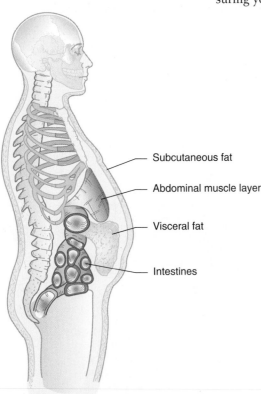

— Subcutaneous fat

— Abdominal muscle layer

— Visceral fat

— Intestines

FIGURE 8.6 **Visceral Fat.** The fat lying deep within the body's abdominal cavity (shown here in cross-section) may pose an especially high risk for metabolic disturbances.

Body Fat Distribution

Body fat or adipose tissue (fatty tissue) is stored in various locations throughout the human body. The majority is stored subcutaneously (under the skin). Subcutaneous fat is the fat that you can see, or the "inch you can pinch." A moderate amount of subcutaneous fat is essential for life because it serves as an insulating layer to conserve body heat and provides shock-absorbent padding if you bang into something or fall down. The fat stored here serves as the main fuel source for long-duration, low- to moderate-intensity exercise. Subcutaneous body fat plays a significant role in reproduction. Sex hormones are fat-soluble and are stored in the body's fat layers. Because of hormones and the ability to bear children, women typically have more of this fat than men. Still, too much can be harmful.

We also store fat deep inside the abdominal cavity under the muscles; this is called intra-abdominal or **visceral fat**. Visceral fat surrounds vital organs like the liver, heart, intestines, and kidneys, as well as hanging, in a separate double flap, off the ends of the stomach like an apron (**FIGURE 8.6**). This apron is known as the **omentum**. Its primary functions include storing fat and lining the abdominal cavity to prevent adhesions. A moderate amount of visceral fat protects the organs it surrounds by absorbing shock and insulating against temperature extremes. But for reasons scientists don't yet fully understand, excess visceral fat—more than fat anywhere else in the body or more than overall obesity—is associated with destructive metabolic abnormalities and harmful health effects. Because it is hidden, you cannot know for sure how much visceral fat you have unless you have a CT scan or MRI—but as you will soon read, you can get a very good idea by measuring your waist.

Several factors determine where we store our fat and how much fat we store, including sex differences, hormones, activity levels, caloric intake, and chronic stress. In the obese and nonobese states, there are characteristic sex differences in the distribution of subcutaneous fat. Nonobese women have relatively more subcutaneous fat in the gluteofemoral (thigh/hip/butt) area than in other subcutaneous regions, whereas in nonobese men the subcutaneous fat is distributed in a uniform fashion. These patterns are determined by secretion of the hormones responsible for the development of secondary sex characteristics. The gender differences are more pronounced in obesity (**FIGURE 8.7**). Obese men usually accumulate fat around the waist. This male obesity is called upper body, central, android, or apple-shaped obesity. Obese women usually accumulate fat in the lower part of the abdominal area and the gluteofemoral region. This female type of obesity is called lower body, peripheral, gynoid, or pear-shaped obesity. The link between gender and regional obesity is not absolute. There are many women (especially after menopause) who have upper body fat distribution, and many men who have lower body fat distribution. Research has indicated that the android pattern is associated with a higher risk of metabolic abnormalities. This is thought to be related to the fact that the android pattern represents more visceral fat storage, whereas the gynoid pattern is more peripheral and away from the internal organs.

We also store more body fat when we consume more calories in food and drink than we burn up. To lose weight, we need to shift that balance and burn up more than we consume. We can accomplish that by consuming fewer calories, burning more, or both. This is the concept behind the energy balance equation, which will be discussed later. Lastly, long-term or chronic stress increases levels of cortisol, which is the second-most abundant hormone in your body. Cortisol boosts glucose levels in your blood, which comes in handy during a fight or flight response in periods of short-term stress. But chronically high levels of cortisol and blood glucose lead to excess production of insulin, a hormone that promotes fat storage—especially in the omentum.

As mentioned earlier, individuals with more visceral body fat have a more adverse metabolic profile and are more vulnerable to a number of health-related complications, like type 2 diabetes and cardiovascular disease, than individuals with more subcutaneous body fat. It is now recognized that visceral fat plays a more significant role in throwing off the hormonal and metabolic processes inside the body.

It is important to understand that fat cells—particularly visceral fat cells—are not passive calorie warehouses, but rather biologically active mini endocrine factories that produce at least 20 different hormones, collectively called *adipokines*. These hormones direct your metabolism and help keep track of your energy stores to control appetite and budget how your body uses energy. Many scientists theorize that excess visceral fat is harmful because of its location near the portal vein, which carries blood from the intestinal area to the liver. Hormones and other substances released by visceral fat, including free fatty acids, enter the portal vein and travel to the liver, where they can influence the production of blood lipids. Visceral fat is directly linked with higher triglycerides, total cholesterol, LDL (bad) cholesterol, and lower HDL (good) cholesterol. Additionally, too many fatty acids coming into the portal vein seem to make the liver produce too much glucose. With so much glucose, the body pumps out more insulin to try to control the high levels of sugar. However, the insulin is absorbed by the omentum so blood sugars remain elevated. Over time, this vicious cycle might contribute to a dreaded condition known as insulin resistance, a major precursor to type 2 diabetes.

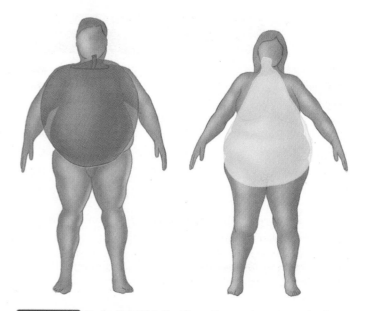

FIGURE 8.7 **Body Fat Distribution.** Men and women who have large body fat deposits centrally located in their waists tend to have a higher risk of diabetes and cardiovascular disease than individuals with the same amount of fat located below the waist. Overweight males typically have central fat deposits (apple-shaped bodies) whereas overweight females often have excess body fat below the waist (pear-shaped bodies).

Waist Circumference

Subcutaneous abdominal fat correlates well with intra-abdominal fat or visceral fat, so for many people, the modest measuring tape provides an easy and reliable way of telling whether additional inches around the waist constitute health risk. To assess waist circumference, locate the upper hip and place a measuring tape in a horizontal plane around the waist while standing (**FIGURE 8.8**). The measurement should be taken at the narrowest point on the torso and made with the abdominal muscles relaxed (not pulled in). Men who have a waist circumference greater than 40 inches (> 102 cm) and women who have a waist circumference greater than 35 inches (> 88 cm) are at higher risk for developing type 2 diabetes, hypertension, and cardiovascular disease.

Many health experts believe that because fat around the waist is so hazardous to heart health, measuring waist circumference may actually provide a more accurate method of assessing overweight and obesity risks than BMI. TABLE 8.3 integrates both BMI and waist circumference to estimate risk status. For BMI classifications of normal, overweight, and class 1 obesity (18.5–24.9, 25.0–29.9, and 30.0–34.9, respective-

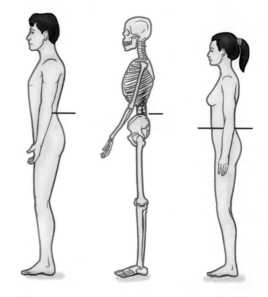

FIGURE 8.8 **Measuring-Tape Position for Waist Circumference in Adults.**

TABLE 8.3	Classification of Overweight and Obesity by BMI and Waist Circumference, and Associated Disease Risk*			
BMI (kg/m²)	Obesity Class	Men ≤ 102 cm (≤ 40 in.) Women ≤ 88 cm (≤ 35 in.)		> 102 cm (> 40 in.) > 88 cm (> 35 in.)
Underweight	< 18.5	—	—	—
Normal†	18.5–24.9	—	—	May increase risk
Overweight	25.0–29.9	—	Increased	High
Obesity	30.0–34.9	I	High	Very high
	35.0–39.9	II	Very high	Very high
Extreme obesity	≥ 40	III	Extremely high	Extremely high

*Disease risk for type 2 diabetes, hypertension, and cardiovascular disease.

†Increased waist circumference can also be a marker for increased risk, even in persons of normal weight.

SOURCE: National Heart, Lung, and Blood Institute. (2000). *The Practical Guide: Identification, Evaluation, and Treatment of Overweight and Obesity in Adults* (NIH Publication No. 00-4084). Washington, DC: U.S. Department of Health and Human Services.

ly), the inclusion of a high waist circumference increases the overall disease risk for type 2 diabetes, hypertension, and cardiovascular disease to a greater degree than BMI by itself. Furthermore, it has been shown that increases or decreases in waist circumference measures, even in the absence of BMI changes, are important predictors of cardiovascular risk factors (Flint et al., 2010).

If you were classified as overweight based on your waist circumference measurement, your focus should be on "waist loss," or losing inches, not necessarily pounds. You can reduce your chances of getting many metabolic diseases by losing a couple of inches. The most promising way to go about losing those inches and significantly reducing the amount of visceral fat you carry around is through increased physical activity (preferably vigorous aerobic exercise), reduced overall daily calorie intake (focus on nutrient-dense foods), and reduced chronic stress levels to diminish the raft of destructive hormones that shoot through your body.

Risk Factors for Diseases and Conditions Associated with Overweight and Obesity

Besides being classified as overweight or obese based on BMI and waist circumference measures, there are risk factors for diseases and conditions associated with overweight and obesity that need to be assessed (TABLE 8.4) (NHLBI, 2000). The

TABLE 8.4	Risk Factors and Conditions to Consider if Overweight or Obese

Risk Factors	Diagnosed Conditions
High blood pressure (hypertension)	Established coronary heart disease
High LDL cholesterol ("bad" cholesterol)	Presence of other atherosclerotic diseases (e.g., peripheral artery disease, symptomatic carotid artery disease)
Low HDL cholesterol ("good" cholesterol)	Type 2 diabetes
High triglycerides	Sleep apnea
High blood glucose (sugar)	Osteoarthritis
Family history of premature heart disease	
Physical inactivity	
Cigarette smoking	

SOURCE: National Heart, Lung, and Blood Institute. (2000). *The Practical Guide: Identification, Evaluation, and Treatment of Overweight and Obesity in Adults* (NIH Publication No. 00-4084). Washington, DC: U.S. Department of Health and Human Services.

treatment algorithm shown in **FIGURE 8.9** graphically identifies the timing of this risk assessment in step 6. According to this treatment guideline, for people who are considered obese (BMI ≥ 30) or overweight (BMI of 25 to 29.9) or who have a high waist circumference (> 40 inches for men and > 35 inches for women) and two or more risk factors (step 7), weight loss is recommended (step 8). It is important to know that even a small weight loss (10 percent of current body mass) or losing a couple of inches around the waist will help lower your risk of developing diseases associated with overweight and obesity. Prevention of weight gain

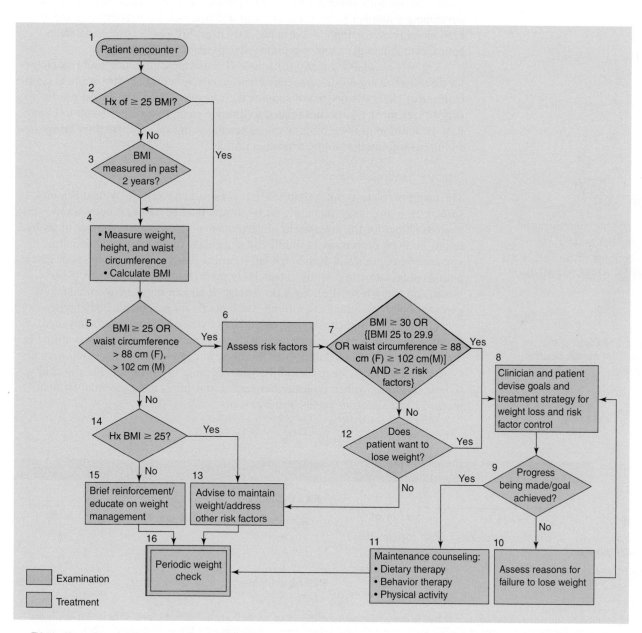

This algorithm applies only to the assessment for overweight and obesity and subsequent decisions based on that assessment. It does not include any initial overall assessment for cardiovascular risk factors or diseases that are indicated.

FIGURE 8.9 **Treatment Algorithm.** This algorithm is used to assess overweight and obesity and to guide health practitioners in the assessment and subsequent treatment planning process. SOURCE: National Heart, Lung, and Blood Institute, (2000). *The Practical Guide: Identification, Evaluation, and Treatment of Overweight and Obesity in Adults* (NIH Publication 00-4084). Washington, DC: U.S. Department of Health and Human Services.

with physical activity and diet is indicated for any individual with a BMI of 25 to 29.9 and two or more comorbidities (TABLE 8.5).

Age and the duration of overweight and obesity can have a powerful harmful impact on developing a chronic disease, particularly in young adults. Approximately 25 to 30 percent of adult obesity cases begin with being overweight during childhood or adolescence (Aprovian, 2010). A history of being overweight in childhood that persists into adulthood is associated with more severe complications of obesity later in life. The steadily increasing incidence of overweight children and teenagers raises concern about the health of these youth as they approach adulthood. As with obese adults, overweight children have an increased risk of developing a number of health conditions and diseases, such as diabetes mellitus, high blood pressure, high blood lipids, fatty liver, orthopedic problems, sleep apnea, eating disorders, and symptoms of depression (FIGURE 8.10).

The process of assessment utilizing BMI, waist circumference, and risk factors for diseases and conditions associated with overweight and obesity can help people realize that change is needed to support their health. These assessment results may suggest treatment approaches related to lifestyle change strategies (refer to Figure 8.9). In addition to these assessments, knowing your body composition brings additional information to the screening profile.

Body Composition

The major problem is not weight itself; it is excessive body fat. Weight is a measure of the entire body, including fat tissue and fat-free tissue. A body composition analysis allows for the assessment of percentage of fat versus percentage of fat-free tissue. Body fat percentage is simply the percentage of fat your body contains. If you are 150 pounds and 10 percent fat, it means that your body consists of 15 pounds of fat and 135 pounds of lean body mass (muscle, bone, organ tissue, blood, and everything else). Your percentage of fat can range between 2 and 70 percent of body weight. Determining cutoff points for acceptable body fat percentages requires first considering essential body fat and storage fat allowances. **Essential body fat** is required for normal physiological functioning and is stored in bone marrow, the heart, lungs, liver, kidneys, intestines, muscles, central nervous system, and other major tissues and organs. Because of hormones and the ability to bear children, women typically have up to four times more essential fat than men—12 to 15 percent versus 3 to 5 percent.

> ④
>
> A body composition analysis allows for the assessment of the percentage of fat versus the percentage of fat-free tissue.

> **Essential body fat** Fat that is required for normal healthy functioning.

TABLE 8.5	A Guide to Selecting Treatment				
	BMI Category				
Treatment	25–26.9	27–29.9	30–34.9	35–39.9	≥ 40
Diet, physical activity, and behavior therapy	With comorbidities	With comorbidities	+	+	+
Pharmacotherapy		With comorbidities	+	+	+
Surgery			With comorbidities	With comorbidities	With comorbidities

Prevention of weight gain with lifestyle therapy is indicated in any patient with a BMI = 25 kg/m², even without comorbidities, while weight loss is not necessarily recommended for those with a BMI of 25–29.9 kg/m² or a high waist circumference, unless they have two or more comorbidities.

Combined therapy with a low-calorie diet, increased physical activity, and behavior therapy provides the most successful intervention for weight loss and weight maintenance.

Consider pharmacotherapy only if a patient has not lost 1 pound per week after 6 months of combined lifestyle therapy.

The + represents the use of indicated treatment regardless of comorbidities.

SOURCE: National Heart, Lung, and Blood Institute. (2000). *The Practical Guide: Identification, Evaluation, and Treatment of Overweight and Obesity in Adults* (NIH Publication No. 00-4084). Washington, DC: U.S. Department of Health and Human Services.

Storage fat is body fat above essential body fat levels that accumulates in adipose tissue (fat cells). Some storage fat is advised for both males and females. Storage fat is needed to protect internal organs from trauma, serve as insulation, and provide an important energy reserve. As an energy storage repository, it provides 3500 calories in every pound of adipose tissue, which is nearly double the calories stored as glycogen. Storage fat accumulates when energy intake (calories consumed) exceeds energy expenditure (calories burned). Desirable storage levels for both men and women are estimated to be between 8 and 20 percent.

Many health experts use the percentage of body fat in assessing health risk. When body fat percentage is used in conjunction with BMI, it can help differentiate people who are overweight because of lean body mass from those who are overweight because of fat. An ideal body fat percentage is one that meets your body's fundamental need for normal physiological functioning and energy needs but does not create health risks (**FIGURE 8.11**). Although there are no perfect criterion standards for ideal body fat percentage, most health experts agree that fat percentages that range from 10 to 25 percent for men and 20 to 30 percent for women are considered to be below average or average risk (American Dietetic Association [ADA], 2009). *Obesity* is the term used to define excessive accumulation of body fat that places individuals at greatest risk. This is usually designated by a body fat percentage that exceeds 25 percent in males and 30 percent in females. Fortunately, even minor fat reduction reduces and improves the conditions associated with obesity.

> **Storage fat** Body fat, above essential levels, that accumulates in adipose tissue.

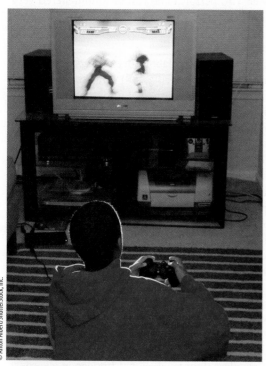

FIGURE 8.10 **Today's Youth.** Many children are following sedentary lifestyles that place them at greater health risks.

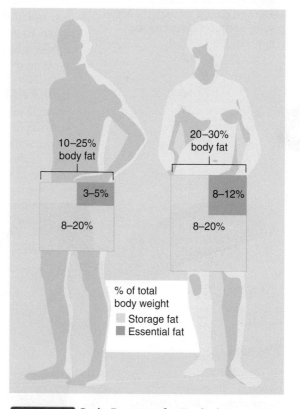

FIGURE 8.11 **Body Fatness of a Typical Man and Woman.** SOURCE: National Institutes of Health. (2009). Weight management: MedlinePlus Medical Encyclopedia. Online: http://www.nlm.nih.gov/medlineplus/ency/article/001943.htm.

ASSESSING BODY COMPOSITION   Direct measurement of body composition in living human beings is not feasible, so various models for indirect estimation of the constituents of the body have been developed. Indirect measurement techniques give estimates of the percentage of body fat, fat-free mass, muscle, bone density, hydration, or other body components. Each method uses one or more measurable body components (such as skinfold thickness and resistance) to make educated predictions about the other components. All of these methods are subject to measurement error and have basic assumptions that do not always hold true. In fact, even the most accurate techniques have measurement errors in the 2 to 4 percent range. According to the National Institutes of Health, no trial data exist to indicate that one method of measuring body fat is better than any other for following overweight and obese individuals to assess the effects of both dietary and physical activity programs. The following sections address three commonly used body composition measurement tools.

Skinfold technique Measure of subcutaneous fat at various body sites using special calipers.

Underwater weighing Technique to measure body fat percentage that requires weighing a person underwater as well as on land.

Bioelectrical impedance Technique to measure body fat percentage that passes a harmless, low-level, single-frequency electrical current through the body using electrodes placed on the wrist and ankle.

SKINFOLD TESTING   The **skinfold technique** is an anthropometric technique that measures subcutaneous fat, the fat located just under your skin throughout your body. This technique requires special calipers and an experienced tester to ensure accuracy and repeatability on future testing. The tester lifts a fold of skin and fat between the thumb and forefinger, pulls it away from the underlying muscle, and then measures the fold (**FIGURE 8.12**). The five most commonly measured sites are the triceps (back of upper arm), subscapular (upper back), suprailiac (just above the hip bone), abdomen (either side of the umbilicus), and the frontal thigh. The values obtained are inserted into an appropriate skinfold formula to calculate body fat percentage. Skinfolds can have a standard error of 3 to 4 percent. Thus, a person with a skinfold estimate of 12 percent body fat may, in actuality, fall between 8 and 16 percent. Skinfold testing is easy to perform and can be administered very quickly and thus is useful as a monitoring device to indicate changes in body composition over time.

UNDERWATER WEIGHING   The most widely used laboratory procedure for measuring body composition is **underwater weighing** (**FIGURE 8.13**). This technique is considered a more precise assessment of body fatness than skinfolds are but requires special equipment and highly trained personnel and is time-consuming. This method uses the *Archimedes principle*, which states that when a body is submerged in water, there is a buoyant counterforce equal to the weight of the water that is displaced. Because bone and muscle are denser than water, a person with a larger percentage of fat-free mass will weigh more in the water and have a lower percentage body fat value. Conversely, fat floats; therefore, a large amount of fat mass will make the body lighter in the water, and have a higher percentage body fat value. This technique provides a density measurement from which the percentage of body fat can be calculated. If each test is performed correctly according to the recommended protocol, the standard error is 1.5 percent.

BIOELECTRICAL IMPEDANCE   In **bioelectrical impedance**, a harmless, low-level, signal-frequency electrical current is passed through your body by electrodes placed on the wrist and an ankle (refer to Figure 8.13). The amount of resistance and the body size are used to calculate body fat percentage. Because body fat contains less water and fewer electrolytes than

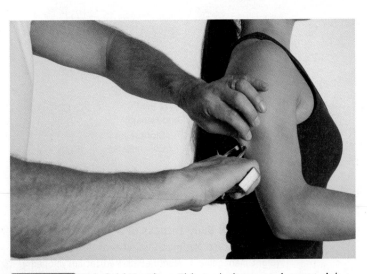

FIGURE 8.12 **Skinfold Testing.** This technique requires special calipers and an experienced tester.

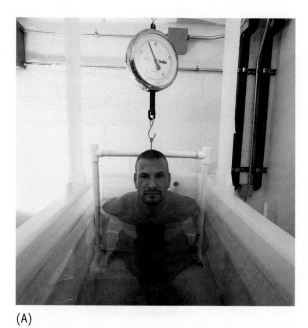

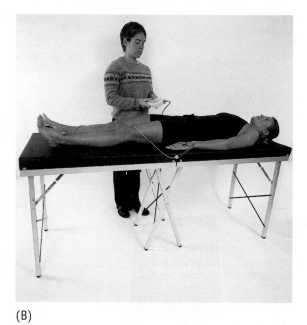

(A)   (B)

FIGURE 8.13 **Measuring Methods.** (A) Body fat is measured using the underwater weighing method. (B) Bioelectrical impedance is another method used to measure body fat.

does lean body mass, it exhibits a greater resistance (impedance) to the flow of an electrical current. If done correctly using properly calibrated equipment, the standard error is 3 percent. Testing is quick and painless.

In summary, further assessment utilizing body composition analysis may significantly add to the criteria used in assessing your health risk related to obesity-related conditions. The next section provides an explanation of your body's intricate mechanism of weight control. Weight control has become an obsession with many in contemporary America. Whether you count the number of people unhappy with their shape, the percentage on a diet, or the billions of dollars spent on diet programs, books, foods, and supplements, the figures all show that our society has become more obsessed with weight in the past decade or two than ever before. Although many still attempt to obtain an ideal body weight to enhance their appearance, a growing number are trying to control their weight because they see it as a serious health problem that needs to be solved.

Maintaining a Healthy Body Weight

Maintaining a healthy body weight should be a simple matter. It demands that we maintain a balance between energy intake and energy output—in other words, balancing calories consumed with calories expended (**FIGURE 8.14**). Because both can be calculated fairly accurately and without elaborate equipment, the conscientious individual should have no problem maintaining a healthy weight. In reality, however, maintaining healthy weight over a lifetime is a constant battle for a majority of Americans. Many factors affect how much or how little food we eat and how that food is processed, or metabolized, by our bodies, and therefore maintaining a healthy body weight can be a challenge. To understand the intricate mechanism of weight control, we examine the relationship between calorie intake and expenditure.

Energy Intake: Hunger, Appetite, and Satiety
Supplying enough energy to support the many functions of the body at work and play is one of the chief functions of food. Energy intake is simply calories consumed

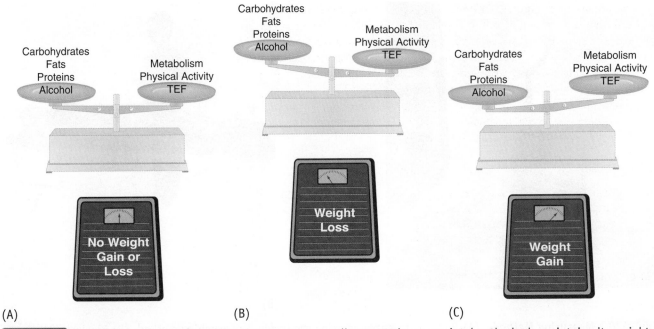

FIGURE 8.14 **Energy Balance Equation.** (A) When energy expenditure equals energy intake, the body maintains its weight. (B) When energy expenditure is greater than energy intake, the body loses weight. (C) When energy expenditure is less than energy intake, the body gains weight.

in the form of macronutrients (protein, carbohydrates, and fats) and alcohol (refer to Figure 8.14). Protein and carbohydrates contain 4 calories per gram and fats 9 calories per gram. Alcohol contains 7 calories per gram, but does not provide any substantial nutrients. To be able to control your food intake (energy intake) and maintain a healthy weight, you need to understand why you feel the need to eat.

Our eating behaviors involve both physiological and psychological factors. Hunger is the physiological need for food. Numerous physiological signals tell us we are hungry, such as an empty or growling stomach, a decrease in blood glucose levels, and alterations in circulating hormones (e.g., increased glucagons and ghrelin and decreased insulin) (**FIGURE 8.15**). Appetite is the psychological desire to eat and is associated with sensory experiences or aspects of food such as the sight and smell of food, emotional cues, social situations, and cultural conventions. Stressful situations often stimulate or repress appetite. Appetite is learned and relates to the desire for specific types of food and eating experiences, instead of food in general. Appetite helps select the quality and balance of food as learned by an individual in his or her environment. Whereas hunger acts as the more basic drive, appetite is more of a reflection of eating experiences. At times we are not hungry but have an appetite (such as seeing a tempting dessert after eating a full meal) or may be hungry but have no appetite (such as when we are sick).

You can use appetite to control hunger when it comes to maintaining a healthy weight. If you wait to eat until you are physiologically hungry, you may eat four or five times the amount you

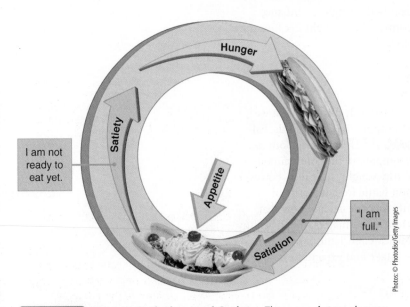

Photos: © Photodisc/Getty Images

FIGURE 8.15 **Hunger, Satiation, and Satiety.** These are internal cues that influence our eating behaviors.

need to fill the necessary nutritional stores. Many people skip meals to try to lose weight and then end up pigging out. It is relatively easy to fight off your appetite but nearly impossible to fight off your hunger. To prevent this situation from occurring, eat nutrient-dense balanced meals every day and avoid allowing yourself to become physiologically hungry by using your appetite to control your hunger.

Satiety is the physiological and psychological feeling of fullness that stops hunger and appetite signals. As was true for hunger and appetite, a number of factors influence the experience of fullness, including stomach distention, elevations in blood glucose and glycogen stores, and alternations in circulating hormones. Fostering a full feeling can be helpful in managing your weight. Here are a few ideas for choosing foods that will help fill your stomach up without filling you out.

- Foods high in water content are known to promote a feeling of fullness. Foods with a high water content and low energy density include fruits, vegetables, low-fat milk, cooked grains, lean meats, fish, poultry, and beans. Dishes such as soups, stews, and some pasta dishes are high in water content and may have low energy density depending on preparation.

- Fiber, like water, has no calories but does add weight to the food; thus, it promotes a feeling of fullness. Fiber is not digested and gives structure or bulk to natural foods such as fruits and vegetables; food high in fiber tends to be very filling.

- Slow down when you eat to allow your stomach time to give a proper "gut check" report to the brain so it can register that you are full.

- Seek out unprocessed foods, which tend to have a low energy density or few calories per weight.

Energy Expenditure: How We Use Calories

Our metabolism is the rate at which the body uses energy (calories) to support all basic functions essential to sustain life, plus all energy requirements for additional activity and digestive processes. There are three components to human metabolism, hence determining our energy needs. These components are the resting metabolic rate, the thermic effect of food, and the thermic effect of activity (**FIGURE 8.16**).

Resting metabolic rate (RMR) is the largest part of total metabolism and accounts for 60 to 75 percent of calories burned in a day. The RMR is usually low per unit of time when compared with energy expenditure while we are active, but because we spend a greater proportion of our time in a rested state, our RMR contributes significantly to total daily energy expenditure. This is the amount of calories needed to run all essential functions and chemical reactions while in a rested and quiet state. The functions included are the respiratory process, the pumping of blood around the body, nerve transmission, producing and transporting substances, cell growth and maintenance, tissue repair, and temperature regulation. RMR is relatively stable for a given individual, but significant differences in RMR can be found when comparing different individuals. Many factors can influence RMR, including the following:

- *Age.* RMR slows with age as a result of a loss in muscle tissue but also because of hormonal and neurological changes. After 20 years of age, RMR declines about 2 percent per decade.

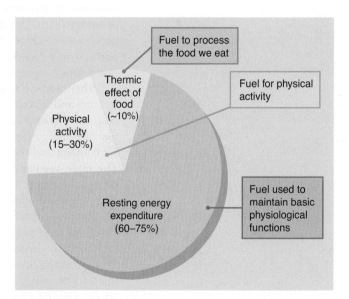

FIGURE 8.16 **Major Components of Energy Expenditure.** The majority of daily expenditure is used to maintain physiological functions. Energy expended by athletes during physical activity and exercise is significant and could equal or exceed the energy needed for maintaining resting energy expenditure. The thermic effect of food is the energy required to digest, absorb, transport, metabolize, and store food.

- *Gender.* Generally, men have faster metabolisms than women because they tend to be larger and have less body fat.
- *Glands.* Thyroxin (produced by the thyroid gland) is a key RMR regulator. The more thyroxin produced, the higher the RMR. If too much thyroxin is produced, RMR can actually double. If too little thyroxin is produced, RMR may shrink to 30 to 40 percent of normal. In some people, the thyroid gland does not function properly, and as a result the organ produces too much or too little thyroid hormone.
- *Muscle-to-fat ratio.* Muscle cells are about eight times more metabolically demanding than fat cells are. So, the greater our proportion of muscle to fat, the faster our metabolic rate.
- *Crash dieting, starving, or fasting.* Starvation or serious abrupt calorie reduction can dramatically reduce RMR by up to 30 percent. Restrictive low-calorie weight loss diets may cause your RMR to drop as much as 20 percent.
- *Infection or illness.* RMR increases because the body has to work harder to build new tissues and create an immune response.
- *Environmental temperature.* If temperature is very low or very high, the body has to work harder to maintain its normal temperature; this increases RMR.
- *Drugs.* Some drugs, such as caffeine and nicotine, increase the RMR.

Thermic effect of food (TEF) The energy expended by our bodies to eat and process (digest, transport, metabolize, and store) food.

Thermic effect of activity (TEA) The energy expended in skeletal muscle contraction and relaxation.

The **thermic effect of food (TEF)** is used to describe the energy expended by our bodies to eat and process (digest, transport, metabolize, and store) food. We expend energy by burning calories. The calories needed to eat and process food are fairly constant, usually about 10 percent of the total calories taken in. For example, a person who consumes 2500 calories per day will expend approximately 250 calories a day to metabolize food. The more calories eaten, the more energy used to digest them, but it's in proportion to total calories. Variance in the type of macronutrients eaten affects TEF. Processing protein requires the greatest amount of energy, with estimates ranging as high as 30 percent. Dietary fat, on the other hand, is so easily processed and stored as body fat that there is little thermic effect, perhaps only 2 or 3 percent. The amount of energy required to process carbohydrates falls between that of protein and fat.

The **thermic effect of activity (TEA)** is the energy costs for skeletal muscle contraction and relaxation. As noted previously, RMR is measured when you are at rest; any physical activity will raise the metabolic activity above the RMR and thus increase energy expenditure. Muscles need energy to contract. The more muscles we contract and the more frequently we contract them, the more calories we burn. Therefore, regular physical activity has a profound effect on human energy expenditure. In general it contributes 15 to 30 percent to the body's total energy output; however, some athletes can actually meet or exceed estimated RMR rates.

Physical activity not only influences burning calories while you are moving but also helps raise your RMR by building extra muscle tissue. Muscle tissue is more metabolically demanding than fat tissue, so you burn more calories even when resting or sleeping. In addition, your metabolic rate remains elevated postactivity. The intensity of your physical activity also affects the magnitude of the postactivity metabolic rate. In fact, many studies suggest a strong correlation between the number of calories burned postexercise or "afterburn effect," also called excess postexercise oxygen consumption (EPOC), and the activity's intensity. A more intense exercise session, compared with a similar less intense exercise session over the same duration, will lead to more oxygen consumed by the body afterward, meaning a higher sustained metabolic rate and thus more calories burned throughout the day.

Although energy intake is easily measured and can be regulated by consulting caloric intake charts, regulating and determining energy output are slightly more complex.

In summary, maintaining a healthy weight is a general matter of energy balance, as illustrated in Figure 8.14. To maintain body weight, energy intake (calories) and energy expenditure must be equal. When calories consumed are greater than energy expended, individuals gain weight. When energy expenditure exceeds caloric intake, weight loss occurs. It is important to remember that all of us from time to time have short-term weight fluctuations. This is normal because it is easy to become dehydrated, leading to losing a couple pounds of water weight within a few days, or because we don't eat exactly the same amount of calories every day or don't do the same level of physical activity every day. However, when weight consistently increases or decreases, we have an energy imbalance, and we need to look into that. In the United States, the energy imbalance is tilted to weight gain for a majority of children and adults.

Causes of Overweight and Obesity

What is becoming increasingly difficult for researchers to explain is why this imbalance in the energy balance equation occurs. Until recently, the major causes of obesity were thought to be behavioral in nature—that is, resulting from excessive energy intake and deficient energy expenditure (people eating too much and exercising too little). This idea led many health professionals, and thus, the public, to believe that excess weight reflects a lack of willpower in people who are overweight and obese. However, recent research provides evidence that obesity is a complex disorder with multiple contributing factors. There is no one cause of obesity. A combination of behavioral, psychological, genetic, physiological, metabolic, hormonal, sociocultural, and environmental factors acting together over time can contribute to weight gain and obesity (**FIGURE 8.17**). Separating one cause from another is not an easy diagnostic task when looking at individuals. For example, obesity tends to run in families, suggesting a genetic link, yet families also share common dietary, physical exercise, and lifestyle habits that may also contribute to obesity.

Genetics determines the "body-weight ballpark" each person is born into. So, there is no denying the fact that biology is at work when it comes to understanding body weight. Genes affect a number of weight-related processes in the body, including influences on fat metabolism and the regulation of certain hormones,

> **5**
>
> Obesity is a complex disorder with multiple contributing factors.

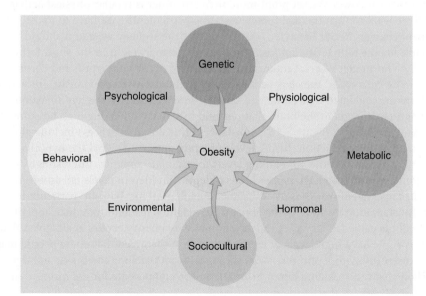

FIGURE 8.17 Multiple Factors Contribute to Obesity. There is no one cause of obesity.

which may affect appetite and contribute to obesity. Several genes have been identified as contributors to obesity, and researchers at the CDC are constructing a human obesity gene map in the hope of finding genetic targets in humans that may lead to the development of new treatments (CDC, 2012a). These genetic discoveries related to obesity are particularly promising for a better understanding of obesity in some individuals who have a genetic tendency to gain weight and store fat.

Although some people may have genes that permit them to become obese, it still is their environment that determines whether they actually do become obese. In other words, while recognizing that genetic differences may predispose an individual toward obesity, it is important to understand that these differences can be overcome by changes in the environment, such as the person being physically active and eating right. So, despite obesity having strong genetic determinants, the genetic composition of the population cannot change rapidly; therefore, the large increase in obesity in our current population must reflect changes in other factors.

Interest in the physiological factors related to obesity focuses on the **set point theory**, which proposes that a regulatory system exists in the human body that is designed to maintain body weight at some fixed level. Similar to other regulated physiological variables in the body (e.g., blood glucose, body temperature) that are maintained within certain limits, the body seeks to protect against pressures to be too heavy or too thin. The level of the body's fat stores is thought to be determined by a mechanism in the brain called the **adipostat**. The adipostat establishes a set point for a fixed amount of body fat just as a thermostat regulates heat according to a preset temperature. The brain maintains this set point by regulating the expenditure or storage of energy until fat stores meet the level determined by the adipostat. A set point above the ideal healthy weight presents a difficult struggle for the obese individual. Unknown to the person who has been diligently dieting, the brain is busily undermining the efforts by working to restore weight to the set point. The adipostat may do this by activating the sensation for hunger so that more calories are consumed or by slowing the metabolism.

Just because our body aggressively maintains a stable amount of body fat at a target level doesn't mean the target level can't be changed. Many health scientists believe that the set point can be changed. If we go back to the analogy of the thermostat, they are saying that the "body fat thermostat" has a dial, and we can turn the dial to a new setting by fine-tuning our lifestyle. The dial of the thermostat is turned by a combination of the type and amount of physical activity we do, the levels of nutrients we eat, and the amount of stress we have in our lives. The lifestyle factor that can lower the set point more than any other is regular physical activity. So, if we want to turn the dial to a new setting permanently, we have to make permanent changes in our lifestyle. This means that the strategy we adopt should be suitable for the long term, not just a strategy for losing weight in the short term.

Two hormones of great interest in the study of obesity are leptin and cortisol. A gene in fat cells called the *ob* gene makes leptin. As discussed previously, our eating patterns are regulated by feeding and satiety centers located in the hypothalamus and pituitary glands in the brain that respond to signals indicating high fat stores and hunger (refer to Figure 8.15). Substances critical to this process include glucose (sugar), insulin, and leptin. Rising levels of leptin appear to signal the hypothalamus to suppress appetite, and falling levels to stimulate appetite. Interestingly, overweight people tend to have higher levels of leptin, and leptin levels fall as weight is lost. This system works as a self-balancing biological mechanism, particularly to prevent starvation by stimulating appetite as weight is lost and to reduce appetite as weight is gained. This raises the question of why obesity occurs at all, given that obese people have high levels of leptin. It has been theorized that obese people may have insensitivity to leptin that stops the signal from reaching the brain, and that the body is overproducing leptin in an attempt to compensate for the insensitivity.

Set point theory A theory that proposes that a regulatory system exists in the human body that is designed to maintain body weight at some fixed level.

Adipostat Brain mechanism that establishes a set point for a fixed amount of body fat.

Cortisol is a hormone produced by the adrenal gland when the body is under stress. Your hypothalamus, via the pituitary gland, directs the adrenal glands to secrete cortisol. Cortisol is released as part of your daily hormonal cycle but can also be released in greater amounts in reaction to acute and chronic stressors—both physical and emotional—as part of the body's fight-or-flight response that is essential for survival. One of the functions of cortisol is to trigger a glucocorticoid effect—helping the body produce blood sugar from proteins. Excess glucose is then used for lipogenesis (fat production). A number of studies have examined the release of cortisol during acute and chronic stress and the physiological effects that this hormone has on the body, especially how it contributes to the deposition of visceral fat, particularly in the abdominal region (Scott, Melhorn, & Sakai, 2012). Many health experts have linked oversecretion of cortisol with obesity and increased fat storage in the body.

Cortisol is thought to affect weight gain and metabolism in a number of ways. Being an inbuilt defense mechanism (fight-or-flight response), it temporarily shuts down certain bodily functions and activates others to deal with the emergency situation. It also increases appetite. Most overweight people can attest to an understanding of "comfort eating" and resultant weight gain during times of stress. It is an evolutionary response to make a person eat, particularly something sweet, to urgently boost blood glucose levels for the energy to either fight or fly from a stressful situation. Similarly, it shuts down or significantly slows down your metabolic rate as your body seeks to preserve its energy supplies. The effect on weight gain from those two factors is obvious. Although it may be possible for a person to have malfunctioning adrenal glands that simply overproduce cortisol, in most cases the real solution is to practice various relaxation and stress-releasing activities or eliminate sources of ongoing stress.

Most cases of obesity occur now in people with normal physiology who live in a sociocultural environment characterized by a sedentary lifestyle and ready access to abundant food. Eating foods high in calories and low in nutrients is common in our daily diets. Food manufacturers know how taste, smell, and texture increase the human appetite, and they engineer food accordingly (Robbins & Nestle, 2011). The increased availability of convenience foods, changes in food preparation, and eating out more often are additional factors that contribute to overeating among Americans and are major contributing factors to Americans consuming 570 more calories a day than they were only a few decades ago (Duffey & Popkin, 2011). A chief culprit behind the calorie increase is calories from sugar-sweetened soft drinks.

In conjunction with an increase in energy consumption is a concurrent decrease in energy expenditure. Everyone who leads a sedentary lifestyle is at risk for obesity. Systematic survey trend data collected over the last couple of decades regularly indicate that the majority of adults are not engaging in the recommended amount of physical activity. Thus, this provides evidence that reduced physical activity, and subsequent decrease in energy expenditure, is a potentially important contributor to obesity.

A sedentary lifestyle and obesity play against each other in a no-win game; that is, lack of physical activity contributes to fat gain, and fat gain makes it more difficult to be physically active. The tendency in the United States is toward an unhealthy weight gain with age. As you age, bone and muscle mass tend to decrease. A sedentary lifestyle accelerates the problem of bone and muscle loss. All physical activity involves muscular movement that requires the expenditure of calories and contributes to lean-tissue maintenance (**FIGURE 8.18**). In other words, body fatness is responsible not only for general weight gain in sedentary individuals, but also for making up more of the lean weight they may have once had.

To summarize, the increased prevalence of overweight and obesity in the United States is largely attributed to an increased consumption of energy-dense and low-nutrient food, which is simultaneously flavorful, pleasurable, and accessible, and a decreased level of caloric expenditure resulting from a sedentary lifestyle. This increase in energy intake and decrease in energy expenditure leads to an unbalancing of the energy equation (refer to Figure 8.14).

A Lifestyle Approach to Achieving and Maintaining a Healthy Weight

A lifestyle approach to weight maintenance focuses on developing a lifelong commitment to a way of life that achieves and maintains a healthy body composition relative to physical and psychological functioning. The most important components in this approach are regular physical activity and eating a healthy nutritious diet. By focusing on these two major components, you will be able to avoid the effects of creeping obesity or the negative consequences of repeated weight gains and losses. You may be currently at a healthy weight; if you are and have a low risk of obesity-related diseases, you ought to read the following as a way to prevent weight gain in the future. If you may be overweight or at risk for an obesity-related condition, and you are ready to make a change, the following will provide essential information to assist you with initial fat loss and maintenance of this loss in the long term. Remember that small victories in weight loss—often as little as 10 percent of total body mass—can result in positive effects on health and well-being, even if an ideal weight remains elusive.

Using the Energy Balance Equation

DETERMINING YOUR ENERGY BALANCE EQUATION   An objective assessment of your average daily energy intake and energy expenditure provides the basis for *unbalancing* the energy equation. To determine your average daily calorie intake, keep a careful daily food intake record. When it comes to healthy eating, it's what you take in over a number of days that counts, not just one day. Withhold judgment regarding your diet until a week's worth of recording food intake has been completed. By avoiding early analysis, you can learn much about your individuality related to your food habits, which is an important aspect of the evaluation process. In addition, your food intake record will provide a more accurate picture of your average daily caloric and nutrient intake. At the same time you are recording your caloric intake you should be recording your daily caloric expenditure. Again, avoid analysis of your daily caloric energy expenditure activities until a week has passed. After determining this important baseline information, you will be able to proceed to develop an effective strategy to achieve a negative energy balance.

UNBALANCING THE ENERGY EQUATION   The best way to create a negative energy balance is through a combination of reduced caloric intake and increased caloric expenditure. The recommended amount of fat loss in a week is 1 pound. This is best accomplished by creating a 3500 weekly calorie deficit or 500 daily calorie deficit (remember, 1 pound of fat equals 3500 calories). Generally, you do not want to attempt to shed more than 1 pound of body fat per week. Increasing the weekly energy deficit above 3500 calories could cause a significant loss of muscle tissue and be counterproductive to your body composition goal of losing body fat. As discussed earlier, although either lowering your caloric intake (dietary modification) or increasing energy expenditure (exercise modification) can be

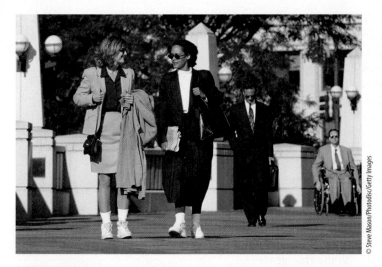

© Steve Mason/Photodisc/Getty Images

FIGURE 8.18 **Get in the Habit.** Regular movement is a good way to burn calories.

A lifestyle approach that includes regular physical activity and a nutritious diet is essential in achieving and maintaining a healthy weight.

effective independently in obtaining the recommended 3500 weekly calorie deficit, a combination of the two produces the best results. In other words, reducing daily caloric intake by 250 calories and increasing daily physical activity by 250 calories will generally produce the best results. As you will discover in the next sections, the advantages of one technique counterbalance the disadvantages of the other. For example, caloric restriction produces a rapid reduction of resting metabolic rate, substantially decreasing energy expenditure, whereas exercise increases resting metabolic rate, thereby negating the dietary effects.

It is important to note that you will not necessarily get bigger using an exercise program when trying to lose fat. For example, if you are losing fat weight through a healthful combination of exercising and eating nutritiously, your actual overall weight may stay constant even as you get leaner and smaller. Why? Because fat loss and muscle gain may occur together. Muscle is much more compact and dense than fat. It actually takes up less space than fat does because of that. That makes sense, right? Fat, on the other hand, is very soft and jelly-like and is a lot less dense than muscle. That means it takes up more space than muscle does. So, although your dress size or pant size may drop, your weight may not.

This lifestyle intervention strategy for fat loss is built on the sound premise that individuals can modify their own behaviors related to managing and maintaining a focus on healthy eating and increased physical activity. However, it is often difficult to motivate people with this sound physiological approach to losing 1 pound of fat per week when they read or hear about such quick fixes as "lose 10 pounds in 1 week" or "lose 30 pounds in 1 month." These ads may lead people to abandon basic fat-loss principles. Rather than defining success solely in terms of general weight loss, a more fitting focus would be on shedding excess body fatness that increases your overall health risk. Any plan to shed excess body fat should include strategies for maintaining or enhancing the level of lean body tissues to provide a more healthy weight. This approach requires a thorough understanding of body fatness and health. This pattern of thinking is consistent with an emphasis on a lifestyle approach that is sustainable and enjoyable.

Physical Activity and Fat Loss

Physical activity is one of the most important components of any fat-loss program (FIGURE 8.19). In addition, accumulated evidence shows that physical activity is the best predictor for achieving and maintaining weight loss (Stehr & von Lengerke, 2012). Therefore, describing the benefits of physical activity related to fat loss and maintenance can provide added incentives to become, or stay, physically active.

PHYSICAL ACTIVITY BURNS CALORIES The immediate function of physical activity in a fat-loss program is simply to increase the level of energy expenditure—helping to unbalance the caloric equation so that there is a greater amount of energy output. Physical activity is the most important way to increase the calories you burn. The calorie-expending effects of physical activity are cumulative and substantial. This means that even mild to moderate increases in physical activity can be beneficial. For example, 40 to 60 minutes of walking expends approximately 350 calories. Performing this activity five times a week would contribute to 1750 calories expended or shedding half a pound of fat. Increasing the intensity or

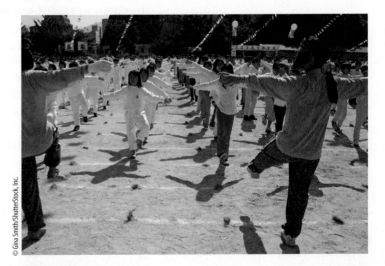

© Gina Smith/ShutterStock, Inc.

FIGURE 8.19 **Opportunities Are Endless.** Physical activity of any kind is generally considered the most important component in a fat-loss program.

duration of physical activity (or participating in a formal exercise program) can further increase the number of calories burned.

PHYSICAL ACTIVITY AMELIORATES OBESITY-ASSOCIATED DISEASES
Physical activity benefits your health even if you don't lose weight. Physical activity has positive effects on blood pressure, blood fat levels, and insulin insensitivity (type 2 diabetes), independent of those produced by weight loss alone.

PHYSICAL ACTIVITY LEADS TO "WAIST LOSS"
Physical activity is the best modifier of visceral fat. Research demonstrates that physical inactivity leads to a significant increase in this potentially dangerous fat, whereas regular amounts of physical activity can lead to significant decreases in such fat over a fairly short time period (Flint et al., 2010). Maintaining a normal waistline by adopting a regular physical activity program and a moderate eating plan helps you avoid midriff weight gain (the apple shape), which puts you at greater risk for diabetes and heart disease.

PHYSICAL ACTIVITY COMPENSATES FOR RMR DECLINE
A well-documented change that occurs during dietary restriction of calories is a considerable reduction in resting metabolic rate. This decline can reach up to 40 percent of RMR after a brief time, significantly reducing overall calorie expenditure by the body. Physical activity increases the metabolic rate both during activity and afterward.

PHYSICAL ACTIVITY MINIMIZES LOSS OF LEAN BODY MASS
Muscle is metabolically active—it requires calories. The more muscle you have, the more calories you need to sustain it, and the more calories you can eat and still lose weight. The use of physical activity in a weight loss program provides protection against a loss of lean tissue routinely seen with diet-only weight loss programs. Aerobic and weight-resistance activities contribute to the conservation of lean tissue in different ways. Aerobic physical activities utilize the oxygen energy system that requires the mobilization and metabolism of the body's fat storage. Weight-resistance activities (weight training) burn calories as well. In addition, weight-resistance activities help stimulate muscular development, preventing significant losses of lean body tissue that generally occur during calorie-restricting diets.

PHYSICAL ACTIVITY SUPPRESSES APPETITE
To some degree, regular physical activity appears to contribute to the normal functioning of the brain's feeding control mechanisms. A sensitive balance between energy expenditure and food intake is apparently not maintained very well in physically inactive people. This lack of precision in regulating food intake may account for some of the increasing obesity observed in the United States (Caudwell et al., 2011). Individuals who are regularly physical active are better able to match daily energy intake with daily expenditure.

PHYSICAL ACTIVITY CAN LOWER SET POINT
The set point theory proposes that a regulatory system exists in the human body that maintains body weight at some fixed level. Instead of a simply genetic determination, set point is now believed to be under control of environmental factors. The environmental factor that can lower set point more than any other is regular, sustained physical activity (Farias, Cuevas, & Rodriguez, 2011). A lower set point can make maintaining a lower percentage of body fat much easier.

PHYSICAL ACTIVITY IMPROVES PSYCHOLOGICAL WELL-BEING
A weight problem or poor body image may contribute to lower self-esteem, guilt, depression, anxiety, and distress. Physical activity can enhance self-esteem and reduce

depression, anxiety, and stress through both physiological and psychological mechanisms. Increased psychological well-being can enhance compliance with a weight loss program as well as helping you to cope with societal pressure.

As you can see, physical activity plays an integral role in a healthy weight loss program. Another key component is healthy eating.

Healthy Eating and Fat Loss

The foundation for any healthy eating plan for fat loss should be built from the *Dietary Guidelines for Americans* and the MyPlate food guidance system. To incorporate their guidelines into a fat-loss program, you must pay particular attention to serving size and to choosing mainly nutrient-dense foods.

FOOD INTAKE MODIFICATION   Using your estimated daily caloric intake, develop a daily caloric plan that reduces your calories by 250 each day. (Avoid daily caloric restriction plans of 1200 calories or less.) As for the diet itself, the cornerstone of any meal plan should be MyPlate, which builds upon and complements the *Dietary Guidelines*. MyPlate recommends a variety of foods, with a notable emphasis on grains, fruits, and vegetables. Moreover, it helps you establish a tolerable, enjoyable, and stable eating pattern that is consistent with a healthy lifestyle approach to fat loss. Finally, the *Dietary Guidelines* advocates the moderation of fat, sugar, and alcohol consumption, all of which are important in weight loss.

Although not designed to be calorie-specific management tools, both MyPlate and the *Dietary Guidelines* are relevant and valuable tools for healthy menu planning related to body fat loss. You just need to pay special attention to the serving size and select nutrient-dense foods.

You can easily choose foods with a high nutrient–calorie benefit ratio by focusing on natural and unrefined foods from the food groups. Avoid refined and processed foods (refined sugar) as much as possible. Because you are encouraged to participate in a regular physical activity program, it is important to maintain an acceptable macronutrient distribution range composed of 45 to 65 percent of your total calories from carbohydrates (preferably complex carbohydrates), 20 to 25 percent from protein, and 10 to 20 percent from fat. Dietary fat is not a terrible thing, but when you are limiting your calories, as on a fat-loss program, the calories are better spent on carbohydrates (to fuel your activity) and protein (to maintain your muscle tissue). Research has shown that, during negative energy balance, slightly more protein (0.5 to 0.7 grams per pound of body weight) is required to maintain muscle mass. Finally, sources of complex carbohydrates, such as grain products and vegetables, not only allow you to feel energetic for longer periods of time, but also are generally higher in other important nutrients.

EATING STYLE MODIFICATION   Obesity is as much a result of how we eat as it is of what we eat. Although what we eat contributes to our fat-loss efforts, so do our eating styles. Eating styles can be hard to change. Correcting problem areas will make a big difference in your success with fat loss. Therefore, it is important to evaluate your eating styles.

EMOTIONAL EATING   One of the primary reasons for keeping a food diary is to have a written record of your moods and the events occurring just prior to eating. How you feel and what's going on around you before you eat are significant; our emotions strongly influence our eating behavior. By keeping an accurate food diary that includes this information, your eating style will become more visible to you. This may include eating when you are stressed or depressed. Once you become aware of the precursors causing unnecessary eating behaviors, you can make a conscious effort to avoid them.

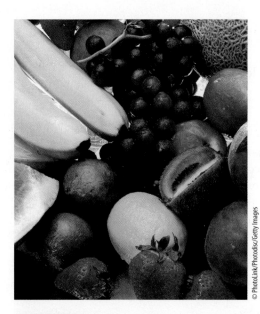

© PhotoLink/Photodisc/Getty Images

FIGURE 8.20 **Rethink Snacks.** Fruits and vegetables make excellent snacks for either maintaining or losing weight.

Body image The picture you have of your body, what it looks like to you, and how you think it looks to others.

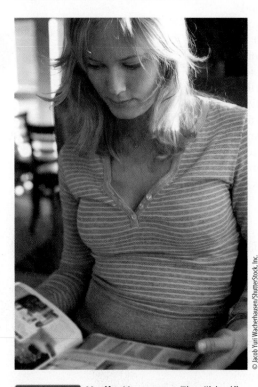

© Jacob Yuri Wacherhausen/ShutterStock, Inc.

FIGURE 8.21 **Media Messages.** The "ideal" body promoted by the fashion industry may influence distorted images in individuals, especially women.

FOCUS ON BODY FAT, NOT WEIGHT   Do not build everything around "losing weight." Too many people focus their dietary restriction program on weight loss and not fat loss. They get up every day and check their weight on the scale. They are depressed if they did not lose anything and elated if they lost weight. You want to focus on losing body fat. You could lose weight and get fatter if you are dieting incorrectly! What matters is your level of body fatness, not your weight.

EAT SMALLER, MORE FREQUENT MEALS   Do not skip meals or go more than 3 to 4 hours without eating. Skipping a meal often leads to bingeing at the next meal, which initiates an up-and-down energy and nutrient pattern. When meals are more than 6 hours apart, plan strategic healthy snacks. You can obtain many nutrients, and energy, by choosing your snacks wisely and eating them in moderation. Include fresh fruits and vegetables and avoid cookies, candies, ice cream, and potato chips (FIGURE 8.20).

EAT SLOWLY   You will probably overeat if you eat too quickly. It takes about 20 to 30 minutes for your stomach to signal the brain that you are full. Put your eating utensil down between bites and chew your food thoroughly.

Body Image and Weight

Most of us are well aware of how much we weigh, and we typically equate our weight with our body image or appearance. **Body image** is the picture you have of your body, what it looks like to you, and how you think it looks to others. This image can be accurate or inaccurate and is often subject to change. The relationship between body image and weight is complicated.

Although you may have a perception of an ideal body weight for appearance, this ideal body weight may or may not be in accord with optimal health. Most research effort has attempted to find an ideal body weight for reducing the risk of disease. An increasing number of Americans, however, attempt to achieve an unrealistic weight and shape based on the fashion industry's ideal body. This "ideal" standard is one of extreme thinness for females and exaggerated muscularity for males. These so-called ideals have been created by the fashion and advertising industry to sell products. For people who try to live up to this standard of "perfection," the defining characteristic for ideal weight and size is perceived body image.

You should not attempt to base your weight or shape on our society's glamour approach. Choosing unrealistic weight loss goals in response to societal ideals can set you up for failure and perpetuate unhealthy choices (FIGURE 8.21). To improve body image, as well as self-esteem, it is important to learn to like ourselves and to take care of ourselves through healthy lifestyle choices that do not emphasize weight loss at the expense of psychological and physical health.

Unfortunately, some people become so focused on their image and body weight that they feel pressured to match the "ideal" portrayed in magazines and on television. This can lead to major discontent with body weight. A negative sign of dissatisfaction with body weight, when basing it on the "ideal" weight portrayed by the mass media, is the development of eating disorders. The term **eating disorder** refers to a wide range of harmful eating behaviors used in an attempt to lose weight or achieve a thin appearance. These dangerous behaviors range from severe restriction of food intake to binge eating and purging.

Eating disorder patterns are far-reaching, affecting more than 7 million women and approximately 1 million men in the United States (National Institute of Mental Health, 2011). Nearly 90 percent of these destructive eating patterns begin before the age of 20, with the majority lasting anywhere from 1 to 15 years. Eating disorders are not the result of a failure of will or behavior; rather, they are real, treatable medical illnesses in which certain maladaptive patterns of eating take on a life of their own. Without treatment, up to 20 percent of people with serious eating disorders die. With treatment, that number falls drastically to 2 to 3 percent. With proper treatment, about 60 percent of people with eating disorders recover. They maintain a healthy weight and feel stronger and more positive about life in general. Anorexia nervosa and bulimia nervosa are the two most severe forms of eating disorders (TABLE 8.6).

Anorexia Nervosa

Anorexia nervosa literally means "loss of appetite." This definition is misleading, in that a person with anorexia nervosa becomes hungry but repudiates the hunger because of an irrational fear of eating and becoming fat. Anorexia nervosa is characterized by a distorted body image, self-starvation, and extreme weight loss.

Because of extreme weight loss, females with anorexia nervosa often suffer from a lack of menstrual periods (amenorrhea) because they have too little body fat. Furthermore, excessive weight loss increases rates of bone loss (osteoporosis), muscle loss, and dehydration. When body fat is severely limited and muscle tissue is lost, the body turns to its organs in a critical search for energy, and the vicious cycle of wasting away continues. Victims lose the ability to function effectively and put themselves in a life-threatening physical condition.

Bulimia Nervosa

Bulimia means to "eat like an ox." Bulimia nervosa is characterized by uncontrollable cycles of binge eating followed by purging through forced vomiting or the abuse of laxatives and diuretics. During a binge, individuals lose control over their eating and may quickly consume large amounts of food—up to 20,000 calories in

Eating disorder Refers to a wide range of harmful eating behaviors used in the attempt to lose weight or achieve a lean appearance.

A negative sign of dissatisfaction with body weight, when basing it on the "ideal" weight portrayed by the mass media, is the development of eating disorders.

TABLE 8.6	Anorexia Nervosa and Bulimia Nervosa Symptoms

Anorexia Nervosa Signs and Symptoms
Anorexia nervosa is characterized by:

- Extreme thinness (emaciation)
- A relentless pursuit of thinness and unwillingness to maintain a normal or healthy weight
- Intense fear of gaining weight
- Distorted body image, a self-esteem that is heavily influenced by perceptions of body weight and shape, or a denial of the seriousness of low body weight
- Lack of menstruation among girls and women
- Extremely restricted eating

Bulimia Nervosa Signs and Symptoms
Bulimia nervosa is characterized by:

- Recurrent and frequent episodes of eating unusually large amounts of food
- Feeling a lack of control over these episodes
- Binge eating followed by behavior that compensates for the overeating such as forced vomiting, excessive use of laxatives or diuretics, fasting, excessive exercise, or a combination of these behaviors
- Chronically inflamed and sore throat
- Swollen salivary glands in the neck and jaw area

SOURCE: Modified from National Institute of Mental Health. (2011). *Eating Disorders* (NIH Publication No. 11-4901). Washington, DC: U.S. Department of Health and Human Services.

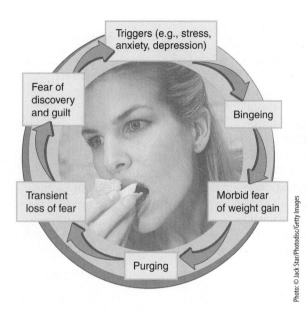

Photo: © Jack Star/Photodisc/Getty Images

FIGURE 8.22 The Binge–Purge Cycle of Bulimia.

a single binge. Bulimic individuals are afraid of being fat and follow the binge with efforts to redress uncontrolled eating by purging the food from their bodies or by fasting (FIGURE 8.22).

The person suffering from bulimia nervosa is usually in a normal weight range but may suffer from weight fluctuations of 10 or more pounds over short periods of time resulting from alternating binges and purging/fasting. This binge–purge cycle puts a tremendous strain on the body. In repeated vomiting, the stomach acid can erode tooth enamel and even the esophagus. Additionally, nutrient deficiencies may occur from vomiting and the use of laxatives.

Compulsive Overeating

Compulsive eaters or those with binge eating disorder are similar to those with bulimia nervosa in that they may eat large amounts of food in a short period of time and exhibit a lack of control regarding their eating. However, compulsive eaters do not purge, and thus they usually become obese, thereby encountering all the health risks of obesity. They may eat continually throughout the day as a means to cope with stress and other emotional issues.

Compulsive Exercising

With an eating disorder, too much exercise, or compulsive exercising, is just another outlet of behavior. Those who have symptoms of compulsive exercising usually have episodes of repeated exercising beyond the requirements of what is considered safe. They will find time at any cost to exercise (including cutting classes and taking off from work) and will work out for hours. The main goal of exercise usually is to burn calories and relieve the guilt from just having eaten or binged, or to give themselves permission to eat ("I can't eat unless I have exercised or know I will exercise"). Compulsive exercise is another way to purge, and afflicted individuals use exercise as another way to cope with their emotions and anxiety about their weight.

Female Athlete Triad

The female athlete triad, or simply the triad, is a combination of three coexistent conditions: disordered eating, amenorrhea, and osteoporosis. The depiction of the triad as a triangle was developed to demonstrate the interrelationship among the three disorders normally considered independent medical conditions (FIGURE 8.23). Alone or in combination, triad disorders can reduce physical performance and have serious medical and psychological consequences.

The triad is most associated with physically active girls and women as well as elite athletes. Females who are most susceptible are those who reach and maintain unrealistically low levels of body weight or body fat or both. The same inner and societal pressures that contribute to the development of eating disorders help initiate the triad. Additional factors that are specific to athletes include sport-related emphasis on body weight and body fat, perfectionism, lack of nutrition knowledge, the drive to excel at any cost, and pressure to lose weight from coaches, judges, and significant others.

Treatment for Eating Disorders

The treatments for disordered eating patterns are complex and most often require professional help. Anorexia nervosa treatment, depending on the duration of the illness, generally begins with medical treatment to address the physical destruction

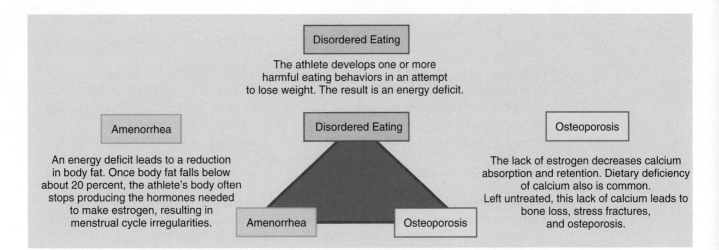

FIGURE 8.23 **The Female Athlete Triad.** The depiction of the triad as a triangle demonstrates the interrelationship among the three disorders normally considered independent conditions.

and to restore the body to a sufficient weight. This generally requires hospitalization. Once health is stabilized, the psychological factors underlying the anorexia nervosa need to be addressed through psychotherapy.

Initial treatment for bulimia nervosa or compulsive eating disorders involves the elimination of the eating pattern. Unlike anorexia nervosa, most bulimia nervosa and compulsive eating disorders do not require hospitalization. They do, however, require professional assistance to uncover the system of thinking that led to the disordered eating. Changing the thinking pattern is necessary for successful treatment.

Self-help and support groups are extremely beneficial adjuncts to treatment by professionals. Family, friends, and support groups all play an important role in helping the person with disordered eating to start and maintain a treatment program.

Physical Activity and Health Connection

Healthy weight management includes a lifelong commitment to a healthy lifestyle. Two elements involved in attaining and maintaining a healthy body weight are eating a nutritious diet and performing regular physical activity. Adequate nutrition and decreased calorie intake are important goals of diet modification for decreasing body fatness. Sufficient physical activity is equally important because it expends excessive fat storage and enhances lean body mass. Moreover, physical activity offsets the harmful effects of a number of morbid conditions that are attributed to excessive body fat storage. The goals of physical activity related to achieving and maintaining a healthy body weight should be based on activities that are enjoyable and can be performed consistently.

concept connections

1 **Achieving and maintaining a healthy body weight has been identified as a major public health challenge in the United States.** Data show that based on the weight-for-height standards developed by the National Institutes of Health (NIH), two-thirds of adult Americans are now overweight, and that number continues to rise. These prevalence rates raise fear because of their implications for Americans' health. According to the NIH and the Centers for Disease Control and Prevention, being overweight or obese increases an individual's risk for developing more than 35 major diseases.

2 **The body mass index (BMI) uses weight and height to produce a number that enables health professionals to gauge risk of weight-related illnesses.** The BMI criterion standards recommended by the National Heart, Lung, and Blood Institute Expert Panel on the Identification, Evaluation, and Treatment of Overweight and Obesity in Adults are as follows: underweight, BMI less than 18.5; normal or healthy weight, BMI of 18.5 to 24.99; overweight or preobesity, BMI of 25.0 to 29.99; and class 1, 2, and 3 obesity, BMI of 30 to 34.99, 35 to 39.99, and 40.0 or greater, respectively. An adult BMI under 18.5 or greater than 25.0 may indicate health risk.

3 **Individuals with more abdominal body fat have a more adverse metabolic profile and an increased risk for type 2 diabetes and cardiovascular disease.** Many scientists theorize that excess visceral fat is harmful because of its location near the portal vein, which carries blood from the intestinal area to the liver. Hormones and other substances released by visceral fat, including free fatty acids, enter the portal vein and travel to the liver, where they can influence the production of blood lipids. Visceral fat is directly linked with higher triglycerides, total cholesterol, LDL (bad) cholesterol, and lower HDL (good) cholesterol.

4 **A body composition analysis allows for the assessment of the percentage of fat versus the percentage of fat-free tissue.** Knowing your body composition brings additional information to the screening profile. When body fat percentage is used in conjunction with BMI, it can help differentiate people who are overweight because of lean body mass from those who are overweight because of fat. Most important, the percentage of fat assists in predicting health risk. An ideal body fat percentage is one that meets your body's fundamental need for normal physiological functioning and energy but does not create health risks.

5 **Obesity is a complex disorder with multiple contributing factors.** There is no one cause of obesity. However, most cases of obesity occur now in people with normal physiology who live in a sociocultural environment characterized by a sedentary lifestyle and ready access to abundant food.

6 **A lifestyle approach that includes regular physical activity and a nutritious diet is essential in achieving and maintaining a healthy weight.** A lifestyle approach to weight maintenance focuses on developing a lifelong commitment to a way of life that achieves and maintains a healthy body composition relative to physical and psychological functioning. This approach requires a lifelong commitment to healthful behaviors that emphasize eating practices and regular physical activities that are sustainable and enjoyable. The goal of maintaining weight through lifestyle efforts is desirable for good physical and psychological health and to avoid the effects of creeping obesity or the negative consequences of repeated weight gains and losses.

7 **A negative sign of dissatisfaction with body weight, when basing it on the "ideal" weight portrayed by the mass media, is the development of eating disorders.** The term *eating disorders* refers to a wide range of harmful eating behaviors used in an attempt to lose weight or achieve a thin appearance. These dangerous behaviors range from severe restriction of food intake to binge eating and purging.

Terms

Adipostat, 186
Bioelectrical impedance, 180
Body image, 192
Eating disorder, 193
Essential body fat, 178
Obesity, 170
Omentum, 174

Overweight, 170
Set point theory, 186
Skinfold technique, 180
Storage fat, 179
Thermic effect of activity (TEA), 184

Thermic effect of food (TEF), 184
Underwater weighing, 180
Visceral fat, 174

making the connection

Leah realizes that what is important is not a weight based on her self-image, but a weight based on healthy physical and psychological functioning. In recognizing these important differences she decides to have a body composition assessment completed. She schedules an appointment with the university wellness center, choosing the skinfold technique. Furthermore, she decides to make an appointment to discuss her self-image with the university's counseling center.

Critical Thinking

1. From the vignette, how would you assess Leah's preoccupation with her weight? What factors influence her concerns about her weight? Do you believe she has an unhealthy obsession with her weight?

2. On your campus, identify and briefly describe the resources available for students regarding healthy weight management and eating disorders.

3. Your housemate, Joan, goes on a new fad diet that was recently reported by a respected national morning TV show. Joan reports that this new diet will allow her to lose 10 pounds by Saturday (6 days from now). Explain to Joan why this fad diet will not work, and if she were to lose the 10 pounds in 6 days, what would likely happen.

4. As a residence hall assistant (RA) you have been asked by your floor to talk about obesity and how as college freshmen they can manage their weight sensibly. In your talk discuss healthy weight, overweight and obesity, body mass index, and the importance of good nutrition and physical activity.

References

American Dietetic Association. (2009). Position of the American Dietetic Association, Dietitians of Canada, and the American College of Sports Medicine: Nutrition and Athletic Performance. *Journal of the American Dietetic Association* 109:509–527.

Aprovian, C.M. (2010). The causes, prevalence, and treatment of obesity revisited in 2009. *American Journal of Clinical Nutrition* 91(1):277S–279S

Caudwell, P., Gibbons, C., Hopkins, M., Naslund, E., King, N., Finlayson, G., & Blundell, J. (2011). The influence of physical activity on appetite control: An experimental system to understand the relationship between exercise-induced energy expenditure and energy intake. *Proceedings of the Nutrition Society* 70(2):171–180.

Centers for Disease Control and Prevention. (2012a). Obesity and genetics: A public health perspective. Online: http://www.cdc.gov/genomics/resources/diseases/obesity/index.htm.

Centers for Disease Control and Prevention. (2012b). Overweight and obesity: Causes and consequences. Online: http://www.cdc.gov/obesity/causes/health.html.

Centers for Disease Control and Prevention. (2012c). U.S. obesity trends 1985–2010. Online: http://www.cdc.gov/obesity/data/trends.html.

Duffey, K.J., & Popkin, B.M. (2011). Energy density, portion size, and eating occasions: Contributions to increased energy intake in the United States, 1977–2006. *PLoS Medicine* 8(6):e1–e8.

Farias, M., Cuevas, A., & Rodriguez, F. (2011). Set-point theory and obesity. *Metabolic Syndrome and Related Disorders* 9(2):e1–e8.

Finkelstein, E.A., Trogdon, J.G., Cohen, J.W., & Dietz, W. (2009). Annual medical spending attributable to obesity: Payer- and service-specific estimates. *Health Affairs* 28:822–831.

Flegal, K.M., Graubard, B.I., Williamson, D.F., & Gail, M.H. (2010). Sources of differences in estimates of obesity-associated deaths from the first National Health and Nutrition Survey (NHANES I) hazard ratios. *American Journal of Clinical Nutrition* 91:519–527.

Flint, A., Rexrode, K., Hu, F., Glynn, R., Caspard, H., Manson, J., Willett, W., & Rimm, E. (2010). Body mass index, waist circumference, and risk of coronary heart disease: A prospective study among men and women. *Obesity Research and Clinical Practice* 4(3):e171–e181.

Jia, H., & Lubetkin, E.L. (2010). Trends in quality-adjusted life-years lost contributed by smoking and obesity: Does the burden of obesity overweight the burden of smoking? *American Journal of Preventive Medicine* 38(2):138–144.

Markey, C. (2010). Why body image is important to adolescent development. *Journal of Youth and Adolescence* 39(12):1387–1391.

National Heart, Lung, and Blood Institute. (2000). *The Practical Guide, Identification, Evaluation, and Treatment of Overweight and Obesity in Adults* (NIH Publication No. 00-4084). Washington, DC: U.S. Department of Health and Human Services.

National Institute of Mental Health. (2011). *Eating Disorders* (NIH Publication No. 11-4901). Washington, DC: U.S. Department of Health and Human Services.

Puhl, R.M., & Heuer, C.A. (2009). The stigma of obesity: A review and update. *Obesity* 17:941–964.

Puhl, R.M., Heuer, C.A., & Brownell, K.D. (2010). Stigma and social consequences of obesity. In Kopelman, P.G., Caterson, I.D., & Dietz, W.H., eds. *Clinical Obesity in Adults and Children*, 3rd ed. Oxford, UK: Wiley-Blackwell. doi: 10.1002/9781444307627.ch3.

Robbins, A., & Nestle, M. (2011). Obesity as collateral damage: A call for papers on the obesity epidemic. *Journal of Public Health Policy* 32:143–145.

Scott, K., Melhorn, S., & Sakai, R. (2012). Effects of chronic social stress on obesity. *Current Obesity Reports* 1(1):16–25.

Stehr, M., & von Lengerke, T. (2012). Preventing weight gain through exercise and physical activity in the elderly: A systematic review. *Maturitas* 71(2):115–121.

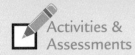

© zulufoto/ShutterStock, Inc.

Achieving Optimal Bone Health

what's the connection?

Julie is a sophomore in college and is concerned about her skeletal health. Her biggest concern is developing osteoporosis, a chronic metabolic disease that causes excessive skeletal weakness and increases her chance for developing bone fractures later in life. Julie watched her grandmother suffer from a broken hip as a result of osteoporosis and therefore is quite aware of its crippling effects. Julie pays close attention to her diet, making sure to fulfill her daily requirements of calcium and vitamin D. Moreover, she has recently been reading about the importance of physical activity and its role in preventing osteoporosis. Julie is interested in "making the connection" by beginning a safe and effective physical activity program to build and maintain a strong skeletal system.

concepts

1. Bones do more than provide structural support; they protect vital organs and support essential metabolic processes.

2. Three types of cells are involved in bone formation and resorption: osteoblasts, osteocytes, and osteoclasts.

3. To maintain bone mass, bone formation must occur at the same rate as bone resorption.

4. Physical activity enhances bone density through both weight-bearing and resistance-training exercises.

5. Osteoporosis is a chronic disease process characterized by progressive bone loss in both males and females.

6. Osteoporosis can be affected by genetic, hormonal, nutritional, and lifestyle factors.

go.jblearning.com/kotecki4e
The website for this book is a great source for supplementary physical health information for both students and instructors. Visit **go.jblearning.com/kotecki4e** to find a variety of useful tools for learning, thinking, and teaching.

Your bones are for life. Look after them and they will carry you far.
—Susan Hampshir

Introduction

Bones play many roles in the body. They provide structure, protect organs, anchor muscles, and store calcium. Each of these roles is a necessary contributor to a healthy and active life. To live well, we must strive to maintain optimal bone health. Like many of our body's tissues, the bones can be affected by disease. A common bone disease affecting many Americans is osteoporosis, which is discussed in detail later in the chapter. Although many therapeutic advances are now available to prevent and treat some bone disorders, others are more difficult to avoid, such as **Paget's disease**, **osteogenesis imperfecta**, and **rickets**, which can lead to a downward spiral in physical health and quality of life, including losing the ability to walk, stand up, or even dress yourself (U.S. Department of Health and Human Services [USDHHS], 2004). Fortunately, we can do much to contribute to our own bone health. By practicing the behaviors of eating nutritious foods, getting regular physical activity, and participating in appropriate medical screenings, Americans of all ages can maintain strong healthy bones. This chapter reviews the physiology and structure of bone, the lifestyle recommendations for preserving healthy bones, and the metabolic osteoporosis and its risk factors, prevention, and detection.

Bone Physiology and Structure

Bone is living tissue and is continuously renewed throughout life. When you are young, your body makes new bone faster than it breaks down old bone. By the time you reach your late 20s, this cycle slows down and you begin to lose slightly more bone than you gain. Bones play a major role in daily metabolic processes: Bones produce cells that contribute to the formation of red and white blood cells and platelets, store fat needed for cellular energy production, and both release and absorb calcium to regulate blood pressure levels.

Bone and cartilage are forms of connective tissue in the human body. **Cartilage** is a semirigid connective tissue that provides firm, flexible support. Bone is a more specialized and harder form of connective tissue (Saladin, 2012). Healthy bone is light, rigid, of high tensile strength, and not brittle. As fetal development begins, the skeleton is made entirely of cartilage. This cartilaginous framework serves as the template for the bone to come later. Mature bone (**FIGURE 9.1**) consists of inorganic bone minerals, calcium, and phosphate precipitates that are incorporated into the organic support material known as osteoid. **Collagen** makes up 95 percent of the osteoid substance (Saladin, 2012).

BONE CELLS   Three types of cells are involved both in bone formation and in **resorption** of mature bone: osteoblasts, osteocytes, and osteoclasts.

Osteoblasts are immature bone cells that deposit new bone around the outside of existing bone. When they are surrounded by mineralized bone, they become mature bone cells and are then called **osteocytes**. **Osteoclasts** digest, or absorb, bony tissue. They remove old bone tissue so that its components can be absorbed into the circulation. This process is known as resorption.

Bone Formation

Although the diameter of bones can change throughout our lifetimes, bones grow in length only while the skeleton develops; this growth usually ends in adolescence. Longitudinal bone growth occurs at the ends of long bones at the epiphyseal plate.

Paget's disease A disease whose precise cause is unknown but that is a consequence of both genetic and environmental factors, such as a viral infection that triggers the osteoblasts to try to repair the damage (infection) by forming new bone. However, the new formation is disrupted, leading to weakness and deformities in the bone.

Osteogenesis imperfecta A disease caused by abnormalities in the collagen matrix within the bone, resulting in a weak structure and the potential for multiple fractures.

Rickets A deficiency of vitamin D (usually seen in children), causing weak bones and deformation as a result of overgrowth of cartilage at the ends of the bones. In adults, this condition leads to softening of the bone, leading to fracture and deformity.

Bones do more than provide structural support; they protect vital organs and support essential metabolic processes.

Cartilage Semirigid connective tissue that provides support.

Collagen The principal substance in connecting fibers and tissues, and in bones.

Resorption The loss of substance (bone, in this case) through physiological or pathological means.

Osteoblasts Bone-forming cells.

Osteocytes Bone cells responsible for the maintenance and turnover of the mineral content of surrounding bone.

Osteoclasts Cells in developing bone that break down unnecessary bone parts.

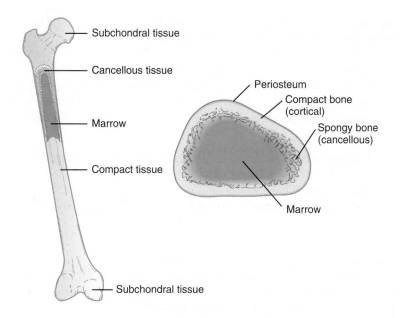

Subchondral tissue

Cancellous tissue

Marrow

Compact tissue

Subchondral tissue

Periosteum
Compact bone (cortical)
Spongy bone (cancellous)

Marrow

The epiphyseal plate is where cartilage synthesis and bone replacement form an area of active growth. Chondrocytes, or chondroblasts (cells like osteoblasts), synthesize the cartilage. Bone replacement, by osteoblasts, begins in the center of the cartilage and proceeds outward (Saladin, 2012). This process of bone formation occurs in layers. As chondrocytes are surrounded and trapped by the cartilage, new chondrocytes replace them on top of the cartilage for continued synthesis of the collagen matrix. The cartilage calcifies, the chondrocytes begin to die off, and the calcified material begins to erode. Osteoblasts move into the area and begin bone replacement. This continuous activity of cartilage synthesis, calcification, erosion, and osteoblast invasion forms the zone of active bone formation (Saladin, 2012).

Chondrocyte activity is greatly influenced by hormones. Growth hormone is considered the major stimulus to bone growth and is an important regulator in the growth of young children. Around puberty, the epiphyseal plates of long bones begin to stop responding to hormonal stimulus (Saladin, 2012). When adult height is reached, the epiphyseal plate is sealed from the marrow by a thin plate of bone. Bone formation is now complete, and the process of bone remodeling begins.

Bone Remodeling

Bone, like the kidneys and heart, is a live tissue that continually remodels itself to maintain **bone mineral density (BMD)** and to repair small damage (microtrauma) and large damage (fractures) that may occur over time. Most individuals reach peak bone mass around the age of 28, at which time BMD is then maintained by a process called **remodeling** (Saladin, 2012).

Remodeling involves the breaking down or removing of old bone (resorption) by osteoclasts, which are large, active cells that live in the central portion of the bone. This is followed up by the activity of cells called osteoblasts, which assist with new bone formation. Basically, as long as everything does its job, the rate of breakdown and buildup maintains itself, and BMD remains optimal. However, any factor that causes greater bone removal than bone building leads to a loss of bone mass, simply because new bone formation can't keep up. This is what accounts for the gradual loss of bone density as a person ages and results in more fragile bones.

This lifelong remodeling process preserves the mechanical integrity of the skeleton. The adult skeleton undergoes bone remodeling 24 hours a day, 7 days a week. Remodeling is under the control of a number of hormones, including estrogens,

Three types of cells are involved in bone formation and resorption: osteoblasts, osteocytes, and osteoclasts.

To maintain bone mass, bone formation must occur at the same rate as bone resorption.

Bone mineral density (BMD) Usually expressed as the amount of mineralized tissue in the scanned area, it is a risk factor for fractures.

Remodeling The ongoing dual processes of bone formation and bone resorption after cessation of growth.

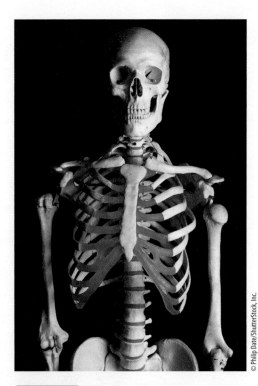

FIGURE 9.2 **Skeleton.** The human skeleton consists of 206 bones, which support your body, protect vital organs, and allow you to move.

androgens, vitamin D, and the parathyroid hormone, which regulates calcium levels in the blood (Baliss et al., 2012).

The same factors that encourage bone formation in young adults affect the maintenance of bone mass during adult years. The most important influences are calcium intake, reproductive hormone status, normal parathyroid gland function, and physical activity. We look in this chapter at how these influences affect the health of your skeleton (FIGURE 9.2).

Nutrition and Physical Activity for Bone Health

To achieve optimal bone health, and to continue to build new bone as you get older, proper nutrition and regular physical activity are necessary.

Nutritional Recommendations

Good nutrition is critical not only for strong bones but also for proper functioning of the heart, muscles, and nerves (FIGURE 9.3). It is important to eat a well-balanced diet containing a variety of foods. Nutrients that are key for bone health are calcium and vitamin D.

CALCIUM REQUIREMENTS   Calcium is a mineral that is necessary for life, yet many Americans do not get the amount of calcium they need every day (National Institutes of Health [NIH], 2012a). Calcium is important to build stronger, denser bones early in life and to keep bones strong and healthy later in life. TABLE 9.1 lists the Dietary Reference Intakes for calcium.

CALCIUM SOURCES   How do you obtain calcium in your daily diet? Many Americans obtain a majority of their calcium by consuming common dairy products such as milk, cheese, and yogurt. Most adults can meet the recommended requirements by drinking three 8-ounce glasses of milk each day in combination with the calcium obtained in their normal daily diet. Low-fat and nonfat dairy products are good choices because of their reduced fat content. Other favorable selections are foods that are fortified with calcium, such as cereal, nonfat milk, and orange juice (USDHHS, 2004). Fruits, vegetables, and grains also provide calcium, but the amount of calcium absorbed varies by the food type. For example, it would take almost 8 cups of spinach to yield the same amount of calcium found in 1 cup of milk (USDHHS, 2004).

For individuals who find it difficult to achieve optimal calcium intake from their daily dietary habits, calcium supplements may be necessary to meet the needed requirements. Two commonly available supplements are calcium carbonate and calcium citrate. Those who take supplements should note that:

- All major forms of calcium are best taken with meals.
- Calcium from supplements is best taken in small doses (500–600 mg at one time).
- Supplements may differ in their absorbability as a result of manufacturing practices (Institute of Medicine [IOM], 2010).
- All calcium sources—food or supplement—reduce the absorption of iron, so calcium and iron supplements should be taken at different times (USDHHS, 2004).

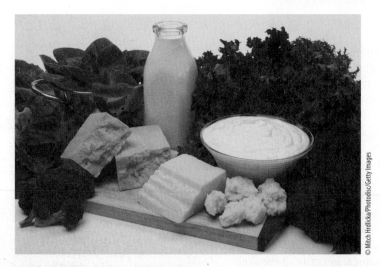

FIGURE 9.3 **Nutritional Recommendations.** Good nutrition is essential for optimal bone health.

TABLE 9.1	Dietary Reference Intakes for Calcium and Vitamin D by Sex and Age

Sex and Age	Calcium RDA (mg/day)	Vitamin D RDA (IU/day)
Males and females, 9–18	1300	600
Males and females, 19–30	1000	600
Males and females, 31–50	1000	600
Males, 51–70	1000	600
Females, 51–70	1200	600
Males and females, > 70	1200	800

To assist in planning a diet containing adequate levels of calcium, TABLE 9.2 provides a list of sources and the percent daily value of calcium they contain.

LACTOSE INTOLERANCE   In some cases, an individual's digestive system may lack the enzyme, lactose, needed to break down milk sugar when consumed, making them lactose intolerant and incapable of ingesting dairy products without intestinal distress. TABLE 9.3 suggests alternative methods for acquiring adequate levels of calcium.

VITAMIN D   Vitamin D is essential to the absorption of calcium and bone health. The link between calcium absorption and vitamin D is comparable to that of a locked door and a key. Vitamin D is the key that unlocks the door and allows calcium to leave the intestine and enter the bloodstream. Vitamin D also helps the kidneys resorb calcium that would otherwise be excreted in the urine. Adults should consume approximately 600 international units (IU) per day of vitamin D (see Table 9.1).

There are two sources of vitamin D: sunlight and dietary intake. Most individuals can obtain adequate levels of vitamin D through exposure to sunlight in the warmer months or exposure of the hands, arms, and face to sunlight for 10 to 15 minutes, two to three times a week. This method is not practical for others, who will therefore need to increase their levels of vitamin D through their diet. Primary food sources include fortified milk and cereals, egg yolk, and fish oils (USDHHS, 2004). To help you make the right choices and obtain the correct amounts, see TABLE 9.4.

BONE ROBBERS   You need not only be aware of nutrients that build strong bones but must also be aware of substances that deplete nutrients from your body, referred to as "bone robbers." Common bone robbers are sodium, protein, and caffeine. A diet high in sodium and protein may cause increased urinary loss and a negative calcium balance. Coffees and colas containing caffeine may be bone robbers of concern today. A diet with a high caffeine intake also causes loss of bone calcium. Recent studies suggest that excessive caffeine intake may contribute to osteoporosis.

Physical Activity Recommendations

You should engage in physical activity throughout your lifetime to promote overall bone health. The foundation of a physical activity regimen for bone health involves the current *Physical Activity Guidelines for Americans*, which states that "adults need at least 150 minutes (2 hours and 30 minutes) of moderate-intensity aerobic activity or 75 minutes (1 hour and 15 minutes) of vigorous-intensity aerobic activity every week or an equivalent mix of moderate- and vigorous-intensity

Physical activity enhances bone density through both weight-bearing and resistance-training exercises.

TABLE 9.2	Selected Food Sources of Calcium	

Food	Calcium (mg)	% Daily Value
Yogurt, plain, low-fat, 8 oz	415	42
Sardines, canned in oil, with bones, 3 oz	324	32
Cheddar cheese, 1½ oz shredded	306	31
Milk, nonfat, 8 fl oz	302	30
Milk, reduced fat (2% milk fat), 8 fl oz	297	30
Milk, lactose-reduced, 8 fl oz	285–302	29–30
Milk, whole (3.25% milk fat), 8 fl oz	291	29
Milk, buttermilk, 8 fl oz	285	29
Mozzarella, part skim, 1½ oz	275	28
Yogurt, fruit, low-fat, 8 oz	245–384	25–38
Tofu, firm, with calcium, ½ cup	204	20
Orange juice, calcium-fortified, 6 fl oz	200–260	20–26
Salmon, pink, canned, solids with bone, 3 oz	181	18
Pudding, chocolate, instant, made with 2% milk, ½ cup	153	15
Cottage cheese, 1% milk fat, 1 cup unpacked	138	14
Tofu, soft, with calcium, ½ cup	138	14
Spinach, cooked, ½ cup	120	12
Ready-to-eat cereal, calcium fortified, 1 cup	100–1000	10–100
Breakfast drink, various flavors and brands, powder prepared with water, 8 fl oz	105–250	10–25
Frozen yogurt, vanilla, soft serve, ½ cup	103	10
Turnip greens, boiled, ½ cup	99	10
Kale, cooked, 1 cup	94	9
Kale, raw, 1 cup	90	9
Ice cream, vanilla, ½ cup	85	8.5
Soy beverage, calcium-fortified, 8 fl oz	80–500	8–50
Chinese cabbage, raw, 1 cup	74	7
Tortilla, corn, ready to bake/fry, 1 medium	42	4
Tortilla, flour, ready to bake/fry, one 6" diameter	37	4
Sour cream, reduced fat, cultured, 2 Tbsp	32	3
Bread, white, 1 oz	31	3
Broccoli, raw, ½ cup	21	2
Bread, whole-wheat, 1 slice	20	2
Cream cheese, regular, 1 Tbsp	12	1

Daily values were developed by the FDA to help consumers compare the nutrient contents among products within the context of a total daily diet. The daily value of calcium is 1000 mg for adults and children aged 4 and older. Foods providing 20% or more of the daily value are considered to be high sources, but foods with a lower percentage also contribute to a healthy diet.

SOURCE: U.S. Department of Agriculture, Agricultural Research Service. (2009). USDA Nutrient Database for Standard Reference, Release 22. Online: http://www.ars.usda.gov/ba/bhnrc/ndl; and National Institutes of Health, Office of Dietary Supplements. (2009). Dietary supplement fact sheet: Calcium. Online: http://dietary-supplements.info.nih.gov/factsheets/calcium.asp#h3; and Heaney, R.P., Dowell, M.S., Rafferty, K., & Bierman, J. (2000). Bioavailability of the calcium in fortified soy imitation milk, with some observations on method. *American Journal of Clinical Nutrition* 71(5):1166–1169.

TABLE 9.3	Tips for Those with Lactose Intolerance

- Seek out and choose dairy and other calcium-rich foods with lower amounts of lactose. Alternative choices might include yogurt with live cultures (which provide bacterial lactase that digests the lactose); hard cheeses like cheddar, Colby, Swiss, and parmesan (the production process for these cheeses breaks down the lactose); and lactose-free or lactose-reduced products (including milk without lactose).
- Gradually increase the amount of lactose-containing foods consumed over a period of weeks to develop the capability to digest lactose.
- Consume nondairy products that contain high levels of calcium, such as fortified soy products or fortified cereal or orange juice.

SOURCE: U.S. Department of Health and Human Services. (2004). *Bone Health and Osteoporosis: A Report of the Surgeon General*, Chapter 7, p. 7. Rockville, MD: U.S. Department of Health and Human Services, Office of the Surgeon General.

TABLE 9.4	Dietary Sources of Vitamin D	
Food	**IUs per Serving**	**% Daily Value**
Cod liver oil, 1 Tbsp	1360	340
Salmon (sockeye), cooked, 3 oz	794	199
Mushrooms, exposed to ultraviolet light, 3 oz (not yet commonly available)	400	100
Mackerel, cooked, 3 oz	388	97
Tuna fish, canned in water, drained, 3 oz	154	39
Milk (nonfat, reduced fat, whole, and fortified), 1 cup	115–124	29–31
Orange juice, fortified, 1 cup (check product label)	100	25
Yogurt, fortified with 20% of the daily value, 6 oz (check product label)	80	20
Margarine, fortified, 1 Tbsp	60	15
Sardines, canned in oil, drained, 2 sardines	46	12
Liver, beef, cooked, 3½ oz	46	12
Ready-to-eat cereal, fortified with 10% of the daily value, ¾–1 cup (check product label)	40	10
Egg, yolk, 1 whole	25	6
Cheese, Swiss, 1 oz	6	2

Daily values were developed by the FDA to help consumers compare the nutrient-rich contents of products within the context of a total diet. The daily value for vitamin D is 600 IUs for adults and children age 4 and older. Food labels, however, are not required to list vitamin D content unless a food has been fortified. Foods providing 20% or more of the daily value are considered to be high sources of a nutrient.

SOURCE: U.S. Department of Agriculture, Agricultural Research Service. (2009). USDA Nutrient Database for Standard Reference, Release 22. Online: http://www.ars.usda.gov/ba/bhnrc/ndl; and National Institutes of Health, Office of Dietary Supplements. (2009). Dietary supplement fact sheet: Vitamin D. Online: http://dietary-supplements.info.nih.gov/factsheets/vitamind.asp.

aerobic activity and muscle-strengthening activities on 2 or more days a week that work all major muscle groups (legs, hips, back, abdomen, chest, shoulders, and arms)" (USDHHS, 2008).

Many studies have investigated the role of physical activity in bone health and report that physical activity is necessary for bone acquisition and maintenance throughout adulthood (**FIGURE 9.4**). Physical activity plays an important role in benefiting bone health specifically because bone mass is responsive to mechanical loads (stress) placed on the skeleton. In other words, bone becomes stronger and denser when you place demands on it, such as when you play a game of tennis or jump rope. Two types of exercise are important for increasing and maintaining bone density: weight-bearing and resistance-training exercises (NIH, 2012b). Weight-bearing exercises include activities in which your muscles and bones work against gravity or in which your lower body bears your body weight (**FIGURE 9.5**). Jogging, walking, and stair climbing are good examples of common weight-bearing activities. Your muscles must be challenged by using weight resistance to improve muscle and bone strength. Evidence suggests that the skeleton responds proactively to resistance training and short bouts of high-load impact, such as jumping for the lower body and weight lifting for the upper body. These types of activities can promote the building of muscle mass as well as the promotion of balance and coordination.

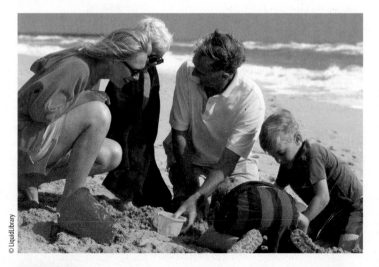

© LiquidLibrary

FIGURE 9.4 Moving for Health. Physical activity at all ages is essential to improve and maintain bone health.

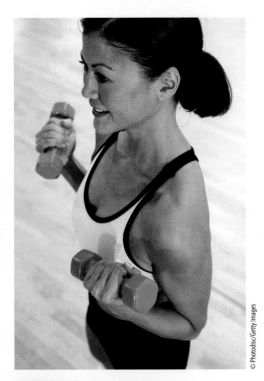

FIGURE 9.5 **Lifting Weights.** Physical activity, particularly weight-bearing exercise, is thought to provide the mechanical stimulus that is important for the maintenance and improvement of bone health.

Unfortunately, research has yet to establish a specific set of exercises for improving bone health, instead offering a set of principles to follow:

- Physical activity affects bone only at the skeletal sites that are stressed (or loaded) by the activity.
- For bone gain to occur, the stimulus must be greater than that which the bone usually experiences. Static loads applied to muscle (such as standing) do not promote increased bone mass.
- Complete lack of activity (e.g., immobility, paralysis, bed rest) causes bone loss.
- General physical activity most days of the week, coupled with weight-bearing, strength-building, and balance-enhancing activities two or more times a week, is effective for promoting bone health in most people.
- Any activity that causes impact (e.g., jumping, skipping) may increase bone mass more than low- to moderate-intensity endurance-type activities.
- Load-bearing physical activities (e.g., jumping) need not be engaged in for long periods of time to provide benefits to skeletal health. Five to 10 minutes of physical activity that incorporates 50 three-inch jumps per day should suffice for most adults.
- Physical activities should include a variety of loading patterns to promote increased bone mass. Be creative in finding ways to add other weight-bearing activities to your daily life. See TABLE 9.5 for a list of weight-bearing exercises for adults.
- Consult a physician or physical therapist if orthopedic conditions or other medical conditions make these physical activity guidelines difficult or unsafe to follow.

TABLE 9.5	Weight-Bearing Exercise for Adults

The best exercise for your bones is weight-bearing activities, which cause muscles and bones to work against gravity. Some examples of weight-bearing exercises include:

Brisk walking	Weight lifting or resistance training
Hiking	Tennis or racquetball
Stair climbing	Field hockey
Jumping rope	Basketball
Jogging or running	Volleyball
Dancing	Soccer
Downhill skiing	Lacrosse
Golf (which includes shouldering the golf bag around for 18 holes)	Yoga (performing the slow, precise Iyengar style or the vigorous ashtanga)

Note: Take a few exercise precautions if you already have low bone mass, osteopenia, or osteoporosis because your fracture risk is higher than normal. Be cautious about trying any exercise with the potential for serious falls, like downhill skiing, and check with your healthcare provider before starting any new exercise program, especially if you're taking medications that slow your coordination or throw off your balance.

SOURCE: Centers for Disease Control and Prevention. (2013). Weight-Bearing Physical Activity. Online: http://www.cdc.gov/nutrition/everyone/basics/vitamins/calcium.html; and the National Institute of Arthritis and Musculoskeletal and Skin Diseases (NIAMS). (2013). Exercise for Your Bone Health. Online: http://www.niams.nih.gov/health_info/bone/bone_health/exercise/default.asp.

Osteoporosis

Osteoporosis, literally meaning "porous bones," is a metabolic disease characterized by excessive skeletal fragility, as noted earlier. Bone loss is so common that most people consider it a normal process of aging. However, osteoporosis is a preventable and unnecessary occurrence in most individuals (USDHHS, 2004).

The onset of osteoporosis occurs most often in women after menopause. As the U.S. population ages, the incidence of osteoporosis will increase, with a subsequent increase in cost to the health care industry. Because osteoporosis is a painful and debilitating disease that can affect a person's quality of life, prevention and early treatment are important issues for all ages. Some changes in bone health are considered permanent; therefore, prevention becomes the primary "cure" for osteoporosis.

Postmenopausal osteoporotic individuals undergo a high rate of bone turnover. Osteoblastic activity cannot meet the rate of osteoclastic bone resorption. Bones are thin and brittle because of the loss of mineralization. The decreased bone mass puts the individual at an increased risk for fracture, most often fractures of the hip, spine, and wrist (**FIGURE 9.6**).

The annual cost of osteoporosis in the United States is estimated to be $18 billion. Currently, 10 million Americans are affected, and 34 million more have low bone mass, placing them at risk for osteoporosis. This cost of osteoporosis is expected to increase over the next decade as a result of the overall aging of the population. Part of the cost of osteoporosis is related to the morbidity of the disease. Only 50 percent of individuals who suffer a hip fracture are able to return home or live independently after injury, and the estimated cost of hip fractures could reach $240 billion by the year 2040 (USDHHS, 2004).

> **Osteoporosis** Literally means "porous bones"; a metabolic disease resulting in bone loss and bones that fracture easily.

Osteoporosis is a chronic disease process characterized by progressive bone loss in both males and females.

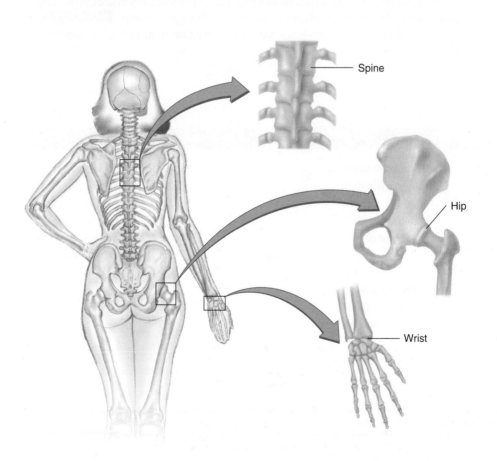

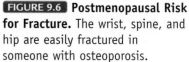

FIGURE 9.6 **Postmenopausal Risk for Fracture.** The wrist, spine, and hip are easily fractured in someone with osteoporosis.

Although the majority (80 percent) of persons affected by osteoporosis are women, one in eight men also suffers from the disease (NIH, 2012a). This rate is expected to increase as men live longer. A majority of American men view osteoporosis solely as a "woman's disease," but many men have lifestyle habits that put them at increased risk later in life when it comes to their mobility and independence. It develops less often in men than in women because men have larger skeletons, their bone loss starts later and progresses more slowly, and they have no period of rapid hormonal change and bone loss (Cawthon, 2011).

Because osteoporosis is often not diagnosed until fractures occur, prevention is considered the most cost-effective approach. Prevention focuses on two main objectives: (1) achieving optimal bone density in the first two to three decades of life, and (2) maintaining bone density and decreasing rate of bone loss in later years. Physical activity and good nutrition are key elements in meeting these preventive strategies.

Risk Factors

The many risk factors that influence osteoporosis (TABLE 9.6) can be grouped into four categories: genetic, hormonal, nutritional, and lifestyle factors.

GENETIC FACTORS   Race, heredity, and gender influence bone fragility. Typically, white and Asian women are at greater risk for developing osteoporosis and related fractures; Hispanic and black women have greater bone mineral density (BMD) and are at less risk for developing osteoporosis (however, they are still at some risk). In addition, women with a family history of osteoporosis are considered to be at increased risk. Daughters of women with spinal fractures generally have lower BMD in the spine. Although most research has focused on the mother's history of osteoporosis, research shows that the father's history also is important. Furthermore, women with relatives who have a dowager's hump (FIGURE 9.7) or have incurred low-trauma fractures have a positive family history of osteoporosis (USDHHS, 2004).

6

Osteoporosis can be affected by genetic, hormonal, nutritional, and lifestyle factors.

| TABLE 9.6 | **Risk Factors for Fracture** |

	Medical conditions:	Medications:
Older age (> 65 years)	• Hyperthyroidism	• Oral glucocorticoids
Fracture after age 45	• Chronic lung disease	• Excess thyroxine replacement
First-degree female relative with a fracture in adulthood	• Endometriosis	• Antiepileptic medications
Self-report health as "fair" or "poor"	• Malignancy	• Gonadal hormone suppression
Current tobacco use	• Chronic hepatic or renal disease	• Immunosuppressive agents
Weight less than 127 lbs.	• Hyperparathyroidism	
Menopause prior to age 45 years	• Vitamin D deficiency	
Amenorrhea	• Cushing's disease	
Lifelong low calcium intake	• Multiple sclerosis	
Excess alcohol consumption	• Sarcoidosis	
Poor vision despite correction	• Hemochromatosis	
Falls		
Minimal weight-bearing exercise		

SOURCE: U.S. Department of Health and Human Services. (2004). *Bone Health and Osteoporosis: A Report of the Surgeon General,* Chapter 10. Rockville, MD: U.S. Department of Health and Human Services, Office of the Surgeon General.

HORMONAL FACTORS Hormonal status greatly influences bone fragility, and menstrual history is a key component. Risk of bone fragility also increases for women after menopause because bone loss accelerates with reduction in estrogen production (Baliss et al., 2012). Hormonal changes of menopause cause the loss of about 10 percent of bone during the first 5 years after menopause and an additional 5 percent during the next 20 years (Recker, 2011). Men with hypogonadism are at special risk for bone loss. (Hypogonadism is a failure of the testes to function normally. It is treated with replacement testosterone therapy.)

Amenorrhea is a condition associated with BMD that may result from excessive exercise or eating disorders. Achieving high bone mineral density is critical during adolescence, but amenorrhea lowers estrogen levels, which can cause a loss of bone mass and increase the risk of osteoporosis later in life. Amenorrhea in young women is of concern because achieving peak bone mass in the second and third decades seems to be an important indicator for lifetime fracture risk. Although physical activity may affect estrogen hormone levels and indirectly affect bone density, low body fat is more likely the culprit.

Estrogen and other sex hormones have been reported to stimulate osteoblastic activity weakly. Estrogens are female sex hormones that are responsible for the development and maintenance of a woman's secondary sex characteristics (development of breasts, for example), and following menstruation, estrogens stimulate the rebuilding of the uterine lining. Ovaries are the primary source of estrogen. Estrogens are probably the most important hormone controlling bone mass loss. Estrogens inhibit bone resorption by modifying osteoclast function. Estrogen replacement therapy is one treatment used to prevent the onset of osteoporosis; however, its many side effects make it an unpopular treatment for many women (USDHHS, 2004).

A condition referred to as *female athlete triad* is chronic overexercising accompanied by disordered eating, amenorrhea, and osteoporosis. Chronic overexercising has been associated with reduced bone mass in premenopausal women. The overexercising and unbalanced diet disrupts the body's hormones enough to impair the influence of estrogens on the skeletal system. Despite the weight-bearing exercise, the lack of estrogen accelerates bone resorption and bone loss.

NUTRITIONAL FACTORS As noted earlier, a general well-balanced diet is recommended, with special attention to adequate calcium and vitamin D.

LIFESTYLE FACTORS People who lead a sedentary lifestyle are at increased risk to suffer from osteoporosis. Children and teenagers who are not physically active do not have the same bone density as active children and teenagers. This makes them more likely to get osteoporosis as an adult. Bones need exercise to become stronger, just as muscles do. Regular exercise, especially resistance or weight-bearing exercise, has been shown to stimulate bone formation and retard bone mass reduction.

Smoking cigarettes, drinking alcohol in excess, and high caffeine intake all affect bone mass negatively. Recent studies have shown a direct relationship between tobacco use and decreased bone density (NIH, 2012a). Women who

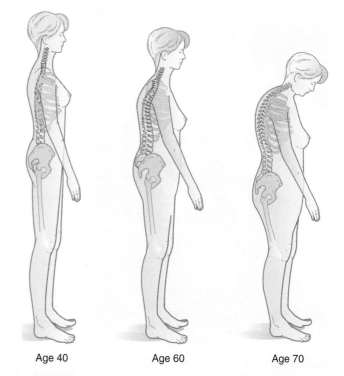

Age 40   Age 60   Age 70

FIGURE 9.7 **Progression of Dowager's Hump.** Women with postmenopausal osteoporosis tend to experience numerous fractures in the bones of their spine (vertebrae) as they age. Eventually these vertebrae can collapse, causing the spine to curve. Such curvature causes loss of height, a tilted rib cage, a dowager's hump, and a protruding abdomen.

Amenorrhea Absence of menstrual periods.

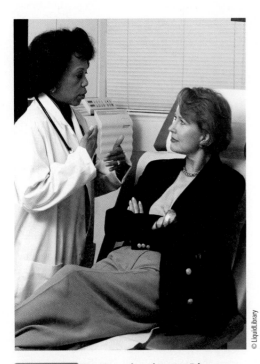

FIGURE 9.8 **An Examination to Diagnose Osteoporosis Can Involve Several Tests.** Before performing these tests, your health care professional will record information about your medical history and lifestyle in an initial physical exam.

Osteopenia Low bone mass.

smoke cigarettes experience an earlier menopause, a higher incidence of vertebral compression fractures, a decreased bone mineral density, and a lower urinary estrogen level. Excessive or heavy alcohol consumption is also detrimental to bones (Maurel et al., 2012). Drinking too much alcohol interferes with the balance of calcium in the body. It also affects the production of hormones, which have a protective effect on bone, and of vitamins, which we need to absorb calcium. Finally, high caffeine intake (more than 3 cups of caffeinated coffee a day) speeds up the excretion of calcium from the body.

Prevention and Detection of Osteoporosis

Osteoporosis diagnosis often begins with a thorough physical examination, which includes an oral history, recording of complaints of height loss, a review of overall nutrition and medication intake, and observations of stature, carriage, and spine curvature (Lewiecki et al., 2012) (FIGURE 9.8). Spinal osteoporosis is often characterized by loss of stature.

BONE MINERAL DENSITY TESTS   BMD tests measure bone density in various body sites: the hip, spine, wrist, finger, kneecap, shinbone, and heel (FIGURE 9.9). A bone density test can detect osteoporosis before a fracture occurs, predict your risk of fracturing in the future, determine your rate of bone loss, and monitor the effect of treatment. The test is conducted at intervals of 1 year.

The BMD tests vary in the type of bone measured (trabecular, cortical, or both), precision (deviation based on multiple measurements, generally represented on a percentage basis as a coefficient of variation), accuracy (variation in quality of bone measured versus real content of bone), and radiation dose (Lewiecki et al., 2012) (TABLE 9.7).

What do your BMD test results mean? A normal bone density is called a "T-score." This means you have the bone density of a normal young adult and have no risk for fractures. The World Health Organization (2007) has established the following mineral density diagnostic criteria for women who have experienced no fragility fractures. These criteria provide a basic diagnostic framework:

- Normal bone mineral density is within 1 standard deviation (SD) of the young adult mean. (*Standard deviation* is a measure of variation in a distribution.)
- **Osteopenia**, or low bone mass, is a bone mineral density between 1 and 2.5 SD of the young adult mean.
- Osteoporosis is defined as a value greater than 2.5 SD below the young adult mean.

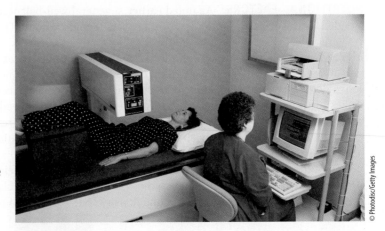

FIGURE 9.9 **Bone Mineral Density Test.** These tests are painless, noninvasive, and safe. Bone density may be measured in the spine, hip, wrist, finger, kneecap, shin bone, or heel depending on the machine used.

TABLE 9.7	Types of BMD Tests	
Acronym	Name	Measures
DXA	Dual-energy X-ray absorptiometry	Spine, hip, or total body
SXA	Single-energy X-ray absorptiometry	Wrist or heel
RA	Radiographic absorptiometry	Uses an X-ray of the hand and a small metal wedge to calculate BMD
DPA	Dual-photon absorptiometry	Spine, hip, or total body
SPA	Single-photon absorptiometry	Wrist
QCT	Quantitative computed tomography	Wrist

Physical Activity and Health Connection

Maintaining optimal bone health requires a lifestyle that includes a balanced diet and a healthy physical activity program. A diet that pays close attention to calcium intake through dairy and other foods is important. If the diet does not contain enough calcium naturally, calcium supplements may be needed.

Bone is a living tissue that responds to exercise by becoming more dense and stronger. Weight-bearing and resistance exercises increase bone mass and density. Therefore, weight-bearing physical activities (e.g., dancing, walking) and resistance activities (e.g., weight lifting, swimming) are essential for improving and maintaining optimal bone health.

concept connections

 Bones do more than provide structural support; they protect vital organs and support essential metabolic processes. Bones contain cells that help form blood cells, store fat, and release and absorb calcium. Bone formation and remodeling are important factors in understanding the development, treatment, and prevention of osteoporosis.

 Three types of cells are involved in bone formation and resorption: osteoblasts, osteo-cytes, and osteoclasts. *Osteoblasts* are immature cells that when surrounded by mature bone cells become *osteocyctes*. *Osteoclasts* absorb bony tissue.

 To maintain bone mass, bone formation must occur at the same rate as bone resorption. Bone remodeling is the lifelong renewal process of the skeletal system. This process allows for bone to be removed and new bone generated. This process of new bone forming at the same rate as resorption is critical because without this balance osteoporosis can take place.

 Physical activity enhances bone density through both weight-bearing and resistance-training exercises. Bone becomes stronger and denser when we place demands on it, such as by jogging or playing tennis. Physical activity is necessary for bone acquisition and maintenance throughout adulthood.

Osteoporosis is a chronic disease process characterized by progressive bone loss in both males and females. Millions of Americans suffer from osteoporosis and the bone fractures that result from it. Optimal physical activity and nutrition habits when young are key elements in an osteoporosis prevention program.

Osteoporosis can be affected by genetic, hormonal, nutritional, and lifestyle factors. Recognizing common osteoporosis risk factors can help you understand effective prevention strategies and is useful in decreasing the incidence and prevalence of osteoporosis.

Terms

Amenorrhea, 211
Bone mineral density (BMD), 203
Cartilage, 202
Collagen, 202
Osteoblasts, 202

Osteoclasts, 202
Osteocytes, 202
Osteogenesis imperfecta, 202
Osteopenia, 212
Osteoporosis, 209

Paget's disease, 202
Remodeling, 203
Resorption, 202
Rickets, 202

making the connection

Julie now knows that, although her bones may seem to be rigid and unchanging, they are actually more like muscles, capable of strengthening with use or weakening without use. Each time a bone is moved, it bends ever so slightly, just enough to stimulate electrical and biochemical changes that stimulate bone formation. The more force, the greater the bending, the greater the stimulus for new bone formation (up to a point). In addition to maintaining the Recommended Daily Intake (RDI) for calcium, Julie knows that a regular physical activity program keeps the density of bone constant or contributes to increased bone mass. Julie now understands that the threat of osteoporosis doesn't just come from a low calcium intake, but from a sedentary lifestyle. She is encouraged to know that by monitoring her dietary habits and participating in a regular weight-bearing physical activity program, she now has the right tools to live strong and live well.

Critical Thinking

1. Like Julie, many people do not understand that both physical inactivity and low calcium intake are key factors in the development of osteoporosis. You have been asked by a local ninth-grade health teacher to explain to her students the importance of physical activity and nutrition in preventing osteoporosis (a condition that is the last thing on most ninth-graders' minds). In 250 words or less, explain their importance.

2. Review the factors that affect osteoporosis (genetic, hormonal, nutritional, and lifestyle). Review your family history to determine whether you are at risk of osteoporosis. Then, select two other factors and, based on your current behaviors, decide which behaviors you could change that would assist in preventing osteoporosis. List them.

3. "Physical activity and nutrition are key elements in achieving optimal bone density during the first 20 to 30 years of life and maintaining bone density throughout life." Provide information that supports that statement.

References

Baliss, L., Mahoney, D., & Monk, P. (2012). Normal bone physiology, remodeling and its hormonal regulation. *Surgery* 30(2):47–53.

Cawthon, P. (2011). Gender differences in osteoporosis and fractures. *Clinical Orthopaedics and Related Research* 469:1900–1905.

Harvey, N., Dennison, E., & Cooper, C. (2010). Osteoporosis: Impact on health and economics. *Nature Reviews Rheumatology* 6:99–105.

Institute of Medicine. (2010). *Dietary Reference Intakes for Calcium and Vitamin D.* Washington, DC: National Academies Press.

Lewiecki, E., Laster, A., Miller, P., & Bilezikian, J.P. (2012). More bone density testing is needed, not less. *Journal of Bone and Mineral Research* 27(4):739–746. doi:10.1002/jbmr.1580.

Maurel, D.B., Boisseau, N., Benhamou, C.L., & Jaffre, C. (2012). Alcohol and bone: Review of dose effects and mechanisms. *Osteoporosis International* 23(1):1–16. doi:10.1007/s00198-011-1787-7.

National Institutes of Health, NIH Osteoporosis and Related Bone Diseases National Resource Center. (2012a). Calcium and vitamin D: Important at every age. Online: http://www.niams.nih.gov/Health_Info/Bone/Bone_Health/Nutrition/default.asp.

National Institutes of Health, NIH Osteoporosis and Related Bone Diseases National Resource Center. (2012b). Exercise for your bone health. Online: http://www.niams.nih.gov/Health_Info/Bone/Bone_Health/Exercise/default.asp.

Recker, R. (2011). Early postmenopausal bone loss and what to do about it. *New York Academy of Sciences* 1240:e26–e30.

Saladin, K.S. (2012). *Anatomy and Physiology: The Unity of Form and Function,* 6th ed. New York: McGraw-Hill.

U.S. Department of Health and Human Services. (2004). *Bone Health and Osteoporosis: A Report of the Surgeon General.* Rockville, MD: U.S. Department of Health and Human Services, Office of the Surgeon General.

U.S. Department of Health and Human Services. (2008). *Physical Activity Guidelines for Americans.* Online: http://health.gov/paguidelines/guidelines/default.aspx.

World Health Organization. (2007). *WHO Scientific Group on the Assessment of Osteoporosis at Primary Health Care Level. Summary Meeting Report.* Geneva, Switzerland: World Health Organization. Online: www.who.int/chp/topics/Osteoporosis.pdf.

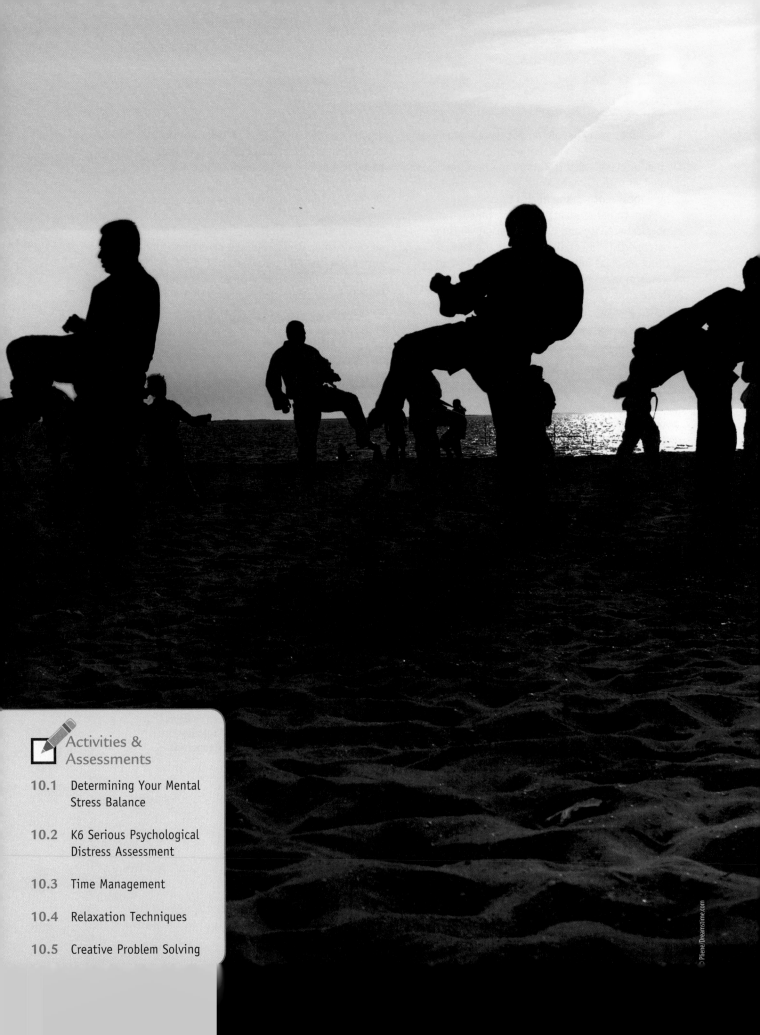

Mental Health and Coping with Stress

10

what's the connection?

Jackson felt anxious and tense as he rehearsed a speech in his dorm room. He had spent two weeks on this English class assignment and now, the day before he was to stand up in front of the class, he was having trouble remembering and delivering his speech. Three days ago he had no trouble reciting the 30-minute presentation in front of the mirror, but now he was fretting about presenting in front of his classmates and instructor. After a number of failed attempts, Jackson decided to take a break and go out for a 45-minute jog. Halfway through the jog, the anxiety and worrying subsided and he began to recite his speech easily in his mind. When Jackson returned to the dorm, his roommate Tim was there. Jackson asked Tim to listen to the speech before they went to the cafeteria for dinner. Jackson was able to deliver his speech flawlessly in front of Tim. He then showered and got dressed for dinner. As they walked to the cafeteria, Jackson told Tim that he planned to jog before presenting his speech because he felt that the exercise had helped him deliver it with a clear head.

concepts

1. People who are physically active tend to have better mental health.

2. Our mental and emotional health are central to the quality of our lives, and both influence our physical health.

3. Maintaining and optimizing our mental and physical health requires making countless adjustments to a variety of life's challenges.

4. Stress is a natural process, and understanding its effects can help you use it to your own advantage.

5. The general adaptation syndrome describes the body's response to stress and the adaptability of the body to maintain homeostasis.

6. The art of stress management is to keep yourself at a level of stimulation that is healthy and enjoyable.

go.jblearning.com/kotecki4e
The website for this book is a great source for supplementary physical health information for both students and instructors. Visit **go.jblearning.com/kotecki4e** to find a variety of useful tools for learning, thinking, and teaching.

Physical fitness is not only one of the most important keys to a healthy body, it is the basis of dynamic and creative intellectual activity.

—Ralph Waldo Emerson

People who are physically active tend to have better mental health.

Introduction

The positive relationship between physical activity and mental health has been well documented (Raglin & Wilson, 2012). The scientific consensus linking physical activity to mental health has resulted in recommendations that exercise should be used for the promotion and maintenance of mental health and in the management of mental health problems (Voss et al., 2011). The consensus is that people who are physically active score higher on important mental health factors such as self-esteem, self-concept, self-worth, body image, and cognitive functioning than do sedentary people (Erickson et al., 2011). Furthermore, physical activity has been shown to be effective in treating people who report symptoms of anxiety, depression, and stress (McAuley et al., 2011).

Improved mental health and its conservation are topics of immense interest among health professionals because of the continuing commonness of mental illness. If you survey the U.S. population during any 12-month span, one in five adults (20 percent) will meet the criteria for having a mental illness, and fully one-fourth of those will have a "serious" disorder that significantly disrupts their ability to function day to day. These prevalence data are based on four major categories of mental illness: anxiety disorders (such as panic and post-traumatic stress disorders), mood disorders (such as major depression and bipolar disease), impulse control disorders (such as attention-deficit/hyperactivity disorder), and substance abuse. In addition, it has been estimated that almost 5 of every 10 people (46 percent) experience a significant mental disorder at some point in their lifetime (Substance Abuse and Mental Health Services Administration [SAMHSA], 2012). Add to this the fact that fewer than half of those in need get treated and you soon realize the scope of the problem. Those who do seek treatment usually do so after a decade or more of delays, during which time they have suffered needlessly.

Another point of interest is that although mental stress is not considered an illness, it can cause specific medical symptoms that are often serious enough to require medical care. In fact, nearly half of all adults suffer adverse health effects from stress, and 60 to 90 percent of all physician office visits have stress-related components (Benson & Proctor, 2003).

Mental illness can afflict anyone, no matter their age, gender, race, or economic status. A mental illness is a disease that causes mild to severe disturbances in thinking, perception, and behavior. If these disturbances significantly impair a person's ability to cope with life's ordinary demands and routines, then he or she should immediately seek proper treatment with a mental health professional. With the proper care and treatment, a person can recover and resume normal activities. As with other chronic conditions, medical science has made incredible progress over the last couple of decades in helping us to understand, cure, and eliminate the causes of mental illness.

Mental health care resources and expenditures for treatment are important considerations when addressing mental illness and its consequences. However, it has been pointed out that, similar to other health problems in which major advances have come from prevention rather than treatment, *preventing* mental health problems is inherently better than having to treat the illness after its onset (U.S. Department of Health and Human Services [USDHHS], 2010). Although there continues to be an insufficient understanding of all of the biological, psychological, and sociocultural effects on mental health and illness, some successful strategies have materialized. A meaningful one includes the choice of a lifestyle that incorporates regular physical activity. Physical activity has the potential not only to enhance mental functioning but also to serve as a protective factor against, as well as provide a treatment modality for, a number of mental disturbances along the mental health continuum (**FIGURE 10.1**).

Many theories have been proposed to explain the positive research findings related to physical activity and mental health along the mental health continuum. To address completely these explanations related to mind and body functioning, we must first begin by looking at mental and emotional health and how they are central to the quality of our lives.

Mental and Emotional Health

Defining mental health is not easy because it encompasses a broad group of values across different cultures and subgroups. The U.S. Department of Health and Human Services (USDHHS) defines **mental health** as a "state of successful performance of mental function, resulting in productive activities, fulfilling relationships with other people, and the ability to adapt to change and to cope with adversity" (USDHHS, 2010). Evident from the definition is that mental health doesn't just occur; we need to pay attention to our mental needs just as we do our physical needs.

Mental health involves such factors as a sense of coherence and insight, moods, self-esteem, and coping ability. It allows us to make informed selections between alternate courses of action. We must use our cognitive abilities to make wise choices based on both previous experience and a willingness to undergo new experiences. An important part of mental health is learning to fully understand and trust the decisions we make. Mental health involves having a mind open to new ideas and concepts. Mental health embodies factors not only of intellect but also of emotions and relationships.

Emotional health calls for understanding our emotions and coping with changes that arise in everyday life. Emotional health encompasses mental states that include feelings or subjective experiences in response to changes in our environment. Joy, disappointment, fear, anxiety, guilt, love, sadness, anger, jealousy, trust, empathy, and compassion describe subjective experiences that are real to us (**FIGURE 10.2** and **FIGURE 10.3**). These emotions play an important role in our overall health.

Everything you think and feel reflects who you are. An *emotion* is a thought linked to a sensation. The thought is usually about the past or the future, but the sensation is in the present. Your mind quickly links this sensation with involuntary and immediate changes in your body function. Our minds and our emotions are interrelated and interdependent. Mental functions do not exist separately from our emotions, and our emotions affect our mental state. Therefore, the terms *mental* and *emotional health* will be used interchangeably in this chapter.

Our mental and emotional health are central to the quality of our lives, and both influence our physical health.

Mental health A "state of successful performance of mental function, resulting in productive activities, fulfilling relationships with other people, and the ability to adapt to change and to cope with adversity" (USDHHS, 2010).

Emotional health Encompasses mental states that include feelings or subjective experiences in response to changes in our environment.

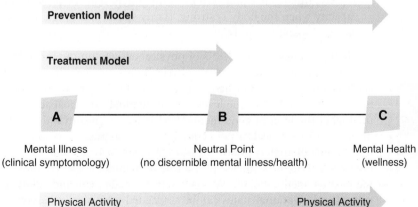

FIGURE 10.1 **The Physical Activity and Mental Health Continuum.** Physical activity has the potential not only to enhance mental functioning but also to serve as a protective factor against—as well as provide a treatment modality for—a number of mental disturbances along the mental health continuum.

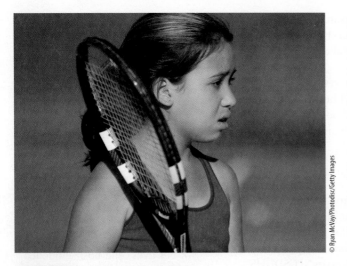

FIGURE 10.2 **Emotional Health.** This includes feelings of sadness and disappointment.

Mind–Body Relationship

Much research related to physical activity has centered on its relationship to physical health. However, holistic health perspectives emphasize mind–body unity and include the complex relationship between mental and physical function as well as the continuum between health and illness (Wipfli et al., 2011). Because of this view, there is currently a great deal of interest in the study of physical activity as it relates to mental health. The line between psychology and biology is becoming increasingly blurred. The physiological parameters of our bodies are constantly eavesdropping on our thoughts and being changed in the process. Similarly, research is now able to substantiate the proposed mental and emotional benefits of habitual physical activity, which include improved intellectual functioning, academic performance, and moods (Erickson et al., 2011). The old paradigm that distinguished between mental and physical health is thus somewhat unsound, in the sense that we now know mental and physical health are highly integrated. Indeed, the USDHHS asserted that it is important to adopt the paradigm that mind and body are inseparable and eliminate the old idea that the mind and body are separate and independent from each other (USDHHS, 2010). The mind–body dualism we speak of today is founded in the classical connection made by the Greeks 24 centuries ago when they considered physical activity and mental health simultaneously.

Mens Sana in Corpore Sana

The Greeks long believed in the mental benefits derived from physical activity. They deemed that a healthy and fit body was positively associated with increased mental and emotional wellness. This was best exemplified by the phrase attributed to Homer: "*Mens* (mind, intellect) *sana* (sound, healthy, sane), *in corpore* (body) *sana*," which translates into "In a sound body is a sound mind." The Greeks maintained that physical activity made the mind more rational and perceptive. During the Golden Age of Greece, regular and vigorous physical activity was engaged in for its contribution to mental as well as physical health.

Former President John F. Kennedy underscored the Greek ideal of *mens sana in corpore sana* when he said:

> Physical fitness is not only one of the most important keys to a healthy body, it is the basis of dynamic and creative intellectual activity. Intelligence and skill can only function at the peak of their capacity when the body is strong. Hardy spirits and tough minds usually inhabit sound bodies.

Many studies on the effects of physical activity on the mental health of physically active versus physically inactive people generally show positive effects (Bertheussen et al., 2011). The invariable findings are that the higher the level of an individual's physical activity, the higher the level of good mental health. Mental health is defined in these studies as feelings of general well-being, positive moods, and fewer bouts of anxiety and depression. The studies conclude that physical activity may indeed play a role in maintaining or promoting positive mental health. We have seen that adequate and enhanced mental and emotional states can be associated with physical activity of the body. Is the reverse true? Can poor mental health states lead to

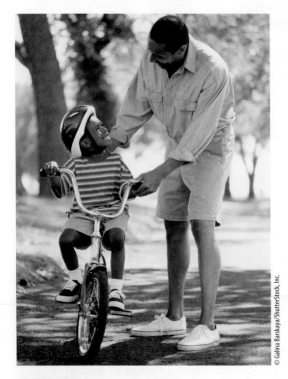

FIGURE 10.3 **Emotional Health.** This also includes feelings of joy and love.

deterioration of the body? A number of research studies seem to indicate that poor mental and emotional states can have an effect on our physical health (Beaula, Carlson, & Boyd, 2011).

Psychosomatic Disease

Psychosomatic disease describes bodily symptoms caused by mental or emotional disturbance. The word *psychosomatic* comes from the Greek words *psyche* (the mind) and *soma* (the body). Numerous studies have confirmed that being emotionally distressed from a number of negative emotions, including chronic anxiety or depression, can lead to physical health problems such as headaches, ulcers, high blood pressure, altered insulin needs, and a suppressed immune system. These physical problems can lead to an increased risk of heart disease, stroke, cancer, and infections. The prevalence of many of these underlying emotions that begin the disease sequence is associated with life-stress circumstances (Mate, 2011). Emotionally, stress can lead to feelings of depression, anxiety, and decreased mental health (McEwen & Gianaros, 2011).

Mental Illness

Mental illness encompasses all diagnosable mental disorders (USDHHS, 2010). These mental disorders are quantified by changes in our thinking, mood, or behavior that lead to impaired functioning. Our focus here is limited to mental health concerns related to anxiety, depression, and stress. These mental problems are the most common experienced by Americans and are influenced by physical activity both as a protective factor and a therapeutic modality.

ANXIETY **Anxiety** is one of the most easily understood and responsive symptoms of mental disorders. Everyone feels anxious from time to time. Anxiety is a normal feeling that each of us experiences when a fear-eliciting situation arises in our environment. These fearful situations can be real or imagined, and the natural physiological response is "fight or flight." Anxiety is inflated worry and tension that sets off the fight-or-flight response. Most of us have felt the pounding of our heart when we think the teacher will call on us for an answer we do not know, or the muscle tension we feel when we think our parents are going to be angry with us over something we have done or not done, or that feeling of lightheadedness before calling someone for a first date. A certain level of anxiety is good because it can spur us on to action. However, it is important that we be able to regulate anxiety, or it may materialize in mood disturbances (depression) and pathological physiological activity (disease).

Experiencing heightened arousal or fear over a sustained period of time can lead to **anxiety disorders**, which are debilitating and disruptive to our health. Anxiety disorders are the most common mental disorders in the United States; five major types include: (1) social anxiety disorder, (2) panic disorder, (3) generalized anxiety disorder, (4) obsessive-compulsive disorder (OCD), and (5) post-traumatic stress disorder (PTSD) (TABLE 10.1).

DEPRESSION **Depression** illustrates a mental disorder mainly noted by alterations in mood. Depression often accompanies anxiety disorders (USDHHS, 2010). Like anxiety disorders, depression can vary in severity and duration. All of us have experienced **depressive reactions** because of a disturbing event in our lives. Depressive reactions encompass the normal depressed feelings, such as sadness, hopelessness, rejection, and worthlessness that arise because of a specific life situation (TABLE 10.2). Fortunately, these deviations do not last long, and they lessen over time. However, when symptoms last for an extended period of time or feature one or more major depressive episodes, the condition may be serious.

Psychosomatic disease Bodily symptoms caused by mental or emotional disturbance.

Mental illness Diagnosable mental disorders that change our thinking, mood, or behavior and lead to impaired functioning.

Anxiety Normal response when a fear-eliciting situation arises.

Anxiety disorders Mental disorders caused by heightened arousal or fear over a sustained period of time.

Depression A mental disorder notable for negative alteration in mood.

Depressive reactions Normal depressed feelings such as sadness and hopelessness.

TABLE 10.1   Kinds of Anxiety Disorders

Condition	Description
Social anxiety disorder (social phobia)	Persistent, intense, and chronic fear of being watched and judged by others and being embarrassed or humiliated by their own actions; an overwhelming and excessive self-consciousness in everyday social situations such as speaking in formal or informal situations, eating or drinking in front of others, or, in its most severe form, being around other people for any reason. Fear may be so severe that it interferes with work, school, and other ordinary activities. Accompanying physical symptoms include blushing, profuse sweating, trembling, nausea, and difficulty talking.
Panic disorder	Unexpected and repeated episodes of intense fear accompanied by physical symptoms that may include chest pain, nausea, heart palpitations or pounding, shortness of breath, abdominal distress, and feeling sweaty, weak, faint, dizzy, flushed, or chilled. Feelings of terror may strike suddenly and repeatedly with no warning. The hands may tingle or feel numb. There may be a smothering sensation, a sense of unreality, or a fear of impending doom or loss of control.
Generalized anxiety disorder	Chronic anxiety and exaggerated worry and tension, even when there is little or nothing to provoke it. Anxiety is often accompanied by fatigue, headaches, muscle tension, muscle aches, difficulty swallowing, trembling, twitching, irritability, sweating, and hot flashes.
Obsessive-compulsive disorder (OCD)	Recurrent, unwanted thoughts (obsessions) and/or repetitive behaviors (compulsions) such as handwashing, counting, checking, or cleaning, often performed with the hope of preventing obsessive thoughts or making them go away. Performing these rituals provides only temporary relief, and not performing them markedly increases anxiety.
Post-traumatic stress disorder (PTSD)	Persistent, frightening thoughts and memories of a prior traumatic experience in which grave physical harm occurred or was threatened and feeling emotionally numb, especially with people to whom one was once close. People with PTSD may experience sleep problems, feel detached or numb, or be easily startled.

SOURCE: Adapted from American Psychiatric Association. (1994). *Diagnostic and Statistical Manual of Mental Disorders: Primary Care Version* (4th ed.). Washington, DC: Author.

TABLE 10.2   Common Symptoms of Depression

Psychological Symptoms	Behavioral Symptoms	Physical Symptoms
Depressed mood	Crying spells	Fatigue
Irritability	Interpersonal confrontation	Reduced or too much sleep
Anxiety/nervousness	Anger attacks/outbursts	Decreased or increased appetite
Reduced concentration	Avoidance of anxiety-provoking situations	Weight loss/gain
Lack of interest/motivation	Social withdrawal	Aches and pains
Inability to enjoy things	Workaholism	Muscle tension
Reduced interest in sex	Tobacco/alcohol/drug use or abuse	Heart palpitations
Hypersensitivity to criticism/rejection	Self-sacrifice/victimization	Burning or tingling sensations
Indecisiveness	Suicide attempts/gestures	
Pessimism/hopelessness		
Feelings of helplessness		
Preoccupation with oneself		
Thoughts of death or suicide		

Dysthymia is a chronic form of depression. Dysthymia is similar to depressive reactions in its symptoms except that the degree of suffering from its unrelenting, seething attack can lead to depressive illness, as well as increasing the susceptibility to **major depression**. Major depression is a serious condition that leads to an inability to function, or even to suicide. Whereas the symptoms in dysthymia are less intense, fewer in number, and longer lasting, major depression is marked by one or more major depressive episodes over a 2-week period.

In general, anxiety and mood disorders are treated by different types of psychotherapy and medication or both that enable many individuals to lead normal, productive lives. The treatment approach depends on both the patient's preference and the severity of the disorder. It is important to have the disorder accurately diagnosed by a trained mental health care professional. If a professional determines that the person's symptoms are the result of an anxiety disorder, the type of disorder or the combination of disorders must be identified, as well as any coexisting conditions, such as depression or substance abuse. For example, at least 50 percent of people who have major depressive disorder also have significant anxiety symptoms.

Maintaining and optimizing our mental health requires making countless adjustments to a variety of life's challenges. Life's challenges are viewed as **stress**. Stress places certain mental and physical demands upon us, and how we adapt to these challenges significantly influences our mental and physical health. Your mind and body are connected, and during stressful times it is important to understand the relationship that exists between them. Emotionally, stress can lead to feelings of anxiety and depression (McEwen & Gianaros, 2011). Just like anxiety and depressive reactions, stress is a normal part of everyone's life and should not be viewed as necessarily bad.

Understanding Stress

We feel stress any time we go through some sort of change in life. All change requires adjustment by the human body. From the moment of our birth to our death, we experience a wide range of personal challenges that result in substantial emotional and physical changes. No particular level of stress is optimal for all people. As you will learn, coping and adapting to the demands of everyday life stressors in an effective manner is of great importance for both mental and physical health (**FIGURE 10.4**).

Decades ago, it was pointed out that "the states of health or disease are the expressions of the success or failure experienced by the human body in its efforts to respond adaptively to environmental challenges" (Dubos, 1965, p. xvii). Those who developed many of today's concepts of stress correctly understood that different life stressors could induce helpful (**eustress**; *eu* is Greek for "good") and harmful (**distress**) outcomes. That is, good health requires the presence of eustress and also the limitation of distress to a level to which the human body can adapt.

Stress and Performance

Stress is a natural process, and understanding its effects can help you use it to your advantage. Stress researchers have long recognized that some stress or stimulation is needed for optimal performance. Yerkes and Dodson describe a phenomenon, known today as the Yerkes–Dodson law, of an inverted U-shaped function between stress and performance (Benson & Proctor, 2003). The **Yerkes–Dodson law** theorizes about the ways health and performance are affected as stress increases. Although the relationship between stress and performance varies from person to person, the general pattern can be expressed by viewing the curve in **FIGURE 10.5** .

The curve is divided into three sections. The far left of the curve represents **hypostress**, not enough stress, which occurs when we lack stimulation. This area is

Maintaining and optimizing our mental and physical health requires making countless adjustments to a variety of life's challenges.

Dysthymia Chronic form of depression.

Major depression Serious condition that leads to inability to function and possibly suicide.

Stress Response that includes both a mental reaction (stressor) and a physical reaction (stress response).

Eustress Helpful or good stress.

Distress Harmful or bad stress.

Yerkes–Dodson law Predicts an inverted U-shaped function between stress and performance.

Hypostress Too little stress or stimulation.

Stress is a natural process, and understanding its effects can help you use it to your own advantage.

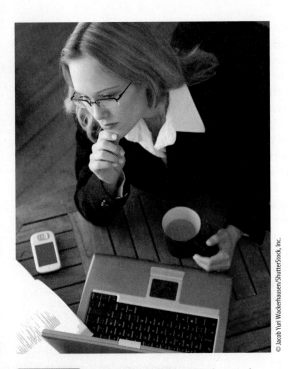

FIGURE 10.4 **Understand Stress.** Coping and adapting to the demands of everyday stressors in an effective manner is of great importance to one's health.

Hyperstress Too much stress; the body begins to decrease in its level of performance.

often referred to as rustout. Rustout is a result of decreased drive and motivation and is caused by lack of challenges in our lives. The middle of the curve represents an area of optimal productivity. This amount of increased stress or stimulation in your life can fuel creativity, create excitement, or physically energize you for important events in your life. This moderate amount of stress can be a motivator toward change and growth that brings forth good results related to our mental and physical health. Moving to the right side of the curve, we find **hyperstress**, or stress beyond that which is optimal. This condition is called burnout, a point where the body begins to decrease its level of performance. Stress becomes unmanageable and out of control at this point and we experience impaired mental and physical capabilities.

Again, no single level of stress is optimal for all people. We are all individual beings with unique requirements. There is no way to predict conclusively how an individual will respond to different stressors. Individual differences in responding to the challenge of stress are products of our experiences, our developmental and environmental influences, and our genetics (McEwen & Gianaros, 2011). Some people may cope well with stress, rising to meet the challenge, and others may be more adversely affected, responding with mental and physical fatigue. And, even when we agree that a particular event is distressing, we are likely to differ from others in our physiological and psychological responses to it.

It has been found that most illness is related to hyperstress and chronic stress. When your resistance resources are overworked, your exhausted body stops functioning smoothly. The signs of hyperstress are so pervasive in our culture that people often fail to recognize them as signs of distress. The signs may show up psychologically, physically, or behaviorally (**FIGURE 10.6**). Psychological signs may include inappropriate anger or intolerance, diminished ability to make priorities and decisions, an inability to concentrate, and a sense of hopelessness or frustration. Physical symptoms may include headaches, aching neck and back, upset stomach, and indigestion.

FIGURE 10.5 **The Effects of Stress on Performance.**

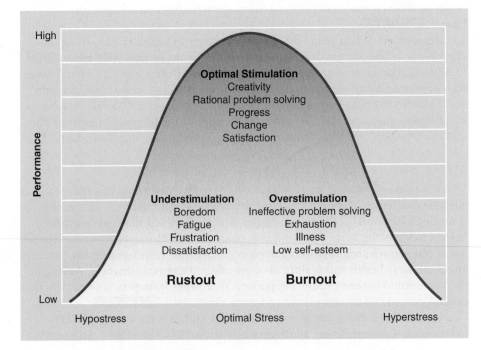

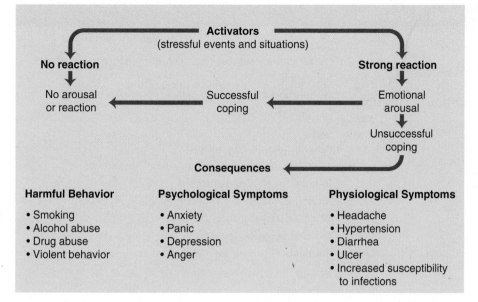

FIGURE 10.6 **Signs and Symptoms of Unsuccessful Coping with Chronic Stress.**

Behavioral signs may include grinding the teeth, biting the fingernails, and over-reacting to minor problems. In summary, stress includes both a mental reaction (stressor) and a physical reaction (stress response).

STRESSORS   The **stressor** itself does not actually create the body's response; the response is your reaction to the stressor. The stress reaction is triggered by our perception of a physical or emotional danger. It is important to underscore that it is our perception of each demand or stressor that makes it stressful or not stressful. What is considered a stressor for one person may not be a stressor for another. For example, the person who loves to mediate disputes and moves from job site to job site would be stressed in a job that was stable and routine, whereas the person who thrives under stable conditions would very likely be stressed in a job where the duties were highly varied. Each individual will have a different response to the same stressor.

Stressors tend to be different not only for different types of people, but also for different ages. As we progress through life, each stage is accompanied by its own distinctive sources of stressors (TABLE 10.3). Our reactions to stressors can be both psychological and physiological. The psychological changes may present themselves as changes in the ways we express our emotions. One of the most frequent undesirable emotional changes is chronic worrying. Worrying too much can lead to variations in mood; you may become depressed, anxious, or irritable. These moods work against you, making finding a solution more difficult. Psychological responses to stressors can be difficult to predict. Your physiological response to stress is much more predictable. A stressor sets into motion a sequence of chemical and nervous system changes that is the same regardless of the type of stressor that initiates it. This sequence has been referred to as the stress response and provides the physical basis for stress.

The Physical Basis of Stress

Hans Selye, a pioneer in stress research, is generally recognized as the father of stress physiology and stress education. Selye coined the word *stress*, which he defined as the "nonspecific response of the body to any demand made upon it" (Selye, 1976). The nonspecificity of the response by the body to any demand was the key factor in the development of Selye's definition of stress. Selye termed this nonspecific response the **general adaptation syndrome (GAS)**. This physical response

Stressor The demand or stimulus that elicits the general adaptation syndrome.

General adaptation syndrome (GAS) The body's response to stress and the adaptability of the body to maintain homeostasis.

The general adaptation syndrome describes the body's response to stress and the adaptability of the body to maintain homeostasis.

TABLE 10.3	Examples of College Student Stressors

Competition

Schoolwork (e.g., difficult, low motivation)

Exams and grades

Poor resources (e.g., library, computers)

Oral presentations/public speaking

Professors/coaches (e.g., unfair, demanding, unavailable)

Choosing and registering for classes

Choosing a major/career

Time

Deadlines

Procrastination

Waiting for appointments and in lines

No time to exercise

Late for appointments or class

Environment

Others' behavior (e.g., rude, inconsiderate, sexist/racist)

Injustice: seeing examples or being a victim of

Crowds/large social groups

Fears of violence/terrorism

Weather (e.g., snow, heat/humidity)

Noise

Lack of privacy

Social

Obligations, annoyances (e.g., family, friends, girl-/boyfriend)

Not dating

Roommate(s)/housemate(s) problems

Concerns about STIs

Self

Behavior (e.g., habits, temper)

Appearance (e.g., unattractive features, grooming)

Ill health or physical symptoms

Forgetting, misplacing, or losing things

Weight/dietary management

Self-confidence/self-esteem

Boredom

Money

Not enough

Bills/overspending

Job: searching for or having interviews

Job/work issues (e.g., demanding, annoying)

Tasks of daily living

Tedious chores (e.g., shopping, cleaning)

Traffic and parking problems

Car problems (e.g., breaking down, repairs)

Housing (e.g., finding/getting, moving)

Food (e.g., unappealing, unhealthful)

---

is based on the principle that your body is constantly attempting to maintain homeostasis (*homeo* = similar, and *stasis* = position), or an internal balance. Maintaining homeostasis requires energy. As mentioned earlier, any situation or force that disturbs the body's homeostasis, or equilibrium, is a stressor.

The GAS describes the body's response to stress and the adaptability of the body to maintain homeostasis. Selye's (1976) research provided evidence that the body goes through a predictable three-stage physiological response to provide energy for the body based on the duration and intensity of the stressor and on whether you are able to cope successfully (**FIGURE 10.7**). The alarm response is an acute, intense, and necessary survival response to a life-threatening stressor. It requires a lot of energy and does not cause harm to the body; rather, it is designed to save lives. In the resistance stage, the body mobilizes energy like in the alarm stage but at a less intense level and over a chronic long-term period. If this adaptation phase continues for a prolonged period of time without periods of relaxation and rest, diseases of maladaptation occur. In the third stage, called exhaustion, the body has run out of its reserve of body energy and immunity. Physical, mental, and emotional resources suffer heavily.

Alarm Reaction

Alarm reaction Immediate response to a stressor that is triggered by any threat to our physical or emotional well-being.

The **alarm reaction** is an immediate, short-duration, high-intensity response to a life-threatening stressor. The reason for this reaction is simple. When a danger or challenge is present, our body reacts in certain ways to protect ourselves. This reaction is part of our human biological makeup. The body follows a typical physiological pattern when reacting to a stressor. When a threat to our well-being is

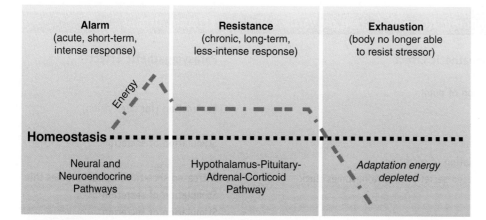

FIGURE 10.7 **The Three Phases of the General Adaptation Syndrome and Three Major Physiological Pathways.** The alarm response is an acute, intense, necessary survival response to a life-threatening stressor. It requires a lot of energy and does not cause harm to the body; rather, it is designed to save our lives. In the resistance stage, the body mobilizes energy like in the alarm stage but at a less intense level and over a chronic long-term period. The body is not at rest and also not in the alarm response. This response occurs from non-life–threatening stressors that are not coped with properly. If this adaptation phase continues for a prolonged period of time without periods of relaxation and rest, diseases of maladaptation occur. In the exhaustion stage, the body has run out of its reserve of body energy and immunity. Physical, mental, and emotional resources suffer heavily.

perceived, a small area of the brain known as the hypothalamus is activated. The hypothalamus stimulates a number of physiological changes, involving activity in both the **autonomic nervous system** (nerve pathways) and the **neuroendocrine system** (nerve and hormonal pathways). These two systems, acting in concert, alter the functioning of almost every part of the body to prepare for immediate vigorous muscle activity. Another term to describe this response to stressors that threaten the body physically is the **fight-or-flight response**.

FIGHT-OR-FLIGHT RESPONSE   The human body has an inborn, "prewired" response for dealing with dangerous situations called the fight-or-flight response. Both fighting and fleeing require the same activities on the part of the body's organs. The stress response is generalized and affects a large number of bodily organs and systems. The term *pathways* is used to describe the routes traveled through the body after a stressor is appraised as threatening or challenging. The three major pathways are (1) the neuro pathway (sympathetic pathway), (2) the neuroendocrine pathway (sympathoadrenomedullary system, or SAM), and (3) the endocrine pathway (hypothalamic-pituitary-adrenal-cortical system, or HPAC). The neuro and neuroendocrine pathways comprise the alarm stage of GAS, and the endocrine pathway comprises the resistance stage of GAS (refer to Figure 10.7).

The actions of the autonomic nervous system (ANS) are the most immediate, sensitive, rapidly acting, and powerful of the body's response to stress. It is called *autonomic* because it can function without conscious thought. The ANS regulates vital internal organs and activities, including circulation, digestion, respiration, and temperature regulation, which are involved in maintaining homeostasis or adjusting to demands of immediate stressors. Two branches of the ANS act to maintain this homeostatic balance, the sympathetic and parasympathetic nervous systems, and they are activated by the hypothalamus. The sympathetic responses are stress responses, whereas the parasympathetic responses are relaxation responses (TABLE 10.4).

Autonomic nervous system
The part of the nervous system that controls smooth muscle, cardiac muscle, and glands; subdivided into sympathetic and parasympathetic.

Neuroendocrine system The hormone-secreting cells of the body; this system is influenced in part by the nervous system.

Fight-or-flight response Response to stressors that challenge the body to respond physically.

| TABLE 10.4 | Effects of the Autonomic Nervous System on Various Visceral Effector Organs |||

Effector	Sympathetic Effect	Parasympathetic Effect
Eye		
Iris (pupillary dilator muscle)	Dilation of pupil	—
Iris (pupillary sphincter muscle)	—	Contraction (for near vision)
Glands		
Lacrimal (tear)	—	Stimulation of secretion
Sweat	Stimulation of secretion	—
Salivary	Decreased secretion; saliva becomes thick	Increased secretion; saliva becomes thin
Stomach	—	Stimulation of secretion
Intestine	—	Stimulation of secretion
Adrenal medulla	Stimulation of hormone secretion	—
Heart		
Rate	Increased	Decreased
Conduction	Increased rate	Decreased rate
Strength	Increased	
Blood vessels	Mostly constriction; affects all organs	Dilation in a few organs (e.g., penis)
Lungs		
Bronchioles (tubes)	Dilation	Constriction
Mucous glands	Inhibition of secretion	Stimulation of secretion
Gastrointestinal tract		
Motility	Inhibition of movement	Stimulation of movement
Sphincters	Closing stimulated	Closing inhibited
Liver	Stimulation of glycogen hydrolysis	—
Adipocytes (fat cells)	Stimulation of fat hydrolysis	
Pancreas	Inhibition of exocrine secretions	Stimulation of exocrine secretions
Spleen	Stimulation of contraction	—
Urinary bladder	Muscle tone added	Stimulation of contraction
Arrector pili muscles	Stimulation of hair erection, causing goosebumps	—
Uterus	If pregnant, contraction If not pregnant, relaxation	
Penis	Ejaculation	Erection (due to vasodilation)

Sympathoadrenal system The second pattern of the fight-or-flight response.

Epinephrine The "fear hormone"; helps supply glucose for increased muscle and nervous system activity.

Norepinephrine The "anger hormone"; helps speed the heart rate and raises blood pressure to provide more oxygen for the body.

Simultaneous to the activation of the neuro axis or the sympathetic nervous system, the second pattern of the fight-or-flight response, called the neuroendocrine or **sympathoadrenal system**, is set in motion. The nerve impulses from the sympathetic branch of the autonomic nervous system reach the core of the adrenal glands (the medulla), resulting in the release of **epinephrine** and **norepinephrine**. Epinephrine is referred to as the "fear hormone" and helps supply glucose to be used for increased muscle and nervous system activity. Norepinephrine is referred to as the "anger hormone" and helps speed up the heart rate and raises blood pressure in an attempt to provide more oxygen for the body. The effects of epinephrine and norepinephrine are similar to those produced by the sympathetic nervous system, except that the effects of the hormones last about 10 times longer (**FIGURE 10.8**).

The sum of the increased activation of the sympathetic nervous system and sympathoadrenal patterns (the fight-or-flight response) is to provide chemicals and hormones that provide huge amounts of energy to permit the person to perform far more strenuous physical activity than normal. This increase in energy needs does not cause harm to the body; rather, it is designed to save our lives. Following

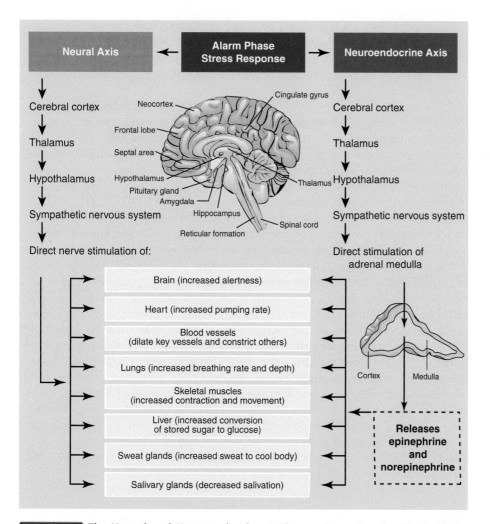

FIGURE 10.8 The Neural and Neuroendocrine Pathways Comprise the Alarm Phase of the General Adaptation Syndrome.

the alarm stage, the body attempts to adapt to the stressor and return to homeostasis. Readjustment occurs if the stressor is removed or properly coped with and body functions return to normal. Physiologically, the **parasympathetic nervous system** is the counterpart to the sympathetic nervous system. The effects of the parasympathetic nervous system are the opposite of the effects of the sympathetic nervous system (refer to Table 10.4). When no danger is perceived or the danger has been coped with successfully, the parasympathetic nervous system releases acetylcholine, a chemical that plays an inhibitory role on the effects of sympathetic stimulation of organs. This is commonly known as the **relaxation response** (**FIGURE 10.9**). The actions of both divisions of the autonomic nervous system must be balanced to maintain homeostasis.

Stage of Resistance

Your body responds to all acute high-intensity stressors, both positive and negative, by trying to get back to normal. After the alarm reaction, a stage of resistance occurs if the stressor is not completely removed or coped with properly. The resistance response also occurs from everyday non-life-threatening stressors that are not coped with properly (refer to Table 10.3). In the resistance stage, the body mobilizes energy like in

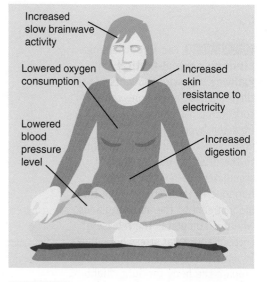

FIGURE 10.9 The Relaxation Response. The relaxation response is important because it allows the body to return to homeostasis following the fight-or-flight response.

the alarm stage but at a less intense level and over a long-term period. The body is not at rest and also not in the alarm response (refer to Figure 10.7). This is the body's response to long-term protection and is also referred to as chronic stress. Prolonged stress without periods of relaxation and rest are responsible for many diseases.

The energy the body requires during this less intense, but extended fight-or-flight response largely comes from the endocrine stress response system, or hypothalamic-pituitary-adrenal-cortical (HPAC) pathway (**FIGURE 10.10**). The emotional perception that you cannot completely cope with a non-life-threatening stressor causes your hypothalamus in the brain to release a hormone called corticotropin-releasing factor (CRF) that triggers the pituitary gland (located near the hypothalamus) to release adrenocorticotropic hormone (ACTH). ACTH circulates in the blood and stimulates the outer shell of the adrenal glands or the adrenal cortex to increase production of hormones called glucocorticoids. **Glucocorticoids** are chemicals responsible for speeding up the body's metabolism and increasing its access to energy storage. One important glucocorticoid is cortisol. Small increases of cortisol during the immediate response to a stressor have positive effects in the body, including providing a quick burst of energy, heightened memory functions, an increase in immunity, and lower sensitivity to pain. However, higher and more prolonged elevated levels of cortisol in the blood stream (like those associated with chronic stress) have negative effects such as impaired cognitive performance, lower immunity, higher blood pressure, increases in blood sugar levels, decreased bone density and muscle tissue, and increased abdominal fat. Increased abdominal fat is associated with many more health problems than is fat deposited in other areas of the body. These health problems include a greater risk of cardiovascular disease, type 2 diabetes, hypertension, hyperlipidemia, and certain cancers. The challenge in this day and age is not to let the HPAC system stay chronically aroused so as to avoid the "toxic chemical cocktail" of corticoid hormones that persist in the body for prolonged periods of time.

Glucocorticoids Chemicals responsible for speeding up the body's metabolism and increasing access to energy storage.

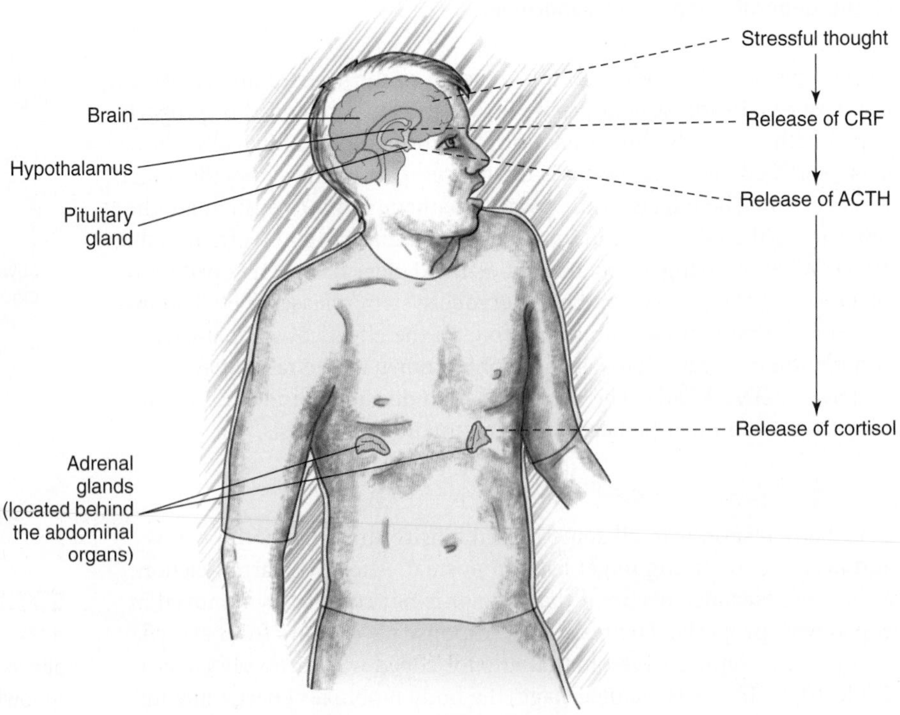

FIGURE 10.10 **The Hypothalamic-Pituitary-Adrenal-Cortical Pathway.** Stressful thoughts trigger the release of a hormone called corticotropin-releasing factor (CRF) from the hypothalamus of the brain. CRF flows in the bloodstream to the pituitary gland, where it stimulates the release of the hormone ACTH. ACTH flows in the bloodstream to the adrenal glands, where it stimulates the release of cortisol and other stress hormones. In acute stress, cortisol helps prepare the body for fight, flight, wound healing, and infection. In chronic stress, cortisol unbalances metabolism and suppresses the immune system.

Brain

Hypothalamus

Pituitary gland

Adrenal glands (located behind the abdominal organs)

Stressful thought

Release of CRF

Release of ACTH

Release of cortisol

Stage of Exhaustion

The stage of exhaustion occurs when the body's adaptation energy resources become depleted and fatigued (refer to Figure 10.7). Prolonged exposure to a stressor can cause the body organs to become weakened and increase the susceptibility to illness (**FIGURE 10.11**). Each person has a breaking point for dealing with stress. In addition to chronic or extended stress, stress research also indicates that the cumulative adjustments required from intermittent and sequential stressors may affect the body over time. Selye (1976) observed that the number of stress responses and readjustments increases the wear and tear on the body, accelerating degenerative disease processes. The ongoing level of demand for adaptation in an individual is called **allostatic load** (*allo* = all, *static* = equilibrium) on that person, and it may be an important contributor to many chronic diseases (McEwen & Gianaros, 2011). The continual setting off of the fight-or-flight response and the resultant efforts of resistance to reestablish equilibrium in the body are increasingly becoming the focal point of research on illness and disease.

> **Allostatic load** The ongoing level of demand for adaptation in an individual.

Stress Management

The art of stress management is to keep yourself at a level of stimulation that is healthy and enjoyable. Life without stimuli would be dull and boring. Life with too many stimuli becomes unpleasant and tiring. The primary purpose for developing stress management techniques is to reduce the potential psychological and physical illnesses that result from too much stress. There are many specific strategies available for managing hyperstress. The specific strategies can be categorized into three basic approaches: (1) the environmental engineering, or "controlling

> The art of stress management is to keep yourself at a level of stimulation that is healthy and enjoyable.

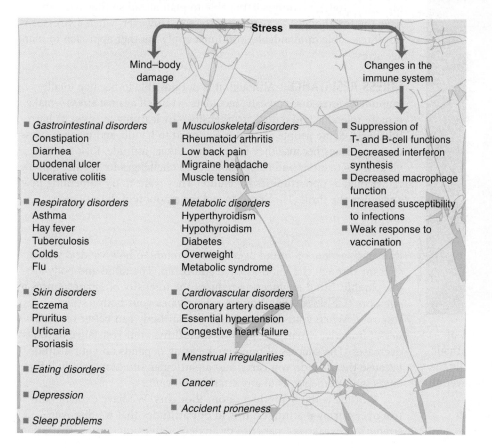

FIGURE 10.11 **The Stress–Illness Relationship.** Stress contributes to illness by causing the mind and body to become exhausted, worn down, and damaged by weakening immunity.

your circumstances," approach; (2) the mind engineering, or "mind over matter," approach; and (3) the physical engineering, or "stress-fit," approach.

These three basic stress approaches can be used singly or in any combination. Different approaches work for different stressors. Additionally, approaches vary among individuals. Before you begin reading about the three basic solutions, it may be helpful for you to have at hand a list of sources of stress in your life. You can then apply a basic approach to your source of stress and select from the wide variety of specific strategies presented at the end of the chapter.

Environmental Engineering

> **Environmental engineering** Stress management approach that attempts to avoid stress in the first place.
>
> **Mind engineering** Stress management approach concerned with reducing the intensity of our emotional responses to stressors.

The **environmental engineering**, "control your circumstances," approach deals with the stressor by attempting to avoid it in the first place. This approach advocates controlling as many environmental circumstances as you can. To accomplish this, you need to analyze the situations in your environment that may lead to foreseeable stressful situations. Keeping a stress diary is a helpful way of finding out what causes you stress and when and where the event occurs. After a few weeks you should be able to analyze this information and plan a change in your environment to avoid the stressor.

For example, lately you have been feeling unprepared and tired for your Friday 8 A.M. economics class, an important class in your major field. Your journal reveals that you have routinely stayed out late with your friends on Thursday evenings and thus not studied for your economics class. You decide to take positive action by changing these circumstances; you make time to study on Thursday evening and get to bed at a reasonable hour. This new course of action leaves you feeling prepared and rested for your economics class.

Recognizing what stressors you can avoid by eliminating interaction with them is a good solution for dealing with a number of stressors. This strategy requires being able to plan ahead so that you can have the forethought to avoid the stressor. However, when a stressor is not foreseeable or avoidable, you must apply another approach to manage stress.

STRESS RESISTANCE   Although it is not possible to become totally immune to stressors, you can "inoculate" yourself against stress—make it more tolerable and reduce its intensity—by learning to resist its harmful effects. Some people are better equipped to handle and manage stress than are others because they have a "risk taker" attitude. Risk takers view new situations and responsibilities as challenges for further growth rather than as opportunities for failure. They want to try something new and enjoy the thrill. They need to feel the emotion of the situation.

Mind Engineering

Mind engineering, or "mind over matter," refers to how we deal with a stressor through the mind–body relationship. The mind and body are inseparable. Mind engineering reduces the intensity of our responses to stressors (**FIGURE 10.12**). Your mind activates your body's stress response. When your mind is healthy, your body can better resist illness. Similarly, when your mind is unhealthy, your resistance to illness decreases. The success of mind engineering depends on your attitude because the attitude you carry into a particular situation greatly influences your perceptions of any stressor or event.

Attitude is the byproduct of our thoughts. We have explicit control over our own attitudes. It is in our attitudes that we discover strength or weakness, patience or anxiety, determination or frustration,

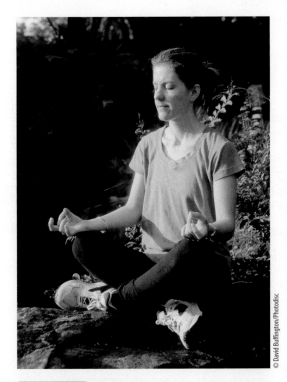

© David Buffington/Photodisc

FIGURE 10.12 **Meditation.** This is a form of mind engineering. Meditation uses a rhythmic activity such as breath awareness to focus the mind, lifting you out of your ordinary level of consciousness into a state of "passive awareness" where the body can deal with stress problems.

when faced with a stressor. Our attitude about what we believe we should be, and the imagined punishment if we fail, determines how we see and react to stressors. When we view stressors positively, we are secure in our knowledge that we can make them beneficial to our growth if we choose. When we view stressors negatively, we are uncertain about our abilities to deal with them effectively and consequently feel that we are not in control.

Are you viewing your stressors in exaggerated terms—taking a challenging situation and making it a disaster? Positive thinking is everything when it comes to managing stress. Most people carry on a silent conversation with themselves, which is referred to as *self-talk*. Positive self-talk offers many stress-reduction benefits. If you think "I know I can ace my chemistry exam," you will have a better chance of success and will have made the stressor a positive one. If you engage in negative self-talk, "I can't pass that chemistry exam," you increase your chances of failure and the stressor becomes negative. As any sailor knows, "It is not the direction of the wind that determines our course so much as how we set our sails"; in sailing parlance, this is known significantly as the *attitude*.

Physical Engineering

The **physical engineering**, "stress-fit," approach is predicated on the fact that it is easier to deal with the stress response when your body is healthy from regular physical activity. Regular physical activity is useful in removing the byproducts that occur as a result of the stress response and in reducing the physiological reactivity of the body to stressors. (**FIGURE 10.13**).

> **Physical engineering** Stress management approach using regular exercise to optimize your stress responses.

EXPENDING EXCESS ENERGY AND BIOCHEMICALS   When the body experiences the fight-or-flight reaction, it provides us with energy via stress hormones and chemicals. The result is that our bodies go into a state of high energy, but there is often nowhere for this energy to be expended, so our bodies stay in a state of arousal for hours. Additionally, the biochemicals that initiated this high state of energy are left to circulate in the body and have the capability for causing illness. During times of high stress, we can benefit from a physical outlet. Physical activity is the most logical way to expend excess energy and throw off its biochemical by-products. When our bodies are in a high state of energy, it is healthful to expend this energy in a brisk walk or run. In addition to enjoying the available energy, the exercise is ridding the body of stress hormones and flushing the excessive biochemical buildup.

Studies show that those who experience stress-related illness, or symptoms of stress, can best reduce or eliminate those symptoms with a program of stress management that includes physical activity. Physical activity reduces many of the physical symptoms associated with stress and illness. A regular physical activity program lowers the resting heart rate and blood pressure and protects against fatigue, reduces digestive problems, and relaxes muscles.

PHYSIOLOGICAL REACTIVITY   The second part of the physical engineering approach deals with the theoretical assumption that higher levels of aerobic fitness are associated with less physiological reactivity to psychosocial stressors. This stress-buffering or inoculation effect occurs as a result of improved physiological functioning of the body. The improved cardiovascular adaptation from aerobic exercise appears to mediate and decrease an individual's physiological reactivity in response to a number of psychosocial stressors (Puterman et al., 2011). In other words, because physical activity provides an almost identical physiological response to that which occurs with mental stress,

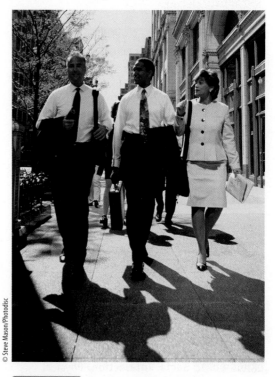

© Steve Mason/Photodisc

FIGURE 10.13 **Physical Engineering.** An excellent way to reduce stress is to take a walk.

strengthening the body to react to physical activity strengthens the body's response to mental stress. Long-term physical activity may adjust the brain's responsiveness to chemicals associated with stress, allowing the brain to deal with stress more efficiently.

The Mental Health Benefits of Physical Activity

You have just read about how physical activity can be therapeutic when it comes to managing stress. Interestingly, the psychological benefits from physical activity across all areas of mental well-being are advocated. There is much speculation, however, about the mechanisms by which physical activity improves mental health. What follows is a brief overview of the most frequently discussed mechanisms. Although these explanations are discussed independently, it is important to understand that they may operate interactively.

Cognitive Behavioral Theory

This explanation maintains that, as a person engages in physical activity and experiences bodily changes, self-efficacy increases. That is, participating in and mastering a specific physical task creates positive feelings because individuals perceive that they can perform activity even in tough situations. This is related to self-efficacy, in which the strength of a belief is enhanced by continued successful execution of a behavior. Feelings of mastery and control are incompatible with negative thoughts (anxiety, depression). Additionally, self-esteem is fostered when you realize that you are doing something that will ultimately benefit you. Participating in physical activity has a positive social value attached to it because it is a health-enhancing activity.

Social Interaction Theory

The buffering effects of social support are well documented when it comes to physical activity. Physical activities that are done with friends and colleagues, or in social settings, can have a net effect of improving mental health (**FIGURE 10.14**). This mental health effect is much more noticeable in groups in which people feel a collective sense of achievement and accomplishment.

Distraction Theory

The solitude experienced when performing physical activities that require a fairly consistent, repetitive motion (bicycling, jogging, hiking) can alter your state of consciousness. The regular breathing and movement associated with these activities may act as a mantra that induces feelings of calmness and tranquility similar to those obtained while practicing meditation. Physical activity provides a distraction, or time-out, from the daily worries of a stressful society. Furthermore, physical activity provides an opportunity for introspective thinking that can stimulate creativity in problem solving.

The Endorphin Hypothesis

The endorphin hypothesis represents the most popular biological explanation, despite questionable evidence. The term **endorphins** is a general classification for important body chemicals that are responsible for enhancing emotions (euphoric feelings) and providing pain relief (analgesic effect). The neurochemical reaction from endorphin release has been shown to increase following physical activity of 20 minutes or more.

Endorphins Body chemicals responsible for enhancing emotions and providing pain relief.

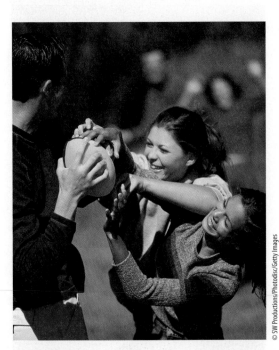

© SW Productions/Photodisc/Getty Images

FIGURE 10.14 **Social Interaction.** Physical activity with friends can improve mental and emotional well-being.

The Thermogenic Hypothesis

During physical activity the body temperature rises. This body-warming effect has been shown to reduce muscle tension, thereby countering the tension that may build up in muscles from stress (e.g., neck, lower back).

The therapeutic benefits of regular physical activity are without rival when it comes to reducing stress and maintaining mental health. The form of physical activity you choose should be enjoyable, noncompetitive, and personally satisfying. Choose activities you like, or they will feel like a chore and you will begin to avoid them. It is also beneficial to have a variety of physical activity outlets.

Quick Relaxation Techniques

Other ways to reduce stress in the body are through certain disciplines that fall under the heading of relaxation techniques. The term *relaxation training* is used in the health literature to refer to various techniques that stimulate the relaxation response (refer to Figure 10.9). The relaxation response is the opposite of the fight-or-flight response to stressful or threatening situations. Just as we are all capable of heightening and sustaining a stress reaction, we have also inherited the ability to put our bodies into a state of relaxation. In this state, all the physiological events in the stress reaction are reversed: breathing and pulse slow, blood pressure declines, and muscles relax. It has been found that relaxing for just 20 minutes each day can be beneficial to both your physical and mental health. Unlike the stress reaction, which is automatic, *the relaxation response needs to be induced by intention*. Fortunately, there are many simple ways to do this. The following relaxation techniques can be practiced by anyone at any time during the day and provide instant relief from stress.

Deep Breathing

Deep breathing is a countermeasure to stress. When stressed, your breathing becomes rapid and shallow, causing an insufficient amount of oxygen to reach your lungs. The goal in deep breathing is to slow and increase the volume of air inhaled, thus providing extra oxygen to the blood. Slowly inhale through your nose, expanding your abdomen before allowing air to fill your lungs. Reverse the process by constricting your stomach and exhaling through your mouth, making a quiet, whooshing sound as you blow out calmly. Continue to take long, slow, deep breaths, focusing on the sound and feeling of breathing. After a few minutes you should become more relaxed. You may want to perform this technique a couple times a day. Deep breathing is a very effective method of relaxation and is the most basic technique used in relaxation training.

Visualization

Visualization is using your imagination to reduce stress. Find a quiet place where you feel comfortable. Sit down and close your eyes, breathing slowly (**FIGURE 10.15**). Next, try focusing on one peaceful thought or on a goal you want to attain. If your mind strays back to the problem causing stress, make yourself return to the peaceful thought for a couple of minutes. Another variation of visualization is to create a picture in your mind of a beautiful place and imagine yourself there, using as many of your senses as you can.

Progressive Muscle Relaxation

Progressive muscle relaxation (PMR) is a simple technique used to induce neuromuscular relaxation by creating an awareness of the difference between muscular tension and a relaxed state. Progressive muscle

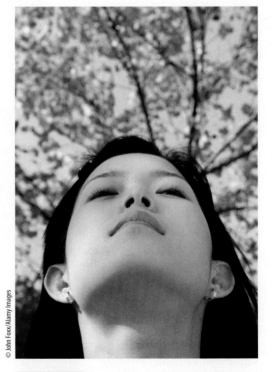

© John Foxx/Alamy Images

FIGURE 10.15 Relaxation. Finding a quiet place where you feel relaxed and can focus on one peaceful thought is important in using visualization.

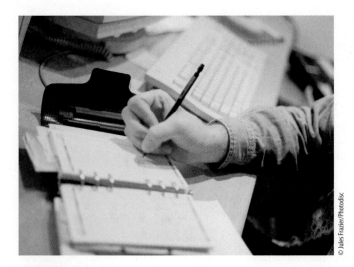

FIGURE 10.16 **Time Management.** Keeping a daily log of how you spend your time is a helpful technique.

relaxation is a two-step process. First, each muscle or muscle group is tensed from 5 to 10 seconds and then relaxed for 15 to 25 seconds. Repeat this procedure at least once; if the area remains tense, repeat up to five times.

Time Management

A major contributor to stress is inadequate time management skills. Despite an image of college life being carefree and fun-filled, college life will probably require more careful and effective utilization of time than a student has ever needed to achieve before. A typical student schedules 15 or more classroom hours a week and is expected to average about 2 hours of preparation for each hour in the classroom. This means that students have at least a 45-hour work week, equivalent to a full-time job. In addition, many students find that they must balance their academic responsibilities with part-time jobs, family, and social responsibilities. Thus, it is not surprising that a common concern among college students is not having enough time to get everything accomplished. The job of being a college student, like most other jobs, can be carried out more effectively with the use of time management techniques that increase your productivity.

ASSESS CURRENT TIME USE A good place to begin is to keep track of how you currently use your time. Assess how you spend your time each day for a week by faithfully keeping a daily log of how you spend your waking hours (**FIGURE 10.16**).

SETTING PRIORITIES Write down your goals and priorities. Divide your goals into essential, important, and trivial. Having a record of how you spend your time allows you to compare your current use of time to essential and important goals and priorities. You need to be spending virtually all of your time on essential and important priorities (**FIGURE 10.17**).

FIGURE 10.17 **Prioritizing Tasks.** Classify tasks from your to-do list according to their urgency and importance and do them in this order: (1) urgent and important; (2) not urgent and important; (3) urgent but not important; and (4) not urgent or important. Move tasks labeled "urgent and not important" to other categories because urgency is a state of mind and makes things seem important even if they are not.

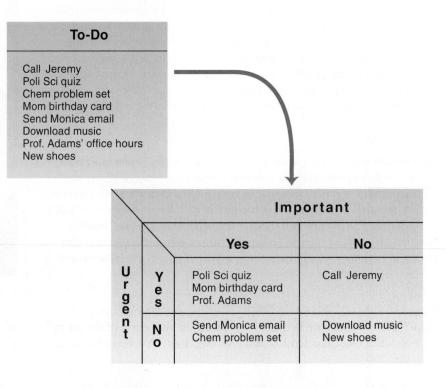

TIME SCHEDULING   One of the best techniques for developing more efficient time-use habits is to prepare a schedule. The following is a flexible way to help establish long-term, intermediate, and short-term goals. A long-term schedule consists of your fixed commitments. These include only obligations you are required to meet every week: classes, job, physical activity, religious activities, organizational meetings. Your immediate schedule consists of a short list of major tasks to be accomplished in the next week: quiz on Monday, ballgame on Wednesday, read 60 pages in history by Friday. Finally, each evening before going to bed, write down on a small card what you must accomplish the next day. Carry this card with you during the day and cross out each item after you accomplish it.

Physical Activity and Health Connection

Our mental and emotional health is essential to the quality of our lives and influences our physical health. The relationship between regular physical activity and mental wellness has been established. Much is known about the physical health benefits of physical activity as it relates to fitness, weight management, and control of a number of chronic disease conditions. Now we can also look at physical activity as an important contributor to mental health and comprehensive stress management strategies. Stress management experts increasingly regard physical activity as one the most healthful ways to reduce stress. People who are physically active tend to have better mental health. Being regularly active increases general feelings of well-being and positive moods, and decreases bouts of anxiety and depression. By engaging your body regularly in physical activity, you prepare it to deal with the physiological strains associated with emotional crises. Your body becomes better able to handle stress and the chemicals that are released during stressful situations. A sound mind and a sound body are equally important to our overall health.

concept connections

1. **People who are physically active tend to have better mental health.** The consensus is that people who are physically active have higher scores on important mental health factors such as self-esteem, self-concept, self-worth, body image, and cognitive functioning than do sedentary people. Furthermore, physical activity has been shown to be effective in treating people who report symptoms of anxiety, depression, and stress.

2. **Our mental and emotional health are central to the quality of our lives, and both influence our physical health.** Holistic health perspectives emphasize mind–body unity and include the complex relationship between mental and physical functioning as well as the continuum between health and illness.

3. **Maintaining and optimizing our mental and physical health requires making countless adjustments to a variety of life's challenges.** Life's challenges are perceived internally as stress. Stress places certain physical and mental demands upon us, and how we adapt to these challenges significantly influences our mental and physical health. Your mind and body are connected, and during stressful times it is important to understand the relationship that exists between them.

4 **Stress is a natural process, and understanding its effects can help you use it to your advantage.** Stress researchers have long recognized that some stress (stimulation) is needed for optimal performance. Yerkes and Dodson describe a phenomenon that is known today as the Yerkes–Dodson law, which predicts an inverted U-shaped function between stress and performance. The Yerkes–Dodson law theorizes about the ways health and performance are affected as stress increases.

5 **The general adaptation syndrome describes the body's response to stress and the adaptability of the body to maintain homeostasis.** Selye's research provided evidence that the body goes through a predictable three-stage physiological response to any kind of stressor: (1) the alarm reaction, when the adrenal glands are activated in an attempt to mobilize the body's energy resources for physical action; (2) the stage of resistance, in which the readjustment occurs; and (3) if the readjustment is not complete, the stage of exhaustion may follow, leading to illness and possibly death.

6 **The art of stress management is to keep yourself at a level of stimulation that is healthy and enjoyable.** Life without stimuli would be dull and boring. Life with too many stimuli becomes unpleasant and tiring. The primary purpose for developing stress management techniques is to reduce the potential psychological and physical illnesses that result from too much stress.

Terms

Alarm reaction, 226
Allostatic load, 231
Anxiety, 221
Anxiety disorders, 221
Autonomic nervous system, 227
Depression, 221
Depressive reactions, 221
Distress, 223
Dysthymia, 223
Emotional health, 219
Endorphins, 234
Environmental engineering, 232
Epinephrine, 228

Eustress, 223
Fight-or-flight response, 227
General adaptation syndrome (GAS), 225
Glucocorticoids, 230
Hyperstress, 224
Hypostress, 223
Major depression, 223
Mental health, 219
Mental illness, 221
Mind engineering, 232
Neuroendocrine system, 227
Norepinephrine, 228

Parasympathetic nervous system, 229
Physical engineering, 233
Psychosomatic disease, 221
Relaxation response, 229
Stress, 223
Stressor, 225
Sympathoadrenal system, 228
Yerkes–Dodson law, 223

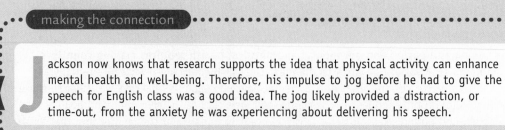

making the connection

Jackson now knows that research supports the idea that physical activity can enhance mental health and well-being. Therefore, his impulse to jog before he had to give the speech for English class was a good idea. The jog likely provided a distraction, or time-out, from the anxiety he was experiencing about delivering his speech.

Critical Thinking

1. Jackson was able to determine that exercising helped relieve the speech anxiety he was having. Review Figure 10.6. Are you experiencing any of the harmful stress symptoms listed? If so, do you think stress is the cause? If yes, what are the specific stressors? What physical activities might you do to help relieve these stressors?

2. Review your list of life stress sources. Next to each source, list whether you would use environmental engineering, mind engineering, or physical engineering to manage the stressor. Would more than one strategy be useful? Do you see physical activity helping to manage the stress in your life? Why or why not?

3. Stressors can be a result of situations present on your campus or in your campus community. Community stressors may be problems such as crime, pollution, lack of recreation facilities, and overcrowded classrooms or residence halls. Identify what you consider to be a major stressor in your campus community. How would you go about changing this stressor?

References

Beaula, J., Carlson, A., & Boyd, J. (2011). Counseling on physical activity to promote mental health: Practical guidelines for family physicians. *Canadian Family Physician* 57(4):399–401.

Benson, H., & Proctor, W. (2003). *The Breakout Principle: How to Activate the Natural Trigger That Maximizes Creativity, Athletic Performance, Productivity and Personal Well-Being*. New York: Simon & Schuster.

Bertheussen, G., Romundstad, P.R., Landmark, T., Kaasa, S., Dale, O., & Helbostad, J. (2011). Associations between physical activity and physical and mental health—A HUNT 3 study. *Medicine and Science in Sports and Exercise* 43(7):1220–1228.

Dubos, R. (1965). *Man Adapting*. New Haven, CT: Yale University Press.

Erickson, K.I., Voss, M.W., Prakash, R.S., Basak, C., Szabo, A., Chaddock, L., Kim, J.S., Heo, S., Alves, H., White, S.M., Wojciki, T.R., Mailey, E., Vieira, V.J., Martin, S.A., Pence, B.D., Woods, J.A., McAuley, E., & Kramer, A.F. (2011). Exercise training increases size of hippocampus and improves memory. *Proceedings of the National Academy of Sciences* 108(7):3017–3022.

Mate, G. (2011). *When the Body Says No: Exploring the Stress–Disease Connection*. Hoboken, NJ: John Wiley & Sons.

McAuley, E., Szabo, A.N., Mailey, E.L., Erickson, K.I., Voss, M., White, S.M., Wojcicki, T.R., Gothe, N., Olson, E.A., Mullun, S.P., & Kramer, A.F. (2011). Non-exercise estimated cardiorespiratory fitness: Associations with brain structure, cognition, and memory complaints in older adults. *Mental Health and Physical Activity*. doi:10.1016/j.mhpa.2011.01.001.

McEwen, B.S., & Gianaros, P.J. (2011). Stress- and allostasis-induced brain plasticity. *Annual Review of Medicine* 62:431–445.

Puterman, E., O'Donovan, A., Adler, N.E., Tomiyama, J., Kemeny, M., Wolkowitz, O.M., & Epel, E. (2011). Physical activity moderates effects of stressor-induced rumination on cortisol reactivity. *Psychosomatic Medicine* 73(7):604–611.

Raglin, J.S., & Wilson, G.S. (2012). Exercise and its effects on mental health. In Bouchard, C., Blair, S.N., & Haskell, W.L., eds. *Physical Activity and Health*, 2nd ed. Champaign, IL: Human Kinetics, Chapter 21, pp.331–344.

Selye, H. (1976). *The Stress of Life*. New York: McGraw-Hill.

Substance Abuse and Mental Health Services Administration. (2012). *Results from the 2010 National Survey on Drug Use and Health: Mental Health Findings* (NSDUH Series H-42, HHS Publication No. (SMA) 11-4667). Rockville, MD: Substance Abuse and Mental Health Services Administration.

U.S. Department of Health and Human Services. (2010). *Healthy People 2020: The Road Ahead*. Online: http://www.healthypeople.gov/hp2020.

Voss, M.W., Nagamatsu, L.S., Liu-Ambrose, T., & Kramer, A.F. (2011). Exercise, brain, and cognition across the life span. *Journal of Applied Physiology* 111(5):1505–1513.

Wipfli, B., Landers, D., Nagoshi, C., & Ringenbach, S. (2011). An examination of serotonin and psychological variables in the relationship between exercise and mental health. *Scandinavian Journal of Medicine and Science in Sports* 21(3):474–481.

Activities & Assessments

© Ron Chapple Studios/Dreamstime.com

Making Informed Decisions About Drug Use

11

what's the connection?

Recently, Jim has realized that his friend and roommate Bill is not handling his drinking of alcohol very well. Whenever they go out to a bar or a club, Bill drinks to get drunk. Furthermore, Jim recognizes that even when they do not go out, Bill still needs to have a few drinks every evening. This has caused Bill to miss class and work as a result of his drinking, as well as to get into trouble with his family and friends. This is making Jim worry about whether Bill has a problem with his drinking and how to approach Bill about this. Jim wonders, "Where can I go for help?"

concepts

1. College students face a conscious choice about whether to drink alcohol, smoke cigarettes, or use other psychoactive drugs while they pursue their degree.

2. Chronic drug use can disrupt the body's normal balance, or homeostasis.

3. Making wise drug use decisions is important.

4. Alcohol misuse and abuse is one of the most significant health-related drug problems in the United States.

5. Cigarette smoking is the most preventable cause of premature death in the United States.

go.jblearning.com/kotecki4e
The website for this book is a great source for supplementary physical health information for both students and instructors. Visit **go.jblearning.com/kotecki4e** to find a variety of useful tools for learning, thinking, and teaching.

College students face a conscious choice about whether to drink alcohol, smoke cigarettes, or use otherpsychoactive drugs while they pursue their degree.

Introduction

Most students are in college for a number of reasons: for an education, to succeed academically, and to get a degree. Students are in college because they are intelligent, certainly smart enough to get into a college and, if they so choose, smart enough to stay there. However, when some students leave school early, it's not because they struggled in the classroom; it may be because they struggled with their choices with psychoactive substance use. Their psychoactive drug use may have resulted in missing classes, performing poorly on tests and assignments, disciplinary issues, or other problems (National Institute on Alcohol Abuse and Alcoholism [NIAAA], 2012).

Nearly all college students face a conscious choice about whether to drink alcohol, smoke marijuana or cigarettes, or use other psychoactive drugs while they pursue their degree. What they choose to do is related to a host of factors, including wanting to have a good time, to fit in or feel more comfortable socially and be accepted, to regulate moods and feelings, to forget about problems or numb out, to relieve emotional or physical pain, or to have a mind-altering experience. However, the use of many psychoactive drugs often creates the opposite effect. Psychoactive drug use can impair alertness and achievement by distorting sensory perception, interfering with memory, and causing a loss of self-control. For example, even occasional use of marijuana affects cognitive development and short-term memory. The major problem with psychoactive drugs is that when people take them, they focus on the immediate desired mental and emotional effects and ignore the potentially damaging mental and physical side effects that can occur. One way or another, the use of psychoactive substances alters the normal functioning of the human body, and in the long run they can cause serious damage.

TABLE 11.1 lists the major types of drugs that affect brain functioning and provides examples of each. Later in the chapter the two most commonly used and abused psychoactive drugs—alcohol and tobacco—are covered. Before discussing these drugs, it is important to examine some general terminology and concepts related to drugs.

Drug Terminology

The word **drug** has many different meanings. For the purpose of this chapter, a *drug* is defined as any absorbed substance, other than food, that changes or enhances any physical or psychological function in the body. This comprehensive definition of a drug includes a variety of substances that many people use for medical or nonmedical purposes. **Drug use** is the taking of a drug for its intended purpose in an appropriate amount, frequency, strength, and manner. The many wonders of modern medicine are based on **drug therapeutics**, the proper use of drugs in treating and preventing diseases and preserving health. For example, a physician prescribes a medication to help fight an infection, reverse a disease process, or restore normal body function, and you follow the directions exactly (TABLE 11.2).

Drug misuse is the unintentional or inappropriate use of prescribed or nonprescribed medicine resulting in the impaired physical, mental, emotional, or social well-being of the user. Continuing with the preceding medication example, taking the medication at the wrong times, not taking all of the medication, or taking too much at one time is drug misuse. As a result, you may not recover as expected, or your condition may worsen.

Drug abuse is a pattern of substance (drug) use leading to significant problems such as failure to attend school, substance use in dangerous situations (driving a car or risky sexual behavior), substance-related legal problems, or continued substance use that negatively affects friends, family, and society. People are more

Drug Any absorbed substance, other than food, that changes or enhances any physical or psychological function in the body.

Drug use The taking of a drug for its intended purpose in an appropriate amount, frequency, strength, and manner.

Drug therapeutics The proper use of drugs in treating and preventing diseases and preserving health.

Drug misuse The taking of a substance for its intended purpose, but not in the appropriate amount, frequency, strength, or manner.

Drug abuse The deliberate use of a substance for other than its intended purpose, in a manner that can damage health or ability to function.

TABLE 11.1	Psychoactive Drugs: Effects on the Body						
Drug Category	Trade or Other Names	Physical Dependence	Psychological Dependence	Tolerance	Possible Side Effects	Overdose Effects	Withdrawal Effects
Stimulants	Caffeine, cocaine (snow, Big C), methamphetamine, crystal meth (crystals), Preludin, Ritalin, Dexadrine or "dex," black beauties, black hollies	Possible	High	Yes	Alertness, euphoria, increased pulse rate and blood pressure, sleeplessness, lack of appetite	Fever, hallucinations, convulsions, death	Prolonged sleep, irritability, depression, anxiety, moodiness, headaches
Depressants	Alcohol, barbiturates (goofballs), Valium, Halcion, Quaalude, GHB, GBL, "roofies" (Rohypnol)	Varies	Varies	Yes	Slurred speech, drunken behavior	Depressed breathing, dilated pupils, coma, death	Depression, anxiety, sleeplessness, convulsions, death
Opiates	Heroin (China white), morphine, codeine-containing products, methadone, Demerol, OxyContin, Vicodin, Darvon, Percodan	Moderate to high	Moderate to high	Yes	Euphoria, sleepiness, depressed breathing, nausea	Slowed breathing, convulsions, coma, death	Teary eyes, watery nose, yawning, tremors, anxiety, abdominal cramps
Marijuana (cannabis)	Pot, hash, hashish oil, Acapulco gold, blunts, buds, Columbo, weed	Unknown	Moderate	Possible	Euphoria, relaxation, increased appetite, distorted time perception	Anxiety, paranoia	Anxiety, depression
Hallucinogens	LSD blotters, mescaline, STP, psilocybin, high doses of PCP, peyote, psychedelic mushrooms, ketamine	None (LSD and mescaline); others, unknown	Unknown	Yes	Euphoria, hallucinations, poor time perception	Anxiety, psychotic behavior	None reported
Inhalants	Gasoline, paint thinners and removers, freon, aerosols, butyl nitrate	None	Possible	No	Euphoria, sleepiness, confusion, slurred speech	Brain, kidney, or liver damage; headaches; death	Anxiety
Drugs with mixed effects	Nicotine, PCP, MDMA (Ecstasy)	Unknown	High (PCP); unknown (MDMA)	Yes	Hallucinations and altered perception	Psychosis, possible death (PCP)	Unknown

SOURCES: Goldberg, R. (2010). *Drugs Across the Spectrum*, 6th ed. Independence, KY: Cengage Learning; and Hanson, G.R., Venturelli, P.J., & Fleckenstein, A.E. (2012). *Drugs and Society*, 11th ed. Burlington, MA: Jones & Bartlett.

TABLE 11.2	Six Tips to Avoid Medication Mistakes

1. **Find out the name of your medication.** Rather than simply letting your doctor write a prescription and send you on your way, be sure to ask the name of the medication.

2. **Ask questions about how to properly use the medication.** Some good questions to ask: What should I do if I forget a dose? Should I take this medication before, during, or after meals? What should the timing be between doses? What side effects might I have? When should I contact my doctor or pharmacist if I have certain side effects? Are there any other medications, food, or activities that I should avoid while using this medication? Should the medication be stored in the refrigerator or at room temperature? Take notes or ask your doctor to write down instructions or other information that is important to know about your medication or condition.

3. **Know what your medication is for.** It is important to understand your medication because you are more likely to use it correctly, more likely to know what to expect from the medication, better able to report what you are using, and better able to report any problems to your doctor and pharmacist.

4. **Read medicine labels and follow directions.** Before you use any medication, you should know when to use it, how much to use, and how long to use it. Be sure to read the medication label every time. In the middle of the night, you could accidentally put drops for your ears into your eyes or give your older child's medicine to the baby if you are not careful about checking the label. Also, read the patient medication information that comes with your prescription thoroughly before using your medication.

5. **Keep all of your health care providers informed about your medications and dietary supplements (including vitamins and herbs).** Make it a habit of showing your list of medications to all health care professionals at every visit to the doctor, pharmacy, and hospital. Include on this list all of your prescriptions and over-the-counter medications as well as dietary supplements including vitamins and herbals. Keeping all of your health care professionals informed about everything that you use will help ensure that you do not use two medicines with the same active ingredient or anything that will interact with something else you are using.

6. **Keep the list of your medications with you at all times and let a loved one know.** Keep a list of your medications and dietary supplements with you at all times, such as in your wallet or purse, and keep a copy in your home. Share a copy of the medication list with a family member or friend or let them know where you keep the list. In an emergency, that person will be able to inform your doctors of the medications and dietary supplements you use.

SOURCE: U.S. Food and Drug Administration. (2010). FDA Consumer Health Information: 6 Tips to Avoid Medication Mistakes. Online: http://www.fda.gov/ForConsumers/ConsumerUpdates/ucm096403.htm.

Psychoactive drug A chemical substance that alters one's thinking, perceptions, feelings, and behavior.

Drug dependence A chronic, progressive, and relapsing disorder that applies to all situations in which drug users develop either a psychological or physical reliance on a drug.

likely to abuse psychoactive drugs than other drugs because of their effects on the mind. A **psychoactive drug** is a chemical substance that alters your thinking, perceptions, feelings, and behavior (refer to Table 11.1). Such drugs include both legal and illegal substances. According to many, alcohol is the most commonly abused psychoactive drug in the United States today (Substance Abuse and Mental Health Services Administration [SAMHSA], 2011).

Drug dependence is used to describe continued use of drugs even when significant problems related to their use have developed. Signs include an increased tolerance or need for increased amounts of a substance to attain the desired effect, withdrawal symptoms with decreased use, unsuccessful efforts to decrease use, increased time spent on activities to obtain substances, withdrawal from social and recreational activities, and continued use of the substance even with awareness of physical or psychological problems encountered because of the extent of substance use (SAMHSA, 2011). TABLE 11.3 lists the diagnostic criteria for substance dependence.

It is generally assumed that no one starts using drugs with the goal of misusing, abusing, or becoming dependent on them; however, it is possible to drift from responsible use to misuse, abuse, or dependence for a number of commonly used drugs. It is also clear that many chronic users eventually do experience problems with drugs and may eventually suffer negative health consequences. Addressing or treating chronic users in terms of their level of involvement is essential in forestalling a number of detrimental health effects. Therefore, it is critical to understand the processes that our bodies and minds undergo with chronic drug use.

TABLE 11.3	Criteria for Drug Dependence Diagnosis

Diagnostic and Statistical Manual IV

A maladaptive pattern of substance use leading to clinically significant impairment or distress as manifested by three (or more) of the following, occurring at any time in the same 12-month period:

- Substance often is taken in larger amounts or over longer period than intended
- Persistent desire or unsuccessful efforts to cut down or control substance use
- A great deal of time is spent on activities necessary to obtain the substance (e.g., visiting multiple doctors, or driving long distances), use the substance (e.g., chain smoking), or recover from its effects
- Important social, occupational, or recreational activities given up or reduced because of substance abuse
- Continued substance use despite knowledge of having a persistent or recurrent psychological or physical problem that is caused or exacerbated by use of the substance
- Tolerance, as defined by either:
  a. need for greater amounts of the substance to achieve intoxication or desired effect; or
  b. markedly diminished effect with continued use of the same amount
- Withdrawal, as manifested by either:
  a. characteristic withdrawal syndrome for the substance; or
  b. the same (or closely related) substance taken to relieve or avoid withdrawal symptoms

International Classification of Diseases, 10th Revision

[ICD-10 research criteria differ from the clinical diagnostic guidelines listed here.] Three or more of the following must have been experienced or exhibited at some time during the previous year:

- Difficulties in controlling substance-taking behavior in terms of its onset, termination, or levels of use
- A strong desire or sense of compulsion to take the substance
- Progressive neglect of alternative pleasures or interests because of psychoactive substance use; increased amount of time necessary to obtain or take the substance or to recover from its effects
- Persisting with substance use despite clear evidence of overtly harmful consequences, depressive mood states consequent to heavy use, or drug-related impairment of cognitive functioning
- Evidence of tolerance, such that increased doses of the psychoactive substance are required to achieve effects originally produced by lower doses
- A physiological withdrawal state when substance use has ceased or been reduced, as evidenced by the characteristic withdrawal syndrome for the substance, or use of the same (or a closely related) substance with the intention of relieving or avoiding withdrawal symptoms

SOURCE: National Institute on Drug Abuse. (2004). Criteria for drug dependence diagnosis.

Chronic Drug Use

Chronic drug use often unsettles the body's normal balance, or homeostasis. The person who continues to use a drug moves to a level of risk one step beyond because each exposure carries with it the possibility that the body's chemical pathways will change to adapt to repeated exposure to the drug. This can be a difficult idea to grasp, but within it lies the foundation for *tolerance, psychological dependence, physical dependence,* and *withdrawal illness.* The following sections define each of these key terms and explain how they are related to the gradual distress of the body. This continuum of involvement with drugs is essential for people to consider as they honestly examine their own drug use and evaluate its possible long-range consequences in terms of quitting or changing drug-related behaviors.

Tolerance

Tolerance, a homeostatic response, is the adaptation of the body to a drug in such a way that repeated exposure to the same dose results in less effect on the body. To counteract the tolerance phenomenon, the individual requires increasing doses

Chronic drug use can disrupt the body's normal balance, or homeostasis.

Tolerance Adaptation of the body to a drug in such a way that repeated exposure to the same dose results in less effect on the body.

to produce the original effect. These increased doses may be dangerous to certain parts of the body, because all body parts do not become equally tolerant to the drug. For example, a higher blood alcohol concentration is thought to be required to diminish a chronically heavy drinker's physical performance as compared with a moderate drinker's performance because the central nervous system is less depressed in the heavy drinker because the nerve tissue has become more tolerant of alcohol. Similarly, the brain and stomach do not adapt well to higher concentrations of alcohol—are not as tolerant to its toxicity—which results in blackouts (not remembering events) and acute stomach irritation and inflammation.

Another example of tolerance occurs with the chemical nicotine, found in cigarettes. Nicotine produces pleasurable feelings that make the smoker want to smoke more; it also acts as a depressant by interfacing with the flow of information between nerve cells. As the nervous system adapts to nicotine, smokers tend to increase the number of cigarettes they smoke and hence the amount of nicotine in their blood. After a while, the smoker develops a tolerance for the drug, which leads to an increase in smoking over time. Eventually, the smoker reaches a certain level and then smokes to maintain this level. Tolerance has been proposed as an important component in understanding substance dependence.

Drug Dependence

Drug dependence, commonly known as drug addiction, is a chronic, progressive, and relapsing disorder that applies to all situations in which drug users develop either a psychological or physical reliance on the drug. **FIGURE 11.1** lists health experts' ratings of how easy it is to become addicted and how difficult it is to stop using various psychoactive drugs. Substance dependence is a strong dependence on a drug typified by three factors: (1) tolerance to a given dose or the need for more and more of the substance, (2) severe withdrawal symptoms, and (3) the loss of control, or the need to consume the substance at all costs. This drug dependence is characterized by a *compulsive and continued use* in spite of adverse health consequences. Drug dependence is based on the concepts of psychological and physical dependence.

PSYCHOLOGICAL DEPENDENCE   **Psychological dependence**, or behavioral dependence, is a craving for a drug for primarily psychological or emotional reasons. The person begins to rely on a drug as a solution to a variety of emotional problems ranging from boredom to relief of anger or frustration. A good example of psychological dependence can be seen in cigarette smokers. Some smokers use the habit to enhance their moods and feelings of competency, whereas others use the habit to reduce their feelings of distress and anxiety. Smoking becomes a means of emotional and psychological support for many smokers and a necessary way of dealing with life. Once this happens, any attempt to quit or reduce smoking results in psychological distress. Psychological cravings for drugs may last for years after quitting.

PHYSICAL DEPENDENCE   **Physical dependence** is the biological adaptation to a drug by the body, in which the drug has become necessary to maintain a balance related to certain body processes. Physical dependence studies investigate the motivational properties of physical withdrawal reactions. At some point the body becomes so completely adapted to the drug that it is a necessity for physiological function. The discomfort experienced during withdrawal of some drugs has long been presumed to be a factor in continued drug intake and addiction. Although physical dependence is not a necessary condition for drug addiction, it may contribute to the total reinforcing impact of some drugs. For example, in many dependent smokers, evidence suggests that the urge to smoke correlates with a low blood nico-

Psychological dependence Craving for a drug for primarily psychological or emotional reasons.

Physical dependence The body's biological adaptation to a drug, in which the drug has become necessary to maintain a balance in certain body processes.

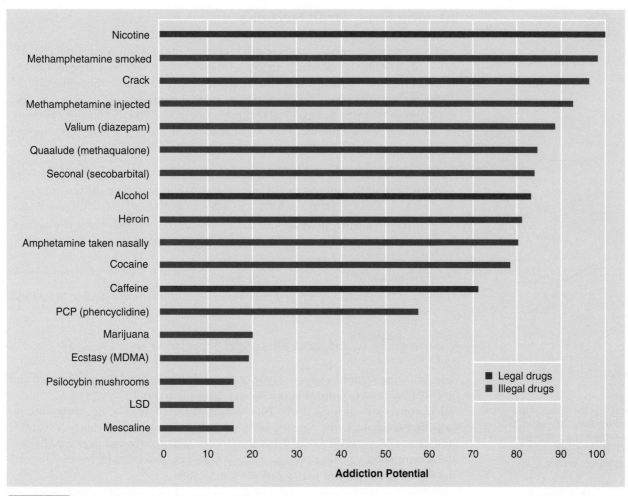

FIGURE 11.1 **The Addiction Potential of Various Drugs.** This chart shows health experts' ratings of the addiction potential of various drugs, with 100 being the highest addiction potential. Note that both legal and illegal drugs can be highly addictive.

tine level, as though the smoker were trying to achieve a certain nicotine level and avoid withdrawal symptoms. Thus, smokers may be smoking to achieve the reward of nicotine effects or to avoid the pain of nicotine withdrawal. When the body has to adapt to the absence of the drug, withdrawal illness develops.

Withdrawal Illness

Withdrawal illness, or *abstinence syndrome*, displays recognizable physical signs and symptoms that result from drug abstinence. Withdrawal illness is a direct result of physical dependence. The signs and symptoms can occur within hours of drug abstinence or take several days to develop. The type and severity vary with the type of drug. For example, the nicotine found in cigarette smoke is a significant physical dependency–producing drug (refer to Figure 11.1).

Discontinuation of nicotine may result in withdrawal illness symptoms—irritability, depression, and dizziness—within hours. The physical distress of the abstinence syndrome may be of sufficient intensity to require medical intervention; it may last from 1 day up to several days (nearly 1 week in the case of alcohol). Once withdrawal sickness subsides, individuals are thought no longer to be physically dependent; however, they still may be psychologically dependent.

Withdrawal illness Recognizable physical signs and symptoms that result from withdrawing drug use.

Making wise drug use decisions is important.

Making Drug Use Decisions

You have reviewed several levels of drug involvement that can occur from chronic drug use. The choices of which drug to use, the amount, and how long to use it are all important individual decisions and should not be made thoughtlessly. Therefore, it is important for you to practice decision-making skills related to taking drugs so that you can make an appropriate response when choosing whether or not to use drugs. Following is a six-stage decision-making strategy that you can use to evaluate your individual drug use (Engs, 2001):

1. Think about the situation and try to understand your reasons for using the drug.
2. Consider all the alternatives to using the drug by examining the reasons and thinking about alternatives for achieving your goals.
3. Attempt to identify potential difficulties associated with each of the alternatives.
4. Consider each alternative in the context of your situation, and select the one that seems best for you.
5. Take action on the alternative you have selected.
6. Assess the results so that you may have more information available to you the next time you are faced with a similar situation.

Commonly Used and Misused Psychoactive Drugs

The following sections examine some of the most familiar and frequently used and misused psychoactive drugs in our society. It is important for you to understand the pharmacology of these drugs. **Pharmacology** is the study of drugs, their sources, how they enter the body, how the body reacts to them, and their short-term and long-term effects on the body. By understanding the positive and negative effects these common drugs have on your body, you will be able to make better-informed decisions related to their use as part of your lifestyle.

Pharmacology The study of drugs, their sources, how they enter the body, how the body reacts to them, and their short-term and long-term effects on the body.

Alcohol and Society

Alcohol misuse and abuse is one of the most significant health-related drug problems in the United States.

Alcohol is the most widely used *psychoactive*, or mood-changing, social drug in the United States. Approximately 50 percent of Americans 12 years and older consume alcoholic beverages on a regular basis, and 14 percent are current infrequent drinkers (SAMHSA, 2011). People drink to relax, reduce self-consciousness and anxiety, celebrate, and have fun, and for social companionship—psychological or emotional benefits that may improve health and well-being. The beneficial effects of moderate alcohol consumption on health are well known and have been studied extensively, as summarized in the 2010 *Dietary Guidelines for Americans* (U.S. Department of Health and Human Services [USDHHS] & U.S. Department of Agriculture [USDA], 2010). Moderate drinking is associated with a lower overall risk of death and a lower risk of diabetes and heart disease among middle-aged and older adults. The guidelines define moderate as an average of up to one alcoholic drink a day for women and up to two drinks a day for men. However, the guidelines don't recommend beginning to drink or drinking more frequently in pursuit of potential health benefits. On the other hand, the detrimental effects of excessive alcohol intake are also well documented, and excessive drinkers should decrease their intake or stop drinking. Excessive alcohol consumption is responsible for approximately 80,000 deaths annually, making it the third leading cause of preventable death in the United States (Centers for Disease Control and Prevention [CDC], 2012a). Excessive alcohol consumption is associated with multiple adverse and social consequences including accidents, violent crime, liver cirrhosis, fetal alcohol spectrum disorder, sexually transmitted infections, and unintended pregnancy. Three in 10 adults drink at excessive levels that put them at risk for alcoholism, liver disease, and other alcohol-related problems (NIAAA, 2010). The estimated economic cost of excessive drinking is more than $220 billion annually (Bouchery et al., 2011).

Alcohol has long been the drug of choice among college students ages 18 to 25. Although it is illegal for anyone under the age of 21 to purchase, possess, or consume alcohol, many college students under age 21 drink alcoholic beverages. College students have notably high rates of heavy drinking compared with the general population. Data from several national surveys indicate that about four in five college students drink and that nearly half of college student drinkers engage in heavy episodic consumption of alcohol. The consequences of excessive and underage drinking affect virtually all college students, campuses, and college communities, whether students choose to drink or not (NIAAA, 2012). TABLE 11.4 lists the consequences of high-risk college drinking.

It is easy to understand why alcohol misuse and abuse is one of the most significant health-related drug problems in the United States. Public health campaigns traditionally urge people to avoid or cut back on their drinking, and appropriately so, because misuse or abuse of alcohol costs the United States in health and social expenditures. Therefore, personal decisions about your alcohol consumption and the associated risks and benefits should be reviewed periodically as part of your health lifestyle strategy.

TABLE 11.4 ▌ Statistical Snapshot of College Drinking

The consequences of excessive and underage drinking affect virtually all college campuses, college communities, and college students, whether they choose to drink or not.

- **Death:** 1,825 college students between the ages of 18 and 24 die from alcohol-related unintentional injuries, including motor vehicle crashes.
- **Injury:** 599,000 students between the ages of 18 and 24 are unintentionally injured under the influence of alcohol.
- **Assault:** 696,000 students between the ages of 18 and 24 are assaulted by another student who has been drinking.
- **Sexual Abuse:** 97,000 students between the ages of 18 and 24 are victims of alcohol-related sexual assault or date rape.
- **Unsafe Sex:** 400,000 students between the ages of 18 and 24 had unprotected sex and more than 100,000 students between the ages of 18 and 24 report having been too intoxicated to know if they consented to having sex.
- **Academic Problems:** About 25 percent of college students report academic consequences of their drinking including missing class, falling behind, doing poorly on exams or papers, and receiving lower grades overall.
- **Health Problems/Suicide Attempts:** More than 150,000 students develop an alcohol-related health problem, and between 1.2 and 1.5 percent of students indicate that they tried to commit suicide within the past year due to drinking or drug use.
- **Drunk Driving:** 3,360,000 students between the ages of 18 and 24 drive under the influence of alcohol.
- **Vandalism:** About 11 percent of college student drinkers report that they have damaged property while under the influence of alcohol.
- **Property Damage:** More than 25 percent of administrators from schools with relatively low drinking levels and over 50 percent from schools with high drinking levels say their campuses have a "moderate" or "major" problem with alcohol-related property damage.
- **Police Involvement:** About 5 percent of four-year college students are involved with the police or campus security as a result of their drinking, and 110,000 students between the ages of 18 and 24 are arrested for an alcohol-related violation such as public drunkenness or driving under the influence.
- **Alcohol Abuse and Dependence:** 31 percent of college students met criteria for a diagnosis of alcohol abuse and 6 percent for a diagnosis of alcohol dependence in the past 12 months, according to questionnaire-based self-reports about their drinking.

SOURCE: National Institute on Alcohol Abuse and Alcoholism. (2012). Snapshot of annual high-risk college drinking consequences. Online: http://www.collegedrinkingprevention.gov/statssummaries/snapshot.aspx.

Measures of Alcohol Consumption

The consumption of alcoholic beverages can have helpful or harmful effects depending on the amount consumed; the pattern of drinking, age, and other characteristics of the person consuming the alcohol; and the specifics of the situation (USDHHS & USDA, 2010).

> **Social drinking** Use of alcohol that consists of an occasional drink or two in the company of friends.
>
> **Moderate drinking** Drinking that causes no problems, either for the drinker or for society; quantified as no more than one drink a day for most women, and no more than two drinks a day for most men.

SOCIAL DRINKING   **Social drinking** is use of alcohol that consists of an occasional drink or two in the company of friends: a glass of champagne at a wedding or on a special occasion, a glass of wine with a special meal, a cold beer after a softball game. This small, infrequent amount of drinking is extremely low risk for harming any body tissue or organ.

MODERATE DRINKING   **Moderate drinking** may be defined as drinking that does not generally cause problems, either for the drinker or society (TABLE 11.5). It should be understood that a given dose of alcohol affects different people differently. Therefore, individuals making the decision to drink must be aware that they are assuming a small inherent risk.

Current recommendations by the *Dietary Guidelines for Americans* state that "those who choose to drink alcoholic beverages should do so sensibly and in moderation—defined as the consumption of up to one drink per day for women and up to two drinks per day for men" (USDHHS & USDA, 2010). A "standard" drink is any drink that contains about 0.6 fluid ounce or 14 grams of "pure" alcohol. A standard drink is defined as 12 fluid ounces of regular beer, 8 to 9 fluid ounces of malt liquor, 5 fluid ounces of wine, or 1.5 fluid ounces of proof or distilled spirits (**FIGURE 11.2**). This current recommendation about moderate drinking by the *Dietary Guidelines* should be acknowledged with the understanding that the guidelines provide many circumstances in which people should not drink alcohol:

- Individuals who cannot restrict their drinking to moderate levels.
- Anyone younger than the legal drinking age. Besides being illegal, alcohol consumption increases the risk of drowning, car accidents, and traumatic injury, which are common causes of death in children and adolescents.

TABLE 11.5	Criteria for Moderate and At-Risk Alcohol Use

Moderate Drinking
Men: ≤ 2 drinks/day*
Women: ≤ 1 drink/day
Over 65 (men and women): ≤ 1 drink/day

At-Risk Drinking
Men: > 14 drinks/week, or > 4 drinks/occasion
Women: > 7 drinks/week, or > 3 drinks/occasion

Alcohol Abuse
Significant impairment or distress in a 12-month period, including
- Failure to meet obligations at work, school, or home
- Recurrent use of alcohol in hazardous situations
- Legal problems related to alcohol
- Continued use despite alcohol-related social or interpersonal problems

Alcohol Dependence
Significant impairment or distress in a 12-month period, including
- Tolerance to alcohol
- Withdrawal symptoms with abstinence from alcohol
- Use of larger amounts over a longer period than intended
- Persistent desire for alcohol (craving)
- Unsuccessful attempts to cut down or control use
- Important social, occupational, or recreational activities given up because of drinking
- Use despite knowledge of alcohol-related problems (denial)

*One drink = 12 g of alcohol, which is the equivalent of 180 mL (6 oz) of wine, 360 mL (12 oz) of beer, or 45 mL (1.5 oz) of 90-proof distilled spirits.

SOURCE: U.S. National Institute on Alcohol Abuse and the American Psychiatric Association.

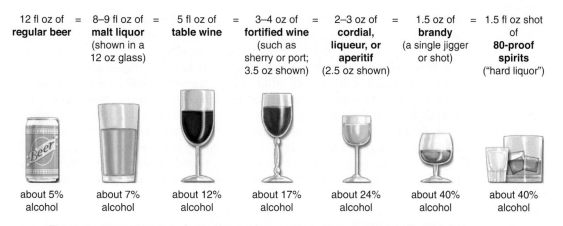

12 fl oz of = 8–9 fl oz of = 5 fl oz of = 3–4 oz of = 2–3 oz of = 1.5 oz of = 1.5 fl oz shot
regular beer   **malt liquor**   **table wine**   **fortified wine**   **cordial,**   **brandy**   of
(shown in a   (such as   **liqueur, or**   (a single jigger   **80-proof**
12 oz glass)   sherry or port;   **aperitif**   or shot)   **spirits**
3.5 oz shown)   (2.5 oz shown)   ("hard liquor")

about 5%   about 7%   about 12%   about 17%   about 24%   about 40%   about 40%
alcohol   alcohol   alcohol   alcohol   alcohol   alcohol   alcohol

The percentage of "pure" alcohol, expressed here as alcohol by volume (alc/vol), varies by beverage.

FIGURE 11.2 **Standard Drink.** In the United States, a "standard" drink is any drink that contains about 0.6 fluid ounce or 14 grams of "pure" alcohol. Although the drinks shown are different sizes, each contains approximately the same amount of alcohol and counts as a single standard drink.
SOURCE: Reproduced from National Institute on Alcohol Abuse and Alcoholism. (n.d.). Rethinking drinking: Alcohol and your health. Online: http://rethinkdrinking.niaaa.nih.gov/whatcountsdrink/whatsastandarddrink.asp.

- Women who are pregnant or who may be pregnant. Drinking during pregnancy, especially in the first few months of pregnancy, may result in negative behavioral or neurological consequences in the offspring. No safe level of alcohol consumption during pregnancy has been established.

- Individuals taking prescription or over-the-counter medications that can interact with alcohol.

- Individuals with certain specific medical conditions (e.g., liver disease, hypertriglyceridemia, pancreatitis).

- Individuals who plan to drive, operate machinery, or take part in other activities that require attention, skill, or coordination or in situations where impaired judgment could cause injury or death (e.g., swimming).

You may be wondering why the recommendation for women is less than that for men. First, women generally have a smaller body size and a lower proportion of water content in which to dilute any alcohol consumed. Second, women have less of a protective stomach enzyme (alcohol dehydrogenase) that breaks down (oxidizes) a portion of alcohol before it enters the bloodstream. Therefore, women will absorb more alcohol into the bloodstream than males of the same weight who have drunk an equal amount of alcoholic beverages. The chemical properties and metabolism of alcohol will be covered in more detail in the alcoholic beverages section later in this chapter.

BINGE DRINKING   Binge drinking differs from social and moderate drinking in terms of the amount of alcohol consumed and the pattern of drinking. Binge drinkers often drink to get drunk and believe that heavy drinking is appropriate and desirable in social situations. The binge is usually planned and will not continue for more than one day. The National Institute on Alcohol Abuse and Alcoholism defines **binge drinking** as a pattern of drinking that brings a person's blood alcohol concentration (BAC) to 0.08 percent or above. This typically happens when men consume five or more drinks, and when women consume four or more drinks, in about 2 hours (NIAAA, 2004). In other words, it is the amount of alcohol consumption that would lead to the presumption of intoxication (drunkenness). Every state considers a person intoxicated and incapable of operating a vehicle safely at this level of intoxication. Furthermore, this high level of intoxication increases

Binge drinking A pattern of drinking that brings a person's blood alcohol concentration to 0.08 percent or above.

the risk for hangovers, fatigue, headaches, shakiness, bloodshot eyes, nausea and vomiting, injuries from accidents, severe impairment of driving, unprotected sex, seizures, brain damage, and death from alcohol overdose.

Most binge drinkers do not feel that they are heavy or high-risk drinkers because they do not drink daily. After a binge, the person will be able to go for days, weeks, or months with little or no drinking before another binge occurs. It is a myth that only daily drinkers have an alcohol problem. Binge drinking is more likely in situations where people drink in groups, where they serve themselves, or where drinking games are involved. Binge drinking is common in college students ages 18 to 24 years, possibly in response to increased freedom in their lives. In the past decade, approximately 40 percent of college students were considered binge drinkers (Johnston et al., 2012).

HEAVY DRINKING **Heavy** or **high-risk drinking** is the consumption of more than 3 drinks on any day or more than 7 per week for women and more than 4 drinks on any day or more than 14 per week for men. Heavy drinking of alcohol results in a significant risk of health consequences, social problems, or both (Table 11.5 and TABLE 11.6). Additionally, for those who drink heavily twice a week, the chances of developing a chronic problem is one in every two people. Chronic abuse of alcohol can lead to a number of serious health conditions (see the section on long-term effects of alcohol), as well as to dependence or alcoholism. *Alcohol dependence*, or *alcoholism*, refers to a disease that is characterized by abnormal alcohol-seeking behavior that leads to impaired control over drinking. Many factors contribute to alcohol dependence, including personality characteristics, stress, family environment, heredity, and the addictive nature of alcohol. Many alcoholics become able to drink ever-larger quantities of alcohol before feeling or appearing drunk. Alcohol users commonly medicate themselves with alcohol, using it, often daily, to help them relax, as a confidence booster, or to avoid withdrawal symptoms.

Alcoholic Beverages

Ethyl alcohol is the common psychoactive ingredient in all alcoholic beverages. It is a direct central nervous system depressant that causes a decreased level of consciousness and decreased motor function. At high concentrations, ethyl alcohol is toxic. It is an anesthetic and can cause autonomic dysfunction leading to death from respiratory depression and cardiovascular failure.

Heavy drinking Consumption of more than 3 drinks on any day or more than 7 per week for women and more than 4 drinks on any day or more than 14 per week for men.

Ethyl alcohol A direct central nervous system depressant that causes a decreased level of consciousness and decreased motor function; the common psychoactive ingredient in all alcoholic beverages.

TABLE 11.6	How Do You Know If You Are Drinking Too Much?

If you are drinking too much, you can improve your life and health by cutting down.

How do you know if you drink too much?

Read these questions and answer yes or no:

- Do you drink alone when you feel angry or sad?
- Does your drinking ever make you late for work?
- Does your drinking worry your family?
- Do you ever drink after telling yourself you won't?
- Do you ever forget what you did while you were drinking?
- Do you get headaches or have a hangover after you have been drinking?

If you answered yes to any of these questions, you may have a drinking problem. Check with your doctor to be sure. Your doctor will be able to tell you whether you should cut down or abstain. If you are an alcoholic or have other medical problems, you should not just cut down on your drinking—you should stop drinking completely. Your doctor will advise you about what is right for you.

SOURCE: National Institute on Alcohol Abuse and Alcoholism. (2001). How to cut down on your drinking. Online: http://pubs.niaaa.nih.gov/publications/handout.htm.

Ethyl alcohol is one of several chemicals in the alcohol family, and is a thin, clear, colorless fluid with a mild, aromatic odor and pungent taste. It is capable of being mixed with water in all proportions and is diffusible through body membranes. Ethyl alcohol contained in beverages is created by fermentation, a process in which the yeast fungus feeds on the sugars or starches in certain plants such as barley or grapes and excretes alcohol along with carbon dioxide. From the cheapest beer to the most expensive wine or after-dinner liqueur, all alcohol is made with the same fermentation process. The different colors, tastes, potencies, and flavors come from the different fruits or vegetables used as well as the additives, by-products, and diluting substances of the fermentation process. The three basic types of alcohol beverages are beer, wine, and distilled spirits (refer to Figure 11.2).

Beer is made from fermented grains and has an alcohol content of approximately 5 percent. Light ("lite") beer, or reduced-calorie beer, has the same percentage of alcohol as regular beer. Wine is made from fermented fruits and has an alcohol content of approximately 12 percent. Some wine drinks, such as wine coolers, have lower alcohol content because of the fruit juice and sugar added to them. Fortified wines, such as port, have alcohol added to them, raising the alcohol content above 12 percent. Finally, distilled spirits, so named because liquid distillation after sugar fermentation increases their alcohol content, originate from sources of starch or sugar, including cereals, molasses from sugar beets, grapes, potatoes, cherries, plums, and other fruits. Distilled spirits (e.g., gin, rum, vodka, whiskey) produce a drink that usually contains 40 to 50 percent alcohol. The alcohol content in distilled spirits is sometimes indicated by degrees of proof, which in the United States is a figure that is twice the percentage of alcohol by volume in a beverage. Thus, 70-proof liquor is 35 percent alcohol. In general, a 12-ounce bottle of beer, a 5-ounce glass of wine, and a 1.5-ounce shot of liquor all contain the same amount of alcohol (0.6 ounce) and therefore have an identical psychoactive effect on the drinker when it comes to intoxication (refer to Figure 11.2).

ALCOHOL AND WEIGHT   Pure alcohol contains about 7 calories per gram, which makes it nearly twice as fattening as carbohydrates or protein (both contain about 4 calories per gram) and only just under the caloric value for fat (9 calories per gram). These calories are considered "empty" calories because they supply no energy value or nutrients; that is, alcohol calories are useless in meeting your body's nutrient needs (TABLE 11.7). Unlike starches and sugars that are converted

---

TABLE 11.7	Calories in Selected Alcoholic Beverages		
Beverage	Approximate Calories per 1 Fluid Ounce*	Example Serving Volume	Approximate Total Calories†
Beer (regular)	12	12 oz	144
Beer (light)	9	12 oz	108
White wine	20	5 oz	100
Red wine	21	5 oz	105
Sweet dessert wine	47	3 oz	141
80-proof distilled spirits (e.g., gin, rum, vodka, whiskey)	64	1.5 oz	96

*Data are from Agricultural Research Service Nutrient Database for Standard Reference, Release 17. Online: http://www.nal.usda.gov/fnic/foodcomp/index.html. Calories are calculated to the nearest whole number per 1 fluid oz.

†The total calories and alcohol content vary depending on the brand. Moreover, adding mixers to an alcoholic beverage can contribute calories in addition to the calories from the alcohol itself.

SOURCE: U.S. Department of Agriculture. (2010). *Dietary Guidelines for Americans*. Washington, DC: Author.

to glucose, glycogen, or fat, alcohol is denatured—mostly in the liver—into carbon dioxide and water. Because an estimated 95 percent of all alcohol we consume is catabolized (the other 5 percent is eliminated through the breath, skin, urine, and feces), it has no direct caloric or nutrient significance. However, many argue that alcoholic beverages indirectly stimulate appetite, decrease physical activity, suppress the basal metabolic rate, and increase consumption of nonalcohol calories from high-calorie unhealthy snacks—all contributing to weight gain. This means that if you want to lose weight, reduce excess body fat, and become physically fit, alcohol is not a good choice.

Alcohol Absorption

When a person drinks alcohol, the alcohol is absorbed primarily by the stomach (20 percent) and small intestine (80 percent) (**FIGURE 11.3**). Because alcohol molecules are small, they are readily absorbed into the blood without being digested. Once the alcohol has been absorbed, it is rapidly carried throughout the body by the blood. A balance occurs such that blood at all points in the system contains approximately the same amount of alcohol. The amount of alcohol in your blood is expressed as **blood alcohol concentration (BAC)**. Blood alcohol concentration is measured in percentages. A simple way to estimate your BAC is shown in (**FIGURE 11.4**).

Alcohol Elimination

The body readily recognizes alcohol in the bloodstream as a toxic substance and begins to remove it from the blood as soon as it reaches the liver. The liver is responsible for eliminating 95 percent of ingested alcohol from the body though an active process of metabolism. The remainder of the alcohol is eliminated through excretion of alcohol in urine, sweat, and breath. Most of the metabolism of alcohol is performed by the enzyme alcohol dehydrogenase (ADH), which is found mostly in the liver. Alcohol dehydrogenase is also found in other tissues of the body, notably in the stomach lining, where it breaks down some of the alcohol before it ever reaches the bloodstream. The ADH enzyme is found

> **Blood alcohol concentration (BAC)** The amount of alcohol in the blood.

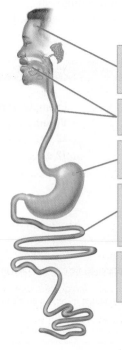

As BAC rises, motor skills, judgment, and reaction times are impaired. If BAC reaches 0.5%, central nervous system function is depressed and coma or death may result.

Small amounts of alcohol are absorbed in the mouth and esophagus as it is swallowed.

Alcohol is readily absorbed in the stomach (approximately 20%), but food will dilute the alcohol and delay its passage into the small intestine.

The small intestine efficiently absorbs most of the alcohol consumed (about 80%). The alcohol then is carried through the bloodstream to all the body's tissues and organs and eventually reaches the liver, where it is metabolized.

The portion of alcohol that is not excreted (about 95%) through sweat, urine, or breath is metabolized by the liver. The liver detoxifies alcohol at a rate of about 0.5 ounce per hour.

FIGURE 11.3 **Alcohol Absorption.** How alcohol is absorbed and metabolized.

in greater quantities and is more active in the stomachs of men than of women—meaning men break down more alcohol before it reaches their bloodstream. The liver can metabolize approximately 0.5 ounce (the equivalent of one drink) per hour. Nothing can be done to speed up this process; cold showers, exercise, black coffee, fresh air, or vomiting will not help. Only time will allow the liver to break down the alcohol in the bloodstream, and unprocessed alcohol circulates through the bloodstream until the liver can process it.

If a person drinks alcohol faster than it can be eliminated from the body, the BAC rises, increasing the toxic effects of ethyl alcohol on the body. There are several important factors that a person can control related to influencing BAC. These include controlling the amount of alcohol consumed and the rate of consumption, and eating before drinking.

AMOUNT OF ALCOHOL As more drinks are consumed, more alcohol is readily available to be absorbed in the blood. It is important to understand the amount of alcohol in each of the three categories of alcoholic beverages. Some people attempt to distinguish among beer, wine, and liquor when explaining their drinking. But, a 12-ounce bottle of beer, a 5-ounce glass of wine, and a 1.5-ounce shot of liquor all contain the same amount of alcohol (0.6 ounce) and therefore have an identical effect on the drinker. The three forms of alcohol have the same potential for intoxication and addiction.

RATE OF CONSUMPTION The rate of drinking affects BAC as a result of a constant rate of alcohol metabolism or elimination by the body. Metabolism of alcohol occurs in the liver. The liver can process about 0.5 ounce (one drink) of alcohol every 1 to 1.5 hours. Because the body metabolizes alcohol at this constant rate, ingesting alcohol at a rate higher than the rate of elimination results in a cumulative effect of increasing BAC.

THE EFFECT OF FOOD The absorption of alcohol is slowed if the stomach contains food. The major reason for this is that alcohol is absorbed most efficiently in the small intestine. The presence of food in the stomach keeps the alcohol from reaching the small intestine. The pyloric valve at the bottom of the stomach remains closed to allow for the digestion of the food in the stomach. Alcohol will still be absorbed through the stomach, but at a much slower rate.

Another factor that significantly influences BAC is body weight. In general, the less you weigh, the more you will be affected by a given amount of alcohol. This is because smaller people have less blood volume than larger people and, therefore, less blood in which to distribute the alcohol. In addition to body weight, body composition also affects the distribution of alcohol. Because alcohol dissolves much more freely in water, a well-muscled individual will be less affected than someone with a higher percentage of fat because fatty tissue does not contain as much water as muscle tissue.

Female

Drinks	Body Weight in Pounds									
	90	100	120	140	160	180	200	220	240	
0	.00	.00	.00	.00	.00	.00	.00	.00	.00	Only safe driving limit
1	.05	.05	.04	.03	.03	.03	.02	.02	.02	Impairment begins
2	.10	.09	.08	.07	.06	.05	.05	.04	.04	Driving skills affected
3	.15	.14	.11	.10	.09	.08	.07	.06	.06	Possible criminal penalties
4	.20	.18	.15	.13	.11	.10	.09	.08	.08	
5	.25	.23	.19	.16	.14	.13	.11	.10	.09	
6	.30	.27	.23	.19	.17	.15	.14	.12	.11	Legally intoxicated
7	.35	.32	.27	.23	.20	.18	.16	.14	.13	Criminal penalties
8	.40	.36	.30	.26	.23	.20	.18	.17	.15	
9	.45	.41	.34	.29	.26	.23	.20	.19	.17	
10	.51	.45	.38	.32	.28	.25	.23	.21	.19	

Your body can get rid of one drink per hour.
One drink = 1.5 oz of 80-proof liquor, 12 oz of beer, or 5 oz of table wine.

Male

Drinks	Body Weight in Pounds								
	100	120	140	160	180	200	220	240	
0	.00	.00	.00	.00	.00	.00	.00	.00	Only safe driving limit
1	.04	.03	.03	.02	.02	.02	.02	.02	Impairment begins
2	.08	.06	.05	.05	.04	.04	.03	.03	Driving skills affected
3	.11	.09	.08	.07	.06	.06	.05	.05	Possible criminal penalties
4	.15	.12	.11	.09	.08	.08	.07	.06	
5	.19	.16	.13	.12	.11	.09	.09	.08	
6	.23	.19	.16	.14	.13	.11	.10	.09	Legally intoxicated
7	.26	.22	.19	.16	.15	.13	.12	.11	Criminal penalties
8	.30	.25	.21	.19	.17	.15	.14	.13	
9	.34	.28	.24	.21	.19	.17	.15	.14	
10	.38	.31	.27	.23	.21	.19	.17	.16	

Your body can get rid of one drink per hour.
One drink = 1.5 oz of 80-proof liquor, 12 oz of beer, or 5 oz of table wine.

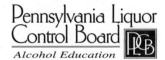

Pennsylvania Liquor Control Board
Alcohol Education

FIGURE 11.4 **Alcohol Impairment—Never Drink and Drive!** SOURCE: "Female Alcohol Impairment Chart" and "Male Alcohol Impairment Chart" from "Blood Alcohol Concentration by Weight and Gender" formulation and computation by the Pennsylvania Liquor Control Board, Bureau of Alcohol Education, and The National Clearinghouse for Alcohol and Drug Information, Substance Abuse, and Mental Health Services Administration.

Immediate Effects of Alcohol

The effects of any drug vary from person to person. The immediate effects of alcohol depend on how much you drink, whether you are used to drinking, your mood, and many other factors such as your weight, sex, and general health status.

Alcohol is considered a **depressant**. Depressants are drugs that produce a slowing of mental and physical activities. When alcohol is absorbed into the circulatory system, its effects are distributed throughout the body. The brain is remarkably sensitive to the effects of alcohol. Alcohol acts on the nerve cells deep in the brain, causing a suppressing effect on the central nervous system. The centers that control cognition, thought, judgment, and speech are depressed with the consumption of one or two drinks. As the blood alcohol concentration increases, depression occurs in the respiratory and spinal cord reflexes. An important correlation exists between the BAC and mental and physical behavior (**FIGURE 11.5**). Five drinks consumed in 2 hours may raise the blood alcohol concentration to 0.10 percent,

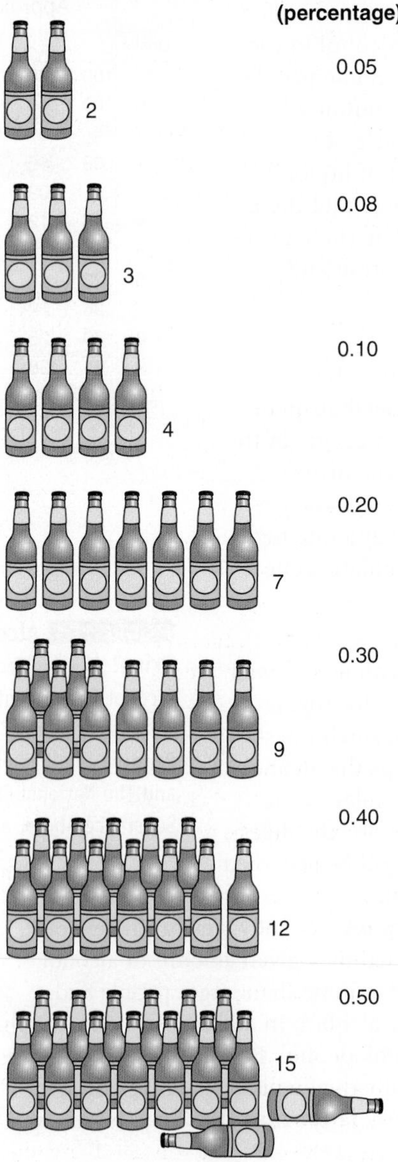

Depressant A drug that produces a slowing of mental and physical activities.

Number of Drinks Consumed in 2 Hours	Alcohol in Blood (percentage)	Typical Effects
2	0.05	Judgment, thought, and restraint weakened; tension released, giving carefree sensation
3	0.08	Tensions of everyday life lessened; cheerfulness
4	0.10	Voluntary motor action affected, making hand and arm movements, walk, and speech clumsy
7	0.20	Severe impairment—staggering, loud, incoherent, emotionally unstable, 100 times greater traffic risk; exuberance and aggressive inclinations magnified
9	0.30	Deeper areas of brain affected, with stimulus response and understanding confused; stuporous; blurred vision
12	0.40	Incapable of voluntary action; sleepy, difficult to arouse; equivalent of surgical anesthesia
15	0.50	Comatose; centers controlling breathing and heartbeat anesthetized; death increasingly probable

FIGURE 11.5 Blood Alcohol Concentration and Physical and Mental Balance.

high enough to be considered legally intoxicated in every state. Signs and symptoms of alcohol use and intoxication include irritability, euphoria, depression, loss of consciousness, impaired short-term memory, inappropriate or violent behavior, loss of balance, unsteady gait, and decreased functioning of the cardiorespiratory system.

ALCOHOL, MEMORY, AND LEARNING   Alcohol inhibits a part of your brain called the hippocampus. This region of the brain is vital to the formation of new memories. If you have alcohol in your system while you are in class or studying, you are less likely to store information in your memory (Montgomery, Ashmore, & Jansan, 2011). Learning and storing memories are complex processes. You are working hard to turn the information you have learned into memories, even after you have stopped thinking about it. Drinking after spending a day in the library will likely negate your hard work.

ALCOHOL AND SLEEP   Sleep is as important for our health as diet and exercise. The average adult needs 8 hours of sleep each night. Yet, most Americans sleep less than 7 hours a night. In fact, one in three adults sleeps 6 or fewer hours each night during the workweek. As a result, many individuals are living with sleep deficits. As our sleep deficit increases, our health and safety decline proportionally. Sleep deprivation causes decreased mental function, reduced reaction time, increased irritability, and hormonal and metabolic changes that mimic the effects of aging. These problems, in turn, can cause driving accidents and on-the-job injuries as a result of human error directly related to fatigue. A few simple lifestyle changes can often ensure better sleeping habits. Most important is getting 8 hours of uninterrupted sleep every night. To help with this, avoid drinking alcohol and caffeinated beverages in the evening. Alcohol consumed within 6 hours of sleep can lead to disruption of valuable rapid eye movement (REM) sleep and often leaves one feeling fatigued and irritable the next morning.

ALCOHOL AND SEXUAL FUNCTION   Despite the fact that, at low doses, alcohol often has a stimulating effect and may help people unwind and socialize, alcohol can have a devastating effect on sexual performance and response. Dehydration from alcohol use leads to less lubrication in the vaginal canal, which increases the potential for painful intercourse and condom breakage. Men are not able to control premature ejaculations when consuming even small amounts of alcohol, and moderate amounts of alcohol result in fewer or no orgasms, a decreased quality of orgasms, difficulty in forming and maintaining erections, and uncertain orgasms.

ALCOHOL POISONING   The dangerous effects of alcohol use can be seen in people who consume large amounts of alcohol relatively quickly. College students frequently engage in this type of drinking behavior, usually in the form of binge drinking. The challenge to drink to your personal limit has become a celebrated observance of college life (**FIGURE 11.6**). In one of the most extensive reports on college drinking, it was found that the majority of students drink "to get drunk" (Kuntsche & Cooper, 2010). Many college students see being drunk as a primary way of socializing.

Drinking to intoxication may result in *alcohol poisoning*, which is a medical emergency that requires immediate attention. Experts estimate that excessive drinking is involved in thousands of student deaths annually. Deadly consequences from alcohol poisoning are usually the result

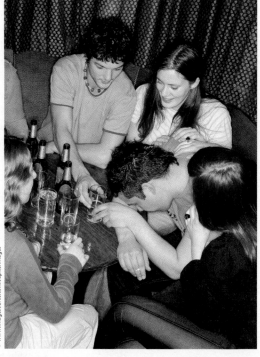

© www.imagesource.com/Jupiterimages

FIGURE 11.6 **Alcohol Poisoning.** College students have notably high rates of drinking compared to the general population and therefore are at higher risk for alcohol-related problems.

of central nervous system and respiratory depression, or of choking to death on vomit after an alcohol overdose. Symptoms of alcohol poisoning are listed in TABLE 11.8 . People who have overdosed on alcohol are unable to help themselves, so it is up to their companions to get assistance. Call for medical attention immediately. Unfortunately, there are no hard and fast rules on how many drinks will result in alcohol poisoning. Generally, a drinker in alcohol poisoning will have a BAC that exceeds 0.25 percent.

UNINTENTIONAL INJURIES   U.S. alcohol-impaired drivers are involved in about 1 in 3 automobile-related deaths (the leading cause of unintentional death in the United States). Even at low blood alcohol concentrations, alcohol impairs your judgment and dulls your reflexes. If you weigh 140 pounds, just two drinks are enough to increase your chances of having a driving accident. You should never operate any type of machinery if you have had alcohol.

Long-Term Effects of Alcohol

Heavy drinking over many years has major toxic effects on the liver, heart, brain, stomach, intestines, and pancreas. These effects increase the risk for developing a number of chronic diseases, including liver disease and cirrhosis, cardiomyopathy and stroke, permanent brain damage, ulcers, pancreas inflammation, and certain forms of cancer (USDHHS, 2010b) (FIGURE 11.7).

Alcohol and Physical Activity

There are some people who believe that physical activity and exercise will offset any detrimental effects of alcohol use. Although moderate drinking the night before physical activity does no real harm, it may limit in a number of ways how well you are able to perform the next day.

Alcohol has various acute and chronic metabolic and physiological effects. You need energy to work out, but the calories from alcohol are unique in that they cannot be stored in the muscles as energy; claims that alcohol provides substantial carbohydrates or energy are false. Alcohol is also a diuretic (it stimulates the production of urine). This increase in urination leads to dehydration and the loss of valuable electrolytes, such as magnesium, calcium, and potassium. These diuretic effects severely impair muscle contraction.

Drinking alcohol the day before or after a workout can also impede your workout performance. Alcohol depletes an important chemical called human

---

TABLE 11.8	**Symptoms of Alcohol Poisoning**

Binge drinking may result in an overdose of alcohol, or alcohol poisoning—a medical emergency that requires immediate attention. It is sometimes hard to tell if someone has only "passed out" or is in serious medical danger. Here are some symptoms of alcohol poisoning:

- Does not respond to being talked to or shouted at
- Does not respond to being pinched, prodded, or poked
- Cannot stand up
- Will not wake up
- Slow, labored, or abnormal breathing
- Skin has a purplish color
- Skin feels clammy
- Rapid pulse rate
- Irregular heart rhythm
- Lowered blood pressure

Pharynx
Cancer of the pharynx is increased 10-fold for drinkers who smoke

Lungs
Lowered resistance is thought to lead to greater incidence of tuberculosis, pneumonia, and emphysema

Heart
Alcoholic cardiomyopathy, a heart condition

Liver
An acute enlargement of the liver, which is reversible, as well as irreversible cirrhosis of the liver

Pancreas
Acute and chronic pancreatitis

Rectum
Hemorrhoids

Osteoporosis
Heavy drinking contributes to bone loss, especially in older women

Testes
Atrophy of the testes

Eyes
Tobacco-alcohol blindness; Wernicke's ophthalmoplegia, a reversible paralysis of the muscles of the eye

Brain
Wernicke's syndrome, an acute condition characterizied by ataxia, mental confusion, and ocular abnormalities; Korsakoff's syndrome, a psychotic condition characterized by impairment of memory and learning ability, apathy, and degeneration of the white brain matter

Esophagus
Esophageal varices, an irreversible condition in which the person can die by drowning in his own blood when the varices open

Stomach
Gastritis and ulcers

Blood and bone marrow
Coagulation defects and anemia

Nerves
Polyneuritis, a condition characterized by loss of sensation

Muscles
Alcoholic myopathy, a condition resulting in painful muscle contractions

FIGURE 11.7 **Long-Term Effects of Alcohol Use.** Because excess alcohol reaches all parts of the body, it causes a wide array of physical problems.

growth hormone (HGH). HGH is part of the muscle-building and repair process and is the body's way of saying that muscle needs to grow. Because of its effects on sleep patterns, alcohol can decrease sleep-related HGH release by as much as 70 percent. Therefore, drinking before or after a workout essentially cancels out most of your hard work.

Tobacco Use: An Enduring Health Threat

Cigarette smoking is the most preventable cause of premature death in the United States.

Although the United States has made significant progress in reducing the number of adult smokers over the last couple of decades, people are still not giving up the habit quickly enough for the country to meet its health goals. Since the U.S. Surgeon General's report in the 1960s about smoking and heart disease, cancer, chronic lower respiratory disease, and other health problems, the nation's smoking rate has fallen dramatically. In the mid-1960s, male smoker rates were well above 50 percent, and approximately one in three women (33 percent) smoked. Currently, less than one in five adults (19.3 percent) smoke cigarettes (males, 21.5 percent; females, 17.3 percent) (CDC, 2011). Although this progress is outstanding, the United States still has a way to go to reach the *Healthy People 2020* goal of reducing smoking to fewer than one in eight adults or 12 percent (USDHHS, 2010a).

Tobacco is still the number one cause of preventable death in the United States. Smoking damages nearly every organ in the body. Annually, approximately 443,000 Americans die (1 in every 5 deaths) as a result of diseases caused by or made worse by smoking, including coronary heart disease, lung cancer and at least nine other cancers, chronic respiratory disease, and stroke (FIGURE 11.8).

Most smokers have a general sense that cigarette smoking is harmful to their health but have difficulty understanding the magnitude of the risk when it comes to the myriad of diseases with which smoking is associated. For many of these people it is important to understand that quitting has an almost immediate impact on a smoker's health. Within minutes, blood pressure and heart rate return to normal. After a few hours, harmful levels of carbon monoxide drop and beneficial levels of oxygen in the blood improve. Within a few weeks or months, respiratory lung function and shortness of breath improve. Over the course of a few years, former smokers can expect to reduce their risk of coronary heart disease, stroke, and cancer.

But cigarette smoking is a tough habit to beat because it is not just a habit but a full-blown addiction to the psychoactive drug **nicotine** (refer to Figure 11.1). In most cases, the decision to start smoking cigarettes is not made by an adult, but rather by a teenager or preteen. Most adult smokers start smoking before reaching the age of 19 (FIGURE 11.9). Currently one in five high school students of all ages (20 percent) are smokers (CDC, 2011). The good news is that recent trends indicate a reduction in the daily use by eighth, tenth, and twelfth graders (FIGURE 11.10).

Smoking is particularly dangerous for teenagers because shortly after initiating the behavior, regular use and dependency can develop. This dependence on smoking can occur in a relatively short time: nicotine addiction can start within a few days of smoking and after just a few cigarettes. Most teenagers believe they will not become dependent or addicted—that they will be able to stop smoking whenever they wish. Their continuation of smoking behavior into adulthood is maintained by

Nicotine A dynamic psychoactive stimulant.

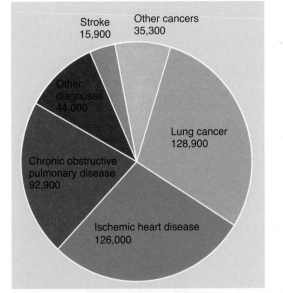

FIGURE 11.8 Roughly 443,000 Annual Deaths Are Attributable to Cigarette Smoking Each Year in the United States. SOURCE: Centers for Disease Control and Prevention. (2008). *Morbidity and Mortality Weekly Report* 57(45):1226–1228. Online: http://www.cdc.gov/nccdphp/publications/aag/osh.htm.

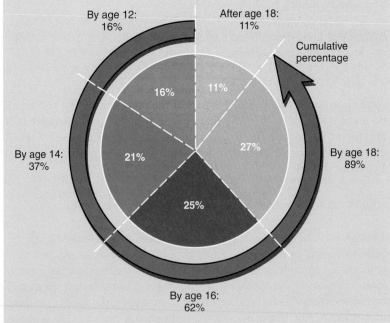

FIGURE 11.9 Age at Which Adults Started Smoking. Most smokers started this habit when they were in their teens or preteens.

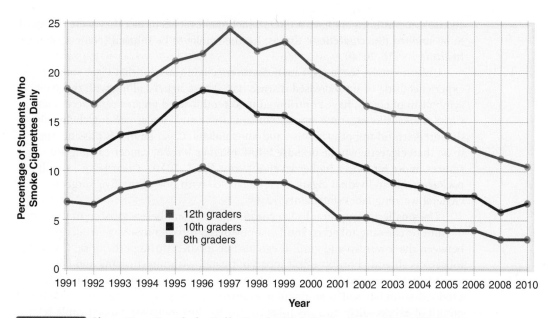

FIGURE 11.10 Cigarettes: Trends in Daily Use by Eighth, Tenth, and Twelfth Graders.

SOURCE: Modified from Johnston, L.D., et al. (2011). *Monitoring the Future National Survey: Results on Drug Use, 1975–2010: Vol. 1, Secondary School Students.* Bethesda, MD: National Institute on Drug Abuse.

a variety of psychological and physiological mechanisms, including familiarity with the act and the events in which it occurs, as well as addiction to nicotine.

The younger a person starts smoking, the more that person will smoke and the longer he or she will do it, all of which leads to greater impairment. Smoking cigarettes doesn't do any part of the body any good, at any time, under any conditions. Although all organs and tissues can be damaged by the toxic chemicals present in cigarette smoke, the developing bodies of teenagers are at particular risk for chemical damage.

Over the past couple of decades, nonsmokers have become increasingly aware that inhaling tobacco smoke from another person's cigarette, cigar, or pipe (secondhand smoke) can pose serious health risks. The process of smoking a cigarette produces three different types of tobacco smoke. The first is mainstream smoke, the smoke directly inhaled through the burning cigarette by the smoker. Second is exhaled mainstream smoke, the smoke breathed out by the smoker from his or her lungs. The composition of mainstream and exhaled mainstream smoke is likely to differ, with some of the compounds in smoke being retained by the smoker or otherwise altered by the process. Third is sidestream smoke, the smoke that drifts from the end of the lit cigarette. **Secondhand smoke**, or environmental tobacco smoke (ETS), consists of exhaled mainstream smoke and sidestream smoke. Prolonged and repeated exposure to secondhand smoke means you are more likely to develop secondhand smoke diseases, including lung cancer, coronary heart disease, asthma, reduced lung function, bronchitis, and pneumonia.

Other forms of tobacco use are not safe alternatives to smoking cigarettes. Many people believe that cigar smoking is a safer choice. Large cigars, cigarillos, and little cigars are the three major types of cigars sold in the United States (CDC, 2012b). Large cigars can measure more than 7 inches in length, and they typically contain between 5 and 20 grams of tobacco. Some premium cigars contain the tobacco equivalent of an entire pack of cigarettes. Large cigars can take between 1 and 2 hours to smoke. Cigarillos are a type of smaller cigar. They are a little bigger than little cigars and cigarettes and contain about 3 grams of tobacco. Little cigars are the same size and shape as cigarettes, often are packaged like cigarettes (20 little cigars in a package), and contain about 1 gram of tobacco. Also, unlike large

Secondhand smoke Exhaled mainstream smoke and sidestream smoke from another person's cigarette, cigar, or pipe. Also known as environmental tobacco smoke (ETS).

cigars, some little cigars have a filter, which makes it seem like they were designed to be smoked like cigarettes—that is, for the smoke to be inhaled (National Cancer Institute [NCI], 2010).

Unfortunately, some cigar manufacturers claim (falsely) that cigar smokers experience little or no increased disease risk. These beliefs, along with the growing symbolism of cigars, have contributed to a trend toward greater cigar acceptance. Cigar smoke, like cigarette smoke, contains toxic and cancer-causing chemicals that are harmful to both smokers and nonsmokers. Cigar smoke is possibly more toxic than cigarette smoke because it has a higher level of cancer-causing substances, more tar, and a higher level of toxins (NCI, 2010). Cigar boxes, smaller packages, and individual cigars must be labeled with one of the five Surgeon General warning label statements (TABLE 11.9).

The smallest group of tobacco consumers uses smokeless tobacco in the form of snuff or chewing tobacco. Snuff is a powdered tobacco that is generally put between the lower lip and gum. It can also be inhaled through the nose. Chewing tobacco is shredded or loose-leaf tobacco, treated with moisturizing and flavoring agents, that is pressed into *plugs* and then placed inside the cheek. Both tobacco products stimulate saliva production, requiring users to spit frequently to clear the mouth of excess saliva and any tobacco that has lost its flavor. Some people refer to smokeless tobacco as "spit tobacco." Approximately 3 percent of all adults 18 and over and 6 percent of high school students currently use smokeless tobacco (CDC, 2012b).

Smokeless tobacco is not a safe alternative to smoking cigarettes. Smokeless tobacco contains more than 2000 chemicals, many of which are potent carcinogens that lead directly to cancer. The strongest association is between smokeless tobacco and oral cancer. Oral cancer risk among regular smokeless tobacco users is *up to fifty times* that of nonusers. The use of smokeless tobacco products leads to nicotine dependence and addiction; the magnitude of nicotine exposure, and its absorption, distribution, and elimination, is similar to smoking cigarettes. Other health effects include gum recession, increased tooth decay, tooth discoloration, bad breath, and a decreased sense of taste, which leads to unhealthy eating habits.

Few behaviors have as many—and as harmful—effects upon a person's health as tobacco use (FIGURE 11.11). The next section examines the composition of

---

TABLE 11.9	Warning Labels on Cigar Products

Health warnings must appear on the principal display panel to ensure warnings are easily seen. Each of the five required warnings must be displayed an equal number of times. Warnings also must be placed on various types of advertising, such as magazines and other periodicals, point-of-purchase displays, and catalogs.

Every cigar package and advertisement requires the following warnings on a rotating basis:

SURGEON GENERAL'S WARNING: Cigar Smoking Can Cause Cancers of the Mouth and Throat, Even If You Do Not Inhale.

SURGEON GENERAL'S WARNING: Cigar Smoking Can Cause Lung Cancer and Heart Disease.

SURGEON GENERAL'S WARNING: Tobacco Use Increases the Risk of Infertility, Stillbirth and Low Birth Weight.

SURGEON GENERAL'S WARNING: Cigars Are Not a Safe Alternative to Cigarettes.

SURGEON GENERAL'S WARNING: Tobacco Smoke Increases the Risk of Lung Cancer and Heart Disease, Even in Nonsmokers.

SOURCE: U.S. Federal Trade Commission. (2001). Nationwide labeling rules for cigar packaging and ads take effect today. Online: http://www.ftc.gov/opa/2001/02/cigarlabel.shtm.

tobacco as a drug, the damaging effects of tobacco on users, why it is habit forming, and how this habit can be defeated.

Constituents of Tobacco Smoke

Tobacco comes from the dried leaves of the native American tobacco plant *Nicotiana tabacum*. Tobacco, in its unprocessed form, contains a number of hazardous chemicals that become increasingly dangerous as it is processed into cigarettes, cigars, or smokeless tobacco forms. The smoke from burning tobacco is the most hazardous to our health. Smoke from burning tobacco consists of a mixture of approximately 4000 chemical substances that are dangerous to living tissue. Within this immense amount of harmful matter, scientists have identified more than 40 chemicals in cigarette smoke that cause cancer. Tobacco smoke is primarily composed of droplets of **tars**, which form 40 percent of the smoke; nicotine, a drug that is poisonous and has addicting qualities; and a dozen gases, including **carbon monoxide**.

TARS Tars are the yellowish-brown solid, sticky materials that are inhaled as part of tobacco smoke. A person who smokes a pack of cigarettes a day will accumulate about 4 ounces of tar in his or her lungs annually. Many tars are deposited on the bronchi, contributing to chronic bronchitis and smoker's cough. Research shows that tobacco tars are *carcinogenic*, or cancer causing. Other chemicals in tobacco tars are co-carcinogens, or stimulate the growth of cancer when combined with other carcinogens.

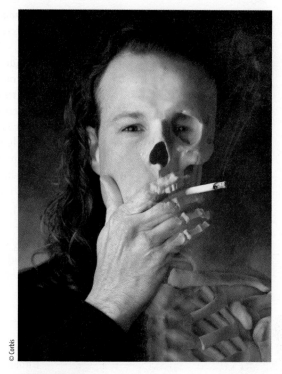

© Corbis

FIGURE 11.11 **Tobacco Use.** Cigarette smoking is the leading cause of preventable death in the United States.

NICOTINE Nicotine is a dynamic psychoactive stimulant. **Stimulants** are drugs that increase central nervous system activity. Nicotine is quickly absorbed into the blood, immediately affecting the brain and the spinal cord as well as the peripheral central nervous system. Nicotine causes a short-term increase in heart rate and blood pressure, and a narrowing or constricting of the peripheral blood vessels and bronchial airways, all of which contribute to an increased workload on the heart.

Nicotine is a powerfully addictive drug (refer to Figure 11.1). This means that the use of nicotine causes changes in the brain that force people to want to use more of the drug. The pharmacological and behavioral processes that reinforce tobacco addiction are similar to those for other addictive drugs. These characteristics include physical dependence and tolerance for the drug, highly controlled or compulsive use, use of the drug to restore psychoactive or physical effects, and predictable withdrawal symptoms when attempts are made to quit (USDHHS, 2010b).

Tars The yellowish-brown solid, sticky materials that are inhaled as part of tobacco smoke.

Carbon monoxide One of the most abundant and poisonous gases in cigarette smoke.

Stimulants Drugs that increase central nervous system activity.

CARBON MONOXIDE Carbon monoxide (CO) is one of the most abundant and poisonous gases in cigarette smoke. Carbon monoxide is an odorless, tasteless, and colorless gas that impairs oxygen transportation to body tissues by competing with oxygen molecules for attachment to the red blood cells. Red blood cells are responsible for carrying oxygen from the lungs to the tissues. Carbon monoxide actually has far greater attachment properties when it comes to binding with the red blood cells than does oxygen. As a result, the capacity of the blood to carry oxygen to the brain, heart, and muscles is diminished. Carbon monoxide also leads to damage of the inner walls of the arteries, a destruction that contributes to plaque buildup and arteriosclerosis.

Smoking and Physical Activity

Many studies have shown that smoking before or during exercise decreases performance as a result of a number of factors. The undesirable effects of carbon monoxide become especially obvious during physical activity. Muscles require more oxygen during physical activity but acquire less from the red blood cells because carbon monoxide has reduced the amount of oxygen the blood can carry. Consequently, muscles tire more quickly.

Smoking also puts an extra burden on the heart and circulatory system. Combined with the effects of decreased oxygen, nicotine's constricting effects on the blood vessels require the heart to work harder to deliver the oxygen. Breathing also becomes hindered as the lungs get irritated and accumulate more mucus from smoking, leading to increased airway resistance. Extra effort to get air in and out of the lungs occurs if a cigarette is smoked within an hour of physical activity. During heavy physical activity, the respiratory muscles are required to work twice as hard for chronic smokers as for nonsmokers.

Quitting Smoking

Quitting smoking is the single most important step that smokers can take to enhance the length and quality of their life (USDHHS, 2010b). Moreover, the health benefits and physical activity benefits of quitting smoking are immediate and substantial for all smokers regardless of age, gender, disease state, or smoking history (FIGURE 11.12).

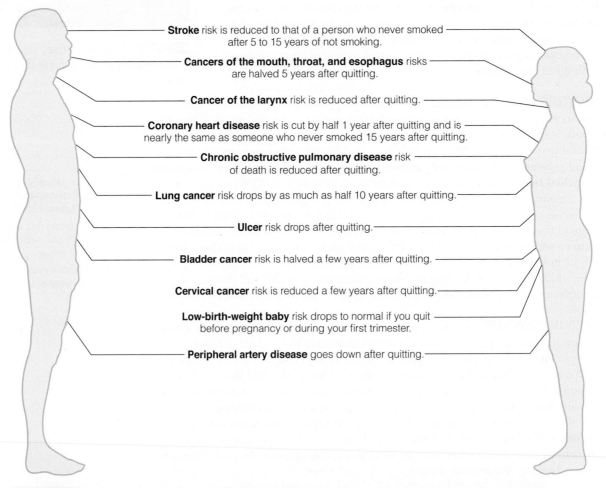

FIGURE 11.12 **The Health Benefits of Quitting Smoking.** The risks of developing many diseases and conditions drop dramatically, in varied lengths of time, after a person quits smoking. SOURCE: Centers for Disease Control and Prevention. (2004). The benefits of quitting. Online: http://www.cdc.gov/tobacco/data_statistics/sgr/2004/posters/benefits/index.htm.

Most people who have quit smoking state that they have done it on their own, without the help of a formal program. Most smokers quit a number of times before achieving long-term abstinence. If you are a present smoker who wants to quit, don't let another day go by (TABLE 11.10). Get help if you need it. Many groups offer programs and free materials to help smokers quit for good (TABLE 11.11). Your college or university health center may also be a good source for help and support.

STAYING TRIM AFTER QUITTING   Most people who quit smoking are concerned about gaining weight. Approximately four of every five people gain weight after quitting smoking, with the average weight gain being about 5 pounds. Changes in eating habits and in the body's processing of food lead to this weight gain.

Smoking suppresses taste-bud awareness and reduces the taste value of food. When people quit smoking they notice an improvement in the taste of food, leading to selection of higher portions and increased helpings. Increasing food consumption may also be an alternate way to deal with stress or a behavioral substitute for the oral satisfaction of smoking.

TABLE 11.10	Quit Tips

1. Don't smoke any number or any kind of cigarette. Smoking even a few cigarettes a day can hurt your health. If you try to smoke fewer cigarettes, but do not stop completely, soon you'll be smoking the same amount again.

   Smoking "low-tar, low-nicotine" cigarettes usually does little good, either. Because nicotine is so addictive, if you switch to lower-nicotine brands you'll likely just puff harder, longer, and more often on each cigarette. The only safe choice is to quit completely.

2. Write down why you want to quit. Do you want
   - to feel in control of your life?
   - to have better health?
   - to set a good example for your children?
   - to protect your family from breathing other people's smoke?

   Really wanting to quit smoking is very important to how much success you will have in quitting. Smokers who live after a heart attack are the most likely to quit for good. They're very motivated. Find a reason for quitting before you have no choice.

3. Know that it will take effort to quit smoking. Nicotine is habit forming. Half of the battle in quitting is knowing you need to quit. This knowledge will help you be more able to deal with the symptoms of withdrawal that can occur, such as bad moods and really wanting to smoke. There are many ways smokers quit, including using nicotine replacement products (gum and patches), but there is no easy way. Nearly all smokers have some feelings of nicotine withdrawal when they try to quit. Give yourself a month to get over these feelings. Take quitting one day at a time, even one minute at a time—whatever you need to succeed.

4. Half of all adult smokers have quit, so you can, too. That's the good news. There are millions of people alive today who have learned to face life without a cigarette. For staying healthy, quitting smoking is the best step you can take.

SOURCE: Centers for Disease Control and Prevention. Tobacco Information and Prevention Source (TIPS). Quit tips. Online: http://www.cdc.gov/tobacco/quit_smoking/how_to_quit/index.htm.

TABLE 11.11	National Groups Are Available to Help You Quit Smoking

American Cancer Society Toll-free number: (800) ACS-2345 Website: http://www.cancer.org	Centers for Disease Control and Prevention (CDC) Office of Smoking and Health Toll-free number: (800) CDC-INFO Website: http://www.cdc.gov/tobacco/quit_smoking/index.htm
American Heart Association Toll-free number: (800) AHA-USA-1 Website: http://www.americanheart.org	National Cancer Institute Toll-free number: (800) 422-6237 (Cancer Information Service) Toll-free number: (877) 448-7848 (help to quit smoking) Website: http://www.cancer.gov
American Lung Association Toll-free number: (800) LUNG-USA Website: http://www.lungusa.org	
American Stroke Association Toll-free number: (888) 4-STROKE Website: http://www.strokeassociation.org	Nicotine Anonymous Toll-free number: (877) 879-6422 Website: http://www.nicotine-anonymous.org
	Smokefree.gov (info on state phone-based quitting programs) Toll-free number: (800) QUITNOW Website: http://www.smokefree.gov

Some researchers believe that the absence of nicotine influences weight gain. First, nicotine causes the liver to release glycogen, raising the blood-sugar level and making the smoker feel satiated; absence of nicotine may factor into ex-smokers' cravings for high-sugar and high-calorie foods. Second, nicotine increases the body's basic metabolic rate, making it easier for the body to expend calories and contributing to a lower body weight.

Research provides compelling evidence that people who participate in an intensive physical activity program are more likely to succeed at quitting smoking and less likely to gain weight than people who did not include physical activity as part of their cessation strategy (USDHHS, 2010b). This is because many people use cigarettes to help them manage their weight, moods, and stress. Clearly, physical activity is a more healthy way to deal with each of these concerns. Moreover, the health benefits derived from avoiding any tobacco use, and the subsequent risk of developing a number of debilitating chronic diseases, overwhelmingly outweigh any small weight gain.

Physical Activity and Health Connection

To develop a high level of physical activity and health in your life, you must address the issue of substance use. We live in a society that believes that some substance use is acceptable. This notion doesn't necessarily complement a physically active or healthy lifestyle. As you increase your understanding of the physical and psychological consequences of alcohol use and cigarette smoking, you can better understand the many negative health consequences related to their use. Your path to being physically active can be significantly impaired by the use of drugs. Before using any drug, remember that you have choices. By making responsible choices that support your goal of being physically active and healthy, you will enhance not only your present quality of life but also your future.

concept connections

 College students face a conscious choice about whether to drink alcohol, smoke cigarettes, or use other psychoactive drugs while they pursue their degree. What they choose to do is related to a host of factors, including wanting to have a good time, to fit in or feel more comfortable socially and be accepted, to regulate moods and feelings, to forget about problems or numb out, to relieve emotional or physical pain, or to have a mind-altering experience. However, the use of many psychoactive drugs often creates the opposite effect. The major problem with psychoactive drugs is that when people take them, they focus on the immediate desired mental and emotional effects and ignore the potentially damaging mental and physical side effects that can occur.

 Chronic drug use can disrupt the body's normal balance, or homeostasis. The person who continues to use a drug moves to a level of risk one step beyond because each exposure carries with it the possibility that the body's chemical pathways will change to adapt to repeated exposure to the drug.

Making wise drug use decisions is important. The choices of which drug to use, how much, and how long are all important individual decisions and should not be made thoughtlessly. It is important for an individual to practice decision-making skills relating to potential substance use so that a well-prepared response is made.

Alcohol misuse and abuse is one of the most significant health-related drug problems in the United States. The consequences of excessive and underage drinking affect virtually all college students, campuses, and college communities, whether students choose to drink or not.

Cigarette smoking is the most preventable cause of premature death in the United States. Smoking damages nearly every organ in the body. Annually, approximately 443,000 Americans die as a result of diseases caused by or made worse by smoking, including coronary heart disease, lung cancer and at least nine other cancers, chronic respiratory disease, and stroke.

Terms

Binge drinking, 251
Blood alcohol concentration
   (BAC), 254
Carbon monoxide, 263
Depressant, 256
Drug, 242
Drug abuse, 242
Drug dependence, 244
Drug misuse, 242

Drug therapeutics, 242
Drug use, 242
Ethyl alcohol, 252
Heavy or high-risk drinking,
   252
Moderate drinking, 250
Nicotine, 260
Pharmacology, 248
Physical dependence, 246

Psychoactive drug, 244
Psychological dependence, 246
Secondhand smoke, 261
Social drinking, 250
Stimulants, 263
Tars, 263
Tolerance, 245
Withdrawal illness, 247

making the connection

Jim makes an appointment with both the college's Counseling and Psychological Services and Health Education Center to speak with professionals and obtain resources for his friend Bill. After learning the best way to approach Bill, Jim sits down with Bill and discusses his concerns about Bill's drinking with him and convinces him to make an appointment with a counselor.

Critical Thinking

1. "I really don't like the taste of liquor that much, but after the first couple of shots, it doesn't taste all that bad. I know I shouldn't drink and I always have a hangover the next day, but, hey, college is stressful and how else can I deal with the stress of getting the grades to keep my scholarship and making my parents happy?" What's your opinion of this person's attitude? Explain why you agree or disagree. If you disagree, how do you think this person can deal with the stress of getting good grades?

2. College campuses often accept money from companies that sell alcoholic beverages—to support athletic events, for example. By allowing these companies to advertise at campus events, the university makes considerable money to enhance the campus environment and provide quality education. What is your campus's policy on allowing alcohol companies to advertise or sponsor events on campus? Do you agree or disagree with this policy?

3. Purchase a popular magazine and count the number of cigarette ads in the issue. In reviewing each of the ads, respond to the following questions:
   a. Who is the ad targeting (young people, older adults, women)?
   b. How is the ad appealing to the target audience (fun, sex)?
   c. What does the ad seem to promise if you smoke their brand of cigarette?

References

Bouchery, E.E., Harwood, H.J., Sacks, J.J., Simon, C.J., & Brewer, R.D. (2011). Economic costs of excessive alcohol consumption in the U.S., 2006. *American Journal of Preventive Medicine* 41(5):516–524.

Centers for Disease Control and Prevention. (2012a). Alcohol and public health. Online: http://www.cdc.gov/alcohol.

Centers for Disease Control and Prevention. (2012b). Economic facts about U.S. tobacco production and use. Online: http://www.cdc.gov/tobacco/data_statistics/fact_sheets/economics/econ_facts.

Centers for Disease Control and Prevention. (2011). Vital signs: Cigarette smoking among adults aged > 18 years—United States, 2005–2010. *Morbidity and Mortality Weekly Report* 60(35):1207–1212.

Engs, R. (2001). *Clean Living Movements: American Cycles of Health Reform*. Westport, CT: Praeger.

Johnston, L.D., O'Malley, P.M., Bachman, J.G., & Schulenberg, J.E. (2012). Monitoring the Future national survey results on drug use, 1975–2010: Volume II, College students and adults ages 19–50. Institute for Social Research, The University of Michigan. Online: http://monitoringthefuture.org.

Kuntsche, E., & Cooper, M.L. (2010). Drinking to have fun and to get drunk: Motives as predictors of weekend drinking over and above usual drinking habits. *Drug and Alcohol Dependence* 110(3):259–262.

Montgomery, C., Ashmore, K.V., & Jansan, A. (2011). The effects of a modest dose of alcohol on executive functioning and prospective memory. *Human Psychopharmacy* 26(3):208–215.

National Cancer Institute, National Institutes of Health, U.S. Department of Health and Human Services. (2010). Cigar smoking and cancer fact sheet. Online: http://www.cancer.gov/cancertopics/factsheet/Tobacco/cigars.

National Institute on Alcohol Abuse and Alcoholism. (2012). Snapshot of annual high-risk college drinking consequences. Online: http://www.collegedrinkingprevention.gov/statsummaries/snapshot.aspx.

National Institute on Alcohol Abuse and Alcoholism. (2010). Rethinking drinking: Alcohol and your health (NIH Publication no. 10-3770). Online: http://rethinkingdrinking.niaaa.nih.gov.

National Institute on Alcohol Abuse and Alcoholism. (2004). NIAAA council approves definition of binge drinking. *NIAAA Newsletter*; No. 3, p. 3. Online: http://pubs.niaaa.nih.gov/publications/Newsletter/winter2004/Newsletter_Number3.pdf.

Substance Abuse and Mental Health Services Administration. (2011). *Results from the 2010 National Survey on Drug Use and Health: Summary of national findings* (NSDUH Series H-41, HHS Publication No. (SMA) 11-4658). Rockville, MD: Substance Abuse and Mental Health Services Administration.

U.S. Department of Health and Human Services. (2010a). *Healthy People 2020: The Road Ahead*. Online: http://www.healthypeople.gov/hp2020.

U.S. Department of Health and Human Services. (2010b). *How Tobacco Smoke Causes Disease: The Biology and Behavioral Basis for Smoking-Attributable Disease: A Report of the Surgeon General*. Atlanta, GA: U.S. Department of Health and Human Services, Centers for Disease Control and Prevention, National Center for Chronic Disease Prevention and Health Promotion, Office on Smoking and Health. Online: http://www.surgeongeneral.gov/library/tobaccosmoke/report/index.html.

U.S. Department of Health and Human Services & U.S. Department of Agriculture. (2010). *Dietary Guidelines for Americans, 2010*. Online: http://www.cnpp.usda.gov/dietaryguidelines.htm.

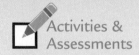

Consumer Health

Crystal's friend Toni constantly asks her to try a new diet pill "guaranteed" to make her lose inches overnight. Toni claims that the pill worked for her and pressures Crystal into trying "just one." Crystal is a bit skeptical and decides to investigate further. She asks Toni for the ingredient list from the product and calls a registered dietitian.

concepts

1. It is important to be a wise health consumer.

2. Fraudulent health products and services cost consumers billions of dollars each year.

3. Health literacy is the degree to which individuals have the capacity to obtain, process, and understand basic health information and services needed to make appropriate health decisions.

4. Being a wise consumer requires knowing and accessing different types of reliable health sources.

5. Everyone will need health care at some time.

go.jblearning.com/kotecki4e
The website for this book is a great source for supplementary physical health information for both students and instructors. Visit **go.jblearning.com/kotecki4e** to find a variety of useful tools for learning, thinking, and teaching.

He who takes medicine and neglects diet wastes the skill of his doctors.
—Chinese proverb

Introduction

Now more than ever, it is important to make sure that you are being a wise health consumer and are getting the most for your money regarding health products and services. The enduring number of myths and misconceptions about health and illness, the promotion and availability of unproven and untested health products, and the ever-increasing perplexity of the health care system have increased the need for health consumers to have specific knowledge and skills to make sound choices, to get full value for their health dollars, and to avoid deceit and fraud. This chapter provides information to help you become more knowledgeable as a consumer of health information, products, and services.

Scope of the Problem

Fraudulent health products and services cost consumers billions of dollars each year. **Fraud** is an intentional act perpetrated to be deceptive in order to gain something of value. **Health fraud** is the deceptive promotion, advertising, distribution, or sale of a product represented as being effective to prevent, diagnose, treat, cure, or lessen an illness or condition, or provide another beneficial effect on health, but that has not been scientifically proven safe and effective for such purposes (Food and Drug Administration [FDA], 2012). In addition to the economic cost, the more serious problem is that health fraud can lead to ineffective or delayed treatment and cause serious or even fatal injuries to its victims.

Promotions for fraudulent health products are everywhere. They are advertised in newspapers and magazines, and on the radio and television. On television, they are even peddled through extensive infomercials, many of which simulate a superficial resemblance to a health/medical program. They accompany products sold in stores, on the Internet, and through mail-order catalogs. They are passed along by word of mouth. Certainly there are individuals who promote products knowing their claims cannot be true, but many people promoting bad products may be unaware of the fraudulent intent of the manufacturer or distributor. Many promoters of fraudulent and misleading products are unwitting victims who themselves have been deceived. They then share misinformation and personal experiences with others.

Common Marketing Techniques

As the Food and Drug Administration (FDA) notes, health fraud marketers often use extremely sophisticated marketing techniques to peddle a useless product. The FDA urges you to take note of marketing tactics used by unscrupulous supplement marketers (**FIGURE 12.1**). The following claims and phrases are "red flags" the FDA advise consumers to look out for when deciding whether to try an unknown or unproven health product (FDA, 2012):

- Miraculous cure
- Quick fix
- Ancient remedy
- New discovery
- Scientific breakthrough
- Secret ingredient
- Natural cure
- Quick and painless cure
- No-risk money-back guarantee

It is important to be a wise health consumer.

Fraudulent health products and services cost consumers billions of dollars each year.

Fraud Intentional act perpetrated to be deceptive in order to gain something of value.

Health fraud Deceptive promotion, advertising, distribution, or sale of a product represented as being effective to prevent, diagnose, treat, cure, or lessen an illness or condition, or provide another beneficial effect on health, but that has not been scientifically proven safe and effective for such purposes.

This suggests that American scientists do not understand that medicines can be derived from plant sources, when, in fact, American researchers often rely on plants as sources of chemicals that have medicinal uses. No scientific evidence is cited to show that the herbs in Panacea have the touted properties. These two sentences, then, contain only value claims; thus, the information may be unreliable.

For centuries, doctors in the Orient have known about the wonders of herbal medicines—nature's botanical cures for human ailments.

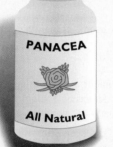

PANACEA

All Natural

Finally, American scientists are recognizing the healthful benefits of these herbs.

SwayCon Pharmaceuticals has developed a capsule that contains everything you need to reduce suffering, enhance health, and regain youthful vigor.

A team of medical experts from three major medical schools in the United States have clinical proof that the ingredients of Panacea are effective! Panacea contains a chemical-free mixture of natural enzymes and exotic herbs that:

- Relieve up to 80% more arthritis pain than aspirin
- Lower blood pressure by up to 20%
- Lower cholesterol by up to 45%
- Reduce lung cancer risk by as much as 50%, even in smokers
- Reduce the risk of heart attack by 75%*

Other remarkable findings:
Taking Panacea for a few months can improve intelligence. R.P., a college student at a large East Coast university, reports, "At the beginning of the fall semester, I started taking three capsules of Panacea a day. My GPA went from a 1.8 to a 3.4! Panacea has helped me get all As!"

Reports are coming into our offices that Panacea acts as a sexual stimulant, increasing potency. S.D., a computer programmer in St. Louis, writes, "Thanks for saving my marriage. Before taking Panacea, my husband complained about my lack of interest in sex. One of my friends told me that Panacea can help. Just a few days after taking the capsules, our marriage turned into a perpetual honeymoon."

Panacea is only available in fine health food stores. Order a three-month supply now, while supplies last!

A PANACEA PILL A DAY KEEPS THE EXPENSIVE DOCTORS AWAY!
* These statements have not been evaluated by the FDA.

This statement has value claims that are not supported with scientific evidence.
No treatment contains everything each person needs to improve his or her health.

"Clinical proof" is a red flag. The medical experts and medical schools where their research has been conducted are not identified.
Objective testing could show the product is neither safe nor effective. The ad should cite the specific effects of the product, including negative ones.

"Chemical-free" is a red flag; all matter, including herbs and other plants, is comprised of chemicals. Furthermore, scientific studies should be cited to provide evidence for these value claims.

A testimonial from an individual is not scientific evidence. This student's G.P.A. may have risen for a variety of reasons. Studies conducted to show that a treatment is useful should contain at least 30 subjects.

"Potency" is a vague and undefined red-flag term. Again, this testimonial is a value claim that is unsupported by scientific evidence.

This is irrelevant information. Where the product is sold has nothing to do with its quality or characteristics. The authors of the ad are simply trying to make their product look superior to other similar products.

This statement gives the impression that consumers have no time to investigate the product thoroughly. It is intended to make consumers think that the product will sell out if they wait, and they will miss out on a good thing. Again, this information is irrelevant.

No scientific evidence is cited that a daily Panacea pill prevents serious illness. Additionally, this statement attacks conventional medical practitioners by implying that they are interested only in making money, which suggests that physicians can't be trusted.

Disclaimer

Conclusion: This ad is merely a collection of value claims that are not supported by scientific research. The ad further attempts to encourage the reader to purchase the product by suggesting that it is better (and less expensive) than conventional therapies. It claims to relieve a wide range of health conditions. The red-flag phrases and testimonials, lack of scientific evidence, and failure to caution consumers about potential hazards of the product all suggest the ad is an unreliable source of health-related information.

FIGURE 12.1 **Value Claims not Supported by Scientific Research.** This ad is merely a collection of value claims that are not supported by scientific research. The ad further attempts to encourage the reader to purchase the product by suggesting that it is better (and less expensive) than conventional therapies. It claims to relieve a wide range of health conditions. The red flag phrases and testimonials rather than scientific evidence, the lack of details concerning the medical experts' credentials, and the lack of caution about the hazards of using the product all suggest the ad is an unreliable source of health-related information.

Other common tactics can be found in `TABLE 12.1`. It is not always easy to spot misleading and fraudulent products or advertising. Marketers often use scientific jargon that can fool people not familiar with the concepts being discussed. Even health professionals sometimes have difficulty separating fact from fiction in fields unrelated to their expertise.

TABLE 12.1	Common Deceptive Marketing Tactics Used to Promote Products
Tactic	**Description**
Bait and switch	One product is focused on, but another is delivered.
False claims (symptom free)	The claim that there are no side effects or symptoms associated with the use of a product.
False expectations	The claim that the product will bring about results that sound too good to be true (they usually are!).
Play upon fears (scare tactics)	Desperation marketing; most effective for people desperately seeking change.
Promise simple solutions to complex problems	"Take a pill and sleep away fat."
Redundancy	Persuade you to purchase a product that might actually bring about advertised results but that is not necessary to achieve those results. An example might be an abdominal assistance contraption. A simple curl-up performed properly will provide the same result for free.
Rarely provide scientific research to support claims (foreign research)	In the United States, the reference is to "European scientists" who have discovered some miracle product. In the rest of the world, claims are that "American scientists" have made the discovery.
Rely on testimonials	It worked for me; therefore, you should believe that it will work for you. Many of the people giving testimonials are being paid by the company to do so, and their objectivity must be questioned.
Criticize the medical establishment (conspiracy)	Marketers tell you that the medical community doesn't want you to know about a product. They claim that there is a vast conspiracy being instigated by the medical community to withhold information from you.
Money-back guarantees	Companies offer money-back guarantees with the knowledge that most people won't take the time or effort to seek their money back. In some cases, it costs more to get your money back than the total amount of money you get back. Additionally, shipping and handling costs are not refunded, which can amount to a significant sum.
Cures or miracles	The manufacturer advertises its product in such a way as to imply that it will cure a disease or work miracles. Then, usually in small print and in a hard-to-find location, it issues a disclaimer that it doesn't intend to imply that the product cures any disease or causes the occurrence of a miracle.
Celebrity endorsements	Companies hire famous spokespersons who tout their product. The hope is that you will connect the product with the celebrity and in some way think that the product had something to do with making this person a celebrity.
Mass media marketing	The product is sold primarily through television, radio, newspaper, and magazine advertisements. You are saturated with ads pushing the product to the point that you come to associate the product with the advertising venue. Certain products are associated with certain television shows. The intent is to get you to believe that the show (and/or actors) supports the product.
Buzzwords (e.g., *secret, rapid*)	The advertising companies use buzzwords to get your attention. They also try to focus your attention on the buzzwords rather than on the product.
Omission of facts	The marketers obscure or completely leave out certain facts that may keep you from purchasing their product. For instance, they may "forget" to tell you that there are certain side effects associated with use of the product. Another common example with weight loss products is when the companies forget to tell you that their product only works when combined with a regular physical activity program and proper nutrition.

TABLE 12.1	Common Deceptive Marketing Tactics Used to Promote Products *(Continued)*

Tactic	Description
For your eyes only	Advertising claims tell you that the product contains secret ingredients known to only a few people. This sometimes means that they don't know what is in the product, or they don't want you to know what is in the product. This method of advertising is meant to make you feel that you are being let in on the secret and are therefore special.
Highly pedigreed	Individuals with multiple degrees from well-known institutions tout a product. Background checks on these individuals sometimes show that the person may never have attended, let alone graduated from, the institution from which he or she claims to have a degree. Another example is where someone is listed as a doctor to lend credence to a marketing claim. In many cases, the doctor is not a medical doctor or has an area of expertise completely unrelated to the product he or she is pushing. One prime example is of a doctor with training in anesthesiology passing himself off as an expert in nutrition.
Express mail	Many companies use express mail to deliver their product to you. One possible reason for doing this is because sending a fraudulent product through the U.S. mail constitutes mail fraud, which is a federal offense. By using express mail, the company skirts this law because it does not apply to nongovernmental mailing agencies.
Sex	It is well known that sex is used to sell just about everything. This also is true in the physical activity and fitness industry. Remember that the product will not enhance your sex life or make members of the opposite sex desire you more just because you use it.

People also rely on personal experience and testimonials in deciding whether a product works. If you feel better after having used a product, you usually associate those sensations with the product. However, many ailments resolve themselves or have symptoms that change frequently. Even serious conditions can have day-to-day variation in intensity. An unscrupulous person can take advantage of this and mislead you into believing a fraudulent product was responsible for the temporary cessation of symptoms. This is the gist of the **placebo effect**. It is what happens when a person takes a product that he or she perceives will help, although it actually has no proven therapeutic effect for his or her particular condition. The treatment itself is known as a placebo, from Latin for "I will please."

Our own naïveté and gullibility often set us up for manipulation by misleading advertisers. People tend to believe what they hear often, and misleading information, particularly about nutrition, is everywhere. As an example, the advertisements promoting the use of shark cartilage supplements to protect against cancer imply that sharks don't get cancer, so they claim that if you take shark cartilage supplements, you won't get cancer. In fact, sharks do get cancer and even get cancer of their cartilage.

Health fraud also is a business that sells false hope. It preys on people who are victims of serious and chronic diseases that have no medical cures, such as HIV/AIDS, Alzheimer's, arthritis, multiple sclerosis, diabetes, and certain forms of advanced cancer. It also thrives on the wishful thinking of those who want shortcuts to weight loss or improvements to personal appearance. It makes enormous profits because it promises quick cures and easy solutions to better health or personal attractiveness.

Health literacy is the degree to which individuals have the capacity to obtain, process, and understand basic health information and services needed to make appropriate health decisions (U.S. Department of Health and Human Services

Placebo effect A physical or emotional change that is not due to properties of an administered substance. The change reflects participants' expectations.

Health literacy Degree to which individuals have the capacity to obtain, process, and understand basic health information and services needed to make appropriate health decisions.

Health literacy is the degree to which individuals have the capacity to obtain, process, and understand basic health information and services needed to make appropriate health decisions.

[USDHHS], 2000). A wide range of competencies is implicated by this definition. Individuals who have proficient health literacy must have the ability to:

- Read and identify credible health information
- Use technology to access health information and services
- Understand numbers in the context of their health care
- Make appointments and fill out forms
- Gather health records and ask appropriate questions of physicians
- Advocate for appropriate care
- Navigate complex health insurance programs

Unfortunately, many people find these tasks challenging. In the only national-level study of health literacy skills conducted to date, the Department of Education's National Assessment of Adult Literacy documented that only 12 percent of U.S. adults are proficient enough in health literacy to understand and use health information effectively (U.S. Department of Education [USDE], 2004) (FIGURE 12.2). This means that nearly 9 out of 10 adults have difficulty using the everyday health information that is commonly available in the media, retail outlets, communities, and health care facilities. Limited health literacy affects an individual's ability to search for and use health information, adopt healthy behaviors, and act on important health alerts, and is associated with poorer health outcomes and higher health care costs (Berkman et al., 2004; USDHHS, 2010).

Healthy People 2020 has included improved consumer health literacy in its objectives and identified health literacy as an important component of health communication and medical product safety (USDHHS, 2010). As noted in *Healthy People 2020*, health information and health care access issues have become more, not less, complex. *Healthy People 2020* states that during the coming decade, the speed, scope, and scale of adoption of health information technology will only increase. This includes the use of social media and emerging technologies that promise to blur the line between expert and peer health information. Monitoring and assessing the impact of these new media, including mobile health, on public health will be challenging.

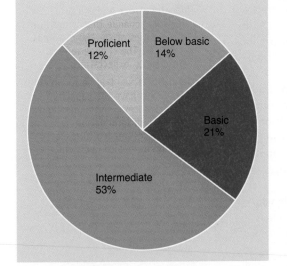

FIGURE 12.2 **Adults' Health Literacy Level.**
SOURCE: Modified from U.S. Department of Education, Institute of Education Sciences. (2004). 2003 National Assessment of Adult Literacy. Online: www .health.gov/communication/literacy/issuebrief/.

Becoming a Wiser Health Consumer

A wise health consumer seeks reliable sources of information, critically evaluates information, selects scientifically proven products, is wary of treatments that lack scientific evidence, selects health care providers with great care, and understands the economic aspects of health care. Today's marketplace is full of health choices. Consumers have certain rights and responsibilities in this marketplace. Among consumers' responsibilities are seeking information before buying, reading and understanding product or service information, and using products correctly and reporting unsafe products.

Surfing the Web for Health Information

You are most likely among the millions of people worldwide who seek health information on the Internet. In 2010, 80 percent of Internet users in the United States searched for a health-related topic online, making it the third most popular online pursuit (Fox, 2011). Only email, which is used by 93 percent of the Internet population, and researching a product or service before purchase (83 percent of users) topped it. There are thousands of reliable websites offering health information to meet your needs. This information can be extremely empowering and beneficial. However, as you probably know, paging Dr. Google can lead you to equally unreliable websites that provide inaccurate or biased medical information. The National Institutes of Health provides the following question and answer list to help you decide whether the information you find on the Internet is likely to be reliable (National Institutes of Health [NIH], 2011):

Who runs the Web site? Any Web site should make it easy for you to learn who is responsible for the site and its information. On the Office of Dietary Supplements (ODS) Web site, for example, the ODS is clearly noted on every major page, along with a link to the site's homepage.

Who pays for the Web site? It costs money to run a Web site. The source of a Web site's funding should be clearly stated or readily apparent. For example, the U.S. government funds Web sites with addresses ending in ".gov," educational institutes maintain ".edu" sites, noncommercial organizations' addresses often use ".org," and ".com" denotes a commercial organization. A Web site's source of funding can affect the content it presents, how it presents that content, and what the owner wants to accomplish on the site.

What is the Web site's purpose? The person or organization that runs a Web site and the site's funding sources determines the site's purpose. Many Web sites have a link to information about the site, often called "About This Site." This Web page should clearly state the purpose of the site and help you evaluate the trustworthiness of the site's information. Although many legitimate Web sites sell health and medical products, keep in mind that the Web site owner's desire to promote a product or service can influence the accuracy of the health information they present. Looking for another source of health information that is independent and unbiased can help you validate the accuracy of the material presented on a Web site.

What is the original source of the Web site's information? Many health and medical Web sites post information that the owner has collected from other Web sites or sources. If the person or organization in charge of the site did not write the material, they should clearly identify the original source.

How does the Web site document the evidence supporting its information? Web sites should identify the medical and scientific evidence that supports the material presented on the site. Medical facts and figures should have references (such as citations of articles published in medical journals). Also, opinions or advice should be clearly set apart from information that is "evidence based" (that is, based on research results). Testimonials from people who said they have tried a particular product or service are not evidence based and usually cannot be corroborated.

Who reviewed the information before the owner posted it on the Web site? Health-related Web sites should give information about the medical credentials of the people who prepared or reviewed the material on the Web site. For example, the ODS Web site contains fact sheets about vitamins, minerals and other dietary supplements. These documents undergo extensive scientific review by recognized experts from the academic and research communities.

How current is the information on the Web site? Experts should review and update the material on Web sites on a regular basis. Medical information needs to be current because medical research is constantly coming up with new information about medical conditions and how best to treat or prevent them. Web sites should clearly post the most recent update or review date. Even if the information has not changed in a long time, the site owner should indicate that someone has reviewed it recently to ensure that the information is still valid.

How does the Web site owner choose links to other sites? Owners of reliable Web sites usually have a policy governing which links to other sites they post. Some medical Web sites take a conservative approach and do not provide links to any other sites; some sites provide links to any site that asks or pays for a link; and others provide links only to sites that have met certain criteria. Checking a Web site's linking policy can help you understand how they choose links to other sites and what they're trying to accomplish by posting those links.

What information about users does the Web site collect, and why? Web sites routinely track the path users take through their sites to determine what pages people are viewing. However, many health-related Web sites also ask users to "subscribe" to or "become a member" of the site. Sites sometimes do this to collect a user fee or select relevant information for the user. The subscription or membership might allow the Web site owner to collect personal information about the user. Any Web site asking you for personal information should explain exactly what the site will and will not do with the information. Many commercial sites sell "aggregate" data—such as what percent of their users take dietary supplements— about their users to other companies. In some cases, sites collect and reuse information that is "personally identifiable," such as your ZIP code, gender, and birth date. Be certain to read and understand any privacy policy or similar language on the site and do not sign up for anything that you do not fully understand.

How does the Web site manage interactions with users? Web sites should always offer a way for users to contact the Web site owner with problems, feedback, and questions. If the site hosts a chat room or some other form of online discussion, it should explain the terms of using the service. For example, the site should explain whether anyone moderates the discussions and, if so, who provides the moderation and what criteria the moderator uses to determine which comments to accept and which to reject. Always read online discussions before participating to make sure that you are comfortable with the discussion and with what participants say to one another.

Reliable Health Organizations

Being a wise consumer requires knowing and accessing different types of reliable health sources.

There are many health agencies, associations, and organizations from which consumers can find reliable health information. Healthfinder.gov provides an extensive list of over 1600 trustworthy government and nonprofit organizations to bring you the best, most reliable health information on the Internet. Visit healthfinder.gov and select "Find Services and Information," and you will find six different categories of health organizations listed: federal agencies, federal clearinghouses, health and human services clearinghouses, nonprofit organizations, professional organizations, and state health and human services. A brief description of each health organization is provided along with contact information and online resources.

Federal Protection

The two agencies in the federal government directed to regulate product worthiness are the Food and Drug Administration (FDA) and the Federal Trade

Commission (FTC). The FDA is an agency within the U.S. Department of Health and Human Services. It consists of six product centers, one research center, and two offices. The FDA is responsible for:

* Protecting the public health by ensuring that foods are safe, wholesome, sanitary and properly labeled, and that human and veterinary drugs, and vaccines and other biological products and medical devices intended for human use are safe and effective
* Protecting the public from electronic product radiation
* Ensuring cosmetics and dietary supplements are safe and properly labeled
* Regulating tobacco products
* Advancing the public health by helping to speed product innovations
* Helping the public get the accurate, science-based information they need to use medicines, devices, and foods to improve their health

If you have a complaint about a product regulated by the FDA, the agency wants to hear about it. It offers a number of ways to report a complaint. Two of the main reporting systems available to consumers are the Consumer Complaint Reporting system and MedWatch. The FDA's Consumer Complaint Coordinators (CCCs), located in FDA offices throughout the United States, will document your complaint about an FDA-regulated product and follow up as necessary. Consumers should report problems to the CCC for their geographic region. A list of CCCs is available on the FDA's website (http://www.fda.gov).

MedWatch is for reporting any adverse events (unexpected side effects) that occur while using human health care products and some other FDA-regulated products such as human drugs (both prescription and over-the-counter), medical devices (e.g., contact lenses, glucose tests, pacemakers, medical X-rays), and special nutritional products (dietary supplements, infant formulas, and medical foods such as nutritional supplements used under medical supervision).

A second governmental agency involved in product safety and regulation is the Federal Trade Commission (FTC). The FTC's mission is to prevent business practices that are anticompetitive or deceptive or unfair to consumers; to enhance informed consumer choice and public understanding of the competitive process; and to accomplish this without unduly burdening legitimate business activity. One of its primary goals is to protect consumers by preventing fraud, deception, and unfair business practices in the marketplace.

The FTC collects complaints about companies, business practices, identity theft, and episodes of violence in the media. Your complaints can help it detect patterns of wrongdoing, and lead to investigations and prosecutions. The FTC enters all complaints it receives into Consumer Sentinel, a secure online database that is used by thousands of civil and criminal law enforcement authorities worldwide. Visit http://www.ftccomplaintassistant.gov to file a complaint with the FTC.

Choosing Dietary Supplements

The majority of adults in the United States take one or more dietary supplements either every day or occasionally in an effort to be well and stay healthy. A **dietary supplement** is a product taken by mouth that contains a "dietary ingredient." Dietary ingredients include vitamins, minerals, amino acids, and herbs or botanicals as well as other substances that can be used to supplement the diet. Dietary supplements come in many forms, including tablets, capsules, powders, energy bars, and liquids. These products are readily available in stores as well as on the Internet (FIGURE 12.3).

Dietary supplements, in general, are not FDA-approved. Under the Dietary Supplement Health and Education Act of 1994 (DSHEA), the dietary supplement or

Dietary supplement A product taken by mouth in tablet, capsule, powder, gelcap, or other nonfood form that contains one or more of the following: vitamins, minerals, amino acids, herbs, enzymes, metabolites, or concentrates.

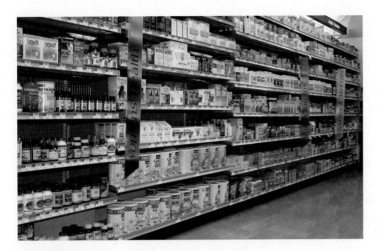

FIGURE 12.3 **Dietary Supplements.** Many different products are marketed to underinformed consumers.

dietary ingredient manufacturer is responsible for ensuring that a dietary supplement or ingredient is safe before it is marketed. Just because you see a supplement product on a store shelf does not mean it is safe or effective. TABLE 12.2 includes information about the safety and effectiveness of some popular herbal supplements. In fact, when a manufacturer makes a structure/function claim on a dietary supplement label it must include a disclaimer that these claims have not been evaluated by the FDA and that the product is not intended to diagnose, treat, cure, or prevent any disease. The FDA (2012) recommends that if you are using or considering using any product marketed as a dietary supplement that you:

- Check with your health care professional or a registered dietitian about any nutrients you may need in addition to your regular diet
- Ask your health care professional for help distinguishing between reliable and questionable information
- Ask yourself if it sounds too good to be true
  - Be cautious if the claims for the product seem exaggerated or unrealistic.
  - Watch out for extreme claims such as "quick and effective" or "totally safe."
  - Be skeptical about anecdotal information from personal "testimonials" about incredible benefits or results obtained from using a product.

Selecting and Effectively Using a Health and Fitness Facility

According to the International Health, Racquet, and Sportsclub Association (IHRSA), there are more than 17,000 health clubs in the United States (ACSM, 2011) (FIGURE 12.4). Many facilities offer safe and attractive places to exercise, but the quality of staff, equipment, and programs vary greatly. It is important to carefully evaluate your fitness center options before making a selection. The American College of Sports Medicine (ACSM) guidelines for selecting and effectively using a health and fitness facility are provided in TABLE 12.3 (ACSM, 2011).

Choosing a Primary Care Provider

Everyone will need health care at some time.

Everyone will need health care at some time. People visit health care professionals for vaccinations, physical exams, and diagnostic tests for treatment when sick. Everyone should have a primary care provider. A **primary care provider** (PCP) is a health care practitioner who sees people who have common medical problems (MedlinePlus, 2012). This person is usually a doctor, but may be a physician assistant or a nurse practitioner. A primary care provider cares for the majority of your nonemergency care, learns your health history, recommends tests and screenings needed to maintain health and detect illness, and notices changes in your health. A primary care provider also coordinates overall care, even if you receive specialty care elsewhere. Your PCP often is involved in your care for a long time, so it is important to select someone with whom you will work well. Selecting a PCP may seem simple, yet many people have little idea how to assess the qualifications of a PCP. When choosing a PCP, the National Library of Medicine (MedlinePlus, 2012) encourages you to ask the following questions:

- Is the office staff friendly and helpful? Is the office good about returning calls?
- Are the office hours convenient to your schedule?

Primary care provider (PCP) A health care practitioner who sees patients with common medical problems.

TABLE 12.2	Popular Herbal Supplements		

		Research Findings	
Supplement	**Common Claims**	**Uses**	**Risks**
St. John's wort	Relieves depression	May reduce mild to moderate depression symptoms; no value for major depression	Can interfere with birth control pills and other prescribed medicines, increase sensitivity to sunlight, and cause stomach upset
Saw palmetto	Improves urine flow	May reduce symptoms of prostate enlargement that are not caused by cancer	May interfere with prostate-specific antigen (PSA) test to detect prostate cancer
Feverfew	Relieves headaches, fever, and arthritis pain	Contains a chemical that may prevent migraines or reduce their severity	May cause dangerous interactions with aspirin or Coumadin (warfarin, a prescribed drug)
Echinacea	Prevents colds and influenza	Does not prevent colds or reduce their severity	May cause allergic response and be a liver toxin
Ginkgo biloba	Enhances memory and sense of well-being; prevents dementia	Weak or inconsistent scientific evidence to support claims	May interfere with normal blood clotting, cause intestinal upset, and increase blood pressure
Ginseng	Enhances sexual, mental, and exercise performance; increases energy; relieves stress and depression	Has no mood-enhancing effects; may reduce risk of respiratory infections and improve blood sugar values of people with diabetes	Can cause "jitters," insomnia, hypertension, and diarrhea and can be addictive; can be contaminated with pesticides and the toxic mineral lead
Yohimbe	Enhances muscle development and sexual performance	Dilates blood vessels but has no beneficial effects on muscle growth or sex drive of humans	Can produce abnormal behavior, high blood pressure, and heart attacks
Guarana	Boosts energy and enhances weight loss	Acts as a stimulant drug	May cause nausea, anxiety, and irregular heartbeat
Kava	Relieves anxiety and induces sleep	Acts as a depressant drug	May cause serious liver damage; do not use when driving

- How easy is it to reach the provider? Does the provider use email?
- Do you prefer a provider whose communication style is friendly and warm, or more formal?
- Do you prefer a provider focused on disease treatment, or wellness and prevention?
- Does the provider have a conservative or aggressive approach to treatment?
- Does the provider order a lot of tests?
- Does the provider refer to other specialists frequently or infrequently?
- What do colleagues and patients say about the provider?
- Does the provider invite you to be involved in your care? Does the provider view your patient–doctor relationship as a true partnership?

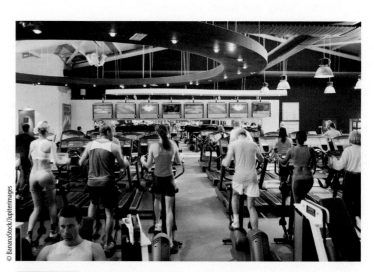

© BananaStock/Jupiterimages

FIGURE 12.4 Selecting a Fitness Facility. Not all facilities are the same—select one that meets your specific needs.

TABLE 12.3	ACSM Information on Selecting and Effectively Using a Health/Fitness Facility

The health/fitness facility should provide a variety of equipment and programs to meet your personal fitness goals and interests. Be sure to establish your exercise/fitness goals before talking to personnel to see if they provide the programs and equipment you seek.

Before Joining

Visit several facilities prior to making your investment. Some facilities offer a trial membership for a day or a week. Before joining, take a tour and ask questions.

Observe the classes and programs. Take into consideration whether the facility is located in an area that is convenient for you. Also, consider the following:

- Does the facility offer the type of exercise or program in which you are interested?
- Do qualified exercise instructors develop the programs?
- Will staff members modify the programs to meet your needs?
- Does the facility offer programs to address medical conditions?
- Does the facility offer programs for the age group in which you are interested?
- Does the facility offer fitness assessments and a personalized exercise program or prescription?

Safety

The staff of the facility should be able to respond to any reasonable emergency situation that threatens the safety of its members. Staff also should provide you with any information regarding potential risks associated with using the facility.

Check for these safety features:

- Does the facility have a posted emergency response evacuation plan?
- Is staff qualified to execute the emergency response evacuation plan?
- Does the facility have automated external defibrillators (AEDs) onsite?
- Is the facility clean and well-maintained?
- Is the facility free from physical or environmental hazards?
- Is the facility appropriately lit?
- Does the facility have adequate heating, cooling, and ventilation?
- Does the facility have adequate parking?

Preactivity Screening

Every adult member should be offered a preactivity screening. Check to see if the facility provides for or adheres to the following:

- Does the facility offer a preactivity screening, such as the PAR-Q, to assess whether members have medical conditions or risk factors that should be addressed by a physician?
- Aside from an initial general health and wellness screening, does the facility have a health and fitness screening method appropriate for the type of exercise you will undertake?
- Does the facility offer fitness assessments?

Special Needs

If you have special needs, it is important to see if the staff of the facility can meet your needs regarding modification of equipment, facilities, and programs.

Personnel and Certification

The facility should have a professional staff that has the appropriate education and training related to their duties.

Professional qualifications should include a college degree in a health-related field such as exercise science, physical education, or kinesiology. Additionally, staff members should hold a certification from a nationally recognized organization such as the American College of Sports Medicine. Any certification should be based on job-related performance criteria, which have been validated by scientific research in the field and analyzed for reliability. Many certification programs do not comply with industry standards. It is important to inquire about how the certification examination was developed and administered and what the prerequisites were for participating in the certification program. Check to make sure the entire staff has credentials and education from credible institutions.

TABLE 12.3	ACSM Information on Selecting and Effectively Using a Health/Fitness Facility *(Continued)*

Checklist for Personnel

- Do staff members have appropriate education, certification, and training recognized by the industry and the public as representing a high level of competence and credibility?
- Is there sufficient staff on site?
- Are staff members easy to recognize?
- Are the staff members friendly and helpful?
- Do staff members receive ongoing professional training?
- Do staff members provide each new member with an orientation to the equipment and/or facility?
- Are the staff members trained in CPR, the use of AEDs, and first aid?
- Are the staff members knowledgeable about your health conditions?
- Can staff help you set realistic exercise goals?

Youth Services

If you are interested in a facility with youth programs, they should be appropriately supervised at all times. In certain parts of the country, background screening, specific training, and licensure are required. Check to make sure that the facility meets your needs regarding childcare and youth programs.

Business Practices

Before signing a contract, consider the following:
- Does the staff pressure you into purchasing a membership?
- Does the membership fee fit into your budget?
- Is there a trial membership program?
- Is there a grace period in which you can cancel your membership and receive a refund?
- Are there different membership options and are all the fees for services posted?
- Does the facility provide you with a written set of rules and policies, which govern the responsibilities of members as well as the facility?
- Does the facility have a procedure to inform members of any changes in charges, services, or policies?

Make sure you read and understand everything before signing a contract. Do not rely on verbal responses. Ask a lot of questions so that you will have accurate information when you are making a decision.

Making an informed decision can help you avoid choosing a facility that does not fit your needs. Selecting a facility with professional and qualified staff, state-of-the-art equipment, and a variety of programs is a sound investment of your money and in your health.

SOURCE: Reprinted with permission of the American College of Sports Medicine. Copyright © 2011 American College of Sports Medicine. This brochure was created and updated by Hank Williford, EdD, FACSM, and Michelle Olson, PhD, FACSM, and is a product of ACSM's Consumer Information Committee. Visit ACSM online at www.acsm.org.

Health Insurance Basics

Health insurance is a formal agreement to provide and/or pay for medical care. The health insurance policy describes what medical services are covered by the insurance company. There are medical services that are not covered and will not be paid by your insurance company. Most college students obtain health insurance as a dependent in a group plan from their parents. Under the Affordable Care Act passed by Congress in 2010, if your parents' plan covers children, your parents can now add or keep you on their health insurance policy until you turn 26 years old. This act is expanding your options for health insurance and making them more affordable.

If you are not on a group insurance option or an employer-sponsored insurance plan, you will need to shop for an individual policy for yourself. Because college students are usually young and healthy, premiums for fairly comprehensive coverage are relatively low. More than half of all colleges offer their own health

| TABLE 12.4 | Consumer Checklist: What to Look for in a Health Insurance Policy |

It can be a challenge to find coverage that meets your health care needs and fits your budget. Health insurance that covers more tends to cost more. Some tips as you are shopping for insurance:

- Do your best to balance the cost (monthly premium) of a policy with the protection it offers.
- Determine what you will have to pay yourself for covered services (deductible, co-insurance, copayments, and out-of-pocket limit).
- Estimate costs for noncovered care (services excluded or limited by the policy) and charges (fees above what the plan recognizes).
- Check whether the plan covers the health care services and medications you require.
- Check whether the plan's health care providers include your current providers, are located conveniently for you, and are high quality.
- Avoid policies that don't have some kind of maximum out-of-pocket limit on covered charges.
- Don't mistake insurance-like products for comprehensive coverage.
- If you have questions, call your state's Department of Insurance or Consumer Assistance Program.

SOURCE: Reproduced from HealthCare.gov. (2012). Consumer Checklist: What to Look for in a Health Insurance Policy. Online: http://www.healthcare.gov/using-insurance/understanding/basics/index.html#ConsumerChecklist:WhattoLookforinaHealthInsurancePolicy.

policies for students, but the coverage varies, so be careful when signing up for a policy. TABLE 12.4 provides a consumer checklist of what to look for in a health insurance policy (HealthCare.gov, 2012).

Physical Activity and Health Connection

The commercial fitness and diet industries offer many unscientific programs and products. To make sure your exercise program is safe and effective, you must be a wise consumer of fitness information and products. The same goes for the diet industry, which is full of unproven programs and products as well. Even though there is a certain degree of governmental oversight of products available to consumers, the best defense against misleading advertising and fraudulent products is being an informed health consumer. Certain products can be dangerous and can lead to ill health. It is important to be vigilant when purchasing any health-related product. Being an educated health consumer will help you be more skillful, sensible, and economically sound in the utilization of health information, products, and services.

concept connections

1 **It is important to be a wise health consumer.** The enduring number of myths and misconceptions about health and illness, the promotion and availability of unproven and untested health products, and the ever-increasing perplexity of the health care system have increased the need for health consumers to have specific knowledge and skills to make sound choices, to get full value of their health dollars, and to avoid deceit and fraud.

2 **Fraudulent health products and services cost consumers billions of dollars each year.** Health fraud is the deceptive promotion, advertising, distribution, or sale of a product represented as being effective to prevent, diagnose, treat, cure, or lessen an illness or condition, or provide another beneficial effect on health, but that has not been scientifically proven safe and effective for such purposes. In addition to the economic cost, the more serious problem is that health fraud can lead to ineffective or delayed treatment and cause serious or even fatal injuries to its victims.

3 **Health literacy is the degree to which individuals have the capacity to obtain, process, and understand basic health information and services needed to make appropriate health decisions.** A wide range of competencies are implicated by this definition. Individuals who have a high level of health literacy must have the ability to read and identify credible health information, use technology to access information and services, understand numbers in the context of their health care, make appointments and fill out forms, gather health records and ask appropriate questions of physicians, advocate for appropriate care, and navigate complex insurance programs and other financial assistance programs.

4 **Being a wise consumer requires knowing and accessing different types of reliable health sources.** There are many health agencies, associations, and organizations from which consumers can find reliable health information. Healthfinder.gov provides an extensive list of over 1600 trustworthy government and nonprofit organizations to bring you the best, most reliable health information on the Internet.

5 **Everyone will need health care at some time.** People visit health care professionals for vaccinations, physical exams, and diagnostic tests for treatment when sick. Everyone should have a primary care provider. A primary care provider (PCP) is a health care practitioner who sees people who have common medical problems. This person is usually a doctor but may be a physician assistant or a nurse practitioner. A primary care provider cares for the majority of your nonemergency care, learns your health history, recommends tests and screenings needed to maintain health and detect illness, and notices changes in your health.

Terms

Dietary supplement, 279
Fraud, 272

Health fraud, 272
Health literacy, 275

Placebo effect, 275
Primary care provider, 280

---

making the connection

Crystal learns that the diet pill contains mostly useless ingredients and a good deal of caffeine. The registered dietitian explains that the caffeine would temporarily increase Crystal's metabolic rate and make her feel nervous, but that the effect would not last long. The impact on Crystal's metabolic rate would not result in a loss of body fat, and could be dangerous for some people. She also tells Crystal that she would have difficulty sleeping after taking the pill. Armed with this information, Crystal feels confident about telling Toni, "Thanks, but no thanks!"

Critical Thinking

1. Like Crystal, we are constantly being bombarded with advertisements about a diet pill or drink that will *guarantee* losing *x* pounds per week. These advertisements are often seen on college and university campuses. As you walk to class, take a look around to see if you notice any of these advertisements. Record what you see. Also review the most recent issue of your college or university newspaper. Are there any ads for fad diets or pills? If so, whom are they targeting?

2. In a popular magazine, find an advertisement that you believe might be misleading or fraudulent. Determine which of the advertising approaches are used to convince readers to purchase the product. What argument would you present to counter the advertising claims?

3. Speculate about why people often fall victim to common physical activity and health misconceptions, frauds, or fallacies.

4. As a critical health consumer, where would you suggest peers go to find valid information on physical activity and health? Give three sources and explain how you determined they were valid.

References

American College of Sports Medicine. (2011). Selecting and effectively using a health/fitness facility. Online: http://www.acsm.org/access-public-information/brochures-fact-sheets/brochures.

Berkman, N.D., DeWalt, D.A., Pignone, M.P., Sheridan, S.L., Lohr, K.N., Lux, L., Sutton, S.F., Swinson, T., & Bonito, A.J. (2004). *Literacy and Health Outcomes* (AHRQ Publication No. 04-E007-2). Rockville, MD: Agency for Healthcare Research and Quality.

Food and Drug Administration. (2012). For consumers: Health fraud scams. Online: http://www.fda.gov/ForConsumers/ProtectYourself/HealthFraud/default.htm.

Fox, S. (2011). Health topics. Online: http://pewinternet.org/Reports/2011/HealthTopics.aspx.

HealthCare.gov. (2012). Insurance basics. Online: http://www.healthcare.gov/using-insurance/understanding/basics/index.html.

MedlinePlus Medical Encyclopedia. (2012). Choosing a primary care provider. Online: http://www.nlm.nih.gov/medlineplus/ency/article/001939.htm.

National Institutes of Health. (2011). How to evaluate health information on the Internet: Questions and answers. Online: http://ods.od.nih.gov/Health_Information/How_To_Evaluate_Health_Information_on_the_Internet_Questions_and_Answers.aspx.

U.S. Department of Education, Institute of Education Sciences. (2004). 2003 National Assessment of Adult Literacy. Online: http://nces.ed.gov/naal.

U.S. Department of Health and Human Services. (2010). *Healthy People 2020*. Online: http://healthypeople.gov/2020.

U.S. Department of Health and Human Services. (2000). *Healthy People 2010*. Online: http://healthypeople.gov/2010.

Activities & Assessments

© Photos.com

Developing Healthy Social and Intimate Relationships

what's the connection?

Mona and Jennifer are roommates in their first year of college. In high school and in college, Mona has a wide circle of friends, is involved in many activities, and has been dating her boyfriend for almost a year now. Jennifer, on the other hand, had a small and very close-knit group of friends in high school. She had a boyfriend in high school, but the relationship ended mutually when they decided to attend colleges in different states. Jennifer stays in touch with her friends using the Internet and has met three new close friends in college. Mona and Jennifer spend time talking about how to make friends. Jennifer says she prefers to have a few close friends and likes not dating right now. Mona is worried that Jennifer does not have enough friends and wonders why she is choosing not to date right now.

concepts

1. Supportive social relationships positively affect our overall well-being and physical health.

2. Social support consists of a wide variety of relationships, including family, friends, romantic partner, acquaintances, work/school relationships, and social networking website relationships.

3. Relationship needs differ between people and can range from a couple of close friends to large social circles. Quality, more than quantity, is the important determinant in social wellness.

4. Intimacy means having a deep, trusting, and emotional connection with another person.

5. Effective communication is critical for developing and maintaining all relationships.

6. A sexual relationship involves two people who mutually consent to become physically intimate and participate in sexual acts such as kissing, caressing, stroking, rubbing, or penetrative behaviors.

go.jblearning.com/kotecki4e
The website for this book is a great source for supplementary physical health information for both students and instructors. Visit **go.jblearning.com/kotecki4e** to find a variety of useful tools for learning, thinking, and teaching.

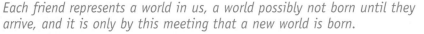

Each friend represents a world in us, a world possibly not born until they arrive, and it is only by this meeting that a new world is born.

—Anaïs Nin

Introduction

Social health, or social wellness, is one of the seven dimensions of health and refers to the quality of our connections with others. Socially healthy people have loving relationships in which they feel valued. Individuals in socially healthy relationships respect the rights of others and provide as well as accept help from others. Building and maintaining healthy relationships with family and friends, as well as communicating needs to others, are important elements in social health. This chapter discusses evidence for the importance of social relationships and the types of relationships, relationship needs, sexuality, intimacy, and communication in relationships.

Positive, supportive social relationships have a tremendous effect on overall well-being and, more specifically, physical health. **Social support** has long been associated with overall wellness and a general sense of satisfaction (**FIGURE 13.1**) (Braveman, Egerter, & Williams, 2011). A myriad of positive effects is found in individuals who have supportive social relationships. For example, positive, supportive relationships have been shown to improve adjustment to college and have been connected with successful completion of college (Busseri et al., 2011). Supportive social relationships also can help decrease overall stress (Chao, 2012).

Social support is related to physical activity in two important ways. First, from a general standpoint, when we have good social relationships, we are more likely to have good physical health (Turncheff et al., 2011). For example, homeless individuals with greater social support also reported better overall physical health (Hwang et al., 2009).

The second relationship suggests that social support for exercise increases the likelihood and maintenance of fitness routines (**FIGURE 13.2**). For example, in a study of college students, Nelson, Kocos, Lytle, and Perry (2009) found that social support was an important facilitator of exercise. For adolescent girls, peer social support increased their physical activity and their perceived ability to deal effectively with barriers (e.g., weather, busy schedule, fatigue) to exercise (Beets, Pitetti, & Forlaw, 2007). Another example involves a sample of Mexican American individuals with diabetes. These individuals expressed that social connection in their walking groups was a powerful motivator to walking (Ingram, Ruiz, Mayorga, & Rosales, 2009).

Many additional studies about the connections between social and physical health examine a range of age, ethnic/racial, and gender groups. With all of this evidence, you are encouraged to find a friend or two to exercise with you. Additionally, you may find that when you are not feeling like working out, your friend can help you. And, when your friend is a bit low on exercise motivation, you can help out your friend.

Social support has a host of other benefits related to health. Overholser and Fisher (2009) found that improving social support may be more effective in managing stress than using medications designed to treat stress-related conditions. Furthermore, individuals who are trying to stop smoking are more likely to succeed when their social support networks provide positive support (Lawhon, Humfleet, Hall, Reus, &

Supportive social relationships positively affect our overall well-being and physical health.

Social health Feelings of being loved, valued, and respected in relationships; includes notions of giving and receiving assistance.

Social support Closeness felt and derived from a variety of relationships, including family, friends, acquaintances, work/school colleagues, and Internet-based relationships.

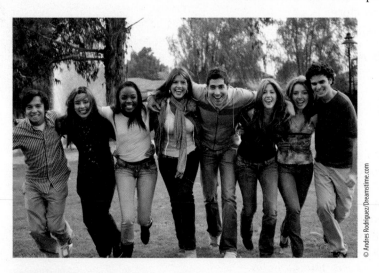

FIGURE 13.1 **Social Relationships.** Positive relationships are essential to our overall well-being.

© Andres Rodriguez/Dreamstime.com

Munoz, 2009). Interestingly, Lawhon et al. (2009) also found that negative messages from social support members regarding smoking cessation were associated with a return to smoking behaviors. These studies looked at a variety of relationships including romantic, peer, close friendship, and family. Thus, social support comes in many forms and has a myriad of positive benefits. Further, negative social support (discouraging messages) can increase the likelihood of unhealthy behaviors.

Social support has several additional benefits, including decreasing stress from moving to a new geographic location (Almeida, Subramanian, & Moihar, 2011). Positive social support has also been shown to reduce the likelihood of drug use and to decrease drug use in current users (Fletcher, Bonell, Sorhaindo, & Strange, 2009). Supportive social relationships have also been linked to reducing the likelihood of bullying behavior (Konishi & Hymel, 2009).

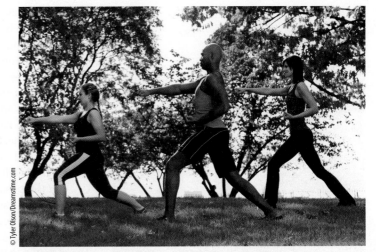

FIGURE 13.2 **Social Support.** Exercising is a great way to combine social and physical wellness.

Take a few minutes to think about whom you turn to when you could use some support, when you need a laugh, or when you want to vent about a tough day. How do you feel after you've shared your experience and received words of comfort and encouragement from your friendships? Now, imagine the reverse of that—your friend comes to you after having a difficult day. The benefits you provide your friends by listening and sharing supportive messages are profound. Being a good friend who listens and provides comfort is an essential part of health.

Relationship Types

Healthy relationships provide the opportunity for you to feel loved and valued as well as afford you the chance to help others. This section examines relationships in terms of closeness/connection, frequency of contact, and setting (in person, work/school, and the Internet) because social support includes a wide variety of relationships. As you read the descriptions of different types of relationships, consider the ways in which your social relationships contribute to your social health, based on the earlier definition of social health.

The specific relationships we each have provide different functions. Our closest, trusted relationships may be our best friends, romantic partners, and/or family members. These relationships provide a refuge, a safe haven. These are the people in whom we confide and share our secrets without fear of being judged; they provide support, allow us to be ourselves, and grant us the opportunity to give back. They are essential to our well-being, and as close, trusted friends, we are essential to our friends' well-being.

Casual acquaintances are those individuals with whom we share common interests or are convenient geographically (such as neighbors at home or in residence halls). These relationships may lend to fun and entertainment, or they may provide us a way to stave off boredom/loneliness, try new activities, or learn new things. They provide the opportunity to get to know another person and may eventually lead to a closer friendship or romantic relationship.

Work and school provide opportunities for close and casual relationships as well. These relationships vary in terms of closeness and provide the bridge of common interests if an increase in closeness is desired. For example, professors, role models, and mentors may provide valuable advice and support as you negotiate starting or advancing in a career. Similarly, classmates and work colleagues

Social support consists of a wide variety of relationships, including family, friends, romantic partner, acquaintances, work/school relationships, and social networking website relationships.

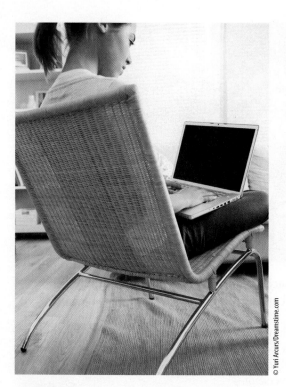

FIGURE 13.3 **Internet Relationships.** Although the computer can be a great way to keep in touch, using it too much has been linked to loneliness.

may provide assistance or may provide you with the opportunity to assist them. They may offer a nice break from the routine of the day at lunchtime, consult about a work- or school-related difficulty, or supply some entertainment or stress relief.

Internet social relationships are very common and have a variety of advantages and disadvantages (**FIGURE 13.3**). Visiting social networking sites such as Facebook is a very popular pastime for many people. Some researchers argue that these websites have positive value in terms of social health. Others argue that using technology to connect with and maintain social relationships can be detrimental to health and well-being (Elphinston & Noller, 2011).

On the positive side, use of social networking sites can increase feelings of connection, decrease feelings of sadness or anxiety, and decrease feelings of social isolation (McEwan, 2011). Use of technology, including social networking websites, has been shown to decrease the distance that so often occurs between friends when they graduate from high school and attend different colleges (McEwan, 2011).

There are downsides to use of social networking websites, however. The seemingly logical assumption is that a person who has "friends" on a social networking site is socially well, or has good social health. However, recent research suggests that these websites have the risk of being misused to the point that loneliness and well-being are affected negatively. For example, relationships formed and maintained on the Internet tend to be weaker compared to relationships formed and maintained with in-person contact (McEwan, 2011). Another potential disadvantage of social networking sites involves the notion of taking the path of least resistance. Although people generally prefer face-to-face connections, they often resort to an option requiring less energy, such as television viewing (Jolin & Weller, 2011). This may be true of Internet usage as well. Imagine you are feeling lonely and tired. What is the easier option: starting the computer or trying to locate a friend to join you for dinner? It is likely that you may choose to watch television or use the Internet rather than calling a friend. Choosing to avoid (through television or the Internet) instead of acting to address those negative feelings may even serve to increase the negative feelings.

One additional risk involves overuse of the Internet, which can decrease communication with family, decrease number of friendships, and even increase feelings of sadness and loneliness (McEwan, 2011). Kim, LaRose, and Peng (2009) found that some individuals use these social networking sites to the point that their in-person relationships are negatively affected. These individuals may actually become lonelier. Overall, it seems that a healthy recommendation involves moderation of use of Internet for social activity. When they are used for recreational or supplemental purposes, social networking websites are likely to have positive effects and enhance your social network.

Finally, consider this note about the technology age in general. Although accessibility is great for maintaining contact with friends and family, it comes with a risk as well. With instant messaging, text messaging, social networking sites, and cell phones, there exists the illusion of instant accessibility and the expectation of immediate response. If a near-immediate response is not received, feelings of sadness, disconnection, anxiety, or even anger can occur. However, the reality is that electronics are far from perfect. Messages can get lost, people may not be online, or they may be very busy and not have a minute to type out a response (for example, when cramming for a midterm exam). Therefore, if you use electronic means to keep in touch, make sure you use positive self-talk during those times when you do not receive instant replies. Remember, your friends may be busy, offline, or having a tough day—they may not be ignoring you.

Various types of relationships provide a variety of functions. Helping a classmate study for a test may provide an internal sense of satisfaction as well as the added benefit of boosting your own academic performance. Getting some advice from a mentor or role model provides you with valuable knowledge while giving your mentor the opportunity to help and feel the sense of satisfaction related to giving back, or altruism. Sharing with a close friend or romantic partner may provide you with feelings of being loved and valued as well as the sense of having helped someone else (FIGURE 13.4).

Relationship Needs

Although we all need some connection with others, the degree and types of relationships we each desire may vary widely. Some individuals may want to focus their attention on a romantic partner, whereas other individuals may want to date casually. Different people are equally satisfied and maintain their social wellness by any number of social network configurations.

Note that some mental health conditions can interfere with the development of social relationships. For example, people with social phobia, Asperger syndrome, and other disorders may express anxiety about relationships or have difficulty using the social skills needed to maintain interpersonal relationships (American Psychiatric Association, 1994). For individuals with these and other mental health concerns that affect relationships negatively, counseling can be very useful in understanding the impact of mental health concerns on social and overall wellness.

Defining Sex and Sexuality

Understanding terminology is critical to good communication and relationships, including sexual relationships.

Sex

Sex can refer to (1) an individual's classification as male or female as determined by the presence of certain anatomic and physiological characteristics, (2) a set of behaviors, and (3) the experience of erotic pleasure.

At the most fundamental biological level, sex refers to the mating of two anatomically distinct individuals, a male and a female, each of whom manufactures specific cells, or gametes, that fuse to become the first cell of a new person. To facilitate the fusion process (called fertilization), males and females of a species possess specific organs and display certain behaviors that are intended to bring about the union of gametes (See the end of this chapter for more on sexual biology).

Often the word *sex* is used to denote aspects of individuals' personal characteristics that are thought to derive from their biological classification. Thus, the biological property of femaleness is associated with the social quality of "femininity," and the biological property of maleness is associated with the social quality of "masculinity." Although most modern dictionaries still define *sex* as having to do with personality characteristics, this concept is more accurately referred to as **gender** to distinguish the fact that it originates in culture rather than biology.

Besides biological classification, sex also is associated with certain behaviors that are defined as sexual. These activities usually involve touching, in various ways, certain anatomic regions of the body, such as the genitalia and breasts, and sexual intercourse.

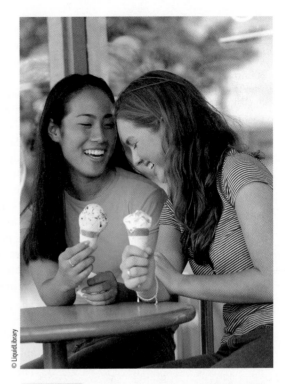
© LiquidLibrary

FIGURE 13.4 **Maintaining Relationships.** Make sure to spend time face-to-face with your friends.

Relationship needs differ between people and can range from a couple of close friends to large social circles. Quality, more than quantity, is the important determinant in social wellness.

Sex An individual's classification as male or female based on (1) anatomic characteristics, (2) a set of behaviors, and (3) the experience of erotic pleasure.

Gender Socialized qualities associated with masculinity or femininity.

Sexuality A person's internal sense of self—thoughts, feelings, attitudes, and behaviors.

Heterosexual individual A person who is attracted to people of the opposite gender.

Lesbian woman A woman who is attracted physically, romantically, and/or emotionally to other women.

Gay man A man who is attracted physically, romantically, and/ or emotionally attracted to other men.

Bisexual individual A person who is attracted to members of both genders.

Sexuality

Sexuality is part of your identity and consists of thoughts, attitudes, feelings, and behaviors. The terms *sex* and *sexuality* have been used interchangeably but differ substantially in meaning. Although most people are aware that sexuality involves more than the sexual acts, it may be helpful to provide definitions for clarity. After all, we are inundated daily with media images and messages that equate sexuality with sexual activity. The Sexuality Information and Education Council of the United States (SIECUS) defines *human sexuality* as, "encompass[ing] the sexual knowledge, beliefs, attitudes, values, and behaviors of individuals" (SIECUS, 2009). Its various dimensions include the anatomy, physiology, and biochemistry of the sexual response system; identity, orientation, roles, and personality; and thoughts, feelings, and relationships.

Another term for sexuality is the *sexual self*, which has several dimensions:

1. The *physical dimension* refers to any region of the body to which an individual gives sexual meaning, including the organs and organ systems we employ to create erotic experiences (the skin, the genitals). It also includes the physical features that define us to ourselves and others as sexual beings.

2. The *psychological dimension* refers to our emotions and our conscious and unconscious beliefs that guide the interpretation of experience. This aspect of sexuality generates strategies for actions that are intended to satisfy our wants and needs.

3. The *social dimension* refers to sexual attitudes and behaviors that affect our interactions with members of the social groups to which we belong.

4. Another aspect of sexuality involves *sexual orientation*, defined as the sex to whom we are physically, romantically, and/or emotionally attracted. People may feel physical attraction to the opposite sex, same sex, or both sexes. People who feel attracted to the opposite sex are called **heterosexual individuals**. People who are attracted to the same sex are referred to as **lesbian women** or **gay men**. The old term, *homosexual*, is not used much anymore because of its history as a negative, or pejorative, label. Finally, people who are attracted to both sexes are referred to as **bisexual individuals**. It is also important to note that genetic, psychological, and sociological research provides *no evidence* for the notion that sexual orientation is chosen or can be changed. People do not choose their sexual orientation. Scientific studies have failed to uncover genetic, hormonal, metabolic, or psychological mechanisms underlying sexual orientation. About 85 to 90 percent of Americans have a sexual orientation to members of the opposite sex (heterosexuals); the rest of the population orients to individuals of either sex (bisexuals) or, more often, exclusively to members of the same sex (lesbians or gays) (Kinsey Institute, 2012). Individuals do not choose their sexual orientation; it develops as a fundamental aspect of a person's personality.

5. The *development dimension* is the evolution of our self throughout our lifetimes. This evolution includes the body, the belief systems, and the ways sex is employed to create and maintain intimacy.

6. The *skill dimension* speaks to the physical and social skills that affect how well we meet our sexual wants and needs.

Sexuality and Culture

There are many determinants of sexuality: biological, cultural, social, familial, and even spiritual. People learn about sexuality from an early age through messages and feedback from others about what is acceptable and not acceptable to say, to do, to wear. Consider television shows, musicians' attire, ads in magazines, the

Internet, television, and messages from friends and family. All of these sources of information (and misinformation) shape our attitudes about sex and sexuality.

Expression of sexuality varies between cultures as well. For example, it may be acceptable for a rock musician to dress in a short skirt in the United States, but some countries have dress requirements that involve covering the body. From an early age, we learn culturally sanctioned ways of expressing sexuality. We internalize these messages and they become part of our sexuality.

Sexuality also is an area over which we have considerable control. Although we each receive many messages about sexuality, we also have some freedom in how we choose to express our sexuality, through dress, mannerisms, and other behaviors and statements. This is not to say than an individual who chooses to dress in tighter or more revealing clothing is more interested in having sex than are individuals who tend to dress more conservatively. Instead, differing ways of dressing may indicate that day's activities (studying versus going out to dance), comfort with one's body, or a simple preference for particular clothes. It is important to reiterate that manner of dress does not equate to a desire or an invitation to sexual advances. It is essential to gain someone's explicit consent before engaging in any form of sexual activity with that person.

Gender Role and Gender Identity

Anatomy and physiology explain the biological basis of gender. Gender identity involves beliefs, attitudes, thoughts, feelings, and social behaviors. While growing up, we learn the behaviors that are acceptable and unacceptable for males and females in our culture (**FIGURE 13.5** and **FIGURE 13.6**). These gender-based behaviors are called **gender roles**. Gender roles influence us from conception onward. When someone is expecting a child, one of the first questions we ask is, "Are you having a boy or a girl?" When a child is born, almost the first thing announced is, "It's a boy!" or "It's a girl!" Gender frequently dictates the clothes that parents purchase for a child, the colors of the child's room, and even hopes/dreams for what the child will accomplish when grown up.

Gender role socialization continues during infancy and through adulthood. Infant girls are dressed in pink or purple whereas infant boys are dressed in blue or green. In childhood, gender role socialization also

> **Gender roles** Behaviors based on sex (male or female).

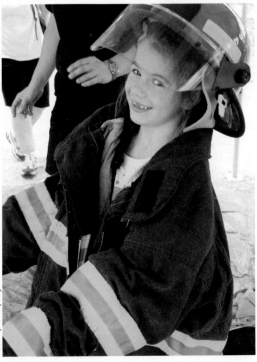

FIGURE 13.6 **Gender Roles.** Not conforming to gender role expectations can be freeing and fun!

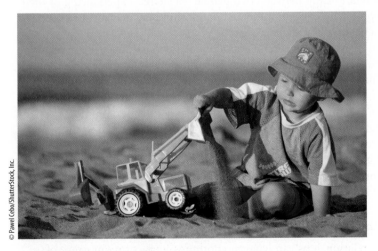

FIGURE 13.5 **Gender Roles.** Children learn gender roles from an early age.

can manifest through gift-giving. Boys often receive trucks, construction toys, or sports toys whereas girls get dolls, clothes, or play kitchens. Fortunately, many people do not live in worlds narrowly defined by gender. In fact, young girls are encouraged to play sports now and boys are given more latitude in play and toys as well.

The term *gender role congruent* means an individual behaves in ways expected of someone of that gender. Seeing a woman wearing a dress is an example of gender role congruency. In the United States, seeing a male dressed in a skirt (unless it's a kilt) is generally an example of gender role incongruence. Through messages from media, family, friends, and social institutions, we develop an understanding of what it means to be a male or female in our culture. Our self-image involves **gender identity**—that awareness of being male or female.

Usually, biological sex matches gender identity. In other words, a person born as a female develops an internal sense of being female. For a small portion of the population (2–3 percent), gender identity does not match biological sex. These individuals, referred to as **transsexual individuals**, often describe feeling like they were born in the wrong body. Thus, their gender identity—their internal sense of sex—does not match their biological sex.

Do not confuse gender identity and sexual orientation. They are two different constructs. **Sexual orientation** is attraction to a particular sex whereas gender identity is the internal feelings, thoughts, and beliefs we have about our gender. It is essential to note that anyone can form intimate and loving relationships, regardless of sexual orientation, gender role, or gender identity.

Developing Positive Intimate Relationships

Intimacy may involve sexual behavior, but intimate relationships occur in many forms, including with friends, family, and romantic partners. It is essential to understand that intimacy does not equate to sexual behavior or romantic relationships only. Intimacy can be felt in any close relationship. Intimacy involves sharing of the self and hearing about the other without worry of being judged or hurt, all of which occur in most close relationships.

Intimacy and sex are erroneously associated perhaps because love and affection are feelings associated with intimacy, and in the United States, there is much confusion between love and sex. Remember that intimacy is a feeling, not an act. It is the quality of a relationship between two people—a shared experiencing of their personal lives. People who have an intimate relationship may or may not choose to express their closeness with sexual activity.

Intimate relationships share certain common characteristics. They are relationships of mutual consent. One person cannot be intimate with another unless both want intimacy. These close relationships tend to grow deeper and richer over time (**FIGURE 13.7**). Meaningful experiences are shared to establish and maintain genuine trust and caring. Intimate relationships carry deep connection but do not result in a merging of personalities. There is connection and still separateness of identities. Finally, intimate relationships involve honesty and respect. Both parties in the relationship are kindly honest. Intimate relationships can withstand challenges and disagreements. The partners in intimate relationships discuss disagreements without use of hurtful language or statements.

Intimacy in Romantic Relationships

Intimate romantic relationships can have an enormous impact on our sense of vitality and well-being. In fact, Saxbe, Repetti, and Nishina (2008) found that women who had happy marriages recovered more quickly from stressful days at work when compared to women in less satisfactory marriages. This finding sug-

---

Gender identity An internal sense or feeling of being male or female.

Transsexual individual An individual whose gender identity does not match his or her biological sex.

Sexual orientation Gender or genders to whom we are physically, romantically, and/or emotionally attracted.

Intimacy means having a deep, trusting, and emotional connection with another person.

gests that a healthy intimate romantic relationship can, in fact, buffer the effects of stress and contribute to improved wellness. When an intimate relationship is flowing smoothly, it can produce rich emotional satisfaction. On the other hand, when an intimate relationship is not going well, those involved can feel lonely, depressed, anxious, or angry. Romantic relationships that are not going well can, at an extreme, interfere with functioning at work or at school.

Cycle of Intimate Romantic Relationships

Before an intimate relationship can develop, the partners have to be open to entering and maintaining it. Some individuals choose not to be involved in an intimate relationship, perhaps because they wish to devote energies to school, work, or self-development, or because they find intimate relationships to be distracting or psychologically threatening at the time. For example, our previous life experiences may result in a fear of emotional closeness. Once we open to a relationship, we likely work on developing and maintaining intimacy with our partner.

Developing and Maintaining Intimacy

At the beginning of a relationship, we do not share much personal information with our new partner. We tend to talk about "safe topics," such as class or work, sports, hobbies, mutual friends, favorite television shows, movies, bands, or politics. As time goes on, we may "test the waters" by sharing information that is more personal. With time, we learn who we can trust with more personal knowledge without fear of being mocked or having our confidence broken.

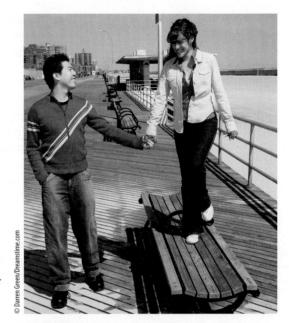

© Darren Green/Dreamstime.com

FIGURE 13.7 **Intimacy.** Intimate relationships take time to develop.

When we begin to share our personal histories, difficulties or challenges, hopes, aspirations, fears, and imperfections, we increase our level of **self-disclosure**. Disclosing this personal information increases our sense of vulnerability. We now entrust the other in the relationship with deeply personal information, information that is not common knowledge to others.

Self-disclosure Sharing of private information.

Intimacy is created and maintained in a cycle of self-disclosure. As we self-disclose, our partner is more likely to self-disclose. By sharing this important information, we communicate trust to our partner. Our partner usually accepts the trust and reciprocates. We do not use shared thoughts and feelings to mock, intimidate, or shame, but instead we treat our partner with respect and kindness. Thus, intimacy progresses as a cycle: self-disclosure, increased trust, increased self-disclosure, increased trust, and so on.

In summary, intimacy is an important component in romantic relationships that may lead to sexual expression of those feelings of trust and safety. However, intimacy also develops in friendships and other relationships. In nonromantic relationships, intimacy is usually expressed in different ways, such as in verbal expressions of appreciation and increasing feelings of trust and safety.

Establishing Commitment

After a period of self-disclosure, in a romantic relationship we may want to develop a commitment. A commitment involves a promise or an action. The involved partners agree to a set of values, terms, and/or conditions in the relationship. A common commitment involves an agreement not to date other people.

Within committed relationships, we have (hopefully) established trust and intimacy. We have agreed upon our expectations and hopes for the relationship. It is important to note that intimate, committed relationships are not free from conflict. When conflict arises, committed partners exhibit respect for each other and dedication to resolve the conflict in a way that is good for both partners. Healthy communication strategies that are useful in resolving conflict are discussed later in this chapter.

Relationship Endings

Everything has a beginning and an end, including close relationships (FIGURE 13.8). The beginning usually involves acquaintanceship and progresses to increasing intimacy. At some point, the relationship may end. Sometimes the formalities of a close relationship continue, but the intimacy dwindles. This decrease in intimacy may occur because of a betrayal; a shift in one partner's goals, hopes, or aspirations; or when one partner decides he or she no longer wants to be involved in a committed relationship.

Another factor associated with endings is lack of support, or even hostility, from the partner's social network. Families may not accept a son's or daughter's choice of a partner. Relationships that involve a partner of a different race, a partner with a mental or physical disability, or a partner of the same sex often face additional biases and hardships based on societal judgments and stigmas. Sometimes family or other social networks exhibit strong (and unfortunate) disapproval, which may result in the ending of the relationship.

Whether a romantic relationship continues or ends can also be affected by the potential of other dating partners or by the desire to be single. If other appealing dating options do not exist, leaving a relationship may feel difficult. In this culture, there is tremendous pressure on and expectations of young people to get married. A relationship can become problematic if there is disrespect, control, or abuse involved. Fear of being alone, worries that you will "never" be able to find another partner, and threats of physical harm can be overwhelming obstacles to leaving a disrespectful or even abusive relationship given the societal pressure to be in a committed relationship.

If you or someone you care about seems to be in a romantic relationship that is unhealthy, encourage that person to get support, but never threaten or shame that person into leaving. Leaving a violent relationship can be complicated. Instead, the person should seek counseling, consult with a shelter for partners in violent relationships, or contact the National Domestic Violence Hotline at (800) 799-SAFE.

Once a relationship ends, its structure usually changes. The relationship usually becomes less intimate and trust may decrease. Time spent together often decreases as well. At the end of relationships, we experience a myriad of feelings, including sadness, loneliness, fatigue, helplessness or hopelessness, anger, resentment, and guilt, to name a few. Some people may even feel relief and hope after a no-longer-satisfying relationship ends.

Most people go through a period of sadness. We may experience physical manifestations of these feelings as well, such as sleep disturbance, change in appetite, decreased concentration, social isolation (withdrawal from friends), and low motivation. When a breakup occurs, remember to take good care of yourself and all aspects of your wellness. Try to stay connected with friends, continue with your other interests, and engage in healthy living activities. If you feel like you cannot cope or manage, consider talking to a professional counselor.

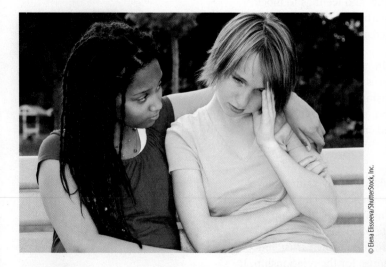

FIGURE 13.8 **Breakups.** The end of a relationship often comes with sadness, but seeking support from friends can help.

© Elena Elisseeva/ShutterStock, Inc.

Relationships and Social Wellness

To maintain good social health, ask yourself how many relationships you want and whether your number is reasonable—if you desire 100 very close friends, that may not be feasible! It takes time and energy to create close, lasting relationships. As noted previously, some people may want many friendships whereas other people may be content with a few close friendships. After eliminating the extremes (none or hundreds), there is no number of relationships that indicates social wellness or a lack of social wellness. That is up to you and depends on what feels right for you.

In addition to number of relationships, ask yourself which kinds of relationships are most important to you. Although the number of relationships is less important for social health, having a wide range of types of relationships is encouraged. You may want just a few close friends and a dating partner, or you may want several close friends and no romantic relationship at present. What is most important is that you feel fulfilled and satisfied with your variety of relationships.

Again, there is no specific number of relationships that indicates social wellness. Thus, after asking yourself which types and how many relationships you want, remember the definition of social health: the ability to interact effectively with others and to help and assist others. Ask yourself if you are, in your relationships, interacting effectively. Are you helping others? And do you ask for assistance when you need it? These are some of the important components of social wellness. The next step in social wellness is maintaining your relationships, which involves healthy communication.

> **I-statements** Statements beginning with "I"; a positive communication skill.
>
> **You-statements** Statements beginning with "you"; a negative communication skill.

Healthy Communication in Relationships

Effective communication is critical for developing and maintaining all relationships and encompasses use of I-statements, emotional regulation, clear and direct communication, and effective/active listening. Different types of relationships involve various levels of self-disclosure; however, these basic communication strategies are useful for relationships at any level. Effective communication skills are essential to relationships (FIGURE 13.9). Communicating clearly, directly, and with respect/concern for the others involved in the relationship are keys to maintaining healthy relationships of all types. For example, you have heard someone say, "If he really loved me, he would know what I need without me telling him." Individuals who know us best may eventually be able to figure out what we want or need, but it is much more effective and easier to communicate directly and clearly what your needs are. The following subsections discuss the four components of effective communication.

Effective communication is critical for developing and maintaining all relationships.

I-Statements

Try to ask for what you want or need by requesting it directly. This communicates respect for yourself and for the other person. **I-statements**, statements that begin with "I . . . ," are a great way to open a conversation and express, appropriately, how you are feeling and what you are hoping for. Conversely, starting a request with, "You should . . ." can sound bossy, demanding, or rude and can undermine healthy relationships. **You-statements** often are experienced as attacks and tend

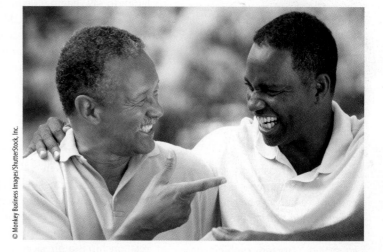

© Monkey Business Images/ShutterStock, Inc.

FIGURE 13.9 **Effective Communication Strategies.** Communication is essential in every relationship.

to set others on the defensive. You-statements can feel blaming and rarely lead to a successful communication experience.

Appropriate Expression of Emotion

The concept of appropriate expression of emotion is also known as emotional regulation and refers to maintaining an appropriate level of emotional expression. For example, if you feel upset and angry, expressing yourself by yelling will most likely not elicit the response you want. But, instead, expressing yourself calmly and identifying the feelings you have will more than likely get you the response you hope for. To illustrate, imagine your response to someone who yells at you for not returning her e-mail compared to your response when a friend says, "I felt worried about you and upset when you did not respond to my e-mail. Is everything OK?"

Clear and Respectful Expression of What You Want and Need

Make sure you specify what you are hoping for. For example, if your friend has not returned your e-mail messages because he didn't think you needed a response, make that request in the future. You might say something like, "I felt worried and upset when you did not respond to my e-mail. In the future, would you please respond, even if it's just a brief, one-sentence reply to my message?" Then, you and your friend can work out the details and compromise.

Effective/Active Listening

Effective communication requires both sending and receiving, both talking and listening. Effective listening is important because the receiver not only takes in the sender's message but also helps to establish the physical and emotional context for the communication. The listener also must communicate to the sender that the sender's message was received. This is called feedback. Some techniques for effective receiving are giving the sender your full attention, making eye contact, listening, being empathetic, being open to receiving the message, giving verbal feedback, acknowledging the sender's feelings, praising the sender's efforts, and being unconditional.

Communication Medium

One final note on relationship communication involves various methods of communication. When you have something important or potentially emotionally laden to say, having a conversation in person—rather than through e-mail or text messaging—is preferred. Most people have been on the receiving end of a "flame mail" in which they feel scolded or like they were getting yelled at for something. Communicating clearly and in person while managing emotions appropriately is preferred because it prevents misunderstandings or makes misunderstandings easier to resolve. Having a conversation also tends to prevent you from e-mailing things you would never have said in person.

A Healthy Sexual Relationship

During your years in college, you will establish many different kinds of relationships. At this time, you most likely will develop close positive intimate relationships. Intimacy means having a deep, trusting relationship and emotional connection with another person and is not an act. People who have developed an intimate relationship may choose to express their closeness with sexual acts. Choosing to have a sexual relationship is a physical way of communicating with someone else (FIGURE 13.10). A **sexual relationship** involves two people who mutually consent to become physically intimate and participate in sexual acts such as kissing, caressing, stroking, rubbing, or

Sexual relationship A relationship in which two people mutually consent to become physically intimate and participate in sexual acts such as kissing, caressing, stroking, rubbing, or penetrative behaviors (penile–vaginal intercourse, anal intercourse, or oral sex).

A sexual relationship is one in which two people mutually consent to become physically intimate and participate in sexual acts such as kissing, caressing, stroking, rubbing, or penetrative behaviors.

penetrative behaviors (penile–vaginal intercourse, anal intercourse, or oral sex). Penetrative sex is not required to make a relationship a sexual one.

Sexual behavior is an instinctive form of physical intimacy. It is most often performed for the purpose of expressing affection and enjoying oneself. When we decide to have sexual contact, we want it to be satisfying for our partner and ourselves. We also need to understand what responsibilities our sexual behavior entails for both our partners and ourselves. Such relationships can be sources of pleasure, happiness, and joy, or pain, sadness, and disappointment. Some of the health risks include unintended pregnancy and being infected with an STI, including HIV/AIDS. In addition, there are emotional consequences of sex. Having sex when you are not ready or because you feel pressured may make you feel "used," guilty, or regretful. Keep in mind that no respectful partner uses pressure or force to engage in sexual relationships. This type of pressure or force to engage in sex is not a healthy and respectful way to engage in a relationship and can lead to fear, anxiety, and mistrust in the relationship for the individual being pressured or forced. A **sexually healthy relationship** is consensual, nonexploitative, honest, mutually pleasurable, safe, and protected from unwanted pregnancy, STIs, and other harm (National Guidelines Task Force, 2004).

In a healthy sexual relationship, both partners have a responsibility to be fully informed when it comes to making their own choices about sexual activity. What you don't know about sex can hurt you and your partner, so you will want to learn as much as you can about related topics and issues. This is true regardless of whether you are sexually active right now, have been in the past, or plan to be in the future. A prerequisite to understanding sexual activity is having a basic knowledge of the female and male sexual anatomy. Once you understand the parts, you can make better sense of how they respond and work together in sexual situations.

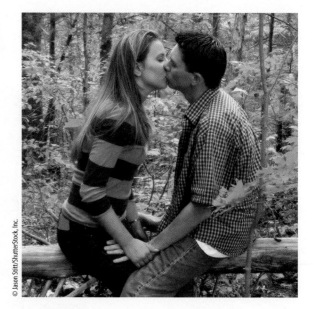

FIGURE 13.10 Sexual Relationship. This is a relationship in which two people mutually consent to become physically intimate and participate in sexual acts such as kissing.

Sexual Anatomy

One of the fundamental roles of sex is biological reproduction. The reproductive role of the male is to produce reproductively capable sperm and to deposit them in the female reproductive tract during sexual intercourse. The reproductive role of the female is to provide reproductively capable eggs, called **ova**, and a safe, nutrient-filled environment in which the fetus develops for the 9 months of pregnancy.

The genetic determination of sexual anatomy also specifies the pattern of male or female steroid hormone production, which in turn affects the **secondary sex characteristics** that distinguish adult males and females: the extent and distribution of facial and body hair, body build and stature, and the appearance of breasts (FIGURE 13.11).

Female Sexual Anatomy

A woman's internal sexual organs consist of two **ovaries**, which lie on either side of the abdominal cavity, the **fallopian tubes**, the **uterus**, and the **vagina**; together these structures make up a specialized receptacle and tube that goes from each ovary to the outside of the body (FIGURE 13.12). The function of the ovaries is to produce fertilizable ova as well as sex hormones, which control the development of the female body type, maintain normal female sexual physiology, and help regulate the course of a normal pregnancy. The fallopian tubes gather and transport the ova that

Sexually healthy relationship A relationship that is consensual, nonexploitative, honest, mutually pleasurable, safe, and protected from unwanted pregnancy, STIs, and other harm.

Ova Eggs.

Secondary sex characteristics Anatomic features appearing at puberty that distinguish males from females.

Ovaries A pair of almond-shaped organs in the female abdomen that produce egg cells (ova) and female sex hormones (estrogen and progesterone).

Fallopian tubes A pair of tube-like structures that transport ova from the ovaries to the uterus; the usual site of fertilization.

Uterus The female organ in which a fetus develops.

Vagina The female organ of copulation, and the exit pathway for the fetus at birth.

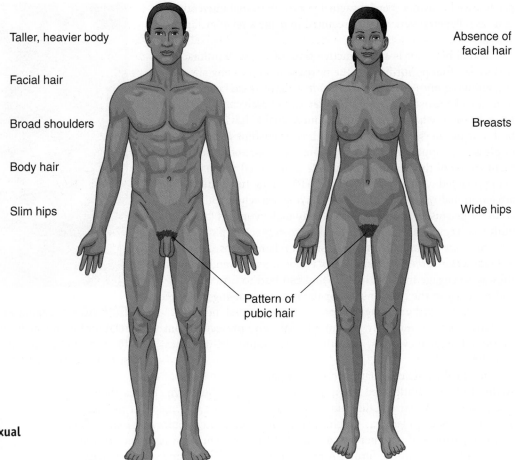

Taller, heavier body

Facial hair

Broad shoulders

Body hair

Slim hips

Absence of facial hair

Breasts

Wide hips

Pattern of pubic hair

FIGURE 13.11 Secondary Sexual Characteristics of Men and Women.

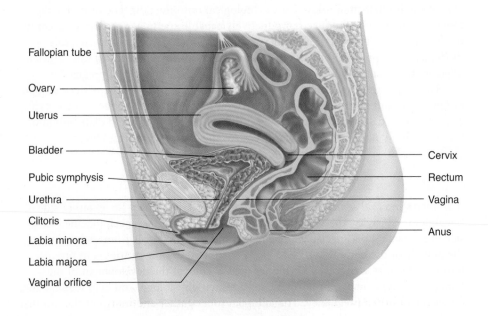

Fallopian tube

Ovary

Uterus

Bladder

Pubic symphysis

Urethra

Clitoris

Labia minora

Labia majora

Vaginal orifice

Cervix

Rectum

Vagina

Anus

FIGURE 13.12 A Cross-Section of the Female Sexual Reproductive System.

are released from the ovaries (about one each month). The fallopian tubes connect to the uterus, an organ about the size of a woman's fist, which is situated just behind the pelvic bone and the bladder (**FIGURE 13.13**). The uterus is part of the passageway for sperm as they move from the vagina to the fallopian tubes to effect fertilization; after fertilization, it provides the environment in which the fetus grows. It is the inner lining of the uterus that is shed each month in menstruation.

The lower part of the uterus is the **cervix**, and the cavity of the uterus is connected to the vagina by means of a small opening called the cervical os. The cervix secretes mucus, which changes in consistency depending on the phase of the menstrual cycle. Some women learn to estimate the time of **ovulation** (ovum release) by examining their cervical mucus.

A woman's external genitals (**FIGURE 13.14**) consist of two pairs of fleshy folds that surround the opening of the vagina and the **clitoris**. The smaller, inner pair of folds is called the **labia minora**, and the larger, outer pair is called the **labia majora**. The clitoris, a highly sensitive sexual organ, is situated above the vaginal opening.

In addition to the primary sex organs, women have secondary sex characteristics, including the **breasts**. The breasts are supplied with numerous nerve endings, which are important in the delivery of milk to a nursing baby. These nerves also make the breasts highly sensitive to touch, and many women find tactile stimulation to be sexually pleasurable. Sexual arousal, tactile stimulation, and cold temperatures can cause small muscles in the nipples to contract, resulting in erection of the nipples.

Male Sexual Anatomy

The principal reproductive role of male sexual organs is to make numerous viable sperm cells and to deliver them into the female reproductive tract during sexual intercourse. The male sexual and reproductive system consists of two **testes**, the

> **Cervix** The lower and narrow end of the uterus.
>
> **Ovulation** Release of an egg (ovum) from the ovary.
>
> **Clitoris** Small, sensitive female organ located in front of the vaginal opening; center of sexual pleasuring.
>
> **Labia minora** A pair of fleshy folds that cover the vagina.
>
> **Labia majora** A pair of fleshy folds that cover the labia minora.
>
> **Breasts** Network of milk glands and ducts in fatty tissue; secondary sex characteristic.
>
> **Testes** A pair of male reproductive organs that produce sperm cells and male sex hormones.

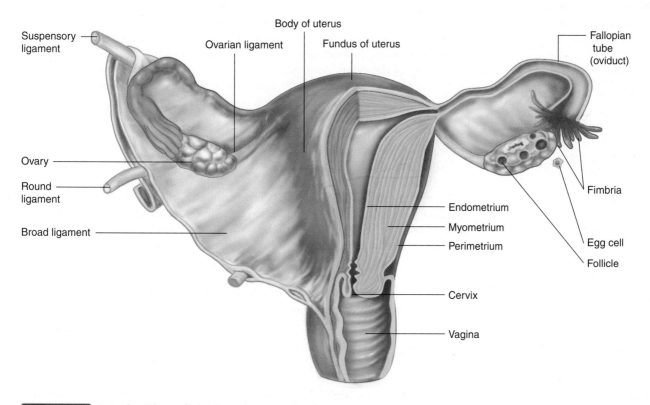

FIGURE 13.13 **Anterior View of the Female Reproductive System.**

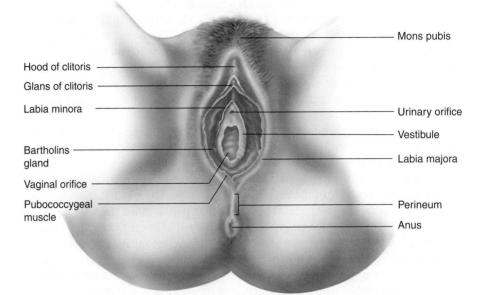

Mons pubis

Hood of clitoris

Glans of clitoris

Labia minora

Bartholins gland

Vaginal orifice

Pubococcygeal muscle

Urinary orifice

Vestibule

Labia majora

Perineum

Anus

FIGURE 13.14 **External Female Sexual Reproductive Organs.**

Penis The male organ of copulation and urination.

Copulation Sexual intercourse.

Seminal vesicles Sac-like structures that secrete a fluid that activates the sperm.

Prostate gland Gland at the base of the male bladder that provides seminal fluid.

Cowper's glands Small glands that secrete drops of alkalinizing fluid into the urethra.

Semen A whitish, creamy fluid containing sperm.

Foreskin A fold of skin covering the tip of the penis.

Circumcision A surgical procedure to remove the foreskin from the penis.

Smegma A foul-smelling, pasty accumulation of skin cells and sebum that collects in moist areas of the genitalia, especially in uncircumcised males.

sites of sperm and sex hormone production; a series of connected sperm ducts that originate at the testes, travel through the pelvis, and terminate at the urethra of the penis; glands that produce seminal fluid; and the **penis**, the organ of **copulation** (**FIGURE 13.15**).

The testes are located in a flesh-covered sac, the scrotum, which hangs outside the male body. In the embryo, the testes develop inside the body, but just before birth they descend into the scrotum. Inside the scrotum, the testes are kept at a temperature a few degrees cooler than the internal body temperature, a condition that is apparently necessary for the production of reproductively capable sperm. One testis is usually a little higher than the other.

When a man ejaculates, sperm are propelled through the sperm ducts and out of the penis by contractions of the smooth muscles that line the ducts and the muscles of the pelvis. As they move out of the male body, the sperm mix with secretions of seminal fluid from the **seminal vesicles**, **prostate gland**, and **Cowper's glands** to form **semen**. The semen, which is the gelatinous milky fluid emitted at ejaculation, contains a mixture of 300 million sperm cells and about 3 to 6 milliliters of seminal fluid. The seminal fluid contributes 95 percent or more of the entire volume of semen.

The penis is normally soft, but when a male becomes sexually aroused, the internal tissues fill with blood and the penis enlarges and becomes erect. All men are born with a fold of skin, the **foreskin**, which covers the end of the penis. For centuries, Jewish and Muslim families have surgically removed the foreskin from male children for religious reasons. This procedure is called **circumcision**. Although there is no clear medical indication that circumcision is beneficial, removal of the foreskin does eliminate the buildup of **smegma**. The belief that circumcision leads to an increase in sexual arousal because it exposes the tip of the penis, and the related belief that circumcision produces an inability to delay ejaculation, are myths. For most men, circumcision has no effect on sexual arousal and sexual activity.

Managing Your Fertility

Most of the time, people engage in sexual intercourse for nonreproductive reasons. This is especially true among young single college students who are more likely to participate in a no-strings relationship in which bonds between young men and

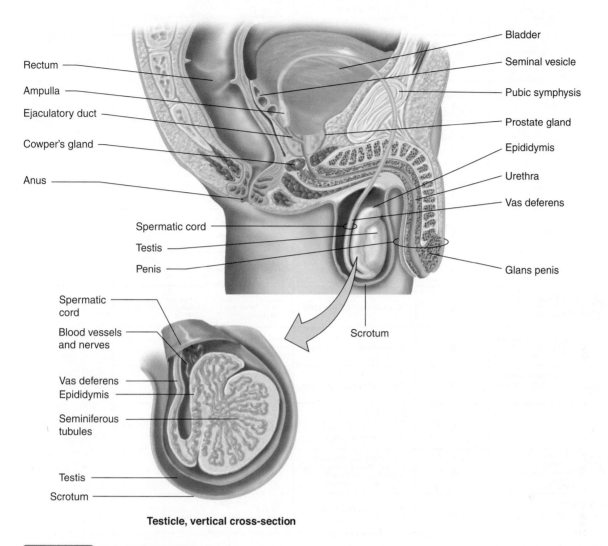

Testicle, vertical cross-section

FIGURE 13.15 **Male Reproductive Organs.**

women are increasingly brief. If you decide to become sexually active you must also take responsibility for managing your fertility and avoiding an unplanned pregnancy. In the United States, almost half of all pregnancies are unintended (Finer & Zolna, 2011). Yet several safe and highly effective methods of birth control (contraception) are available to prevent unintended pregnancy. **FIGURE 13.16** provides a list of FDA-approved products for birth control. Talk to your health care provider about the best method for you.

Some things to consider when choosing a birth control method: your health, how often you have sex, how many sexual partners you have, if you want to have children in the future, if you will need a prescription or if you can buy the method over-the-counter, and the number of pregnancies expected per 100 women who use a method for one year. No one product is best for everyone. The only sure way to avoid pregnancy is not to have sexual contact with a member of the opposite sex (abstinence).

Physical Activity and Health Connection

Relationships can be a source of joy or a source of stress. Either way, relationships contribute substantially to physical health. If your relationships are going well, including exercise as a part of your social time can be an even more effective

Most Effective ↑

Least Effective ↓

Methods	Number of pregnancies expected per 100 women*	Use	Some Risks
Sterilization Surgery for Women	less than 1	Onetime procedure Permanent	• Pain • Bleeding • Infection or other complications after surgery • Ectopic (tubal) pregnancy
Surgical Sterilization Implant for Women	less than 1	Onetime procedure Waiting period before it works Permanent	• Mild to moderate pain after insertion • Ectopic (tubal) pregnancy
Sterilization Surgery for Men	less than 1	Onetime procedure Waiting period before it works Permanent	• Pain • Bleeding • Infection
Implantable Rod	less than 1	Inserted by a healthcare provider Lasts up to 3 years	• Changes in bleeding patterns • Weight gain • Breast and abdominal pain
IUD Copper	less than 1	Inserted by a healthcare provider Lasts up to 10 years	• Cramps • Bleeding • Pelvic inflammatory disease • Infertility • Tear or hole in the uterus
IUD w/ Progestin	less than 1	Inserted by a healthcare provider Lasts up to 5 years	• Irregular bleeding • No periods • Abdominal/pelvic pain • Ovarian cysts
Shot/Injection	6	Need a shot every 3 months	• Bone loss • Nervousness • Bleeding between periods • Abdominal discomfort • Weight gain • Headaches
Oral Contraceptives (Combined Pill) "The Pill"	9	Must swallow a pill every day	• Nausea • Rare: high blood pressure, • Breast Tenderness blood clots, heart attack, • Headache stroke
Oral Contraceptives (Progestin only) "The MiniPill"	9	Must swallow a pill every day	• Irregular bleeding • Nausea • Headache • Dizziness • Breast tenderness
Oral Contraceptives Extended/Continuous Use "The Pill"	9	Must swallow a pill every day.	• Risks are similar to other oral contraceptives (combined) • Light bleeding or spotting between periods
Patch	9	Put on a new patch each week for 3 weeks (21 total days). Don't put on a patch during the fourth week.	• Exposure to higher average levels of estrogen than most oral contraceptives
Vaginal Contraceptive Ring	9	Put the ring into the vagina yourself. Keep the ring in your vagina for 3 weeks and then take it out for one week.	• Vaginal discharge • Discomfort in the vagina • Mild irritation • Risks are similar to oral contraceptives (combined)
Diaphragm with Spermicide	12	Must use every time you have sex.	• Irritation • Urinary tract infection • Allergic reactions • Toxic shock
Sponge with Spermicide	12-24	Must use every time you have sex.	• Irritation • Hard time removing • Allergic reactions • Toxic shock
Cervical Cap with Spermicide	17-23	Must use every time you have sex.	• Irritation • Abnormal Pap test • Allergic reactions • Toxic shock
Male Condom	18	Must use every time you have sex. Except for abstinence, latex condoms are the best protection against HIV/AIDS and other STIs.	• Allergic reactions
Female Condom	21	Must use every time you have sex. May give some protection against STIs.	• Irritation • Allergic reactions
Spermicide Alone	28	Must use every time you have sex.	• Irritation • Allergic reactions • Urinary tract infection
Emergency Contraception — If your primary method of birth control fails			
Plan B Plan B One Step Next Choice	7 out of every 8 women who would have gotten pregnant will not become pregnant after taking Plan B, Plan B One-Step, or Next Choice	Swallow the pills within 3 days after having unprotected sex.	• Nausea • Fatigue • Vomiting • Headache • Abdominal pain
Ella	6 or 7 out of every 10 women who would have gotten pregnant will not become pregnant after taking Ella.	Swallow the pill within 5 days after having unprotected sex.	• Headache • Menstrual pain • Nausea • Tiredness • Abdominal pain • Dizziness

*effectiveness of the different methods during typical/actual use (including sometimes using a method in a way that is not correct or not consistent)   http://www.fda.gov/birthcontrol

FIGURE 13.16 **Birth Control Guide.** SOURCE: Reproduced from U.S. Food and Drug Administration. (2012). Birth Control Guide. Online: http://www.fda.gov/forconsumers/byaudience/forwomen/vcmii8465.htm.

use of your time. You get to socialize, receive support if you're not in the mood to exercise, and strengthen your relationship through emotional connection and shared activity. Thus, combining social and physical activity can lead to improved overall well-being. On the other hand, if (when) you experience stress in a relationship, physical activity can help mitigate the impact of that stress. In fact, physical exercise has positive effects on mood management and on reducing stress.

concept connections

1. **Supportive social relationships positively affect our overall well-being and physical health.** Social support has long been associated with overall wellness and a general sense of satisfaction. A myriad of positive effects is found in those individuals who have supportive social relationships. For example, positive supportive relationships have been shown to improve adjustment to college and are connected with successful completion of college. Supportive social relationships also can help decrease overall stress.

2. **Social support consists of a wide variety of relationships, including family, friends, romantic partner, acquaintances, work/school relationships, and social networking website relationships.** You can think of relationships in terms of closeness/connection, frequency of contact, and setting (in person, work/school, and the Internet). Healthy relationships provide the opportunity to feel loved and valued as well as afford the chance to help others.

3. **Relationship needs differ between people and can range from a couple of close friends to large social circles. Quality, more than quantity, is the important determinant in social wellness.** Although we all need some connection with others, the degree and types of relationships we each desire may vary widely. Some of us may want to focus attention on a romantic partner whereas other individuals may want to date casually. Different people are equally satisfied and maintain social wellness by any number of social network configurations.

4. **Intimacy means having a deep, trusting, and emotional connection with another person.** Intimacy may involve sexual behavior, but intimate relationships occur in many different forms. It is essential to understand that intimacy does not equate to sexual behavior or romantic relationships only. We can feel intimacy in any close relationship. Intimacy involves sharing of the self and hearing about the other without worry of being judged or hurt, all of which occur in most close relationships.

5. **Effective communication is critical for developing and maintaining all relationships.** Different types of relationships involve various levels of self-disclosure; however, basic communication strategies are useful for relationships at any level. Effective communication skills are essential to relationships. Communicating clearly, directly, and with respect/concern for the others involved in the relationship is key to maintaining healthy relationships of all types.

6. **A sexual relationship involves two people who mutually consent to become physically intimate and participate in sexual acts such as kissing, caressing, stroking, rubbing, or penetrative behaviors.** Sexual behavior is an instinctive form of physical intimacy. It is most often performed for the purpose of expressing affection and enjoying oneself. When we decide to have sexual contact, we want it to be satisfying for our partner and ourselves. We also need to understand what responsibilities our sexual behavior entails for both our partners and ourselves. Such relationships can be sources of pleasure, happiness, and joy, or pain, sadness, and disappointment. Some of the health risks include unintended pregnancy and being infected with a sexually transmitted infection (STI), including HIV/AIDS.

Terms

Bisexual individual, 294
Breasts, 303
Cervix, 303
Circumcision, 304
Clitoris, 303
Copulation, 304
Cowper's glands, 304
Fallopian tubes, 301
Foreskin, 304
Gay man, 294
Gender, 293
Gender identity, 296
Gender roles, 295
Heterosexual individual, 294

I-statements, 299
Labia majora, 303
Labia minora, 303
Lesbian woman, 294
Ova, 301
Ovaries, 301
Ovulation, 303
Penis, 304
Prostate gland, 304
Secondary sex characteristics, 301
Self-disclosure, 297
Semen, 304
Seminal vesicles, 304

Sex, 293
Sexuality, 294
Sexual orientation, 296
Sexual relationship, 300
Sexually healthy relationship, 301
Smegma, 304
Social health, 290
Social support, 290
Testes, 303
Transsexual individual, 296
Uterus, 301
Vagina, 301
You-statements, 299

making the connection

Both Mona and Jennifer are satisfied with their social groups and their preferred ways of making friends. They also each have social networks that suit them—from large to small groups of friends. Which student has greater social wellness? Based on the information in this chapter, Mona and Jennifer both have good social health. Mona has a wide range of friends, a few close and intimate friends, and a boyfriend. Jennifer has a few close and intimate friends, prefers not to date right now, and feels good about her choices. After reading this chapter and then talking with her roommate using I-statements, effective listening skills, and emotional regulation skills, Mona now understands that she and Jennifer have different, though equally healthy, relationship needs. Mona is glad she is making friends at her new college instead of just relying on connections with her high school friends through the Internet, and she understands that Jennifer prefers to have a small number of friends. In fact, they decide to start working out at their college fitness facility together to improve their social and physical wellness.

Critical Thinking

1. Consider your relationship portfolio for a moment. What types of relationships do you have and when do you seek out each relationship? Which of your friends or relationships seek you out for advice, comfort, a laugh, or help? Do you want to diversify your relationship portfolio—add more people?

2. What are you doing to maintain intimacy (trust, deep emotional connection) in your relationships?

3. Do you feel respected in your friendships and romantic relationship? What might need to change in your relationships?

4. Think about the messages you receive— from family, teachers, friends, and media— about sex and sexuality. Are there any messages you do not agree with about how men and women "should" act? What can you do to live more in harmony with your own gender role beliefs?

5. Using the tips for effective communication, think about a disagreement you had with a friend. Did you and that friend use effective communication skills? Did you feel heard by that friend? Consider talking with a friend with whom communication is not as effective. Try to establish a plan for effective communication if you have a disagreement again.

References

Almeida, J., Subramanian, S.V., & Moinar, B.E. (2011). Is blood thicker than water? Social support, depression and the modifying role of ethnicity/nativity status. *Journal of Epidemiology and Community Health* 65:51–56.

American Psychiatric Association. (1994). *Diagnostic and statistical manual of mental disorders (DSM-IV)*. Arlington, VA: Author.

Beets, M.W., Pitetti, K.H., & Forlaw, L. (2007). The role of self-efficacy and referent specific social support in promoting rural adolescent girls' psychical activity. *American Journal of Health Behavior* 31:227–237.

Braveman, J.P., Egerter, S., & Williams, D.R. (2011). The social determinants of health: Coming of age. *Annual Review of Public Health* 32:381–398.

Busseri, M.A., Rose-Krasnor, L., Pancer, S.M., Pratt, M.W., Adams, G.R., Birnie-Lefcovitch, S., Polivy, J., & Wintre, M.G. (2011). A longitudinal study of breadth of activity involvement and transition to university. *Journal of Adolescence* 21(2):512–518.

Chao, R.C. (2012). Managing perceived stress among college students: The roles of social support and dysfunctional coping. *Journal of College Counseling* 15(1):5–21.

Elphinston, R.A., & Noller, P. (2011). Time to face it! Facebook intrusion and implications for romantic jealousy and relationship satisfaction. *Cyberpsychology, Behavior, and Social Networking* 14(11):631–635.

Finer, L.B., & Zolna, M.R. (2011). Unintended pregnancy in the United States: Incidence and disparities. *Contraception* 84(5):478–485.

Fletcher, A., Bonell, C., Sorhaindo, A., & Strange, V. (2009). How might schools influence young people's drug use? Development of theory from qualitative case-study research. *Journal of Adolescent Health* 45:126–132.

Hwang, S., Kirst, M., Chiu, S., Tolomiczenko, G., Kiss, A., Cowan, L., & Levinson, W. (2009). Multidimensional social support and the health of homeless individuals. *Journal of Urban Health* 86:791–803.

Ingram, M., Ruiz, M., Mayorga, M.T., & Rosales, C. (2009). The animadora project: Identifying factors related to the promotion of physical activity among Mexican Americans with diabetes. *American Journal of Health Promotion* 23:396–402.

Jolin, E.M., & Weller, R.A. (2011). Television viewing and its impact on childhood behaviors. *Current Psychiatry Reports* 13(2):122–128.

Kim, J., LaRose, R., & Peng, W. (2009). Loneliness as the cause and effect of problematic Internet use: The relationship between Internet use and psychological well-being. *CyberPsychology and Behavior* 12:451–455.

Kinsey Institute. (2012). Gender and sexual orientation. Online: http://kinseyconfidential.org/resources/gender-sexual-orientation.

Konishi, C., & Hymel, S. (2009). Bullying and stress in early adolescence: The role of coping and social support. *Journal of Early Adolescence* 29:333–356.

Lawhon, D., Humfleet, G.L., Hall, S.M., Reus, V.I., & Munoz, R.F. (2009). Longitudinal analysis of abstinence-specific social support and smoking cessation. *Health Psychology* 28:465–472.

McEwan, B. (2011), Hybrid engagement: How Facebook helps and hinders students' social integration, in Laura A. Wankel & Charles Wankel (eds.), *Higher Education Administration with Social Media (Cutting-Edge Technologies in Higher Education, Volume 2)* United Kingdom: Emerald Group Publishing Limited, pp. 3–23.

National Guidelines Task Force. (2004). *Guidelines for Comprehensive Sexuality Education: Kindergarten–12th Grade*, 3rd ed. New York: Sexuality Information and Education Council of the United States. Online: http://www.nsba.org/SHHC/SearchSchoolHealth/GuidelinesforComprehensiveSexualityEducatonKindergartenthrough12thGrade3rdEdition.aspx.

Nelson, M.C., Kocos, R., Lytle, L.A., & Perry, C.L. (2009). Understanding the perceived determinants of weight-related behaviors in late adolescence: A qualitative analysis among college youth. *Journal of Nutrition Education and Behavior* 41:287–292.

Overholser, J.C., & Fisher, L.B. (2009). Contemporary perspectives on stress management: Medication, meditation, or mitigation. *Journal of Contemporary Psychotherapy* 39:147–155.

Saxbe, D.E., Repetti, R.L., & Nishina, A. (2008). Marital satisfaction, recovery from work, and diurnal cortisol among men and women. *Health Psychology* 27:15–25.

Sexuality Information and Education Council of the United States. (2009). Consensus Statement on Adolescent Sexual Health and Human Sexuality. Online: http://www.siecus.org/index.cfm?fuseaction=Page.viewPage&pageId=494&parentID=472.

Turncheff, C.E., Serbin, L.A., Martin-Storey, A., Stack, D.M., Ledingham, J., & Schwartzman, A.E. (2011). Predicting adult physical outcomes from childhood aggression, social withdrawal and likeability: A 30-year prospective longitudinal study. *International Journal of Behavioral Medicine* 18(5):5–12.

Protecting Your Cardiovascular System

14

what's the connection?

Sky knows that cardiovascular disease (CVD) is the number one killer in the United States. He understands that CVD is not one single disease or condition. His father was diagnosed last year with coronary heart disease at age 45, and his grandfather died of a stroke 2 years ago. Sky wants to avoid following in their footsteps. Sky, however, does not fully understand what each of these medical terms mean or what causes them. Sky knows that the more he understands about the various types of CVD and the destruction they can inflict on the body, the more inclined he will be to take steps to prevent or control them.

concepts

1. Cardiovascular disease is a group of different illnesses that affect your heart and blood vessels.

2. Atherosclerosis is the main underlying disease responsible for CVD morbidity and mortality.

3. Coronary heart disease is most commonly the result of atherosclerosis narrowing the two coronary arteries (the ones that supply the muscles of the heart).

4. Stroke occurs when vital oxygen-rich blood flow to the brain fails.

5. High blood pressure is the third leading cause of death for CVD.

6. The six major modifiable CVD risk factors are cigarette smoking, physical inactivity, high blood fats, high blood pressure, being overweight/obese, and diabetes mellitus.

7. The three major unmodifiable CVD risk factors are increasing age, male gender, and heredity/race.

go.jblearning.com/kotecki4e
The website for this book is a great source for supplementary physical health information for both students and instructors. Visit **go.jblearning.com/kotecki4e** to find a variety of useful tools for learning, thinking, and teaching.

All parts of the body which have a function if used in moderation and exercised in labors in which each is accustomed, become thereby healthy, well developed and age more slowly, but if unused they become liable to disease, defective in growth and age quickly.

—Hippocrates

Introduction

This chapter is about protecting your cardiovascular system—your internal superhighway to life. There is a great deal we can do to keep our cardiovascular system healthy through regular aerobic exercise. Even so, diseases of the cardiovascular system—the heart and blood vessels—remain the number one killer in the United States today. But there is good news: there are many other things you can do to reduce your risk of developing cardiovascular disease (CVD), and the earlier you get started, the better. This chapter explains the major types of CVD and the conditions and lifestyle factors that put you at risk for CVD. Most important, it explains the steps you can take to protect your heart and blood vessels to maintain your internal superhighway to life.

Understanding Cardiovascular Disease

The term *cardiovascular*—a long name for one of the most important body systems—refers to the heart (*cardio*) and blood vessels (*vascular*). More simply, your cardiovascular system is the network that connects your heart and blood vessels. Think of it as a delivery system of highways and roads that allow oxygen-rich blood to reach every organ and tissue in your body. Every minute of every day, millions of blood cells travel through about 60,000 miles of blood vessels to truck oxygen and nutrients to every cell and haul away cellular waste products. Most of us take the sheer efficiency and complexity of our body's internal transport plan for granted until we suffer from either a malfunction in the mighty heart muscle or a clogged artery along one of the main routes of the far-flung transportation system.

Cardiovascular disease (CVD) is not a single disease or condition. It is a group of different illnesses that affect your heart and blood vessels. In fact, some types of CVD can even cause other types of CVD. More than 1 in 3 Americans (more than 105 million) have one or more forms of diagnosable heart and blood vessel disease (Centers for Disease Control and Prevention [CDC], 2012b). CVD—the leading cause of death in the United States—accounts for more than one-third (33.6 percent) of all deaths (CDC, 2012b). **FIGURE 14.1** shows the percentage of deaths from the major forms of CVD. Coronary heart disease is the number one killer, accounting for slightly less than one-half of all CVD deaths each year. Stroke is the next biggest killer, followed by high blood pressure, heart failure, and diseases of the arteries.

You may not fully understand what each of these CVD terms mean or how harmful they can be to your health. However, understanding the various types of CVD is vital. By knowing more about the different types of CVD and the destruction they can inflict on your body, you will be more inclined to take steps to prevent or control them.

Cardiovascular disease (CVD)
A group of different illnesses that affect your heart and blood vessels.

Cardiovascular disease is a group of different illnesses that affect your heart and blood vessels.

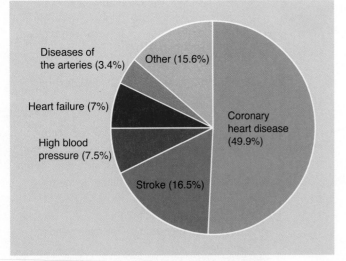

FIGURE 14.1 **Deaths from Cardiovascular Disease.** Breakdown of deaths from cardiovascular disease in the United States. SOURCE: Data from Miniño, A.M., Murphy, S.L., Xu, J., & Kochanek, K.D. (2011). Deaths: Final Data for 2008. *National Vital Statistics Reports* 59(10): 1–21. Online: http://www.cdc.gov/nchs/data/nvsr/nvsr59/nvsr59-10.pdf.

Furthermore, you will gain a greater appreciation for how the different types interact to affect your health.

The most widespread form of cardiovascular disease starts with damage to the blood vessels. The main process by which the blood vessels become damaged is through a progressive narrowing and hardening of their inner walls—a disease process known as **atherosclerosis**. Most people are unfamiliar with this common disease process.

Atherosclerosis: The Enemy Within

Atherosclerosis comes from the Greek words *athero* (meaning "paste") and *sclerosis* (meaning "hardness"), which is an accurate description of the "hardening" of this artery-clogging "paste" (plaque) that occurs on the insides of the arteries. Atherosclerosis is a slow, progressive disease that typically starts in early adulthood and develops gradually over decades. As the arterial plaque builds up, it can eventually clog our large or medium-sized arteries, making them stiff and inflexible. The exact cause of atherosclerosis is not known. However, according to current thinking of scientists, this complex, progressive, artery-clogging disease develops in the following four stages (FIGURE 14.2).

First, atherosclerosis is thought to begin with an injury (lesion) to the innermost layer of the artery (endothelium) (see Figure 14.2A). Such injuries are thought to be caused mainly by high blood pressure, high amounts of certain fats (LDL) in the blood, high amounts of sugar in the blood resulting from insulin resistance or diabetes, and tobacco smoke. These injuries create areas where higher levels of low-density lipoprotein (LDL) cholesterol can be trapped. As LDL accumulates in the arterial wall, it undergoes chemical changes and signals to endothelial cells to latch onto white blood cells (immune cells) circulating in the blood.

Second, these immune cells penetrate the inner lining and trigger an inflammatory response, devouring the LDLs, to become fat-laden "foam cells." The lesions now appear as a "fatty streak"—a yellow streak running along the major arteries (see Figure 14.2B). The streak is filled with fatty deposits, such as cholesterol; smooth muscle cells; and white blood cells called macrophages (an immune system "scavenger" cell that tries to remove the fat deposition from the artery wall and whose secretions stimulate the growth of smooth muscle cells to aid repair). This fatty streak or plaque by itself does not cause any symptoms but, over time, can grow and form a fibrous cap leading to the development of a more advanced form of atherosclerosis called **fibrous plaque**. The buildup of fibrous plaque is thought to occur from a chronic inflammatory response in the walls of arteries, in large part because of the accumulation of macrophage white blood cells. Hypertension and hyperlipidemia are key factors in this process, and both are discussed later in the chapter.

The third stage is when a fibrous plaque (atheroma) forms in the inner layer of the artery (see Figure 14.2C). The plaque consists of large numbers of smooth muscle cells and macrophages filled with cholesterol. The

> **Atherosclerosis** A vascular disease in which plaque buildup occurs inside of the arteries.
>
> **Fibrous plaque** An advanced form of atherosclerosis that occurs from a chronic inflammatory response in the walls of arteries.

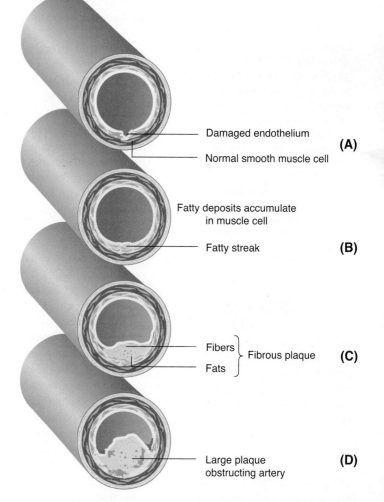

Damaged endothelium — Normal smooth muscle cell **(A)**

Fatty deposits accumulate in muscle cell — Fatty streak **(B)**

Fibers ⎫ Fibrous plaque **(C)**
Fats ⎭

Large plaque obstructing artery **(D)**

FIGURE 14.2 Progression of Athersclerosis. The development of atherosclerotic plaque inside an artery can eventually block blood flow, causing serious problems such as heart attack, stroke, or even death.

Atherosclerosis is the main underlying disease responsible for CVD morbidity and mortality.

Arteriosclerosis A vascular disease in which the arteries harden and lose elasticity.

Blood clot Blood that has been converted from a liquid state to a solid state. Also called a thrombus.

Coagulation Process by which a blood clot forms.

Coronary heart disease (CHD) Disease of the heart caused by the atherosclerotic narrowing of the two coronary arteries (arteries that supply blood to the muscles of the heart).

Angina pectoris Chest pain caused by coronary heart disease.

Ischemia Decreased blood flow to an organ, usually the result of the constriction or obstruction of an artery.

Myocardial infarction Death of, or damage to part of, the heart muscle resulting from insufficient blood supply.

Stroke A rapid loss of brain functions caused by a loss of oxygen-rich blood flow to the brain. Also known as a brain attack.

Coronary heart disease is most commonly the result of atherosclerosis narrowing the two coronary arteries (the ones that supply the muscles of the heart).

Stroke occurs when vital oxygen-rich blood flow to the brain fails.

macrophages become increasingly ineffective at fat removal and undergo cell death, accumulating at the site. This leads to fibrous plaque growth into the space inside the artery where the blood is flowing. Over time, when the fibrous plaque grows large enough, it begins to narrow the artery. Additionally, when the fibrous plaque forms inside the walls of an artery, it can restrict the artery's ability to dilate (widen) so that more blood can flow through when needed. This "hardening" of the arteries results in the condition known as **arteriosclerosis**.

The last stage of atherosclerosis occurs when the fibrous plaque ruptures or cracks as a result of substances released from the macrophage cells that eventually destabilize the fibrous cap. This rupture or crack provokes a strong clotting reaction from the blood and can result in a **blood clot**. A blood clot is blood that has been converted from a liquid state to a solid state; they are also called thrombi (*thrombus* is the singular form). The process by which a blood clot forms is termed **coagulation**. If the resulting blood clot is so large that it suddenly and completely blocks blood flow, a downstream organ or tissue may be damaged or die from a lack of oxygen (see Figure 14.2D).

Atherosclerosis can affect any artery in the body, including arteries in the heart, brain, arms, legs, and pelvis, and it is the main item responsible for CVD morbidity and mortality. Different diseases can develop based on which arteries are affected. Atherosclerosis can lead to serious problems, including heart attack, stroke, or even death.

Coronary Heart Disease

Of all the major cardiovascular diseases, **coronary heart disease (CHD)** is the greatest killer (refer to Figure 14.1). More than 11 percent of the adult U.S. population suffers from CHD (CDC, 2012b). Based on current estimates, 1 in 2 men and 1 in 3 women will eventually develop CHD at some point in their lives.

CHD is most commonly the result of atherosclerosis narrowing the two coronary arteries (the ones that supply blood to the muscles of the heart) (**FIGURE 14.3**). When your coronary arteries are narrowed or blocked, oxygen-rich blood can't reach your heart muscle. As less blood reaches the heart, it can't function normally, and this may cause anything from chest pain to a fatal heart attack.

Angina pectoris, or simply *angina*, is the main symptom of CHD and is characterized by severe chest pain. This pain, caused by a shortage of blood to the heart muscle, or **ischemia**, is usually felt on the left side of the chest or sometimes in the left arm or shoulder. Angina can occur when blood circulation to the heart is not sufficient to meet the heart's increased needs, such as during physical activity or acute emotional arousal. For example, running up a flight of stairs or becoming angry or hostile can contribute to angina. Angina may be a warning sign of a pending heart attack.

The medical term for heart attack is **myocardial infarction**. An infarct is an area of dead or dying tissue. A myocardial infarction is the death of heart muscle tissue from a lack of blood supply (refer to Figure 14.3). A heart attack is a frightening event that requires immediate medical attention. Therefore, it is important to learn the warning symptoms of a heart attack and what steps to take. TABLE 14.1 lists the warning symptoms for a heart attack. If you experience any of the symptoms of a heart attack or are with someone who does, call 9-1-1 or your local emergency operator immediately and follow their instructions. Every minute counts when it comes to getting treatment for heart attacks. Fast action saves lives.

Stroke

Stroke is the second leading cause of CVD death and the fourth leading cause of death in the United States (refer to Figure 14.1). **Stroke**, or "brain attack," occurs when vital oxygen-rich blood flow to the brain fails. Deprived of its blood sup-

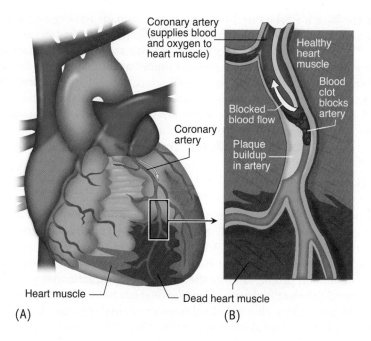

FIGURE 14.3 Coronary Heart Disease. (A) Overview of a heart attack and coronary artery showing damage (dead heart muscle) caused by a heart attack. (B) Cross-section of the coronary artery with plaque buildup and a blood clot. SOURCE: National Heart, Lung, and Blood Institute. (2012). What is coronary heart disease? Online: http://www.nhlbi.nih.gov/health/health-topics/heartattack.

ply, even for a few minutes, the affected parts of the brain may be damaged or destroyed, leading to a rapid loss of brain functions. There are two broad categories of stroke: those caused by a blockage of blood flow (ischemic), and those caused by bleeding (hemorrhage).

Ischemic strokes are caused by a blockage of a blood vessel in the brain or neck (carotid artery disease) and are responsible for 80 percent of all strokes (National Institute of Neurological Disorders and Stroke [NINDS], 2012). These blockages stem from three conditions: the formation of a blood clot (thrombus) within a blood vessel of the brain or neck; the movement of a blood clot (embolism) from another part of the body; or a severe narrowing (stenosis) of an artery in or leading to the brain (NINDS, 2012).

Hemorrhage strokes occur when blood seeps from a hole in the wall of a blood vessel. There are two types of hemorrhagic strokes: **cerebral hemorrhage** and **subarachnoid hemorrhage**. Cerebral hemorrhage occurs when a defective artery in the brain ruptures, flooding the surrounding tissue with blood. A subarachnoid hemorrhage occurs when a blood vessel on the surface of the brain ruptures and bleeds into the space between the brain and the skull.

Ischemic strokes Strokes caused by a blockage of a blood vessel in the brain or neck.

Hemorrhage strokes Strokes caused by blood that seeps from a hole in the wall of a blood vessel.

Cerebral hemorrhage Bleeding within the brain as the result of a defective artery in the brain that ruptures, flooding the surrounding tissue with blood.

Subarachnoid hemorrhage Bleeding from a blood vessel on the surface of the brain as the result of a defective blood vessel between the brain and the skull.

TABLE 14.1	Heart Attack Warning Signs

Chest Pain or Discomfort: Discomfort in the center or left side of the chest that lasts more than a few minutes or goes away and comes back. May feel like pressure, squeezing, fullness, or pain. May also feel like heartburn or indigestion.

Other Upper Body Pain or Discomfort: May be felt in one or both arms, the back, shoulders, neck, jaw, or upper part of the stomach (above the belly button).

Shortness of Breath: May be the only symptom, or it may occur before or along with chest pain or discomfort. May occur when resting or during easy activities.

Other Possible Symptoms: May include breaking out in a cold sweat, feeling unusually tired, nausea, or light-headedness. Any sudden new symptom or change in usual symptoms also should be a concern.

SOURCE: Reproduced from National Heart, Lung, and Blood Institute. (2012). Heart attack: Know the symptoms. Take action. Online: http://www.nhlbi.nih.gov/health/public/heart/mi/heart_attack_wallet_card.htm.

The effects of a stroke vary from person to person, depending on the type of stroke and the area of the brain affected (**FIGURE 14.4**). A stroke can cause paralysis and affect sight, touch, movement, and cognitive abilities. Like a heart attack, a stroke is a medical emergency that requires immediate attention. The message to remember is "Stroke strikes fast. You should too. Call 9-1-1." Therefore, it is important to know the symptoms of a stroke. TABLE 14.2 lists the symptoms of a stroke. If you experience any of the symptoms of a stroke or are with someone who does, don't wait to call 9-1-1 or your local emergency operator, and follow their instructions. Fast action significantly reduces disability and saves lives.

High Blood Pressure

High blood pressure (HBP), or hypertension, is the third leading cause of death for CVD (refer to Figure 14.1). HBP affects about 1 in 3 adults—an estimated 68 million people in the United States—but because there are no symptoms, more than 1 in 5 don't know they have it (CDC, 2011a). Furthermore, nearly 3 in 10 adults, or 60 million people, fall into the category of **prehypertension**—a condition in which blood pressure is elevated above normal but not to the level considered to be hypertensive. Once elevated blood pressure occurs, it usually lasts a lifetime. If uncontrolled, it can lead to many serious health problems, including heart attack and stroke, congestive heart failure, peripheral vascular disease, kidney damage, and blindness.

Blood pressure is a measure of the force of blood pushing against the walls of arteries as blood travels through the circulatory system. Pressure is created when the heart contracts and pumps blood into the arteries. It is recorded as two numbers: the **systolic pressure** over the **diastolic pressure**. Systolic pressure is the pressure as the heart beats, and diastolic pressure measures the pressure when the heart relaxes between beats. As we go through the day, our blood pressure just naturally raises and lowers depending on a lot of conditions. But when it stays elevated over time, you have **high blood pressure**. HBP usually causes no symptoms. Even if HBP does cause symptoms, the symptoms are usually mild and nonspecific. Thus, HBP is labeled the "silent killer." People with HBP typically do not know their blood pressure is elevated until they have their blood pressure measured.

5

High blood pressure is the third leading cause of death for CVD.

Prehypertension Blood pressure elevated above normal but not to the level considered to be hypertensive.

Blood pressure Measure of the force of blood pushing against the walls of arteries as blood travels through the circulatory system.

Systolic pressure Blood pressure as the heart beats.

Diastolic pressure Blood pressure when the heart relaxes between beats.

High blood pressure (HBP) Blood pressure that stays elevated over time. Also known as hypertension.

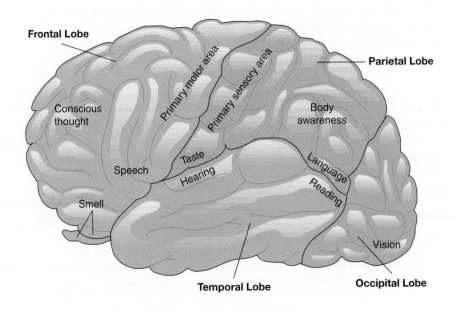

FIGURE 14.4 Areas of the Brain Potentially Affected by a Stroke.

TABLE 14.2	Public Health Education Message for Stroke

The National Institute of Neurological Disorders and Stroke (NINDS) developed the *"Stroke strikes fast. You should, too. Call 9-1-1"* message to create a strong sense of urgency and establish a clear, actionable idea—to act quickly, and call 9-1-1 if stroke is suspected. The symptoms are:

- Sudden **NUMBNESS** or weakness of face, arm, or leg, especially on one side of the body
- Sudden **CONFUSION**, trouble speaking, or understanding speech
- Sudden **TROUBLE SEEING** in one or both eyes
- Sudden **TROUBLE WALKING**, dizziness, loss of balance, or coordination
- Sudden **SEVERE HEADACHE** with no known cause

SOURCE: National Institute of Neurological Disorders and Stroke, National Institutes of Health. Know stroke. Online: http://stroke.nih.gov.

Measuring Blood Pressure

Correct blood pressure measurements are essential to diagnosing and treating high blood pressure. When you are preparing for a blood pressure measurement, you should follow the tips listed in TABLE 14.3 . Blood pressure is measured using a **sphygmomanometer**. The sphygmomanometer is attached to a blood pressure cuff. The blood pressure cuff is wrapped around the upper part of your arm, and a stethoscope is placed over the artery just below the cuff (FIGURE 14.5). Air is pumped into the cuff until pressure stops the flow of blood through the artery. The pressure in the cuff is gradually reduced as the air is released. The measure of the blood's pressure as it starts flowing through the vessel again is known as systolic pressure; this is the higher of the two numbers stated in a blood pressure reading. The air continues to be released from the cuff until no pulse is audible, indicating that the blood is flowing normally through the artery; this is known as the diastolic pressure. The measures are expressed in units of millimeters of mercury and are recorded as the systolic pressure over the diastolic pressure, for example, 110/70.

Sphygmomanometer Instrument that measures blood pressure.

Classification of Blood Pressure

TABLE 14.4 provides a classification of blood pressure for adults ages 18 and older. The classification is based on the average of two or more properly measured, seated blood pressure readings on each of two or more office visits. An acceptable blood pressure for an adult is lower than 120/80. Adult blood pressure levels between 120 and 139 systolic or 80 and 89 diastolic are classified as "prehypertensive." This means the blood pressure is elevated above normal but not to the level considered to be hypertensive. Having this condition puts you at higher risk for developing hypertension, is considered unsafe, and calls for lifestyle changes and

TABLE 14.3	Tips for Having Your Blood Pressure Taken

- Don't drink coffee or smoke cigarettes 30 minutes before having your blood pressure measured.
- Before the test, sit for 5 minutes with your back supported and your feet flat on the ground. Rest your arm on a table at the level of your heart.
- Wear short sleeves so your arm is exposed.
- Go to the bathroom prior to the reading. A full bladder can change your blood pressure reading.
- Get two readings—taken at least 2 minutes apart—and average the results.
- Ask the doctor or nurse to tell you the blood pressure reading in numbers.

SOURCE: National Heart, Lung, and Blood Institute. Your guide to lowering high blood pressure. Online: http://www.nhlbi.nih.gov/hbp/index.html.

FIGURE 14.5 **Measuring Blood Pressure.** The inflatable cuff, which is wrapped around the upper arm, squeezes the brachial artery tightly so blood cannot pass. The systolic reading is taken when turbulent blood sounds can first be heard in this artery, indicating the strength of the pressure against the artery wall when the ventricle contracts and can push the blood through the constricted artery. If the blood pressure is high, it will force the blood vessel to open sooner (at a higher reading) than if the blood pressure is low. The diastolic reading is taken when the turbulent blood sounds stop, indicating the strength of the pressure against the artery wall when the ventricle relaxes, the artery is no longer constricted, and the blood is flowing freely.

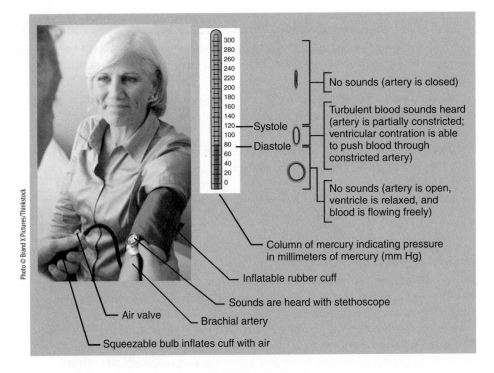

Photo © Brand X Pictures/Thinkstock

Primary hypertension
Hypertension in which the cause is unknown.

Secondary hypertension
Hypertension caused by a specific disorder of a particular organ or blood vessel.

regular monitoring. If your blood pressure level is above 140 systolic or 90 diastolic, you are classified as having HBP or being hypertensive.

The causes of HBP vary. Two forms of high blood pressure have been described: primary (or essential) hypertension, and secondary hypertension. **Primary hypertension** accounts for between 90 and 95 percent of all cases. Although the cause of primary hypertension is not known, it tends to develop gradually over the years. Certain traits, conditions, or habits may raise your risk for HBP. These include older age, race (blacks), overweight or obesity, gender, unhealthy lifestyle habits, genetics, a family history of HBP, chronic stress, and having prehypertension.

Secondary hypertension means that the hypertension is secondary to (caused by) a specific disorder of a particular organ or blood vessel, such as the kidney, adrenal gland, or aortic artery. Five to 10 percent of high blood pressure cases are caused by an underlying condition. Secondary hypertension may appear suddenly and cause higher blood pressure than does primary hypertension.

TABLE 14.4	Categories for Blood Pressure Levels in Adults* (measured in millimeters of mercury)		
	Blood Pressure Level (mm Hg)		
Category	Systolic (top number)		Diastolic (bottom number)
Normal	Less than 120	and	Less than 80
Prehypertension	120–139	or	80–89
High blood pressure			
• Stage 1	140–159	or	90–99
• Stage 2	160 or higher	or	100 or higher

*For those not taking medicine for high blood pressure and not having a short-term illness. These categories are from the National High Blood Pressure Education Program. Adults are those age 18 years and older.

SOURCE: Modified from National Heart, Lung, and Blood Institute. (2005). What is high blood pressure? Online: http://www.nhlbi.nih.gov/hbp/detect/categ.htm.

Although HBP usually cannot be cured, in most cases it can be prevented or controlled. You can do several things to keep your blood pressure healthy. These include maintaining a healthy weight, getting regular physical activity, following a nutritious diet, monitoring salt intake, not smoking, drinking alcoholic beverages only in moderation, and managing stress. If you develop HBP, you can help lower your blood pressure by making healthy changes in your lifestyle. If lifestyle changes don't work, you may also need to take prescribed medication pills. When your blood pressure is brought under control, you might be required to continue your medication to keep your blood pressure in check. Either way, you need to control your high blood pressure throughout your life.

Heart Failure

Heart failure, also called congestive heart failure (CHF), is a life-threatening condition in which the heart's function as a pump to deliver oxygen-rich blood to the body is inadequate to meet the body's needs. CHF happens when the heart's weak pumping action causes a buildup or "backup" of fluid called congestion in your lungs, legs, ankles, and other body tissues. This can result from previous heart attacks, coronary artery disease, high blood pressure, arrhythmia (irregular heartbeat), heart valve disease (from rheumatic fever or other causes), cardiomyopathy (disease of the heart muscle), congenital heart defects (heart defects at birth), and alcohol and drug abuse.

Heart failure develops slowly over time as the pumping of the heart grows weaker. A person may go years without symptoms. It is also a very common condition. Nearly 6 million people in the United States have heart failure, and it results in about 300,000 deaths annually (refer to Figure 14.1). Generally, CHF is treatable using many different therapies that ease the workload on the heart, including lifestyle changes, medicines, and surgery.

Diseases of the Arteries

Peripheral arterial disease (PAD) and *peripheral vascular disease (PVD)* are terms used to describe a blood vessel disease that affects any of the blood vessels outside of the heart and brain. The three most common examples of PAD are carotid artery disease (which affects arteries in the neck leading to the brain), lower extremity arterial disease (which affects arteries of the legs), and renovascular disease (which affects the arteries of the kidney). The most common cause of PAD is atherosclerosis. Between 8 and 12 million Americans have PAD.

Cardiovascular Disease Risk Factors

Extensive epidemiological research identifies a number of factors that increase your risk of developing the various types of CVD. They are classified as either major risk factors or contributing risk factors based on their strength of association with CVD. Major risk factors are those that research shows drastically increase risk of CVD. Contributing factors are related to CVD, but to a much lesser extent than major risk factors are. The more risk factors you have, the greater your chance of developing CVD. Additionally, the stronger the association of each risk factor, the greater the risk of developing CVD.

The American Heart Association identifies nine major risk factors and three contributing risk factors for CVD. Six major risk factors, along with three contributing risk factors, can be controlled by lifestyle changes or treated by medications. They include cigarette smoking, physical inactivity, high blood fats, high blood pressure, being overweight/obese, diabetes mellitus, stress, alcohol use, and diet. Three major risk factors that cannot be changed are age, sex, and heredity.

> **Heart failure** A life-threatening condition in which the heart's function as a pump to deliver oxygen-rich blood to the body is inadequate to meet the body's needs. Also called congestive heart failure.
>
> **Peripheral arterial disease (PAD)** A blood vessel disease that affects any of the blood vessels outside of the heart and brain.

The six major modifiable CVD risk factors are cigarette smoking, physical inactivity, high blood fats, high blood pressure, being overweight/obese, and diabetes mellitus.

Risk Factors You Can Change

Cigarette Smoking

Cigarette smoking is directly associated with 20 percent of all deaths from CVD. It contributes to cardiovascular disease in several ways. Cigarette smokers tend to have increased levels of low-density lipoprotein cholesterol (LDL-C) and reduced levels of high-density lipoprotein cholesterol (HDL-C). Additionally, blood clotting increases. Together, these factors contribute to a buildup of plaque in the arteries. Cigarette smoking also impairs lung function, reducing stamina and the ability to tolerate exercise. The carbon monoxide in smoke depletes the oxygen available to the heart, lungs, and other tissues and forces the heart to work harder to supply sufficient oxygen to the body. Nicotine, the psychoactive stimulant in tobacco, accelerates the heart rate and constricts arteries, leading to an increase in blood pressure. The heart must pump harder to compensate, but this additional workload requires more oxygen, which is unavailable because of the presence of carbon monoxide. The great news is that quitting smoking, regardless of how long or much you have smoked, decreases your risk of CVD rapidly.

Physical Inactivity

Lack of physical activity has clearly been shown to be a major risk factor for cardiovascular disease. Regular aerobic exercise strengthens the heart muscle and blood vessels, improving the ability of the cardiovascular system to transfer blood and oxygen to all parts of the body efficiently. In addition to its direct effect on the heart and blood circulation, regular exercise decreases other CVD risk factors in the following ways:

- Improves blood lipid profile by decreasing LDL-C and increasing HDL-C
- Lowers blood pressure by maintaining elasticity of the arteries
- Helps with weight loss by decreasing body fat percentage
- Increases insulin sensitivity to cell receptor sites and treats insulin resistance, a condition that increases the chance of developing type 2 diabetes and CVD
- Controls stress

Many of the chronic diseases of the cardiovascular system result from physical inactivity. A more comprehensive list of the primary and secondary benefits of the biological mechanisms by which exercise contributes to preventing CHD are listed in TABLE 14.5 .

High Blood Fats

The levels of several types of fat found in the blood are considered a primary risk factor for CVD. These fatty substances include cholesterol and triglycerides. The medical term for elevated levels of fats (lipids) in the blood is **hyperlipidemia**.

Cholesterol is a fatty waxlike substance in your blood, naturally manufactured by the liver or consumed in certain foods. It is needed for your body to function normally, and the liver makes enough for your body's needs. The problem is that when there is too much cholesterol in your blood—because of diet and the rate at which cholesterol is processed by the liver—it can build up in the walls of the arteries and form plaque. Cholesterol can't dissolve in the blood and therefore needs some assistance to travel throughout the bloodstream. It has to be transported to and from the cells by carriers called **lipoproteins** (which are made up of proteins and fats). Two major classes of lipoproteins exist: **low-density lipoprotein (LDL)** and **high-density lipoprotein (HDL)**.

Low-density lipoprotein, or LDL, is known as "bad" cholesterol because it plays a role in the development of plaque in the arteries. When there is too much LDL

Hyperlipidemia The medical term for elevated levels of fats (lipids) in the blood.

Cholesterol Fatty waxlike substance in your blood, naturally manufactured by the liver or consumed in certain foods and needed by the body to function normally.

Lipoprotein A protein that transports fat through the bloodstream.

Low-density lipoprotein (LDL) Known as "bad" cholesterol because it plays a role in the development of plaque in the arteries.

High-density lipoprotein (HDL) Known as "good" cholesterol because it gives some protection against atherosclerosis by carrying excess cholesterol back to the liver for processing where it can be removed from the body.

TABLE 14.5	Biological Mechanisms by Which Exercise May Contribute to the Primary and Secondary Prevention of Coronary Heart Disease

Maintain or increase myocardial oxygen supply

- Delay progression of coronary atherosclerosis (possible)
- Improve lipoprotein profile (increase HDL-C/LDL-C ratio, decrease triglycerides) (probable)
- Improve carbohydrate metabolism (increase insulin sensitivity) (probable)
- Decrease platelet aggregation and increase fibrinolysis (probable)
- Decrease adiposity (usually)
- Increase coronary collateral vascularization (unlikely)
- Increase epicardial artery diameter (possible)
- Increase coronary blood flow (myocardial perfusion) or distribution (possible)

Decrease myocardial work and oxygen demand

- Decrease heart rate at rest and submaximal exercise (usually)
- Decrease systolic and mean systemic arterial pressure during submaximal exercise (usually) and at rest (usually)
- Decrease cardiac output during submaximal exercise (probable)
- Decrease circulating plasma catecholamine levels (decrease sympathetic tone) at rest (probable) and at submaximal exercise (usually)

Increase myocardial function

- Increase stroke volume at rest and in submaximal and maximal exercise (likely)
- Increase ejection fraction at rest and during exercise (likely)
- Increase intrinsic myocardial contractility (possible)
- Increase myocardial function resulting from decreased "afterload" (probable)
- Increase myocardial hypertrophy (probable); but this may not reduce CHD risk

Increase electrical stability of myocardium

- Decrease regional ischemia or at submaximal exercise (possible)
- Decrease catecholamines in myocardium at rest (possible) and at submaximal exercise (probable)
- Increase ventricular fibrillation threshold due to reduction of cyclic AMP (possible)

Likelihood that effect will occur for an individual participating in endurance-type training—for 16 weeks or longer, at 65 to 80 percent of functional capacity, for 25 min or longer per session (300 kcal), for three or more sessions per week—ranges from unlikely, possible, likely, probable, to usually.

HDL-C = high-density lipoprotein cholesterol; LDL-C = low-density lipoprotein cholesterol; CHD = coronary heart disease; AMP = adenosine monophosphate.

SOURCE: Haskell, W.L. (1995). Physical activity in the prevention and management of coronary heart disease. *Physical Activity and Fitness Research Digest* 2(1):8–9. President's Council on Physical Fitness and Sports, Department of Health and Human Services.

circulating in the blood, it can begin to build up on the artery walls, which can lead to atherosclerosis. Therefore, you want to keep your LDL low. High-density lipoprotein, or HDL, is known as "good" cholesterol because it gives some protection against atherosclerosis. It appears to scour the walls of blood vessels, cleaning out excess cholesterol. It then carries excess cholesterol back to the liver for processing where the cholesterol can be removed from the body. Therefore, you want your HDL to be high. To remember the difference, think of the *H* in HDL as standing for "healthy" cholesterol, and the *L* in LDL as standing for "lethal."

Triglycerides, another form of fat present in the blood, also appear to promote atherosclerosis in association with high levels of cholesterol. Elevated triglycerides can be the result of overweight/obesity, physical inactivity, cigarette smoking, excess alcohol consumption, and a diet very high in carbohydrates (60 percent of calories or higher).

You can't feel or see high cholesterol or high triglycerides. The only way to know for sure is by having a blood lipid profile test. A blood lipid profile test measures several different forms of cholesterol and triglycerides. It is recommended that healthy adults with no other risk factors for heart disease be tested with a fasting lipid profile once every 5 years. If you have other risk factors or have had a high cholesterol level in the past, you should be tested more regularly. It is important that you know your numbers. TABLE 14.6 provides the classifications for total cholesterol, LDL, HDL, and triglycerides.

TABLE 14.6	Classification of Total, LDL, and HDL Cholesterol (mg/dL) and Recommended Levels for Adults
Total Cholesterol	
< 200	Desirable
200–239	Borderline high
≥ 240	High
LDL Cholesterol	
< 100	Optimal
100–129	Near optimal/above optimal
130–159	Borderline high
160–189	High
≥ 190	Very high
HDL Cholesterol	
< 40	Low
≥ 60	High
Triglycerides	
< 150	Normal
150–199	Borderline high
200–499	High
≥ 500	Very high

SOURCE: National Heart, Lung, and Blood Institute. (2005). *Third Report of the Expert Panel on Detection, Evaluation, and Treatment of High Blood Cholesterol in Adults* (NIH Publication No. 05-3290). Online: http://www.nhlbi.nih.gov/health/public/heart/chol/wyntk.htm.

If you are wondering how to lower blood fats, there is a group of therapeutic lifestyle changes (TLCs) recommendations put forth by the National Cholesterol Education Program (NCEP) for living a heart-healthy lifestyle (National Heart, Lung, and Blood Institute [NHLBI], 2004). The lifestyle changes include modifying your diet (i.e., eating low amounts of saturated fat and cholesterol [TLC Diet]), participating in regular physical activity, and managing your weight. The TLC Diet guidelines include eating according to the following guidelines:

- Less than 7 percent of the day's total calories come from saturated fat.
- Twenty-five to 35 percent of the day's total calories come from fat.
- Consume less than 200 milligrams of dietary cholesterol a day.
- Limit sodium intake to 2400 milligrams a day.
- Consume just enough calories to achieve or maintain a healthy weight and reduce your blood cholesterol level.

High Blood Pressure

Having uncontrolled high blood pressure, or hypertension, is a major risk factor for many forms of CVD but is also a type of CVD. High blood pressure has far-reaching and serious health consequences related to CVD. For one thing, it accelerates the development of atherosclerosis in blood vessels, which in turn makes high blood pressure worse and further increases the risk of other cardiovascular complications. High blood pressure forces your heart to work harder than normal, making it more susceptible to a number of injuries. Fortunately, HBP also is one of the most preventable and treatable types of cardiovascular disease.

You can take several steps to keep your blood pressure healthy (TABLE 14.7). These steps include maintaining a healthy weight; being physically active; following a healthy eating plan that emphasizes fruits, vegetables, and low-fat dairy foods; choosing and preparing foods with less salt and sodium; and, if you drink alcoholic

TABLE 14.7	Nine Things You Can Do to Control Blood Pressure

1. *Lose weight if you are overweight and maintain a healthy weight.* Limit portion sizes, especially of high calorie foods, and try to eat only as many calories as you burn each day—or less if you want to lose weight.

2. *Eat heart healthfully.* Follow an eating plan that emphasizes fruits, vegetables, and low-fat dairy products and is moderate in total fat and low in saturated fat and cholesterol.

3. *Reduce salt and sodium intake.* Read food labels to choose canned, processed, and convenience foods that are lower in sodium. Limit sodium intake to no more than 2400 mg, or about 1 teaspoon's worth, of salt each day. Avoid fast foods that are high in salt and sodium.

4. *If you drink alcoholic beverages, do so in moderation.* For men, that means a maximum of 2 drinks a day, for women, a maximum of 1.

5. *Become more physically active.* Work up to at least 30 minutes of a moderate-level activity, such as brisk walking or bicycling, each day. If you don't have 30 minutes, try to find 2 15-minute periods or even 3 10-minute periods for physical activity.

6. *Quit smoking.* Smoking increases your chances of developing a stroke, heart disease, peripheral arterial disease, and several forms of cancer.

7. *If you are pregnant, make sure you are under a doctor's care.* High blood pressure is a major cause of complications in pregnancy.

8. *Talk with your health care professional.* Ask what your blood pressure numbers are and what they mean.

9. *Take medication as prescribed.* If you need medication, make sure you understand what it's for and how and when to take it and then take it as your doctor recommends.

SOURCE: National Heart, Lung, and Blood Institute, National High Blood Pressure Education Program. Your guide to lowering high blood pressure. Online: http://www.nhlbi.nih.gov/hbp/index.html.

beverages, drinking in moderation (NHLBI, 2005). If you develop high blood pressure, your doctor may prescribe medications along with the lifestyle steps noted previously to help bring it under control (CDC, 2011b).

Being Overweight/Obese

Evidence continues to accumulate that obesity is associated with significant morbidity and mortality and, in particular, that it is an independent risk factor for cardiovascular disease. More specifically, individuals with disproportionate amounts of excess fat located primarily around the abdomen (visceral adiposity) are at significantly greater risk for CVD. Abdominal obesity is one of the primary clinical signs of **metabolic syndrome**, a term used to describe a cluster of specific disorders that, when they occur together, may significantly increase a person's risk of developing cardiovascular disease or type 2 diabetes.

Metabolic syndrome is not a disease or a disorder per se, but rather a term used to alert you and your health care provider to a group of important warning signs that something may be metabolically wrong and needs to be addressed. According to the National Cholesterol Education Program/Adult Treatment Panel III (NHLBI, 2004), you have metabolic syndrome if you have at least three of the following five abnormalities and/or medical conditions:

> **Metabolic syndrome** Term used to alert you and your health care provider to a group of important warning signs that something may be metabolically wrong and needs to be addressed. Also called insulin resistance.

- Elevated waist circumference (excessive fat tissue in and around the abdomen):
  - Men: > 40 inches
  - Women: > 35 inches
- Elevated triglycerides:
  - Men and women: > 150 mg/dL, or taking medication for elevated triglyceride levels
- Reduced HDL cholesterol or taking medication to treat low HDL cholesterol:
  - Men: < 40 mg/dL
  - Women: < 50 mg/dL
- Elevated blood pressure, or taking medication for elevated blood pressure levels:
  - Men and women: > 130/85 mmHg

- Elevated fasting glucose (signifying insulin resistance, the inability of the body to utilize glucose efficiently):
  - Men and women: > 100 mg/dL, or taking medication for elevated blood glucose levels

Considered individually, each factor may not seem particularly serious. When you put them together, however, health risks for type 2 diabetes rise dramatically. All of the factors that comprise metabolic syndrome are interrelated. However, the dominant underlying risk factor for this syndrome appears to be abdominal obesity because it is a risk for high triglyceride levels, low HDL cholesterol, high blood pressure, and **insulin resistance**. Insulin resistance is a generalized metabolic disorder in which the body can't use insulin efficiently. This is why metabolic syndrome is also called insulin resistance syndrome. Insulin resistance is very hard to measure, but it is known to be a dangerous precursor to type 2 diabetes.

Insulin resistance is when the body's cells no longer respond as they should to insulin (a hormone that helps move blood sugar into cells where it is used), so the body compensates by secreting even more insulin. Most people with insulin resistance secrete enough insulin to maintain nondiabetic glucose levels. Eventually, some of them do develop type 2 diabetes, but damage is already occurring long before diabetes appears. Whether or not they develop diabetes, the majority of people with insulin resistance are at significantly increased risk for heart attack, stroke, and other cardiovascular diseases. Currently, more than one in three adults meets the criteria for metabolic syndrome (Mozumda & Liguori, 2011).

In summary, insulin resistance occurs when insulin is unable to do its job of transferring sugars from the blood stream into the muscle and fat cells. Glucose buildup in your blood stream usually follows, gradually leads to type 2 diabetes, and increases your risk of cardiovascular disease. Therefore, insulin resistance is a medical condition waiting to explode; it will always have a measured impact of severity. Everyone who has type 2 diabetes has resistance to insulin, although everyone who has resistance to insulin does not have diabetes—yet.

A clinical diagnosis of the metabolic syndrome is not sufficient, by itself, to assess the risk of CVD. To evaluate and manage global CVD risk in clinical practice properly, it is important to take into account the risk associated with traditional risk factors, as well as the potential additional contribution of abdominal obesity/insulin resistance and related complications. This global risk is referred to as cardiometabolic risk.

Cardiometabolic risk is a measure of your risk for developing diabetes and CVD and is a good gauge of overall health (American Diabetes Association [ADA], 2012). Cardiometabolic risk combines classical risk factors (smoking, elevated cholesterol, hypertension, and diabetes) with emerging markers such as intra-abdominal obesity and insulin resistance.

Diabetes Mellitus

Having uncontrolled diabetes or pre-diabetes dramatically raises your risk for many cardiovascular diseases. Adults with diabetes are two to four times more likely to have heart disease or suffer a stroke. In fact, CVD is the leading cause of death among diabetic patients: two out of every three people with diabetes die from heart disease or stroke. Making this link between diabetes and heart disease and stroke is essential because the rates of diabetes continue to rise at alarming speeds; the number of Americans with diabetes has tripled in the last 30 years (CDC, 2012b).

In 2011, nearly 26 million children and adults in the United States (1 in 12 or 8.3 percent of the country's population) had diabetes (CDC, 2012a). As bad as these numbers are, they are not the worst part of this alarming statistic. Approximately one-fourth of these people are unaware they have this chronic and disabling disease.

Insulin resistance Generalized metabolic disorder in which the body can't use insulin efficiently.

Cardiometabolic risk Measure of your risk for developing diabetes and CVD and a good gauge of overall health.

In addition, another 79 million adults (35 percent) have **pre-diabetes**, a condition in which individuals have blood glucose or A1c levels higher than normal but not high enough to be classified as diabetes (CDC, 2012a). Pre-diabetes is a condition that increases the risk of developing type 2 diabetes as well as heart disease and stroke. The good news is that studies have shown that people with pre-diabetes who lose weight and increase their physical activity can prevent or delay type 2 diabetes and, in some cases, return their blood glucose levels to normal.

Diabetes is a group of diseases marked by high levels of blood glucose resulting from defects in insulin production, insulin action, or both. **Insulin**, a hormone secreted by the pancreas, is needed by muscle, fat, and the liver to metabolize glucose. Diabetes is diagnosed by identifying high levels of blood glucose (hyperglycemia). Not all people who have insulin-regulating difficulties have clinical diabetes. Diabetes is also related to conditions in which glucose regulation is impaired. In pre-diabetes, impaired glucose tolerance (IGT), impaired fasting glucose (IFG), or both exist. With IFG, blood sugar levels are elevated after an overnight fast but not to levels high enough to be classified as clinical diabetes. With IGT, blood glucose levels are elevated after a glucose tolerance test but, again, not at levels high enough to be classified as clinical diabetes.

There are two main types of full-blown clinical diabetes: type 1 and type 2. **Type 1 diabetes**, once known as juvenile diabetes or insulin-dependent diabetes, is a chronic (lifelong) disease in which the pancreas produces little or no insulin to control blood sugar levels properly. This form of diabetes is the result of an autoimmune disease that occurs when the insulin-producing beta cells in the pancreas are gradually destroyed and eventually fail to produce insulin. Although type 1 diabetes develops most often in children and young adults, the disease can be diagnosed at any age. Type 1 diabetes has no cure, though it can be managed. With proper treatment, people who have type 1 diabetes can expect to live longer and healthy lives. Type 1 diabetes accounts for between 5 percent and 10 percent of all diagnosed diabetes in the United States.

Type 2 diabetes, or what was once known as adult-onset or non-insulin-dependent diabetes, accounts for 90 to 95 percent of all diagnosed cases of diabetes. The increase in cases of type 2 diabetes is largely a result of the epidemic of obesity, a major risk factor for developing this type of diabetes (about 80 percent of people with type 2 diabetes are overweight). The connection is so strong that some health experts have coined the term "diabesity."

Type 2 diabetes allows for sufficient production of insulin, but the body's cells have become resistant to it. As mentioned earlier, this can lead to a condition known as insulin resistance, when body cells become less responsive to insulin. Although your genes, increasing age, and certain medications can all contribute to the development of insulin resistance, being overweight (specifically abdominal obesity) and not getting enough exercise are the major causes.

Fortunately, it is possible to prevent and delay the onset of type 2 diabetes by participating in a regular physical activity program and maintaining a healthy weight. The positive biological mechanism of physical activity in diabetes prevention comes from its role in improving insulin sensitivity and reducing the incidence of being overweight or obese. With improved insulin sensitivity, cells in the body do not require as much insulin to regulate blood sugar levels. Physical activity also increases energy expenditure, thereby reducing the likelihood of a positive energy balance occurring with resultant weight gain. However, physical activity has a beneficial effect on insulin sensitivity in normal as well as insulin-resistant populations, even if you do not lose weight. Therefore, you can conclude that physical training is an important, if not essential, factor in the treatment and prevention of insulin insensitivity.

Many people with type 2 diabetes can control their blood glucose levels by following a healthy diet (plenty of fruits, vegetables, whole grains) and exercise

Pre-diabetes Condition in which your blood sugar level is higher than normal but not high enough to be classified as type 2 diabetes.

Diabetes Group of diseases marked by high levels of blood glucose resulting from defects in insulin production, insulin action, or both.

Insulin A hormone secreted by the pancreas that is needed by muscle, fat, and the liver to metabolize glucose.

Type 1 diabetes A chronic (lifelong) disease in which the pancreas produces little or no insulin to control blood sugar levels properly.

Type 2 diabetes A medical condition in which the body produces sufficient insulin, but the body's cells have become resistant to it.

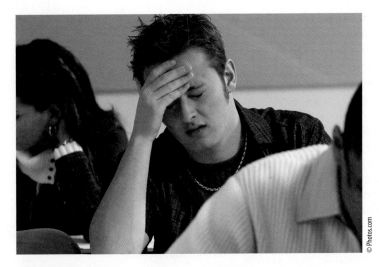

FIGURE 14.6 **Effect of Stress.** Chronic stress may contribute to CVD.

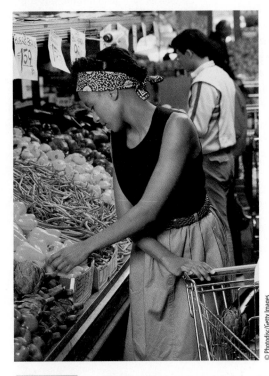

FIGURE 14.7 **A Healthy Diet.** A diet rich in fruits and vegetables may decrease the risk of CVD.

The three major unmodifiable CVD risk factors are increasing age, male gender, and heredity/race.

program, losing excess weight, and taking any diabetes medications as recommended. Whereas some people who have type 2 diabetes can manage their blood sugar with diet and exercise alone, many need diabetes medications or insulin therapy.

Contributing CVD Factors

Chronic Stress

Stress is a given in our society today. The ordinary events at home, on the job, and even at leisure can trigger stress responses as we try to maintain ourselves in an increasingly complex set of circumstances. We may not be able to get away from stress, but we can learn to deal with it. Research has not yet revealed exactly how stress affects the heart, but there appears to be a relationship between the occurrence of a heart attack, for instance, and a person's stress level, risky behaviors (e.g., cigarette smoking, diet), and socioeconomic status (**FIGURE 14.6**). For instance, you may develop high blood pressure as a result of stress, or you may respond to stress by overeating or smoking.

Alcohol Use

Drinking too much alcohol can raise blood pressure, contribute to high levels of triglycerides in the blood, and lead to obesity. Each is associated with increased risk for cardiovascular disease.

Diet and Nutrition

An overall healthy diet can help lower blood pressure and cholesterol levels, prevent obesity, reduce the likelihood of diabetes, and limit all contributing factors to CVD. A healthy diet includes eating plenty of fruits and vegetables, lowering or cutting out added salt or sodium, and eating less saturated fat and cholesterol (**FIGURE 14.7**).

Risk Factors You Cannot Change

Increasing Age

The risk of CVD increases as we get older. In fact, about four of every five deaths caused by heart disease occur in people older than 65 years. As we age, our hearts tend not to work as efficiently. The heart's walls may thicken and arteries may narrow and harden, making the heart less able to pump blood to the muscles of the body. Because of these changes, the risk of developing cardiovascular disease increases with age. However, you can significantly slow down the aging process by choosing a heart-smart lifestyle.

Male Sex

Overall, men are more likely than women are to develop CVD. Current theory speculates that male hormones (androgens) increase risk, whereas female hormones (estrogens) protect against atherosclerosis. But the difference in risk narrows after women reach menopause. Menopause brings changes in the level of fats in a woman's blood. LDL cholesterol appears to increase while HDL decreases in postmenopausal women as a direct result of estrogen deficiency. Elevated LDL and lowered

HDL increase the progression of atherosclerosis. After the age of 65, the risk of heart disease is about the same between the sexes when other risk factors are similar.

Heredity and Race

There appears to be a hereditary tendency toward heart disease and atherosclerosis. For example, if your parents or siblings had a heart or circulatory problem before age 55, then you are at greater risk for heart disease than is someone who does not have that family history. Medical conditions that increase risk (including high blood pressure, diabetes, and obesity) also may be passed from one generation to another.

Race/ethnicity is also a consideration. CVD risk is higher among African Americans, Mexican Americans, American Indians, native Hawaiians, and some Asian Americans compared to Caucasians. Some of this difference is explained by higher rates of obesity and diabetes in certain groups. African Americans are likely to develop high blood pressure more than any other racial or ethnic group, and often to a greater extent, though scientists have yet to determine the exact reason why this is true. Again, despite your family history, you can significantly reduce your hereditary risk for CVD by choosing a heart-smart lifestyle.

In summary, you can do a lot to protect your cardiovascular system and lower your risk of developing cardiovascular disease. You now understand that many of the risk factors for CVD are under your control. By taking simple small steps in your life and knowing your numbers, you can prevent CVD and live a healthier life.

Physical Activity and Health Connection

Lack of physical activity is clearly shown to be a major risk factor for cardiovascular disease. Conversely, participation in regular physical activity helps to strengthen the function of all components of your cardiovascular system. This is important not only in terms of cardiovascular efficiency, but also in terms of disease protection. In addition to its direct effect on the heart and blood circulation, regular exercise decreases other major CVD risk factors: it improves your blood lipid profile by decreasing LDL-C and increasing HDL-C; it lowers blood pressure by maintaining elasticity of the arteries; it helps with weight loss by decreasing body fat percentage; it increases insulin sensitivity to cell receptor sites and treats insulin resistance; and it helps control stress.

concept connections

1 **Cardiovascular disease is a group of different illnesses that affect your heart and blood vessels.** In fact, some types of CVD can even cause other types of CVD. One in three Americans (more than 105 million) has one or more forms of diagnosable heart or blood vessel disease. CVD—the leading cause of death in the United States—accounts for more than one-third of all deaths.

2 **Atherosclerosis is the main underlying disease responsible for CVD morbidity and mortality.** Atherosclerosis is a slow, progressive disease that typically starts in early adulthood. As we get older, arterial plaque can build up and can eventually clog our arteries, making them stiff and inflexible. It can affect any artery in the body, including arteries in the heart, brain, arms, legs, and pelvis. As a result, different diseases may develop based on which arteries are affected.

3 **Coronary heart disease is most commonly the result of atherosclerosis narrowing the two coronary arteries (the ones that supply the muscles of the heart).** When your coronary arteries are narrowed or blocked, oxygen-rich blood can't reach your heart muscle. As less blood reaches the heart, it can't function normally, and this may cause anything from chest pain to a fatal heart attack. Based on current estimates, one in two men and one in three women will eventually develop CHD at some point in their lives.

4 **Stroke occurs when vital oxygen-rich blood flow to the brain fails.** Deprived of its blood supply, even for a few minutes, the affected parts of the brain may be damaged or destroyed, leading to a rapid loss of brain functions. Stroke is the second leading cause of CVD death and the third leading cause of death in the United States.

5 **High blood pressure is the third leading cause of death for CVD.** HBP affects about 1 in 3 adults, or 68 million people, in the United States, but because there are no symptoms, more than 1 in 5 don't know they have it. Furthermore, nearly 3 in 10 adults, or 60 million people, fall into the category of prehypertension—a blood pressure elevated above normal but not to the level considered to be hypertensive. Once elevated blood pressure occurs, it usually lasts a lifetime. If uncontrolled, it can lead to many serious health problems, including heart attack and stroke, congestive heart failure, peripheral vascular disease, kidney damage, and blindness.

6 **The six major modifiable CVD risk factors are cigarette smoking, physical inactivity, high blood fats, high blood pressure, being overweight/obese, and diabetes mellitus.** There is a lot you can do to protect your cardiovascular system and lower your risk of developing cardiovascular disease. By taking simple small steps in your life and knowing your numbers, you can prevent CVD and live a healthier life.

7 **The three major unmodifiable CVD risk factors are increasing age, male sex, and heredity/race.** The risk of CVD increases as we get older, men are more likely than are women to develop CVD, and there appears to be a hereditary tendency toward heart disease and atherosclerosis.

Terms

Angina pectoris, 314
Arteriosclerosis, 314
Atherosclerosis, 313
Blood clot, 314
Blood pressure, 316
Cardiometabolic risk, 324
Cardiovascular disease
 (CVD), 312
Cerebral hemorrhage, 315
Cholesterol, 320
Coagulation, 314
Coronary heart disease
 (CHD), 314
Diabetes, 325
Diastolic pressure, 316

Fibrous plaque, 313
Heart failure, 319
Hemorrhage strokes, 315
High blood pressure (HBP), 316
High-density lipoprotein
 (HDL), 320
Hyperlipidemia, 320
Insulin, 325
Insulin resistance, 324
Ischemia, 314
Ischemic strokes, 315
Lipoprotein, 320
Low-density lipoprotein
 (LDL), 320

Metabolic syndrome, 323
Myocardial infarction, 314
Peripheral arterial disease
 (PAD), 319
Pre-diabetes, 325
Prehypertension, 316
Primary hypertension, 318
Secondary hypertension, 318
Sphygmomanometer, 317
Stroke, 314
Subarachnoid hemorrhage, 315
Systolic pressure, 316
Type 1 diabetes, 325
Type 2 diabetes, 325

making the connection

Sky has learned that there are nine major risk factors and three contributing risk factors for cardiovascular disease (CVD). Six major risk factors, along with three contributing risk factors, can be controlled by lifestyle changes or treated by medications. They are cigarette smoking, physical inactivity, high blood fats, high blood pressure, obesity, diabetes mellitus, stress, alcohol use, and diet. Three major risk factors that cannot be changed are age, sex, and heredity. Although Sky can't completely control every risk factor, there are many that he can control. The internal satisfaction of knowing that there is much he can do to reduce his risk of developing cardiovascular disease is a huge relief.

Critical Thinking

1. Make a list of all six major modifiable risk factors that increase your chance of getting CVD. Which risk factors pertain to you? How can you modify or change any of these risk factors?

2. A risk factor of cardiovascular disease is family history. Family history of CVD does not guarantee that you will get the disease; neither does it cancel out the importance of a healthy lifestyle. A family history of CVD does predispose you to the disease, so it is important for you to determine your family CVD history. Construct a family tree by listing your biological parents, siblings, grandparents (maternal and paternal), and aunts and uncles (maternal and paternal). Next to each name, list the CVD disease and the age at which it was discovered. Your family may be helpful with this activity. After completing your tree, you may want to share it with your family and discuss prevention efforts.

3. Elena is a 21-year-old college student who is very studious. Because her studies are her number one priority (she wants to go to graduate school), Elena finds it difficult to make time to maintain a healthy lifestyle, despite knowing how important it is. Although Elena is not a regular smoker, she has a tendency to smoke when under stress (studying for finals) and frequently eats nonnutritious snacks. Elena was active in high school sports, but she does not seem to find time for sports now that she is in college. As a matter of fact, she has gained about 15 pounds, although she would not be considered overweight. What can you suggest to help Elena reduce her risk of cardiovascular disease?

References

American Diabetes Association. (2012). The Cardio-metabolic Risk Initiative. Online: http://professional.diabetes.org/ResourcesForProfessionals.aspx?cid=60379.

Centers for Disease Control and Prevention. (2011a). High blood pressure: Prevention. Online: http://www.cdc.gov/bloodpressure/prevention.htm.

Centers for Disease Control and Prevention. (2011b). Vital signs: Prevalence, treatment, and control of hypertension—United States, 1999–2002 and 2005–2008. *Morbidity and Mortality Weekly Report* 60(4):103–108.

Centers for Disease Control and Prevention. (2012a). Diabetes data and trends. Online: http://apps.nccd.cdc.gov/DDTSTRS/default.aspx.

Centers for Disease Control and Prevention. (2012b). Heart disease and stroke prevention: Addressing the nation's leading killers. Online: http://www.cdc.gov/nccdphp/publications/AAG/dhdsp.htm.

Miniño, A.M, Murphy, S.L., Xu, J., & Kochanek, K.D. (2011). Deaths: Final data for 2008. *National Vital Statistics Reports* 59(10). Online: http://www.cdc.gov/nchs/data/nvsr/nvsr59/nvsr59_10.pdf.

Mozumda, A., & Liguori, G. (2011). Persistent increase of prevalence of metabolic syndrome among U.S. adults: NHANES III to NHANES 1999–2006. *Diabetes Care* 34(1):216–219.

National Heart, Lung, and Blood Institute, National Institutes of Health. (2004). *Third Report of the Expert Panel on Detection, Evaluation, and Treatment of High Blood Cholesterol in Adults (Adult Treatment Panel III)*. Online: http://www.nhlbi.nih.gov/guidelines/cholesterol/index.htm.

National Heart, Lung, and Blood Institute, National Institutes of Health. (2005). Your guide to lowering high blood pressure. Online: http://www.nhlbi.nih.gov/hbp.

National Institute of Diabetes and Digestive and Kidney Diseases. (2012). Diabetes prevention program. Online: http://diabetes.niddk.nih.gov/dm/pubs/preventionprogram.

National Institute of Neurological Disorders and Stroke, National Institutes of Health. (2012). Brain basics: Preventing strokes. Online: http://www.ninds.nih.gov/disorders/stroke/preventing_stroke.htm.

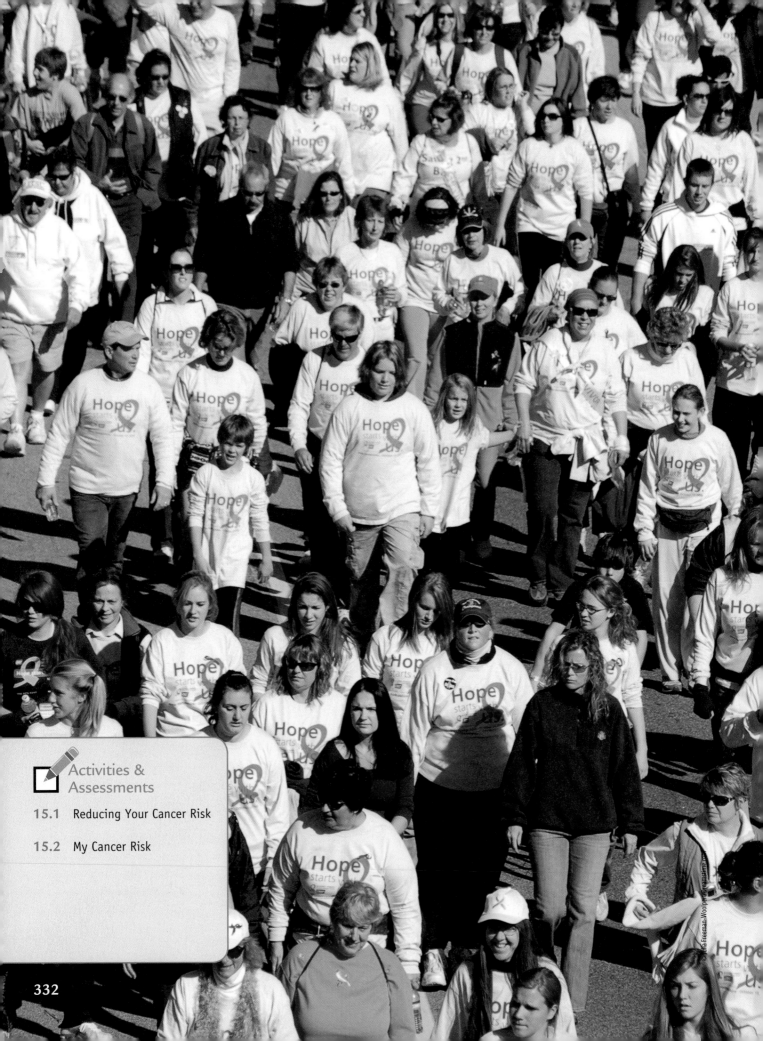

Reducing Your Cancer Risk

15

what's the connection?

Katrina has been smoking cigarettes for the past couple of years. She believes that cigarettes are harmful to her health long term but presently savors the immediate and instant pleasure that comes from smoking. Katrina believes she will be able to quit smoking once she graduates from college. Last week, Katrina's uncle was diagnosed with lung cancer. His diagnosis came just weeks after her mother's first cousin was diagnosed with colon cancer. Katrina is upset and concerned by these diagnoses of cancer. She wonders whether these cancers could have been prevented. Katrina sets out to learn as much as she can about what causes cancer.

concepts

1. Cancer is potentially the most preventable and curable of the life-threatening diseases facing us today.

2. *Cancer* is the term given to a complex group of diseases characterized by the uncontrolled growth and spread of abnormal cells.

3. Health education professionals utilize the concept of prevention based on three types: primary, secondary, and tertiary.

4. Research scientists estimate that between 50 and 75 percent of cancer deaths in the United States are preventable by altering our behaviors.

5. Cancer screening and early detection of cancer can play important roles in cancer survival rates.

6. Currently, two in every three cancer patients survive 5 years or longer after diagnosis and treatment.

go.jblearning.com/kotecki4e
The website for this book is a great source for supplementary physical health information for both students and instructors. Visit **go.jblearning.com/kotecki4e** to find a variety of useful tools for learning, thinking, and teaching.

An ounce of prevention is worth a pound of cure.
—Henry de Bracton

Introduction

Cancer is a chilling word. Almost everyone knows someone who got very ill or died from cancer. The lifetime risk of being diagnosed with cancer is not warming either. One in two men and one in three women will hear the words "you have cancer" in their lifetime. More than 1.6 million Americans will receive news of a cancer diagnosis this year, and more than half a million will die from some form of cancer (American Cancer Society [ACS], 2012b). Cancer is the second most common cause of death in the United States, accounting for nearly one of every four deaths (**FIGURE 15.1**). Despite these grim statistics, the news about cancer is not all dreadful.

Preventing cancer is possible. Dr. John R. Seffrin, CEO of the American Cancer Society, states, "Cancer is potentially the most preventable and curable of the life-threatening diseases facing us today" (Mackay, Jemal, Lee, & Parkin, 2006). This statement is based on tremendous advances in cancer research over the past couple of decades. Scientists now understand that cancer is a continuum that can be interrupted at many stages, from susceptibility to initiation to clinically detectable disease.

Research scientists estimate that between 50 and 75 percent of cancer deaths in the United States are preventable by translating current knowledge related to a few controllable behavioral risk factors for cancer into actual practice (National Cancer Institute [NCI], 2012). More good news is that early detection, diagnosis, and treatment have dramatically improved the survival odds of someone with a cancer diagnosis. Today, more than 2 out of 3 cancer patients (67 percent) survive 5 years or longer after diagnosis and treatment—up considerably from 30 years ago when the number was 1 in 2 (ACS, 2012b). The National Cancer Institute (2012) estimates that an additional 20 to 30 percent of all cancer deaths could be prevented with earlier diagnosis and treatment. More and more Americans are doing the things that prevent cancer, such as not smoking, eating a healthy diet, being physically active, and getting regular screening examinations by a health care professional. That's why, for the first time in many decades, cancer rates are decreasing. The cancer death rate has dropped in the United States nearly 20

Cancer is potentially the most preventable and curable of the life-threatening diseases facing us today.

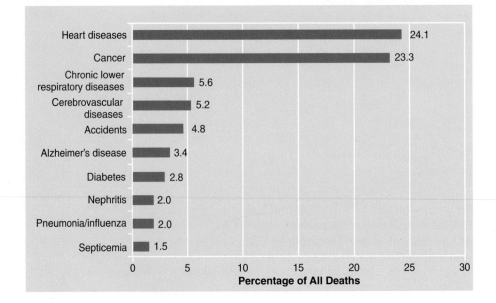

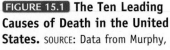
The Ten Leading Causes of Death in the United States. SOURCE: Data from Murphy, S.L., Jiaquan, X., & Kochanek, K.D. (2012). Deaths: Preliminary data for 2010. *National Vital Statistics Reports* 60(4): 1–67.

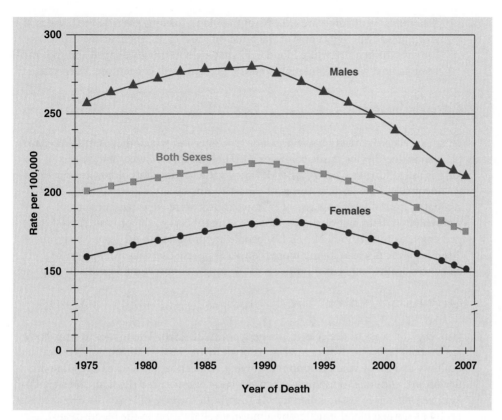

FIGURE 15.2 **Death Rates for All Cancers, 1975–2007.** SOURCE: Reproduced from National Cancer Institute, National Institutes of Health, Department of Health and Human Services. (2011 December). *Cancer Trends Progress Report—2007 Update.* Bethesda, MD: Government Printing Office. Online: http://progressreport.cancer.gov.

percent in recent years, largely because of better prevention and treatment (FIGURE 15.2) (NCI, 2012).

The immediate goal of this chapter is to replace fear with understanding. Only then can the task of practicing cancer prevention and early detection be effectively implemented. Let's begin with defining cancer. You have heard the word *cancer* many times; however, very few people understand the disease and how it develops.

Defining Cancer

Cancer is the term given to a complex group of diseases characterized by the uncontrolled growth and spread of abnormal cells. There are at least one hundred different types of cancer, differing in their cause, type of cell or organ affected, symptoms, and treatment. For example, breast cancers are different from colon cancers, and lung cancers are different from skin cancers. It is possible to divide these numerous cancer diseases into four broad groups on the basis of the type of tissue from which the cancer cells arise. The four major categories are the following:

- *Carcinomas:* Carcinomas are the most common types of cancer and derive from epithelial tissue that lines external and internal body surfaces. Carcinomas of the breast, prostate, lung, and colon are the most common examples. About 80 to 90 percent of all cancers are carcinomas.
- *Sarcomas:* Sarcomas are tumors made up principally of connective tissue cells found in the supporting tissues of the body such as bones (osteosarcoma), muscles (myosarcoma), fat (liposarcoma), and cartilage (chondrosarcoma). About 2 percent of all cancers are sarcomas.
- *Lymphomas:* Lymphomas are cancers that affect cells that play a role in the immune system and primarily represent cells involved in the lymphatic system of the body. About 5 percent of all cancers, the most common being Hodgkin's disease, are lymphomas.

Cancer is the term given to a complex group of diseases characterized by the uncontrolled growth and spread of abnormal cells.

Cancer A complex group of diseases characterized by the uncontrolled growth and spread of abnormal cells.

• *Leukemias:* Leukemias are cancers of the blood-forming parts of the bone marrow, the soft spongy center of the bone. In most cases, the marrow produces too many immature white blood cells that are abnormally shaped and that prohibit normal blood circulation About 4 percent of all cancers are leukemias.

Cancer Statistics

Most cancers are named for the organ or type of cell in which they start—for example, cancer that begins in the colon is called colon cancer; cancer that begins in the lung is called lung cancer. **FIGURE 15.3** shows the leading sites of new cancer cases (incidence) and the leading causes of cancer deaths by site expected in 2012. An estimated 1.6 million new cases of invasive cancer were expected in men and women. More than half of all new cancers were cancers of the prostate, breast, lung, and colon/rectum. A total of 577,190 people are projected to die from cancer in 2012, with the diseases killing more than 1500 people each day. More than half of all cancer deaths will be from cancers of the lung, colon/rectum, breast, and prostate.

Origins of Cancer

Cancer is a disease of the cells in the body (**FIGURE 15.4**). The tissues in your body are made of cells (small structural units of all living things). Normal cells divide and multiply and know when to stop multiplying. Cancer happens when cells that are not normal continue to multiply when the body doesn't need them to, and they form lumps or masses of tissue called **tumors** (except in the case of leukemia where cancer prohibits normal blood function by abnormal cell division in the bloodstream).

Not all tumors are cancerous or malignant; in fact, most are noncancerous or benign. **Benign** tumors have well-defined boundaries, grow at a relatively slow pace, and demonstrate limited growth. They are rarely life-threatening, unless the tumor compresses the surrounding tissue against a hard surface in the body. For example, a benign brain tumor that compresses brain tissue against the skull can result in paralysis, loss of hearing or sight, dizziness, and other ailments.

Tumors When cells that are not normal continue to multiply and form lumps or masses.

Benign Refers to a noncancerous tumor that has a well-defined boundary, grows at a relatively slow pace, and demonstrates limited growth.

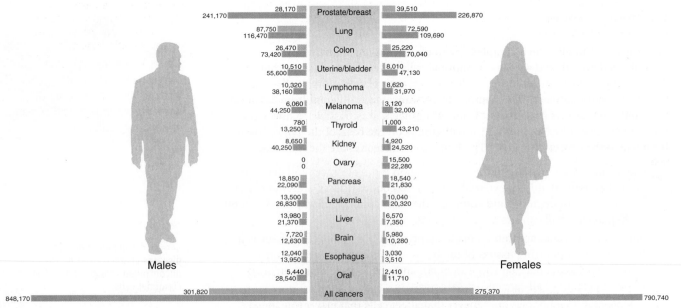

FIGURE 15.3 **U.S. Cancer Incidence and Mortality, 2012.** SOURCE: Data from American Cancer Society. (2012). *Cancer Facts and Figures 2012.* Atlanta, GA: Author.

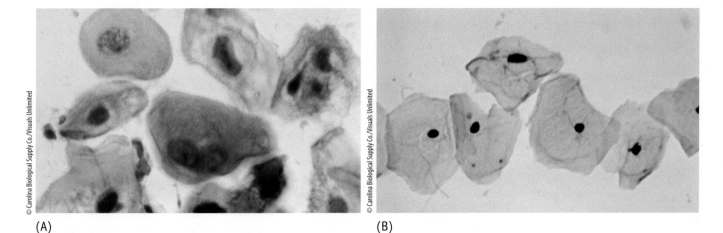

(A)   (B)

FIGURE 15.4 **Normal and Cancer Cell Differences.** (A) Dysplastic cells. (B) Normal cells.

Malignant tumors are usually faster growing and can be fatal. They usually have irregular boundaries and invade the surrounding tissue instead of pressing it aside. Most important, this primary tumor also sheds cells that travel through the bloodstream and lymphatic system, starting new tumor growth (secondary tumor) at other locations in the body (**FIGURE 15.5**). This process is called **metastasis**. The cancerous cells can establish a cancer in tissue that is different from the original cancer.

Approximately 90 percent of all cancer deaths are not because of the primary tumor itself, but rather because of the effects of the metastatic spread of the disease. For example, a patient with colon cancer may actually die from liver failure after the cancer has spread to that organ. The condition is then called metastatic colon cancer to the liver. Some parts of the body are more likely than others to become sites of metastatic cancer or secondary tumors, including the liver, bones, brain, lungs, and lymph nodes.

The ability of cancer cells to invade surrounding tissue and to metastasize makes early detection vital. Some common cancers are easier to treat and cure if they are found early. If the tumor is found when it is still small and has not yet spread, curing the cancer can be straightforward. However, the longer the cancerous tumor goes unnoticed, the greater the chance that the cancer will spread or metastasize. Treating metastatic cancer is much more challenging.

Cancer does not develop all at once in a cell. Several changes must occur in the genetic information (i.e., DNA) carried in a single cell before it can become a cancer cell and multiply into a tumor. The change is triggered by a gradual accumulation of damage or **mutations** to the genes involved in cell division over time. Each mutation pushes the cell further along to uncontrolled growth. Mutations are caused by both external (lifestyle, chemicals, radiation, and infectious organisms) and internal (inherited mutations, hormones, immune conditions, and mutations that occur from metabolism) factors. These factors may act independently or together to initiate or promote the development of normal cells into cancer cells, a process called **carcinogenesis**.

Ninety to 95 percent of cancers develop because of complex interactions between our bodies, our lifestyles, our environment, and our genetic makeup. These cancers are considered to be sporadic. People with **sporadic cancer** did not inherit cancer-causing mutations from their parents. Instead, certain cells in their body developed mutations that led to cancer as a result of growing older, tobacco, sunlight, ionizing radiation, certain chemicals, some viruses and bacteria, certain hormones, alcohol, poor diet, lack of physical activity, and being overweight (NCI, 2006). These causes of cancer, or, more correctly, the risk factors associated with the development of cancer, are addressed in the next section.

Malignant Refers to a cancerous tumor that has a tendency to invade and destroy nearby tissue and spread to other parts of the body.

Metastasis The spread of cancer from one part of the body to another. Cells in the metastatic (secondary) tumor are the same as those in the original (primary) tumor.

Mutation Damage to the genes involved in cell division.

Carcinogenesis Process by which normal cells are transformed into cancer cells.

Sporadic cancers Cancer that develops because of complex interactions between our bodies, our lifestyles, our environment, and our genetic makeup.

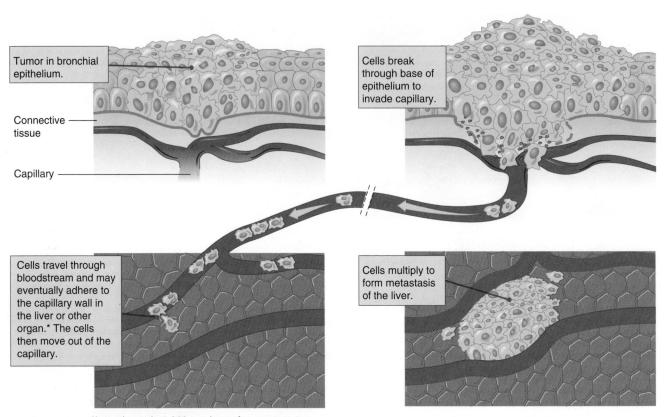

Tumor in bronchial epithelium.

Connective tissue

Capillary

Cells break through base of epithelium to invade capillary.

Cells travel through bloodstream and may eventually adhere to the capillary wall in the liver or other organ.* The cells then move out of the capillary.

Cells multiply to form metastasis of the liver.

*Less than 1 in 1,000 survive to form metastases.

FIGURE 15.5 **How Cancer Cells Multiply and Spread.** Cancer cells secrete chemicals that destroy the substances holding tissues together. As these tissues break down, cancer cells move from their original site, enter the blood and lymph, and travel to other parts of the body.

Heredity cancer Cancer that develops as a result of inheriting a cancer-causing mutation from parents. Also known as a cancer susceptibility gene.

Cancer susceptibility gene The type of genes involved in cancer.

About 5 to 10 percent of cancers develop as a result of an inherited susceptibility. People with **hereditary cancer** inherit a mutated gene from their parents. Every cell in the person's body contains the mutation or cancer susceptibility gene. A **cancer susceptibility gene** does not increase the risk for every type of cancer, and not everyone who is born with a mutated gene will develop cancer; risks vary according to the exact mutation that was inherited. Many other factors affect the risk of cancer in someone born with a gene mutation, including exposure to various environmental factors. But people who have inherited a mutation are one step closer to cancer than those who have not. Hereditary cancer tends to occur at an earlier age than the sporadic form of the same cancer, so screening and risk-lowering recommendations for cancer may be different and may begin at an earlier age for members of a family with an inherited gene mutation. TABLE 15.1 lists a number of cancer susceptibility genes.

Levels of Prevention

Health education professionals utilize the concept of prevention based on three types: primary, secondary, and tertiary.

Scientists now understand that cancer is a continuum that can be interrupted at many stages from susceptibility to initiation to clinically detectable disease. Most cancers are slow to start and take upward of 10 to 20 to 40 years to grow to a detectable stage. If they go undetected or if their growth is not stopped, death may result. This is called the "natural history of cancer." The goal of cancer prevention depends on the stage of health or disease of the individual. Health education professionals think about prevention on three types or levels: primary, secondary, and tertiary.

TABLE 15.1	Cancer Susceptibility Genes

Abnormalities (mutations) in these genes can be inherited. Each abnormal gene contributes to the development of cancer in a specific organ.

Gene	Organ Affected
Breast cancer	
BRCA1	Breast, ovary
BRCA2	Breast
p53	Breast, brain
Colon cancer	
MSH2	Colon, uterus
MSH1	Colon, uterus
PMS1, PMS2	Colon, other
APC	Colon
Melanoma	
MTS1 (CDKN2)	Skin, pancreas
CDK4	Skin
Prostate cancer	
HPC1	Prostate
MSR1	Prostate
AR	Prostate
CYP1	Prostate
SRD5A2	Prostate

Primary prevention includes actions that keep the disease process or health condition from becoming established in the first place by elimination of causes of the disease (reducing known risk factors) or increasing resistance to disease. Focusing on risky behaviors rather than specific diseases is crucial because one risk factor can result in or worsen several major diseases and conditions. For example, physical inactivity plays a major role in certain cancers, cardiovascular disease, type 2 diabetes, high blood pressure, obesity, and osteoporosis. Alcohol misuse and abuse contributes not only to cancer of the liver, but also dementia (neurologic damage and memory loss), cirrhosis, and injuries and death resulting from accidents and violence. Unsafe sexual practices can lead to cervical cancer, HIV/AIDS, other sexually transmitted infections, and unwanted pregnancies.

Secondary prevention aims at early detection of asymptomatic disease through preventive screenings and tests. Routine screenings can identify a previously undiagnosed condition or potential risk of a condition early in the disease process before it becomes symptomatic. For example, screening mammography is recommended every 1 to 2 years for women aged 40 and older to detect breast cancer. Screening examples for cardiovascular risk factors include testing for high blood pressure or high blood lipids. Secondary prevention allows primary care medical professionals to intervene early with treatments to control the disease before it progresses. When coupled with lifestyle changes, these treatments are much more effective. Unfortunately, many Americans do not routinely follow some basic health screening recommendations.

Tertiary prevention is treatment for a person who is symptomatic and ill and is typically offered by medical specialists. Examples for cancer include surgery, chemotherapy, and radiation therapy. Examples to treat coronary heart disease include bypass angioplasty or surgery. The methods are designed to limit the physical and social consequences of disease or injury after the disease has occurred or becomes symptomatic. However, these methods are extremely expensive and, more often than not, fail to restore people to the same health status they enjoyed before acquiring the disease.

Primary prevention Actions that keep the disease process or health condition from becoming established in the first place by eliminating causes of disease (reducing known risk factors) or increasing resistance to disease.

Secondary prevention Early detection of asymptomatic disease through preventive screenings and tests.

Tertiary prevention Treatment for a person who is symptomatic and ill that is typically offered by medical specialists.

Research scientists estimate that between 50 and 75 percent of cancer deaths in the United States are preventable by altering our behaviors.

Cancer Risk Factors

Learning what causes cancer and what the risk factors are is the first step in cancer prevention or primary prevention. Many cancer risk factors can be avoided, thus reducing the likelihood of developing cancer in the first place. Research scientists estimate that between 50 and 75 percent of cancer deaths in the United States are preventable by simply altering our behaviors (NCI, 2012). **FIGURE 15.6** summarizes research on the percentage of all cancer deaths based on different causes. Tobacco use is the most preventable cause of cancer death. For the overwhelming majority of people who do not use tobacco, dietary choices, weight control, and physical activity are the most important determinates of risk. Further decreases in cancer risk could be achieved by avoiding specific infections, including practicing safer sex, protection from excessive sun exposure, and reducing and/or eliminating alcohol consumption.

It is important to understand that the preventable percentage varies considerably by specific cancer. For example, approximately 90 percent of lung cancer deaths could be avoided by not smoking, whereas most studies have found no link between cigarette smoking and breast cancer. The risk factors for common types of cancer are provided in TABLE 15.2.

Tobacco

Avoiding tobacco in all forms is the most significant risk factor we can reduce. Cigarette smoking is directly responsible for approximately 30 percent of all cancer deaths annually in the United States (NCI, 2012). Smoking causes about 90 percent of lung cancer deaths in men and almost 80 percent in women (FIGURE 15.7). Compared to nonsmokers, men who smoke are about 23 times more likely to develop lung cancer, and women who smoke are about 13 times more likely to develop lung cancer than are women who do not smoke (U.S. Department of Health and Human Services [USDHHS], 2004). Lung cancer is the leading cause of cancer death in both men and women (refer to Figure 15.3). Smoking is also responsible for most cancers of the larynx, oral cavity and pharynx, esophagus, and bladder. In addition, it is a cause of kidney, pancreatic, cervical, and stomach cancers.

What makes cigarette smoking cause cancer are chemical ingredients known as carcinogens. **Carcinogen** literally means "cancer-causing." Cigarette smoke contains more than 60 carcinogens that damage important genes that control the growth of cells, causing them to grow abnormally or to reproduce too rapidly (USDHHS, 2004).

Carcinogen Chemical that damages cells and causes cancer.

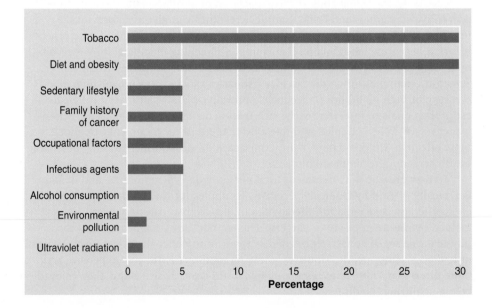

FIGURE 15.6 **Percentage of All Cancer Deaths Linked to a Specific Risk Factor.** SOURCE: Data from Harvard Center for Cancer Prevention. (1996). *Harvard Report on Cancer Prevention. Volume 1: Causes of Cancer.* Netherlands: Springer.

TABLE 15.2	Risk Factors for Common Cancers

Lung Cancer

* Tobacco smoke (smoking cigarettes is by far the leading risk factor for lung cancer)
* Secondhand smoke (if you don't smoke, breathing in the smoke of others)
* Radon
* Asbestos

Breast Cancer

* Aging (roughly 2 out of 3 invasive breast cancers are found in women age 55 or older)
* Genetic risk factors (roughly 5–10 percent of breast cancer cases are thought to be hereditary)
* Family history of breast cancer
* Personal history of breast cancer
* Race and ethnicity (white women are slightly more likely to develop breast cancer than are African American women)
* Dense breast tissue
* Certain benign breast conditions
* Menstrual periods (women who started menstruating at an early age [before age 12] and/or went through menopause at a later age [after age 55])
* Not having children or having them later in life
* Recent oral contraceptive use
* Using postmenopausal hormone therapy
* Not breast-feeding
* Alcohol
* Being overweight or obese
* Lack of physical activity

Prostate Cancer

* Age (two out of three prostate cancers are found in men over the age of 65)
* Race/ethnicity (prostate cancer occurs more often in African American men than in men of other races)
* Nationality (prostate cancer is most common in North America, northwestern Europe, and Australia)
* Family history
* Diet (men who eat a lot of red meat or high-fat dairy products)
* Obesity
* Physical inactivity

Colorectal Cancer

* Age (more than 90 percent of people diagnosed with colorectal cancer are over age 50)
* Personal history of colorectal polyps or colorectal cancer
* Personal history of inflammatory bowel disease
* Family history of colorectal cancer
* Inherited syndromes
* Diet (high in red meats [beef, lamb, or liver] and/or processed meats [hot dogs and some luncheon meats])
* Physical inactivity
* Obesity
* Smoking
* Heavy alcohol use

Skin Cancer

* Excessive exposure to ultraviolet radiation
* Multiple moles (nevi) or atypical mole
* Fair complexion
* Family history

SOURCES: Data from The National Cancer Institute. Cancer Causes and Risk Factors. Online: http://www.cancer.gov/cancertopics/prevention-genetics-causes/causes; Centers for Disease Control and Prevention. Cancer Risk Factors. Online: http://www.cdc.gov/cancer/dcpc/prevention/other.htm; and American Cancer Society. Learn About Cancer. Online: http://www.cancer.org/cancer/index. Accessed April 12, 2012.

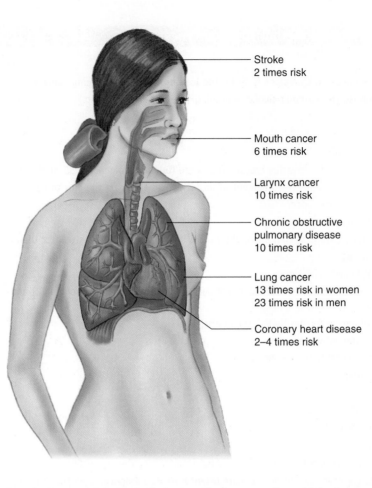

Stroke
2 times risk

Mouth cancer
6 times risk

Larynx cancer
10 times risk

Chronic obstructive
pulmonary disease
10 times risk

Lung cancer
13 times risk in women
23 times risk in men

Coronary heart disease
2–4 times risk

FIGURE 15.7 **The Risk of Smoking Cigarettes.** A smoker has a greater risk of developing certain diseases than does a nonsmoker. SOURCE: Centers for Disease Control and Prevention (2009 December). Health effects of cigarette smoking. Online: http://www.cdc.gov/tobacco/data_statistics/fact_sheets/health_effects/effects_cig_smoking/index.htm; U.S. Department of Health and Human Services. (1989). *Reducing the health consequences of smoking: 25 years of progress. A report of the surgeon general.* Rockville, MD: Office of Smoking and Health.

Carcinogens in cigarettes include cyanide, benzene, formaldehyde, methanol, ammonia, and acetylene. Quitting smoking significantly reduces the risk of developing and dying from cancer. This benefit increases the sooner a person quits and the longer a person remains smoke free.

Smokeless tobacco—snuff and chewing tobacco—is not a safe alternative. These types of tobacco contain 28 carcinogens, with the most harmful carcinogens being the tobacco-specific nitrosamines. Smokeless tobacco users increase their risk for cancer of the oral cavity (**FIGURE 15.8**). Oral cancer can include cancer of the lip, tongue, cheeks, gums, and the floor and roof of the mouth.

FIGURE 15.8 **Gruen Von Behrens, After Using Smokeless Tobacco.** Gruen began using smokeless (spit) tobacco at age 13, and by age 17 he had oral cancer and a 25 percent chance of survival. Formerly a star baseball player, Gruen no longer plays sports, and, after 40 operations, he is still missing his lower teeth and jawbone. Gruen is now a spokesperson for the Oral Health America's National Spit Tobacco Education Program (NSTEP), warning audiences of the dangers of using smokeless tobacco.

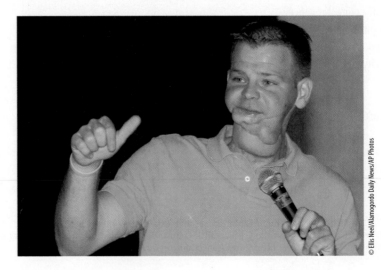

Diet

Some foods contribute to an increase in some cancers; other foods decrease the risk. A number of studies have linked a diet high in animal fat, such as red meat (especially if it is processed), with an increase in cancers of the breast, colon, and prostate (FIGURE 15.9). A diet high in fat may also contribute to increased caloric intake, which contributes to obesity, a risk factor for many types of cancer.

Although cancer can affect many different parts of the body, the foods that prevent cancer and deter cancer growth are mostly foods of plant origin. You do not need to become a vegetarian, but you are encouraged to fill your plate with a variety of vegetables, fruits, whole grains, and legumes (e.g., beans, lentils, chickpeas) (FIGURE 15.10) and (FIGURE 15.11). These foods all contain important nutrients and other cancer-fighting substances such as antioxidants (which help repair damaged cells) and phytochemicals that strengthen immune function and destroy cancer-causing substances before they cause harm. The American Cancer Society (2012a) encourages everyone to eat a healthy diet, with an emphasis on plant foods, and has issued the following guidelines for cancer prevention related to nutrition.

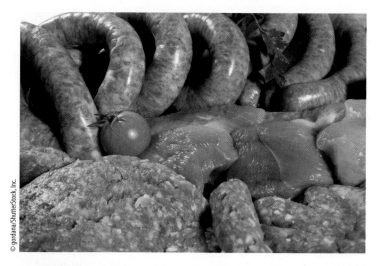

FIGURE 15.9 **Diet and Cancer.** Limit how much processed meat and red meat you eat to reduce your cancer risk.

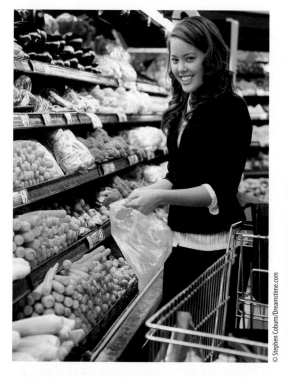

FIGURE 15.10 **Diet and Cancer.** Eat at least 2 ½ cups of vegetables and fruits each day to reduce your cancer risk.

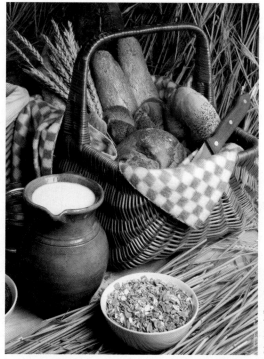

FIGURE 15.11 **Diet and Cancer.** Choose whole grains instead of refined grains products to reduce your cancer risk.

Choose foods and drinks in amounts that help you get to and maintain a healthy weight.

- Read food labels to become more aware of portion sizes and calories. Be aware that "low-fat" or "nonfat" does not necessarily mean "low-calorie."
- Eat smaller portions when eating high-calorie foods.
- Choose vegetables, whole fruit, and other low-calorie foods instead of calorie-dense foods such as French fries, potato and other chips, ice cream, donuts, and other sweets.
- Limit your intake of sugar-sweetened beverages such as soft drinks, sports drinks, and fruit-flavored drinks.
- When you eat away from home, be especially mindful to choose food low in calories, fat, and added sugar, and avoid eating large portion sizes.

Limit how much processed meat and red meat you eat.

- Limit your intake of processed meats such as bacon, sausage, lunch meats, and hot dogs.
- Choose fish, poultry, or beans instead of red meat (beef, pork, and lamb).
- If you eat red meat, choose lean cuts and eat smaller portions.
- Prepare meat, poultry, and fish by baking, broiling, or poaching rather than by frying or charbroiling.

Eat at least 2½ cups of vegetables and fruits each day.

- Include vegetables and fruits at every meal and for snacks.
- Eat a variety of vegetables and fruits each day.
- Emphasize whole fruits and vegetables; choose 100 percent juice if you drink vegetable or fruit juices.
- Limit your use of creamy sauces, dressings, and dips with fruits and vegetables.

Choose whole grains instead of refined grain products.

- Choose whole-grain breads, pasta, and cereals (such as barley and oats) instead of breads, cereals, and pasta made from refined grains, and brown rice instead of white rice.
- Limit your intake of refined carbohydrate foods, including pastries, candy, sugar-sweetened breakfast cereals, and other high-sugar foods.

Obesity

In the United States, overweight and obesity contribute to between 15 and 20 percent of all cancer-related mortality (NCI, 2012). Cancers of the breast, endometrium (the lining of the uterus), kidney, colon, pancreas, esophagus, and gallbladder have been shown to be strongly linked to excess body fat (American Institute for Cancer Research [AICR], 2007). Several other types of cancer—including liver and certain leukemias—have been linked to obesity in some studies, but more research is needed to confirm this connection. Excess weight raises cancer risk in different ways. The biological mechanisms of being overfat that affect cancer risk include an increase in the level of several hormones, decreased immune function, and increased cell proliferation and growth. In addition to the amount of body fat, the location of it affects cancer risk. Abdominal fatness increases the risk of some cancers more than others, colon cancer in particular (**FIGURE 15.12**).

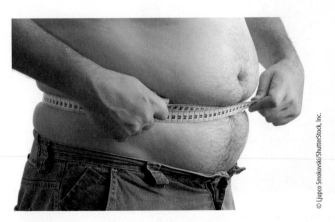

FIGURE 15.12 **Impact of Obesity.** Abdominal fat is a risk factor for some cancers.

© Ljupco Smokovski/ShutterStock, Inc.

The concern about excess visceral fat tissue—the fat that accumulates in and around abdominal organs—is that it is directly related to insulin and elevated insulin levels and inflammation throughout the body, which has been linked to cancer and heart disease. Insulin is a very powerful cellular growth factor and it affects cancer cells (Khandekar, Cohen, & Spiegelman, 2011).

Sedentary Lifestyle

A number of scientific studies indicate that physical activity may reduce the risk of several types of cancer, including cancers of the colon, breast, prostate, lung, and endometrium (Eheman et al., 2012). Physical activity acts in a variety of ways to reduce cancer risk (**FIGURE 15.13**). Regular physical activity aids in reducing the risk of cancer through its effect on maintaining a healthy body weight. Physical activity and weight control are strongly associated with the concept of energy balance. Physical activity is believed to reduce the risk of colon cancer by accelerating the digestive process, reducing the length of time that the bowel lining is exposed to potential fecal carcinogens. In addition, physical activity protects against colon cancer by reducing insulin resistance, thus diminishing chronic inflammation. It can lower levels of estrogen and testosterone, which is important because having high levels of these hormones can increase cancer risk for breast, endometrial, and prostate cancers. Finally, regular physical activity may also stimulate and strengthen your immune system, which may then scavenge abnormal cells more effectively.

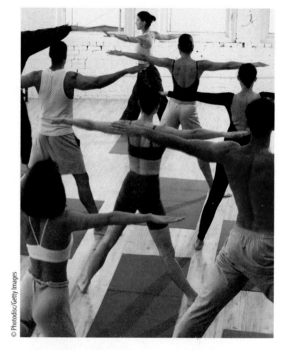

FIGURE 15.13 **Avoid a Sedentary Lifestyle.** Regular physical activity is important in reducing cancer risk.

Infectious Agents

Cancer is not infectious (contagious)—you can't catch it from someone who has it—but being infected with some viruses and bacteria may increase the risk of developing cancer. These include the following:

- *Human papillomavirus (HPV)*. Certain types of HPV are the main cause of cervical cancer. HPV can also cause less common cancers such as cancers of the vulva, vagina, and penis.
- *Hepatitis B and hepatitis C viruses*. Hepatitis B and C virus infections are a major risk factor for liver cancer.
- *Human T-cell leukemia/lymphoma virus (HTLV-1)*. HTLV-1 is a virus that infects T cells (a type of white blood cell) and can cause leukemia and lymphoma.
- *Human immunodeficiency virus (HIV)*. HIV is the virus that causes AIDS. People infected with HIV are at an increased risk for specific cancers, such as Kaposi's sarcoma, non-Hodgkin's lymphoma, and invasive cervical cancer.
- *Epstein-Barr virus (EBV)*. EBV was the first human virus to be implicated directly in carcinogenesis. EBV is associated with some types of cancer, such as Burkitt's lymphoma and cancers of the mouth.
- *Human herpes virus 8 (HHV8)*. HHV8 is a associated with Kaposi's sarcoma.
- *Helicobacter pylori*. The *Helicobacter pylori* bacterium infection is a risk factor for stomach cancer.

You can reduce your risk of exposure to these infections by behavioral changes, including practicing safer sex. For example, condom use during sex can significantly reduce your risk of exposure to HPV, HIV, and hepatitis B. Safer sex practices are particularly vital for young adults because the highest-risk age group for sexually transmitted infections is between the ages of 15 and 24. Additionally,

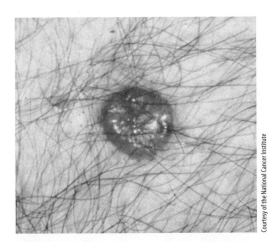

(A)

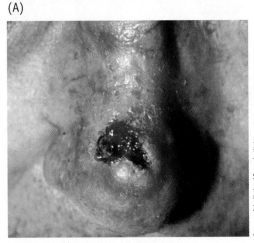

(B)

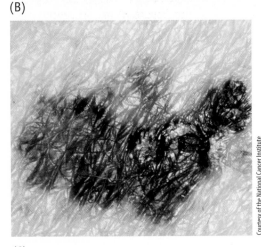

(C)

FIGURE 15.14 **Skin Cancers.** (A) Squamous cell carcinoma looks like a red rounded mass or a flat sore, as shown in this photo. (B) This basal cell carcinoma is a raised lesion with central depressions that bleed and crust over. (C) Lesions of malignant melanoma are usually characterized by irregular borders with red, white, blue or blue-black spots. Some portions may be raised.

two cancer-preventive vaccines have been licensed by the U.S. Food and Drug Administration: hepatitis B vaccine and Gardasil, the human papillomavirus (HPV) vaccine. The hepatitis B vaccine prevents infection with the hepatitis B virus, which may cause some forms of liver cancer. Gardasil (quadrivalent human papillomavirus recombinant vaccine) prevents infection with HPV types 16 and 18, which cause 70 percent of cervical cancers.

Alcohol

The consumption of alcoholic beverages is causally related to cancers of the mouth, pharynx, larynx, and esophagus, with the risk most pronounced among smokers and those who consume the most alcohol (Gentry, 2011). Further, there is evidence that suggests a link between alcoholic beverage consumption and cancer of the liver and breast.

There are many possible explanations for how alcohol causes cancer. It is likely that it causes different types of cancer in various ways. It could be that alcohol causes cancer itself by increasing the level of some hormones such as estrogen, testosterone, and insulin. Unusually high levels of estrogen increase the risk of breast cancer. Alcohol may also be carcinogenic because of the way it is metabolized by the liver into acetaldehyde. Acetal-dehyde causes liver cells to grow faster than normal. These regenerating cells are more likely to pick up changes in their genes that could lead to cancer. Finally, alcohol could make other cells more susceptible to carcinogens. For example, alcohol makes it easier for the tissues of the mouth and throat to absorb the cancer-causing chemicals in tobacco. Whatever the cause, reducing the amount of alcohol you drink can sharply reduce your cancer risk. Research shows that even moderate drinkers—two drinks a day for men and one drink a day for women—have an increased risk of developing certain cancers.

Ultraviolet Radiation

Ultraviolet (UV) radiation comes from the sun, sunlamps, and tanning beds or booths. Overexposure to the sun is the main cause of skin cancer (**FIGURE 15.14**). One in five Americans will develop skin cancer in the course of a lifetime (Stern, 2010). There is no such thing as a safe or healthy tan, whether it is from exposure to the UV rays of the sun or the UV rays of a tanning bed. To minimize the risk of skin cancer follow the simple guidelines in   TABLE 15.3 .

Family History

Knowing your family history of cancer is important to properly assess your risk for certain types of cancer. Approximately 5 to 10 percent of cancers are inherited. People may inherit defective or mutant genes that lead to a greater risk of developing specific cancers (Table 15.1). Let your doctor know if a certain type of cancer runs in your family. Together, you can determine an appropriate screening plan and more accurately assess your risk.

Environmental Factors

Certain chemicals and substances, including arsenic, asbestos, uranium, vinyl chloride, ionizing radiation, ultraviolet rays, X-rays, and coal tar derivatives, are carcinogens. Follow safety precautions at work and at home to avoid or reduce contact with unsafe substances. Check with

TABLE 15.3	**What You Need to Know About Skin Cancer**

Doctors encourage people of all ages to limit their time in the sun and to avoid other sources of UV radiation.

- It is best to avoid the midday sun (from mid-morning to late afternoon) whenever possible. You also should protect yourself from UV radiation reflected by sand, water, snow, and ice. UV radiation can penetrate light clothing, windshields, and windows.
- Wear long sleeves, long pants, a hat with a wide brim, and sunglasses with lenses that absorb UV.
- Use sunscreen. Sunscreen may help prevent skin cancer, especially sunscreen with a sun protection factor (SPF) of at least 15. But sunscreens cannot replace avoiding the sun and wearing clothing to protect the skin.
- Stay away from sunlamps and tanning booths. They are no safer than sunlight.

SOURCE: National Cancer Institute. (2012). What you need to know about skin cancer. Online: http://www.cancer.gov/cancertopics/wyntk/skin.

local environmental protection professionals about possible hazards in your community.

Acquiring this knowledge regarding cancer causation is merely the beginning of the prevention process; you need to translate this knowledge into action. If everyone practiced everything known about reducing the risk of getting cancer in the first place, up to 75 percent of all cancers could be prevented. Equally as important is the fact that more cancer patients could be cured of their cancer if it was detected at an earlier stage before cancer cells have metastasized. Most cancers, when diagnosed early when there is relatively less malignant potential, are more responsive to treatment.

Cancer Screening and Early Detection of Cancer

An important role in increasing cancer survival rates is cancer screening and early detection of cancer. **Cancer screening** refers to checking for cancer in people who have no symptoms of the disease. TABLE 15.4 provides a summary of the Centers for Disease Control and Prevention screening recommendations for people who are at average risk and without any specific symptoms for these cancers. TABLE 15.5 explains how to perform a testicular self-examination, and FIGURE 15.15 demonstrates how to perform a breast self-examination. It is important to have cancer screening tests at the appropriate age. However, people at an increased risk for certain cancers may want to start at an earlier age. Cancer screening tests can also include checking to see if you have an inherited cancer-related gene mutation.

Although screening tests can help detect cancer malignancies in their earliest stages, it is important to be alert for early warning signs in functions of the body that may indicate that cancer is developing. Recognizing possible symptoms of cancer and taking prompt action leads to an earlier diagnosis. The American Cancer Society developed an easy way to recognize the seven warning signs of cancer that uses the acronym CAUTION (TABLE 15.6). These signs aren't a cancer diagnosis, but are warning signs suggesting that you may want to seek out your health care professional to determine whether you have the condition. Screening and early detection of cancer enable doctors to diagnose cancer in its early stages, which can improve patients' potential for a cure.

Treating Cancer

Today, most cancers that are not prevented can be treated successfully, resulting in long-term survival—two in every three cancer patients survive 5 years or longer after diagnosis and treatment (NCI, 2012). Many believe this cure rate could

5

Cancer screening and early detection of cancer can play an important role in cancer survival rates.

Cancer screening Checking for cancer in people who have no symptoms of the disease.

6

Currently, two in every three cancer patients survive 5 years or longer after diagnosis and treatment.

TABLE 15.4	Cancer Screening Tests

The Centers for Disease Control and Prevention supports screening for breast, cervical, and colorectal (colon) cancers as recommended by the U.S. Preventive Services Task Force.

Breast Cancer Screening

- **Mammogram.** A mammogram is an X-ray of the breast. Mammograms are the best method to detect breast cancer early when it is easier to treat and before it is big enough to feel or cause symptoms. Having regular mammograms can lower the risk of dying from breast cancer. If you are age 50 to 74 years, be sure to have a screening mammogram every two years. If you are age 40–49 years, talk to your doctor about when and how often you should have a screening mammogram.
- **Clinical breast exam.** A clinical breast exam is an examination by a doctor or nurse, who uses his or her hands to feel for lumps or other changes.
- **Breast self-exam.** A breast self-exam is when you check your own breasts for lumps, changes in size or shape of the breast, or any other changes in the breasts or underarm (armpit).

Which tests to choose: Having a clinical breast exam or a breast self-exam has not been found to decrease risk of dying from breast cancer. Keep in mind that, at this time, the best way to find breast cancer is with a mammogram. If you choose to have clinical breast exams and to perform breast self-exams, be sure you also get regular mammograms.

Cervical Cancer Screening

- The **Pap test** (or Pap smear) looks for precancers, cell changes on the cervix that might become cervical cancer if they are not treated appropriately. You should start getting regular Pap tests at age 21, or within three years of the first time you have sex—whichever happens first.
- The **HPV test** looks for the virus (human papillomavirus) that can cause these cell changes. The HPV test may also be used to screen women age 30 years or older, or women of any age who have unclear Pap test results.

Colorectal Cancer Screening

The U.S. Preventive Services Task Force recommends colorectal cancer screening for men and women ages 50–75 using high-sensitivity fecal occult blood testing (FOBT), sigmoidoscopy, or colonoscopy. (The decision to be screened after age 75 should be made on an individual basis. If you are older than 75, ask your doctor if you should be screened.)

High-Sensitivity FOBT (Stool Test)

There are two types of FOBT. One uses the chemical guaiac to detect blood. The other, a fecal immunochemical test (FIT), uses antibodies to detect blood in the stool. You receive a test kit from your health care provider. At home, you use a stick or brush to obtain a small amount of stool. You return the test kit to the doctor or a lab, where the stool samples are checked for the presence of blood.

How often: Once a year.

Flexible Sigmoidoscopy

For this test, the doctor puts a short, thin, flexible, lighted tube into your rectum. The doctor checks for polyps or cancer inside the rectum and lower third of the colon.

How often: Every 5 years.

Colonoscopy

This is similar to flexible sigmoidoscopy, except the doctor uses a longer, thin, flexible, lighted tube to check for polyps or cancer inside the rectum and the entire colon. During the test, the doctor can find and remove most polyps and some cancers. Colonoscopy also is used as a follow-up test if anything unusual is found during one of the other screening tests.

How often: Every 10 years.

SOURCE: Reproduced from Centers for Disease Control and Prevention. (2012). Cancer prevention and control: Cancer screening tests. Online: http://www.cdc.gov/cancer/dcpc/prevention/screening.htm.

be even higher if the early detection tests presently known were put into practice, leading to earlier diagnosis and treatment (NCI, 2012).

Treatment plans vary a great deal depending on how advanced the cancer is and what type it is. Most treatment plans include surgery, radiation, and chemotherapy. Surgery can remove tumors or as much of the cancerous tissue as possible. It is often performed in conjunction with chemotherapy or radiation therapy. Chemotherapy is a type of cancer treatment that uses drugs to eliminate cancer cells. Unlike surgery, chemotherapy affects the entire body, not just a specific part. It works by targeting rapidly multiplying cancer cells. Unfortunately, other types of cells in our bodies also multiply at high rates, such as hair follicle cells and the cells that line our stomachs. This is why chemotherapy can cause side effects including hair loss and an upset stomach. Radiation therapy uses certain types of ionizing radiation to shrink tumors or eliminate cancer cells. It works by damaging cancer cells' DNA, making them unable to multiply.

TABLE 15.5	**Testicular Self-Examination**

A testicular self-examination (TSE) is an examination of the male testicles. The testicles (also called the testes) are located in the scrotum—the bag of skin hanging behind the penis.

Why TSE Is Performed

TSE is a simple and effective way for men to recognize the early signs and symptoms of testicular cancer. Cancer of the testes is a relatively rare form of cancer, accounting for approximately 1% of cancers in American men. However, testicular cancer is one of the most frequently occurring types of cancer in men ages 15 to 35. Performing a TSE can help you become familiar with what is normal for you. Then, if you notice a change, you will be warned to notify your health care provider. If it is caught early, testicular cancer is one of the most curable forms of cancer.

How Do I Perform a TSE?

A TSE is simple to perform and can quickly become a part of your routine. A TSE should be performed once a month during or after a warm bath or shower, when the heat causes the scrotal skin to relax, making it easier to find anything unusual.

- Examine each testicle separately with both hands. Place your thumbs on top of the testicle and the pads of your fingers under and behind the testicle.

- Gently slide or roll the skin of scrotum across each testicle between the thumbs and fingers, checking for lumps or irregularities. Do not rub. Examine the entire area of the testicle. The surface of each testicle should feel firm or smooth, but not rock hard, and should be absence of lumps or tenderness.

- Feel the side of testicle closest to the body for the epididymis (cord-like, comma-shaped structure or tube on the top and back of each testicle that stores and transports sperm). Do not confuse the epididymis with an abnormal lump. The most common tumor to feel for is about the size of a pea, on the front or side of the testicle.

- Stand naked in front of a mirror and look for any swelling in the skin of the scrotum or unusual contours in the groin. It is normal for a man's testicles to be different sizes and for one to hang lower than the other.

Notify Your Health Care Provider

- If you notice a lump, enlargement, tenderness, or other unexplained changes in your testicles, talk to your health care provider right away. Lumps are not always cancerous. The change may be a sign of infection in the testicle or a testicular torsion. If you have any doubts, see your health care provider.

SOURCE: Adapted from MedlinePlus Medical Encyclopedia. (2012). Testicular Self-Examination. Online: http://www.nlm.nih.gov/medlineplus/ency/article/003909.htm; American Cancer Society. (2012). Do I Have Testicular Cancer? Online: http://www.cancer.org/cancer/testicularcancer/moreinformation/doihavetesticularcancer/do-i-have-testicular-cancer-self-exam; and the Testicular Cancer Resource Center. (2012). How to Do a Testicular Self Examination. Online: http:// http://tcrc.acor.org.

Physical Activity and Health Connection

Scientific evidence is accumulating that regular physical activity is associated with a reduced risk of some cancers. The evidence for decreased cancer risk with increased physical activity is most convincing with colon and breast cancers. To a lesser degree of certainty, studies show a reduction for prostate, lung, and endometrial cancers. Regular physical activity aids in reducing the risk of cancer from being overweight because weight control and physical activity are strongly associated with the concept of energy balance. Physical activity has also been shown to lower levels of certain hormones that may accelerate the rate at which cancer cells grow and divide.

Breast self-examinations should be done once a month so you become familiar with the usual appearance and feel of your breasts. Familiarity makes it easier to notice any changes in the breast from month to month. Early discovery of a change from what is "normal" is the main idea behind the BSE. The outlook is much better if you detect cancer in an early stage.

If you menstruate, the best time to do a BSE is 2 or 3 days after your period ends, when your breasts are least likely to be tender or swollen. If you no longer menstruate, pick a day such as the first day of the month, to remind yourself it is time to do a BSE.

Here is one way to do a BSE.

1 Stand before a mirror. Inspect both breasts for anything unusual, such as any discharge from the nipples or puckering, dimpling, or scaling of the skin.

The next two steps are designed to emphasize any change in the shape or contour of your breasts. As you do them, you should be able to feel your chest muscles tighten.

FIGURE 15.15 **Breast Self-Examination.**

2 Watching closely in the mirror, clasp your hands behind your head and press your hands forward.

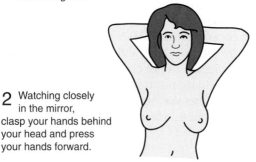

3 Next, press your hands firmly on your hips and bow slightly toward your mirror as you pull your shoulders and elbows forward.

Some women do the next part of the exam in the shower because fingers glide over soapy skin, making it easy to concentrate on the texture underneath.

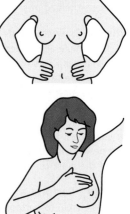

4 Raise your left arm. Use three or four fingers of your right hand to explore your left breast firmly, carefully, and thoroughly. Beginning at the outer edge, press the flat part of your fingers in small circles, moving the circles slowly around the breast. Gradually work toward the nipple. Be sure to cover the entire breast. Pay special attention to the area between the breast and the underarm, including the underarm itself. Feel for any unusual lump or mass under the skin.

5 Gently squeeze the nipple and look for discharge. (If you have any discharge during the month—whether or not it is during BSE–see your doctor.) Repeat steps 4 and 5 on your right breast.

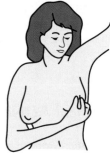

6 Steps 4 and 5 should be repeated lying down. Lie flat on your back with your left arm over your head and a pillow or folded towel under your left shoulder. This position flattens the breast and makes it easier to examine. Use the same circular motion described earlier. Repeat the exam on your right breast.

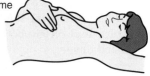

TABLE 15.6	Cancer's Seven Warning Signs

You can remember the following signs easily by knowing that they are a CAUTION—these signs do not necessarily mean you have cancer but that you should see your health care provider to evaluate the sign.

Change in bowel or bladder habits

A sore that does not heal

Unusual bleeding or discharge

Thickening or lump in breast or elsewhere

Indigestion or difficulty in swallowing

Obvious change in a wart or mole

Nagging cough or hoarseness

concept connections

1. **Cancer is potentially the most preventable and curable of the life-threatening diseases facing us today.** This statement is based on tremendous advances in cancer research over the past couple of decades. Research scientists estimate that between 50 and 75 percent of cancer deaths in the United States are preventable by translating current knowledge related to a few controllable behavioral risk factors for cancer into actual practice. The other good news is that early detection, diagnosis, and treatment have dramatically improved survival odds of those with cancer diagnoses. Today, more than two out of three cancer patients (67 percent) survive 5 years or longer after diagnosis and treatment—this rate is up considerably from 30 years ago when the number was one in two.

2. *Cancer* **is the term given to a complex group of diseases characterized by the uncontrolled growth and spread of abnormal cells.** There are at least one hundred different types of cancer, differing as to their cause, type of cell or organ affected, symptoms, and treatment. For example, breast cancers are different from colon cancers, and lung cancers are different from skin cancers.

3. **Health education professionals utilize the concept of prevention based on three types: primary, secondary, and tertiary.** Primary prevention includes actions that keep the disease process or health condition from becoming established in the first place by eliminating causes of disease (reducing known risk factors) or increasing resistance to the disease. Secondary prevention aims at early detection of asymptomatic disease through preventive screenings and tests. Routine screenings can identify a previously undiagnosed condition or potential risk of a condition early in the disease process before it becomes symptomatic. Tertiary prevention is treatment for a person who is symptomatic and ill and is typically offered by medical specialists. The methods are designed to limit the physical and social consequences of disease or injury after it has occurred or become symptomatic.

4. **Research scientists estimate that between 50 and 75 percent of cancer deaths in the United States are preventable by altering our behaviors.** Tobacco use is the most preventable cause of cancer death. For the overwhelming majority of people who do not use tobacco, dietary choices, weight control, and physical activity are the most important determinates of risk. We can achieve further decreases in cancer risk by controlling specific infections, including practicing safer sex, protecting ourselves from excessive sun exposure, and reducing and/or eliminating alcohol consumption.

5. **Cancer screening and early detection of cancer can play an important role in cancer survival rates.** *Cancer screening* refers to checking for cancer in people who have no symptoms of the disease. It is important to have cancer screening tests at the appropriate age. However, people at an increased risk for certain cancers may want to start at an earlier age. Cancer screening tests can also include checking to see whether you have an inherited cancer-related gene mutation.

6. **Currently, two in every three cancer patients survive 5 years or longer after diagnosis and treatment.** Many believe that this cure rate could be even higher if the early detection tests presently known were put into practice, leading to earlier diagnosis and treatment. Treatment plans vary a great deal depending on how advanced the cancer is and what type it is. Most treatment plans include surgery, radiation, and chemotherapy.

Terms

Benign, 336
Cancer, 335
Cancer screening, 347
Cancer susceptibility gene, 338
Carcinogen, 340

Carcinogenesis, 337
Heredity cancer, 338
Malignant, 337
Metastasis, 337
Mutation, 337

Primary prevention, 339
Secondary prevention, 339
Sporadic cancer, 337
Tertiary prevention, 339
Tumors, 336

making the connection

Katrina has learned much about the causes of cancer. In so doing, she has gained an appreciation for the ways in which simple lifestyle changes would help her significantly reduce her own risk of developing cancer. She understands that she needs to break her smoking habit immediately. In addition, she now knows that eating a nutritious diet, maintaining a healthy weight, and getting regular physical activity will not only help her obtain optimal health now but also pave the way for further reducing her cancer risk. Katrina decides to stop smoking first. She prepares for quitting by beginning to self-monitor her smoking habit. She records the number of cigarettes she smokes a day and when she smokes them. Katrina also signs up for a smoking cessation class offered by the university's health education center.

Critical Thinking

1. Make a list of all the modifiable risk factors that increase your chance of getting cancer. Order the list from the highest to lowest risk. Which risk factors pertain to you? How can you modify or change these risk factors?

2. Family history is a risk factor for cancer. A family history of cancer does not guarantee that you will get the disease, and neither does it cancel out the importance of a healthy lifestyle (not smoking, good dietary habits, and regular physical activity). A family history of cancer does predispose you to the disease; therefore, it is important for you to determine your family cancer history. Construct a family tree by listing your biological parents, siblings, grandparents (maternal and paternal), and aunts and uncles (paternal and maternal). Next to each name, list the type of cancer and the age at which it was discovered. Your family may be helpful with this activity. After completing your tree, you may want to share it with your family and discuss prevention efforts (include cancer screenings and early detection methods).

3. Do you have any family members or friends like Katrina who would like to quit smoking? If yes, go online to the American Cancer Society website and search for ways to quit smoking. After completing this activity, sit down and share the information with the individual trying to quit smoking.

References

American Cancer Society. (2012a). ACS guidelines on nutrition and physical activity for cancer prevention. Online: http://www.cancer.org/Healthy/ EatHealthyGetActive/ACSGuidelinesonNutrition PhysicalActivityforCancerPrevention/ nupa-guidelines-toc.

American Cancer Society. (2012b). *Cancer Facts and Figures 2012*. Atlanta, GA: Author.

American Institute for Cancer Research. (2007). Food, nutrition, physical activity, and the prevention of cancer: A global perspective. Online: http://www.aicr.org/research/research_science _expert_report.html.

Eheman, C., Henlye, J., Ballard-Barbash, R., Jacobs, E.J., Schymura, M.J., Noone, A., Pan, L., Anderson, R.N., Fulton, J.E., Kohler, B.A., Jemal, A., Ward, E., Plescia, M., Ries, L.A., & Edwards, B.K. (2012, March 28). Annual report to the nation on the status of cancer, 1975–2008, featuring cancers associated with excess weight and lack of sufficient physical activity. *Cancer* 118(9):2338–2366.

Gentry, R.T. (2011). Alcohol and cancer epidemiology. *Alcohol and Cancer*. Editors: Zakari, S., Vasilious, V., & Guo, M. New York, NY: Springer Publishing.

Khandekar, M.J., Cohen, P., & Spiegelman, B.M. (2011). Molecular mechanisms of cancer development in obesity. *Nature Cancer Reviews* 11:886–895.

Mackay, J., Jemal, A., Lee, N., & Parkin, M. (2006). *The Cancer Atlas*. Atlanta, GA: American Cancer Society.

National Cancer Institute. (2006). What you need to know about cancer. NIH Publication No. 06-1566. Online: http://www.cancer.gov/cancertopics/ wyntk/cancer/page1.

National Cancer Institute, National Institutes of Health, Department of Health and Human Services. (2012). *Cancer Trends Progress Report— 2009/2010 Update*. Bethesda, MD: Government Printing Office. Online: http://progressreport .cancer.gov.

Stern, R.S. (2010). Prevalence of a history of skin cancer in 2007: Results of an incidence-based model. *Archives of Dermatology* 146(3):279–282.

U.S. Department of Health and Human Services. (2004). The health consequences of smoking: A report of the surgeon general. Online: http:// www.surgeongeneral.gov/library/reports/ smokingconsequences/index.htm.

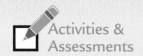

Activities &
Assessments

16

Preventing Sexually Transmitted Infections

what's the connection?

Jeremy has a close friend, Christina, whom he loves very much. Jeremy has never been closer to anyone than he is to Christina. They attend the same college and get along well. Jeremy and Christina are best friends, and they have a close intimate relationship, but Jeremy wants to have a sexual relationship to show the depth of his love. Christina values the emotional intimacy she has with Jeremy but is not sure she is ready for sex or that she even wants to include physical intimacy and intercourse in their relationship. She feels uncomfortable discussing her feelings about these issues with Jeremy.

concepts

1. A pathogen or infectious agent is a biological agent that causes disease or illness to its host.

2. Sexually transmitted infections are infections that are spread primarily through person-to-person sexual contact.

3. There are many reasons for the high rates of sexually transmitted infections in the United States.

4. Abstinence from sexual activity is the most effective behavior for eliminating your risk of contracting a sexually transmitted infection.

5. *Safer sex* is a general term used to describe methods for reducing the chance that you will contract or spread sexually transmitted infections.

go.jblearning.com/kotecki4e
The website for this book is a great source for supplementary physical health information for both students and instructors. Visit **go.jblearning.com/kotecki4e** to find a variety of useful tools for learning, thinking, and teaching.

What marvels there are in so small a creature.
Antonie Van Leeuwenhoek

Introduction

Many young people away at college are out of the family home and away from parental supervision for the first time in their lives and may choose to explore their newfound freedom with high-risk behaviors. One such high-risk behavior can be engaging in potentially unsafe sexual situations. Conceivably that is why sexually transmitted infection (STI) rates are so much higher among teenagers and young adults than they are with any other age group. According to the Centers for Disease Control and Prevention (CDC), 19 million new cases of STIs occur every year, half of them being among 15–24 year olds (CDC, 2012b). In fact, one in four college students today will contract some kind of STI during their time at school. Furthermore, 80 percent of individuals with an STI experience no noticeable symptoms, so they or their partner could be transmitting an infection without even knowing it. Although treatment is available for all STIs, not all are curable. If you choose to be sexually active, it is important to know your risks for STIs. Being knowledgeable about the infectious disease process is a start to preventing STIs.

Understanding Infectious Diseases

A **pathogen** or infectious agent is a biological agent that causes disease or illness to its host. Because of their small size, pathogens are sometimes called microorganisms or microbes. Of the many microbes found in nature, only a relatively small proportion cause disease in humans. There are five major types of pathogenic microbes: bacteria, viruses, fungi, protozoa, and helminths. In addition, a new class of infectious agents, the prions, has recently been recognized. An **infection** results when a pathogen invades and begins growing within a host. **Infectious disease** results only if and when, as a consequence of the invasion and growth of a pathogen, tissue function is impaired. To understand how to prevent infectious disease we must first understand how it is spread. The **chain of infection** is a way of describing how disease is transmitted from one living organism to another.

Chain of Infection

The six links in the chain of infection are the pathogen or causative agent, reservoir, portals of exit, modes of transmission, portals of entry, and a new or susceptible host (**FIGURE 16.1**). The movement of a pathogenic agent through the various links explains how diseases spread. If one of the links in the chain is broken, the spread of infection cannot take place.

Pathogen

Link one is that the pathogen must be present. A few characteristics influence when a pathogen will be transmitted to a host, whether it will produce disease, the severity of the disease, and the outcome of the infection. **Infectivity** refers to the ability of a pathogen to establish an infection or the minimum number of infectious particles to cause disease. For example, the infectivity of tuberculosis is low and the infectivity of smallpox is high. **Pathogenicity** refers to the ability of a microbe to induce disease. Because the smallpox virus can produce disease fairly easily, it is considered to have high pathogenicity. **Virulence** refers to the seriousness or severity of the disease. HIV, which causes AIDS, produces a much more serious infection than the common cold. Through mutation, some pathogenic agents can become more virulent. For example, recent research suggests that HIV is becoming more virulent (Herbeck et al., 2012).

A pathogen or infectious agent is a biological agent that causes disease or illness to its host.

Pathogen A biological agent that causes disease or illness to its host; also known as an *infectious agent*

Infection Results when a pathogen invades and begins growing within a host.

Infectious disease Results only if and when, as a consequence of the invasion and growth of a pathogen, tissue function is impaired; the consequence of impaired tissue function.

Chain of infection Describes how disease is transmitted from one living organism to another.

Infectivity The ability of a pathogen to establish an infection or the minimum number of infectious particles to cause disease.

Pathogenicity The ability of microbe to induce disease.

Virulence The seriousness or severity of the disease.

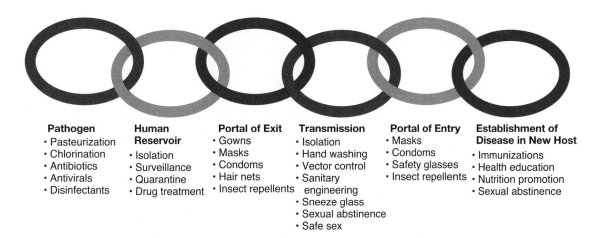

Pathogen
- Pasteurization
- Chlorination
- Antibiotics
- Antivirals
- Disinfectants

Human Reservoir
- Isolation
- Surveillance
- Quarantine
- Drug treatment

Portal of Exit
- Gowns
- Masks
- Condoms
- Hair nets
- Insect repellents

Transmission
- Isolation
- Hand washing
- Vector control
- Sanitary engineering
- Sneeze glass
- Sexual abstinence
- Safe sex

Portal of Entry
- Masks
- Condoms
- Safety glasses
- Insect repellents

Establishment of Disease in New Host
- Immunizations
- Health education
- Nutrition promotion
- Sexual abstinence

FIGURE 16.1 **Chain of Infection.** Chain of infection model showing disease prevention and control strategies.

Reservoir

The principal habitat where a specific infectious agent lives and multiplies and from which it may spread to cause disease is called the **reservoir**. The bodies of people already infected are the most common reservoir for many infections. Diseases for which the reservoir resides in animals are called **zoonoses**. Nonliving things like water, food, and soil can also be reservoirs for infectious agents, but they are called **vehicles** (not infected hosts) because they are not alive.

Portals of Exit

For pathogenic agents to cause diseases they must leave their reservoirs. This will include any body opening on an infected person, such as mouth, nose, eyes, mucus membranes, and an open wound of the skin (**FIGURE 16.2**). **Portals of exit** vary from disease to disease. Natural portals of exit and diseases that use them are the respiratory tract (cold and flu), the urogenital tract (STIs like gonorrhea, syphilis, herpes, and HIV), and the digestive tract (hepatitis A or staphylococcal food poisoning).

Transmission

This link is the mechanism by which an infectious agent is spread through the environment to another person. The two principle methods are direct transmission and indirect transmission. **Direct transmission** implies the immediate transfer of the disease agent between the infected and susceptible individuals by direct contact such as touching, kissing, sexual intercourse, or direct droplet spread by sneezing, coughing, or spitting from a distance of one meter or less. **Indirect transmission** is when infectious agents travel by means of nonhuman materials and are of three types—airborne, vector-borne, or vehicle-borne. In airborne transmission, the agent is carried from the source to the host suspended in air particles. With vector-borne diseases, a live carrier, usually an arthropod such as mosquitos, fleas, or ticks, transmits the agent indirectly. Vehicle-borne diseases are carried by inanimate objects, such as food or water, blood, or items like handkerchiefs, or from sharing cups, water bottles, eating utensils, and toothbrushes.

Portals of Entry

Pathogens can enter the body at sites called **portals of entry** (refer to Figure 16.2). As with portals of exit, there are three primary portals of entry that allow pathogenic agents to enter the bodies of uninfected people. These are the respiratory system, the digestive system, and the reproductive system. The most common site of

Reservoir Principal habitat where a specific infectious agent lives and multiplies and from which it may spread to cause disease.

Zoonoses Diseases for which the reservoir resides in animals

Vehicles Nonliving things like water, food, and soil can also be reservoirs for infectious agents.

Portals of exit Any body opening on an infected person that allows a pathogenic agent to leave their reservoir such as mouth, nose, eyes, mucus membranes, and an open wound of the skin.

Direct transmission Immediate transfer of the disease agent between the infected and susceptible individuals by direct contact such as touching, kissing, sexual intercourse, or by direct droplet spread by sneezing, coughing, or spitting from a distance of one meter or less.

Indirect transmission Travel of infectious agents by means of nonhuman materials and are of three types—airborne, vehicleborne, or vectorborne.

Portals of entry How pathogens enter the body.

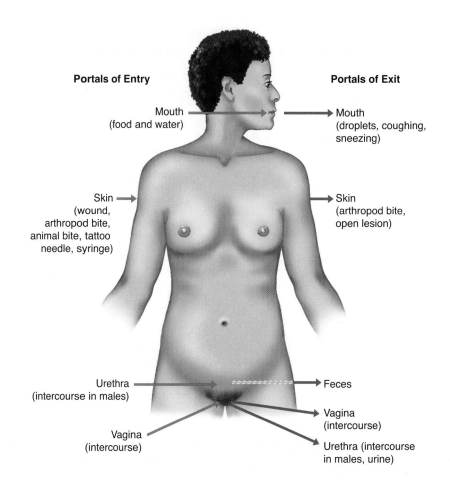

Portals of Entry

Mouth
(food and water)

Skin
(wound,
arthropod bite,
animal bite, tattoo
needle, syringe)

Urethra
(intercourse in males)

Vagina
(intercourse)

Portals of Exit

Mouth
(droplets, coughing,
sneezing)

Skin
(arthropod bite,
open lesion)

Feces

Vagina
(intercourse)

Urethra (intercourse
in males, urine)

FIGURE 16.2 **Portals of Entry and Portals of Exit.**

entry for STIs is the urethra in males and the vagina in females, but the throat and the rectum may also provide entry.

A New Host

A new or susceptible **host** is an uninfected person who can become infected. Different individuals are not equally susceptible to infection, for a variety of reasons. Some factors arise from outside the individual—for example, poor personal hygiene, or poor control of reservoirs of infection in the environment. Factors such as this increase the *exposure* of susceptible hosts to infectious agents, which makes the disease more likely to develop. Some factors arise from inside the individual—for example, not being vaccinated; poor nutritional status; diseases like HIV/AIDS, which suppress immunity; and poorly developed or immature immunity.

Understanding the chain of infection is important in order to identify accessible targets for control strategies (refer to Figure 16.1). For example, direct person-to-person transmission may be inhibited by proper hygiene and sanitary conditions as well as education. Infection by a pathogen or development of a pathogen within a host may be prevented by vaccination. Finally, drugs may be used to prevent infection or suppress the disease process.

The Body's Defense Mechanisms

The human body has two separate general **defense mechanisms** for preventing infectious diseases (**FIGURE 16.3**). Some of these mechanisms are referred to as *nonspecific*

> **Host** An uninfected person who can become infected.
>
> **Defense mechanisms** The body's primary defense against infectious disease.

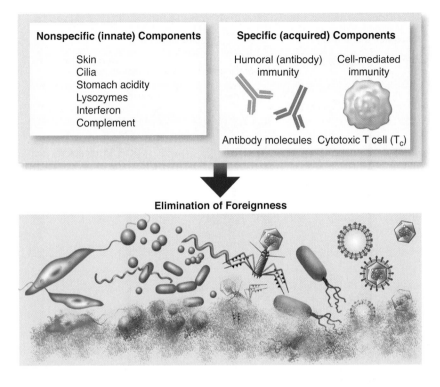

Nonspecific (innate) Components

Skin
Cilia
Stomach acidity
Lysozymes
Interferon
Complement

Specific (acquired) Components

Humoral (antibody) immunity   Cell-mediated immunity

Antibody molecules   Cytotoxic T cell (T_c)

Elimination of Foreignness

FIGURE 16.3 Nonspecific and specific components of the immune system protect against foreignness.

defenses because they operate against a wide range of pathogens. Other mechanisms are referred to as *specific defenses* because they target particular pathogens and pathogen-infected cells.

Nonspecific Mechanisms

Nonspecific mechanisms are the body's primary defense against disease. One of the most powerful barriers between you and pathogens is your skin. Your skin protects you from infection by making a barrier that bacteria, viruses, and other infectious agents can't get through. Other ways skin protects you from disease include its role in alerting the immune system to the presence of harmful organisms, producing and excreting antibacterial substances, and supporting the growth of healthy bacteria. Another anatomical barrier is the nasal passages of the respiratory system. The nasal passages are lined with specialized cells that produce mucus, a sticky, thick, moist fluid that helps filter the air. Filtering prevents airborne bacteria, viruses, and other potentially disease-causing particles from entering the lungs, where they may cause infection. Other natural openings also are protected by a variety of physiological deterrents. For example, tears continually flush debris from the eyes.

Specific Mechanisms

When these nonspecific mechanisms fail, the body initiates a second, specific line of defense. This specific immune response enables the body to target particular pathogens and pathogen-infected cells for destruction via the immune system. Your immune system is composed of different cells, tissues, and organs that work in tandem with each other to eliminate the pathogens inside you. The cells that are directly involved in the process of immune response are the white blood cells, also known as leukocytes. Some white blood cells respond to a broad range of foreign invaders and attack and destroy them, in what is called a *nonspecific response*

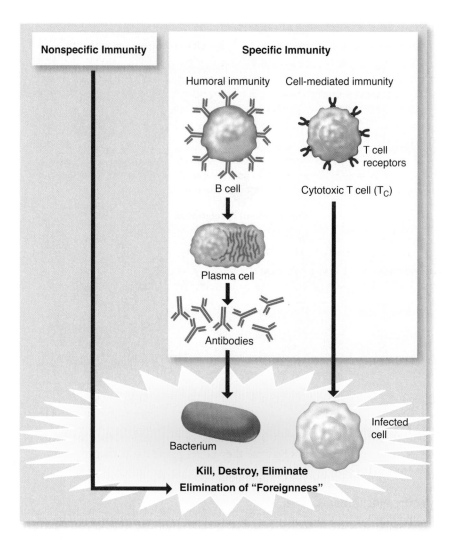

FIGURE 16.4 **Nonspecific and specific immunity.**

(FIGURE 16.4). Other white blood cells mount a *specific response* in which they recognize and attack specific pathogens. These white blood cells are subdivided further into two major types: the B cells and the T cells. Both B cells and T cells carry customized molecules that allow them to recognize and respond to their specific targets (refer to Figure 16.4).

Immunization

Immunization is the process whereby a person is made immune or resistant to an infectious disease, typically by the administration of a vaccine. Vaccines stimulate the body's own immune system to protect the person against subsequent infection or disease. Vaccines prevent disease in the people who receive them and protect those who come into contact with unvaccinated individuals. Vaccines help prevent infectious diseases and save lives. Vaccines are responsible for the control of many infectious diseases that were once common. Several STIs can be effectively prevented through pre-exposure vaccination with widely available vaccines, including hepatitis A, hepatitis B, and human papillomavirus.

Sexually Transmitted Infections

Sexually transmitted infections (STIs) are spread primarily through person-to-person contact. STI, rather than sexually transmitted disease (STD), is a slightly more precise term because the infection comes first and is what needs to be prevented. Furthermore, the word "disease," as in STD, implies a clear medical problem, with some obvious symptom. But many of the most common STIs have no signs or symptoms in infected women and men, or they have mild signs and symptoms that are easily overlooked. So the sexually transmitted virus or bacteria can be described as creating infection, which may or may not result in a disease.

There are more than 25 different infectious bacteria, viruses, and parasites that are transmitted through sexual contact (TABLE 16.1). Many STIs are spread through infected body fluids, such as semen, pre-cum fluids, vaginal secretions, and blood. They also can be spread through contact with infected skin or mucous membranes, such as sores in the mouth. The most common conditions they cause are trichomoniasis, genital warts, chlamydia, herpes, gonorrhea, hepatitis B, syphilis, and HIV/AIDS (TABLE 16.2). These conditions can include a range of symp-

> **Sexually transmitted infection (STI)** An infection that is spread primarily through person-to-person sexual contact.

Sexually transmitted infections are infections that are spread primarily through person-to-person sexual contact.

TABLE 16.1	**Common Sexually Transmitted Infections**

Infectious Agent	STI	Symptoms	Treatment
Human immunodeficiency virus	HIV/AIDS	Flulike symptoms followed by any of a number of diseases characteristic of immunodeficiency	HIV antiretroviral drug treatment; opportunistic infections can be treated to some degree
Human papillomavirus	Genital warts	Usually occur within 1 to 3 months: small, dry growths on the genitals, anus, cervix, and possibly mouth	Podofilox, Sinecathechins, and Imiquimod to treat warts; vaccination for HPV
Hepatitis virus	Hepatitis B	Low-grade fever, fatigue, headaches, loss of appetite, nausea, dark urine, jaundice	Interferon, Lamivudine, Adefovir dipivoxil, Baraclude; vaccination for hepatitis B
Herpes simplex virus	Genital herpes	Usually occur within 2 weeks: painful blisters on site(s) of infection (genitals, anus, cervix); occasionally itching, painful urination, and fever	Antiviral medications such as Zovirax, Famvir, and Valtrex relieve symptoms
Chlamydia trachomatis	Chlamydia	Usually occur within 3 weeks: Infected men have a discharge from the penis and painful urination or defecation; women may have a vaginal discharge but often are asymptomatic	Antibiotics
Neisseria gonnorrhoeae	Gonorrhea	Usually occur within 2 weeks: discharge from the penis, vagina, or anus; painful urination or defecation or intercourse; pain and swelling in the pelvic region; genital and oral infections may be asymptomatic	Antibiotics
Treponema pallidum	Syphilis	Usually occur within 3 weeks: a chancre (painless sore) on the genitals, anus, or mouth: secondary stage, skin rash (if left untreated); tertiary stage includes diseases of several body organs	Antibiotics
Trichomonas vaginalis	Trichomoniasis	Yellowish-green vaginal discharge with an unpleasant odor; vaginal itching; occasionally painful intercourse	Metronidazole
Phthirus pubis	Pubic lice	Usually occur within 5 weeks: intense itching in the genital region; lice may be visible in pubic hair; small white eggs may be visible on pubic hair	A lice-killing shampoo (called pediculicide)
Sarcoptes scabiei	Scabies	Tiny, itchy lesions caused by mites burrowing into the skin	Topical insecticides

TABLE 16.2	Estimated Yearly Number of STIs in the United States

In the United States, an estimated 19 million new cases of STIs are reported each year. This table shows the incidence and prevalence of some of the most common STIs.

STI	Incidence*	Prevalence†
Chlamydia	1,307,893	‡
Gonorrhea	309,341	‡
Syphilis	13,774 (reported)	‡
Herpes (HSV)	‡	45,000,000§
Hepatitis B (HBV)	40,000	800,000 to 1.4 million
Genital warts (HPV)	6,000,000	20,000,000
Trichomoniasis	2,300,000	‡
HIV/AIDS	47,129	1.2 million

* Estimated number of annual new cases.

† Estimated number of people currently infected.

‡ No data available.

§ Nationwide, estimated number of people age 12 or older who have had genital HSV infection.

SOURCE: Data from Centers for Disease Control and Prevention. (2012). Trends in Reportable Sexually Transmitted Diseases in the United States, 2010. Online: http://www.cdc.gov/std/stats10/default.htm./trends.htm.

There are many reasons for the high rates of sexually transmitted infections in the United States.

toms. STIs can be serious, painful, and may have long-term effects, especially if undetected and left untreated.

Of course, STIs are a concern for anyone—male or female. However, if you happen to be female and your goal is to have children, or more children at some point, then be aware that a clean bill of health free from STIs will better help you reach your goal. For example, each year untreated STIs cause infertility in at least 24,000 women in the United States, and untreated syphilis in pregnant women results in infant death in up to 40 percent of cases. In fact, STIs are such a concern when it comes to women's health that the Centers for Disease Control and Prevention [CDC] has released a fact sheet on 10 ways STIs impact women differently from men (TABLE 16.3).

Despite the fact that a great deal of progress has been made in STI preventive efforts over the past couple of decades, the United States continues to have the highest rates of STIs in the industrialized world. More than 19 million new cases of STIs are reported each year in the United States, with almost half of them occurring in people ages 15 to 24, even though they account for only one-fourth of the sexually active population (CDC, 2012b). In fact, one in two sexually active youth will have contracted an STI by the age of 24. There are many reasons for the high rates of STIs.

Failure to Inform

From a personal and moral responsibility perspective, if a person knows that he or she is infected with an STI, it is that person's duty to inform his or her partner. Does this always occur in reality? No. Although failure to disclose the existence of an STI may result from shame, embarrassment, or dishonesty, sometimes it is because a person truthfully does not know that he or she is infected, either because the individual has no symptoms or because he or she does not recognize the meaning of the symptoms. If a person has an incurable STI, the use of safer sex practices

TABLE 16.3	Ten Ways STDs Impact Women Differently from Men

1. A woman's anatomy can place her at a unique risk for an STD, compared to a man.
- The lining of the vagina is thinner and more delicate than the skin on a penis, so it's easier for bacteria and viruses to penetrate.
- The vagina is a good environment (moist) for bacteria to grow.

2. Women are less likely to have symptoms of common STDs—such as chlamydia and gonorrhea—compared to men.
- If symptoms do occur, they can go away even though the infection may remain.

3. Women are more likely to confuse symptoms of an STD for something else.
- Women often have normal discharge or think that burning/itching is related to a yeast infection.
- Men usually notice symptoms like discharge because it is unusual.

4. Women may not see symptoms as easily as men.
- Genital ulcers (like from herpes or syphilis) can occur in the vagina and may not be easily visible, whereas men may be more likely to notice sores on their penis.

5. STDs can lead to serious health complications and affect a woman's future reproductive plans.
- Untreated STDs can lead to pelvic inflammatory disease, which can result in infertility and ectopic pregnancy.
- Chlamydia (one of the most common STDs) results in few complications in men.

6. Women who are pregnant can pass STDs to their babies.
- Genital herpes, syphilis, and HIV can be passed to babies during pregnancy and at delivery.
- The harmful effects of STDs in babies may include stillbirth (a baby that is born dead), low birth weight (less than five pounds), brain damage, blindness, and deafness.

7. Human papillomavirus (HPV) is the most common sexually transmitted infection in women, and is the main cause of cervical cancer.
- Although HPV is also very common in men, most do not develop serious health problems.

The Good News

8. Women typically see their doctor more often than men do.
- Women should use this time with their doctor as an opportunity to ask for STD testing, and not assume STD testing is part of their annual exam. Although the Pap test screens for cervical cancer, it is not a good test for other types of cancer or STDs.

9. There is a vaccine to prevent HPV, and available treatments for other STDs can prevent serious health consequences, such as infertility, if diagnosed and treated early.

10. There are resources available for women to learn more about actions they can take to protect themselves and their partners from STDs, and where to receive testing and treatment.
- **Health care providers**—A doctor or physician can provide patient-specific information about STD prevention, protection, and tests.
- **1-800-CDC-INFO (232-4636)**—Operators can provide information about local STD testing sites and put callers in touch with trained professionals to answer questions about STDs.
- **http://FindSTDTest.org**—This website provides users with locations for HIV and STD testing and STD vaccines around the United States.
- **http://www.cdc.gov/std**—The CDC's website includes comprehensive information about STDs, including fact sheets on STDs and Pregnancy (http://www.cdc.gov/std/pregnancy) and STDs and Infertility (http://www.cdc.gov/std/infertility).

SOURCE: Reproduced from Centers for Disease Control and Prevention. (April 2011). 10 ways STDs impact woman differently from men. 2011. Online: www.cdc.gov/nchhstp/newsroom/docs/STDs-Women-042011.pdf.

is even more essential. Safer sex practices are things you do to lower your risk not only of getting an STI, but also of transmitting it to another person; these practices are discussed in more detail at the end of the chapter.

Multiple Sexual Partners

In our society, there is a large pool of unmarried, sexually active people because many individuals become active in late adolescence. This group consists of those who delay marriage until their mid- to late 20s and early 30s, or later, and those who are divorced or widowed and have subsequent sexual partners. Twenty percent of unmarried adults report having more than one sexual partner in the previous year. Slightly more than one in four (27 percent) of American college students have more than one sexual partner a year.

False Sense of Security

Condoms help prevent transmission of many STIs, but the use of contraceptive measures tends to decrease the use of condoms. Additionally, the availability of antibiotics to cure many bacterial STIs has made many people less fearful of contracting an STI. They believe that as long as there is a cure for bacterial infections, there is nothing to worry about. However, STIs caused by viruses cannot be cured.

Absence of Signs and Symptoms

Some STIs have very mild or no symptoms, which permits a worsening of the infection and the possibility of unknowingly passing it to others. For example, most women infected with chlamydia have no symptoms and may not know they have it. People infected with the human immunodeficiency virus (HIV) can have mild or no symptoms for years yet still be infectious.

Untreated Conditions

Some individuals lack sufficient knowledge of the signs and symptoms of STIs to know that they are infected. Those who are not accustomed to seeking health care, or who cannot afford it, are less likely to seek treatment for an infection. Furthermore, many individuals with STIs do not comply with treatment regimens. When medications are not taken for the required length of time, an infection may not be completely eradicated even though symptoms may disappear, and people who do not complete treatment may still be infectious.

Impaired Judgment

The use of drugs, including alcohol, can increase the risk of transmitting STIs because people with impaired judgment do not stop to think about using condoms. Also, people in an impaired state may be more likely to have sex with someone they do not know; this also means they know nothing of their partner's sexual and drug history.

Lack of Immunity

Some STI-causing organisms, especially viruses, can escape the body's immune defenses, causing individuals to remain infected and to transmit the infection. This may permit reinfection and it also makes the development of vaccinations difficult to impossible.

Value Judgments

Unlike nearly all other kinds of infections, STIs are associated with sinfulness, dirtiness, condemnation, shame, guilt, and disgust. These negative attitudes keep people from getting checkups, contacting partners when an STI has been diagnosed, and talking to new partners about previous exposures.

Denial

With respect to contracting an STI, many people think "It can't happen to me" or "This person is too nice to have an STI" or "This isn't the type of person who would have an STI." Because there are no vaccinations against the infectious agents that cause sexually transmitted infections, the only way to prevent them is for sexually active individuals who are not in monogamous (lifelong single-partner) sexual relationships to assume responsibility for protecting themselves and their partners. This means becoming aware of the signs and symptoms of the common STIs and seeking treatment when such signs occur. It means that sexually active people who have more than one partner within a year should obtain periodic (about every 6 months) STI checkups. It also means knowing about and practicing safer sex.

Dealing directly and responsibly with STIs is not always easy. However, we owe it to ourselves and the people we care about to be responsible. Some of these infections may lead to major illness, particularly for women and their unborn babies. STIs can cause pelvic inflammatory disease, tubal pregnancy, sterility, certain types of cancer, or blindness. Some last a lifetime. There are more than 65 million people living with incurable STIs in the United States (CDC, 2012b). A few can be fatal. AIDS, genital warts, herpes, syphilis, and hepatitis have all been known to contribute to conditions that cause death.

Sexually Transmitted Viral Infections

STIs transmitted by viruses include HIV, herpes, human papillomavirus (HPV; genital warts), and hepatitis B. These STIs are the most difficult to eradicate because they have no cure. However, many of their symptoms can be alleviated with treatment. Additionally, there are vaccines available to help prevent both HPV and hepatitis B.

HIV Infection and AIDS

The acquired immunodeficiency syndrome (AIDS) was first recognized in 1981 and has since become a major worldwide pandemic. AIDS is caused by the **human immunodeficiency virus (HIV)**. By leading to the destruction or functional impairment of cells of the immune system, notably CD4+ T cells, HIV progressively destroys the body's ability to fight infections and certain cancers. An HIV-infected person is diagnosed with AIDS when his or her immune system is seriously compromised and manifestations of HIV infection are severe. The CDC currently defines AIDS in an adult or adolescent age 13 years or older as the presence of one of 26 conditions indicative of severe immunosuppression associated with HIV infection, such as *Pneumocystis carinii* pneumonia (PCP), a condition extraordinarily rare in people without HIV infection (CDC, 1999). Most other AIDS-defining conditions are also opportunistic infections that rarely cause harm in healthy individuals. A diagnosis of AIDS also is given to HIV-infected individuals when their CD4+ T-cell count falls below 200 cells per cubic millimeter (mm^3) of blood. Healthy adults usually have CD4+ T-cell counts of 600 to 1500 cells per mm^3 of blood. In HIV-infected children younger than 13 years, the CDC definition of AIDS is similar to that in adolescents and adults, except for the addition of certain infections commonly seen in pediatric patients with HIV (CDC, 2011b).

At the end of 2010, an estimated 1.2 million persons in the United States were living with diagnosed and undiagnosed HIV infection (CDC, 2012a). Approximately 47,000 newly diagnosed HIV infections occurred in the United States in 2010, with nearly 79 percent of them among men. Of the new infections, among males, approximately 77 percent were from male-to-male sexual contact and 12 percent from heterosexual contact (**FIGURE 16.5**). Of the new infections

Human immunodeficiency virus (HIV) The virus that causes AIDS; it causes a defect in the body's immune system by invading and then multiplying within the white blood cells.

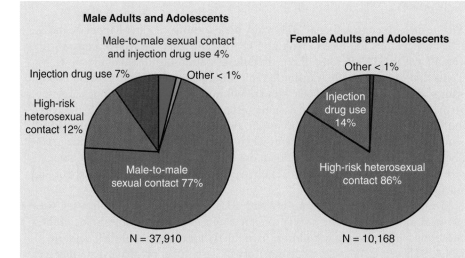

FIGURE 16.5 Exposure Categories of Adults and Adolescents Who Received Diagnosis of HIV/AIDS, 2010. SOURCE: Reproduced from Centers for Disease Control and Prevention. (2012). HIV/AIDS in the United States. Online: http://www.cdc.gov/hiv/resources/factsheets/us.htm.

among females, 86 percent were from high-risk heterosexual contact and 14 percent from injection drug use. Minority groups in the United States have also been disproportionately affected by the epidemic. Blacks represent approximately 14 percent of the U.S. population, but accounted for 44 percent of new infections in 2010. The CDC estimates that nearly 18,000 people with AIDS died in 2010, and nearly 620,000 people with AIDS have died since the epidemic began in the early 1980s.

Methods of Transmission

HIV is transmitted exclusively via blood, semen (which contains small amounts of blood), and vaginal fluids. The virus is not transmitted by touching the skin or clothes of an infected person, by saliva, by shared toilets, or by air, food, or water that has been touched by an infected person. Indeed, hardly any HIV transmission has been found among family members who live in intimate contact with HIV-infected hemophiliacs who received the virus from HIV-contaminated blood products used to treat their hereditary bleeding disorder.

HIV is a **retrovirus**, which means that once it gains entry to a cell it incorporates itself into the host cell's DNA. This allows HIV to manufacture many copies of itself, which eventually infect neighboring cells. Because HIV incorporates itself into host cells, it cannot be eliminated from an infected person's body. HIV infections are lifelong.

Within a few weeks of becoming infected with HIV, individuals usually experience flu-like symptoms from which they eventually recover. Their immune systems are still intact, and they produce copious antibodies to HIV. The mounting of an immune response in the early phases of an HIV infection provides the basis for HIV testing. Nearly all of the tests for HIV infection detect antibodies to HIV. A positive result ("seropositive") indicates that a person has been exposed to sufficient quantities of HIV particles to mount an immune response. The first stage of HIV infection is known as silent infection.

Some HIV-infected individuals will progress to the second stage of infection, symptomatic infection. The first signs of AIDS are usually mononucleosis-like symptoms (swollen lymph glands, fever, night sweats) and possibly headaches and impaired mental functioning caused by HIV infection of the brain. As the disease progresses, individuals often suffer weight loss, infections on the skin (shingles) or the throat ("thrush"), and one or more opportunistic infections, perhaps including cancer.

Retrovirus A type of virus (such as the one that causes AIDS) that can invade cells and integrate its own genetic information into chromosomes.

Because there is now no way to rid the body of HIV and hence cure AIDS, the best treatment available to infected individuals is to treat the opportunistic infections that result from immune suppression. In addition, some attempts have been made to slow the replication of the virus. Because many viral diseases have been conquered by vaccination, much effort has gone into developing vaccines against HIV, so far without success. The only effective way to control the spread of AIDS is to prevent the transfer of HIV from person to person. This is accomplished by using condoms, reducing exposure to infected individuals, and avoiding casual sex.

Genital Herpes

Genital herpes is caused by the herpes simplex virus, or HSV. Various strains of HSV can cause cold sores on the mouth ("fever blisters") (**FIGURE 16.6**), skin rashes, mononucleosis, and lesions on the penis, vagina, or rectum. Each year up to 500,000 adults acquire a genital herpes infection (CDC, 2012b). Up to 8 out of 10 American adults have oral herpes, and about 1 out of 4 American adults have genital herpes. Millions of people do not know they have herpes because they never had, or noticed, the herpes symptoms.

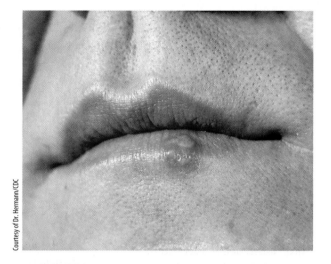

Courtesy of Dr. Hermann/CDC

FIGURE 16.6 **Herpes.** A cold sore is common among people infected by herpes simplex virus.

Genital herpes An infection caused by the herpes simplex virus, or HSV.

Genital herpes infections are caused most frequently by the viral strain HSV-2. Oral herpes is caused most frequently by HSV-1. However, both HSV-2 and HSV-1 can cause genital and oral infections with virtually identical symptoms. Thus, people with oral herpes can transmit the infection to partners via oral sex. Once a person has been infected, oral HSV-1 infections tend to recur much more frequently than do oral HSV-2 infections. Conversely, genital HSV-2 infections tend to recur more frequently than genital HSV-1 infections. Oral herpes can occur without sexual contact; however, genital herpes cannot occur without some form of sexual contact: vaginal, anal, or oral or through masturbation.

A herpes lesion on the genitals usually appears within 2 to 20 days after contact with the virus. Transmission of the virus via bed linen, clothing, towels, toilet seats, and hot tubs is highly unlikely. The major symptoms of a genital herpes infection are the presence of one or more blisters, which eventually break to become wet, painful sores that last about 2 or 3 weeks; fever; and occasionally pain in the lower abdomen. Eventually, these initial symptoms disappear, but the herpes virus remains dormant in certain of the body's nerve cells, permitting periodic recurrences of the symptoms, called "flare-ups," at or near the site(s) of the initial infection. Stress, anxiety, improper nutrition, sunlight, and skin irritation can bring on flare-ups.

There is no cure for herpes. Infected individuals remain so for life. Antiviral medications, such as Zovirax (acyclovir), Famvir (famciclovir), and Valtrex (valacyclovir hydrochloride), can minimize the duration and severity of the symptoms of an initial infection or a flare-up.

Herpes is extremely contagious when a sore is present. People with open lesions should avoid sex with others until the lesions disappear. Even if no sore is present, transmission is possible, although much less likely, through the "shedding" of viral particles from the skin.

Because the herpes virus remains in the body, and because flare-ups are a persistent possibility, some people believe that infected persons can never be sexually active. This is not true. People with herpes can learn to manage the condition. In many instances, after one or two episodes, they can recognize an oncoming flare-up because they get a tingling sensation, itching, pain, or numbness at the site of the initial infection. This can be a signal to refrain from sexual contact. If used appropriately, this signal can protect against the spread of herpes.

Because genital herpes is associated with a risk of cervical cancer, women with herpes are especially urged to have annual Pap smears to ascertain the condition of the vagina and cervix.

Genital Warts

Genital warts (condylomata acuminata) are hard, cauliflower-like growths that appear in men on the penis, in women on the external genitals and cervix, and in both sexes in the anal region (**FIGURE 16.7**). Warts are caused by several of the approximately 60 varieties of **human papillomavirus (HPV)**. When HPV infects skin cells and cells of the genital tract, it causes them to multiply, thus forming the wart. Genital warts usually appear about 3 months after contact with an infected person. They can be removed by coating the wart with a liquid containing podophyllin, which dries the wart. In severe cases, wart removal is accomplished by freezing the warts with liquid nitrogen or removing them with laser surgery.

Infection with many varieties of HPV is often more of a nuisance than it is dangerous. However, HPV types 16, 18, 31, 33, and 35 are linked to cervical cancer. These high-risk HPVs may also be linked to increased risk of cancers of the vulva, anus, and bladder.

In June 2006, the first vaccine to prevent four major subtypes of cervical genital HPV was licensed for use in the United States. The vaccine is called Gardasil, and it protects women against HPV subtypes 6 and 11, which cause 90 percent of genital warts, and 16 and 18, which together cause 70 percent of cervical cancers in American women. The vaccine is claimed to be between 95 and 100 percent effective. It is approved for use in the United States for girls and women aged 9 to 26 years. The vaccine may be less effective in women who are already sexually active because they may have already been infected with HPV. In October 2009, the U.S. Food and Drug Administration approved use of the vaccine Gardasil for the prevention of genital warts due to HPV types 6 and 11 in boys and men ages 9 through 26.

Hepatitis B

Hepatitis B is a disease of the liver caused by the **hepatitis B virus** (HBV). HBV is transmitted sexually and in blood, similar to HIV transmission, whereas other types of hepatitis are transmitted in fecally contaminated food. HBV is more easily transmitted than HIV is, and it is estimated that between 800,000 and

Genital warts Hard, cauliflower-like growths that appear in men on the penis, in women on the external genitals and cervix, and in both sexes in the anal region.

Human papillomavirus (HPV) Infection of the skin cells and cells of the genital tract that causes them to multiply, thus forming warts. There are approximately 60 varieties of HPV that cause warts.

Hepatitis B virus A virus that is transmitted sexually and in blood, similar to HIV transmission.

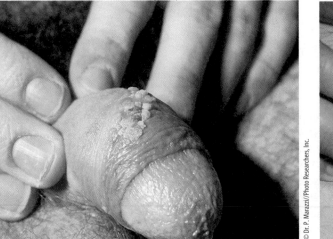
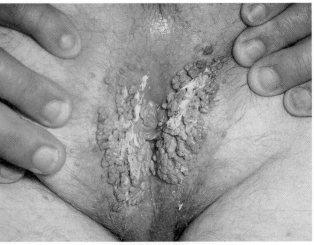

(A)   (B)

FIGURE 16.7 **Genital Warts.** These warts can appear on the penis (A) or in the vaginal area (B).

1.4 million people in the United States are infected with HBV (refer to Table 16.2). You are at increased risk of contracting HBV if you are sexually active, have unsafe sex, have sex with more than one partner, have another STI, work in health care, or share needles. You can also contract HBV if you are exposed to an infected person's blood via cuts or open sores. Although it is very rare in the United States, you can contract HBV through transfusions of infected blood or blood products.

There is no cure for HBV; however, an HBV vaccine is available, and everyone is advised to be vaccinated—especially children, health care workers, and others who are at high risk of exposure (sexually active). The CDC recommends HBV vaccination for infants and young adults before they become sexually active.

Sexually Transmitted Bacterial Infections

STIs transmitted by bacteria include chlamydia, gonorrhea, and syphilis. In contrast to viral STIs, bacterial STIs can be cured with antibiotics. However, if not treated promptly and properly, bacterial infections can have devastating health consequences.

Chlamydia

Chlamydia is caused by the bacterium *Chlamydia trachomatis*, which specifically infests certain cells lining the mucous membranes of the genitals, mouth, anus, and rectum, the conjunctiva of the eyes, and occasionally the lungs. The chlamydial bacteria bind to cell surfaces and induce the host cells to engulf them. After gaining entrance to the cell, these organisms resist a host cell's defenses and eventually "steal" from the host cell the biochemical compounds required for their own survival. The chlamydial organisms use the stolen nutrients to reproduce and multiply, and ultimately the host cells die. In as many as half of all cases, chlamydia occurs simultaneously with gonorrhea.

One reason that chlamydial infections are so prevalent is that infected individuals often have extremely mild or no symptoms. Thus, infected individuals can unknowingly transmit the infection to new sex partners. When symptoms do occur, they include pain during urination in both men and women (dysuria) and a whitish discharge from the penis or vagina. Symptoms generally appear within 7 to 21 days of infection.

An infection caused by chlamydia can be readily treated with antibiotics if diagnosed early. Left untreated, the chlamydial bacteria can multiply and cause inflammation and damage the reproductive organs in both sexes. In men, untreated chlamydia can result in inflammation of the epididymis (**epididymitis**), characterized by pain, swelling, and tenderness in the scrotum and sometimes by mild fever. In women, untreated chlamydia can lead to **pelvic inflammatory disease (PID)**.

Gonorrhea

Gonorrhea, also known as "the clap" or "the drip," is caused by the bacterium *Neisseria gonorrhoeae*. Gonorrheal organisms specifically infect the mucous membranes of the body, most often the genitals, reproductive organs, mouth and throat, anus, and eyes. *N. gonorrhoeae* cannot survive on toilet seats, doorknobs, bed sheets, clothes, or towels. Transmission in adults almost always occurs by genital, oral, or anal sexual contact; infection of the eyes occurs by hand (often through self-infection).

Although the bacteria causing them are quite different, the symptoms of gonorrheal and chlamydial infections are very similar. Like chlamydia, many people infected with gonorrheal organisms do not develop symptoms and their infections go unnoticed. If the infection progresses, men may develop epididymitis and

Chlamydia An infection caused by the bacterium *Chlamydia trachomatis*, which specifically infests certain cells lining the mucous membranes of the genitals, mouth, anus, and rectum.

Epididymitis Inflammation of the epididymis (structure that connects the vas deferens and the testes).

Pelvic inflammatory disease (PID) Infection of the female reproductive organs; specifically, the uterus, fallopian tubes, and pelvic cavity.

Gonorrhea Sexually transmitted infection caused by the bacterium *Neisseria gonorrhoeae*.

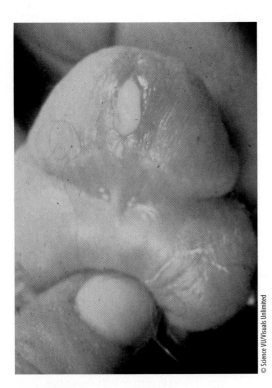

© Science VU/Visuals Unlimited

FIGURE 16.8 **Pus-Containing Discharge from the Penis as a Result of Gonorrhea.**

Syphilis Sexually transmitted infection caused by spirochete bacteria (*Treponema pallidum*).

Chancre The primary lesion of syphilis, which appears as a hard, painless sore or ulcer, often on the penis or vaginal tissue; pronounced "shanker."

women may develop infections of the uterus, fallopian tubes, and pelvic region. Such infections may cause sterility. When symptoms appear, they include painful urination in both sexes and a yellowish discharge from the penis or vagina (FIGURE 16.8). Occasionally, there is pain in the groin, testes, or lower abdomen. The first symptoms of gonorrhea usually appear within 7 to 10 days of exposure.

Gonorrhea can be treated with antibiotics. However, new antibiotic-resistant strains of the organism are constantly evolving. In nearly half of all cases of gonorrhea, chlamydia also is present. Individuals undergoing diagnosis for gonorrhea should also be tested for chlamydia.

Syphilis

Syphilis is caused by a spiral-shaped bacterium called *Treponema pallidum*. These organisms are transmitted from person to person through genital, oral, and anal contact, and also can be acquired from blood. Syphilis can also be transmitted from a mother to her unborn fetus, perhaps as early as the 9th week of pregnancy.

The first noticeable sign of syphilis is a painless open sore called a **chancre** (pronounced "shanker"), which can appear any time between the first week and third month after infection (FIGURE 16.9). If the infection is not treated within that period, the chancre will heal and the disease will enter a secondary stage, characterized by a skin rash, hair loss, and the appearance of round, flat-topped growths on most areas of the body. Left untreated, the signs of the secondary stage also disappear, and the infection enters a symptomless (latency) period during which the syphilis organisms multiply in many other regions of the body. In the final, tertiary stage, the disease damages vital organs, such as the heart or brain, causing severe symptoms and leading to death. Syphilis can be treated with antibiotics at any stage of the infection.

Other Sexually Transmitted Infections

Other STIs include *Trichomoniasis vaginalis*, an infection caused by a parasitic protozoan; pubic lice, an infection caused by parasites; and scabies, an infection caused by tiny mites.

FIGURE 16.9 **A Syphilitic Chancre of the Penis.** These painless sores can occur on the genital or anal areas, lips, tongue, breast, or fingers. They are characteristic of the first stage of syphilis.

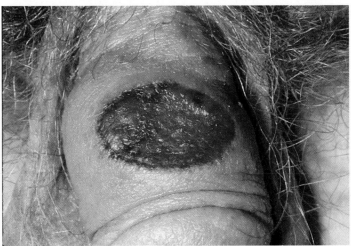

© Biophoto Associates/Photo Researchers, Inc.

Trichomonas Vaginalis

Trichomonas vaginalis is a one-celled organism that burrows under the vaginal mucosa to cause trichomonas, or trick. Symptoms tend to occur only in women (vaginal itching and a cheesy, odorous discharge from the vagina), but the organisms can survive in the urethra of the penis and under the penile foreskin. A man who harbors these organisms can infect other partners or even reinfect the partner who transmitted the organisms to him. Medications can eliminate these infections, and it is essential for both partners to undergo treatment.

Pubic Lice

Pubic lice (*Phthirus pubis*), also known as "crabs," are barely visible insects that live on hair shafts primarily in the genital-rectal region and occasionally on hair in the armpits, beard, and eyelashes. The organisms' claws are specifically adapted for grasping hairs with the diameter of pubic and axillary hair, which differs in diameter from the shafts of scalp hair. Thus, pubic lice are not usually found on the head. (Scalp hair is the ecological niche of the head louse, *Pediculus humanus capitis*.)

Lice feed on blood taken from tiny blood vessels in the skin, which they pierce with their mouths. Some people are sensitive to the bites and may experience itching, which is often the main symptom of infestation. The lice can also be seen; they look like small freckles. The eggs of lice are enclosed in small white pods (called "nits"), which attach to hair shafts. The presence of nits is also a sign of infestation.

Transfer of lice is via physical—usually sexual—contact. They can also be transmitted via contact with objects on which eggs might have been laid, such as towels, bed linens, and clothes. An infestation of pubic lice can be eliminated by washing the pubic hair with liquids or shampoos containing agents that specifically kill lice (pyrethrins, piperonyl butoxide, and gamma benzene hydrochloride). All of an infected person's clothes, towels, and bed linens should also be washed with cleaning agents made specifically for killing lice.

Scabies

Scabies is an infestation of certain regions of the skin by extremely small (invisible to the naked eye) mites, *Sarcoptes scabiei*. The mites burrow into the skin, where they live and lay eggs. The tiny lesions produced by the mites often cause intense itching, which is the major sign of a scabies infection. The mites produce tiny burrows across skin lines, which often go unnoticed. Occasionally, an infestation produces small round nodules. The mites tend to live in the webs between the fingers, on the sides of fingers, and on the wrists, elbows, breasts, abdomen, penis, and buttocks. Rarely do mites live on the face, neck, upper back, palms, or soles.

Scabies can be transmitted both sexually and nonsexually. All that is required is close personal contact. The itching and physical symptoms often take several weeks to appear. Scabies can be treated with topical agents that kill the mites and their eggs.

Preventing Sexually Transmitted Infections

College students choose to abstain from sexual activity—the most effective behavior for eliminating the risk of contracting a STI—for many reasons including waiting for the right partner, waiting until they are ready for a sexual relationship, and wanting to focus on school. However, for others, abstinence is not acceptable. Next in line is a long-term monogamous sexual relationship with an uninfected partner. However, monogamy is not fail-safe because some seemingly trustworthy

> **Trichomonas vaginalis** A protozoan that causes trichomoniasis; symptoms of infection include a foul-smelling, foamy-white or yellow-green discharge that irritates the vagina.
>
> **Pubic lice** Small insects that live in hair in the genital–rectal region.
>
> **Scabies** Infestation of the skin by microscopic mites (insects).

Abstinence from sexual activity is the most effective behavior for eliminating your risk of contracting a sexually transmitted infection.

sexual partners have been known to have a sexual relationship with others. If a person is unwilling or unable to maintain a monogamous relationship, limiting the number of partners reduces the chances of contracting an STI. Your STI risk is higher if you have had many sex partners, have had sex with someone who has had many partners, or have had sex without using condoms.

With regard to the partners you have, you can lower your risk by delaying having sex with them until you know them well enough to assess their risk as sexual partners. This includes knowing your partner's sexual history, including all high-risk activities in which your partner may have engaged. Often this kind of information is difficult to gain early in a relationship because exchanging information about sexual histories requires a level of trust that takes some time to develop. Until you have this knowledge, it is important to protect yourself by using a condom. All men and women who are sexually active should accept as standard practice the use of condoms with new partners, even if some other form of contraceptive is being used.

Using Latex Condoms

The condom's primary purpose is to keep bodily fluids of different people separate. This helps prevent STIs that are transmitted mainly through contact with sexual fluids, such as semen and vaginal lubricant. Latex (a synthetic form of rubber) condoms can protect you during contact between the penis, mouth, vagina, or rectum. The pores of a latex condom are too small for some organisms that cause STIs to penetrate. Condom use substantially reduces your risk for contracting the following STIs: HIV infection, HSV infection, hepatitis B, gonorrhea, and chlamydial infection (CDC, 2011a).

According to the Centers for Disease Control and Prevention, the failure of condoms to protect against STI/HIV transmission usually results from inconsistent or incorrect use rather than product failure (CDC, 2011a). Inconsistent or nonuse can lead to STI acquisition because transmission can occur with a single sex act with an infected partner. Incorrect use diminishes the protective effect of condoms by leading to breakage, slippage, or leakage. Incorrect use more commonly entails a failure to use condoms throughout the entire sex act, from start (of sexual contact) to finish (after ejaculation). The Centers for Disease Control and Prevention (2011a) provides the following directions for consistent and correct condom use (see also **FIGURE 16.10**).

Consistent Use

- Use a new condom for every act of vaginal, anal, and oral sex—throughout the entire sex act (from start to finish).

Correct Use

- Before any genital contact, put the condom on the tip of the erect penis with the rolled side out.
- If the condom does not have a reservoir tip, pinch the tip enough to leave a half-inch space for semen to collect. While holding the tip, unroll the condom all the way to the base of the erect penis.
- After ejaculation and before the penis gets soft, grip the rim of the condom and carefully withdraw. Then, gently pull the condom off the penis, making sure that semen doesn't spill out.
- Wrap the condom in a tissue and throw it in the trash where others won't handle it.
- If you feel the condom break at any point during sexual activity, stop immediately, withdraw, remove the broken condom, and put on a new condom.

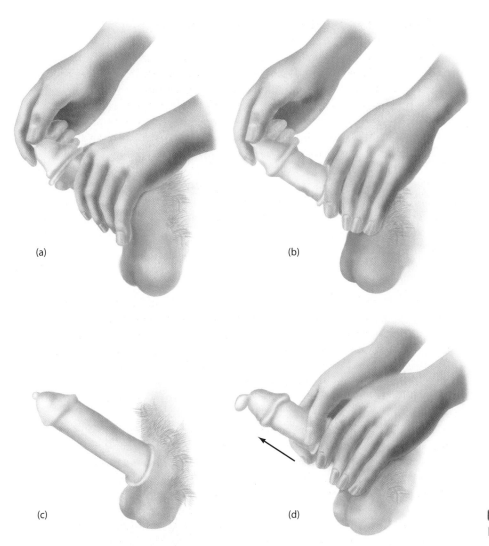

(a)

(b)

(c)

(d)

FIGURE 16.10 **How to Put on and Remove a Condom.**

- Ensure that adequate lubrication is used during vaginal and anal sex, which might require water-based lubricants. Oil-based lubricants (e.g., petroleum jelly, shortening, mineral oil, massage oils, body lotions, cooking oil) should not be used because they can weaken latex, causing breakage.

Practicing Safer Sex

Safer sex is a general term used to describe methods for reducing the chance that you will contract or spread STIs. Using a condom every time you have sexual intercourse is an example of safer sex. It is important to realize that it is possible to contract an STI even without penetrative sex (TABLE 16.4). Safer sex also involves talking with your partner (FIGURE 16.11). The stigma associated with STIs is a great hindrance to prevention efforts. Viewing STIs in moral terms—that is, associating them with dirtiness and immorality—makes people reluctant to think and talk about them.

Judgmental attitudes also make talking about STIs difficult. To have to tell a partner that you have an STI, or even to say that you once had an infection and are now perfectly OK, can bring feelings of guilt and shame, which can lead to avoiding the discussion altogether. Similarly, to ask about a partner's previous STIs may be interpreted as an accusation that the person is "loose" or immoral. To avoid feeling embarrassed or avoid the risk of offending a sexual partner, people are

Safer sex is a general term used to describe methods for reducing the chance that you will contract or spread sexually transmitted infections.

Safer sex General term used to describe methods for reducing the chance that you will contract or spread sexually transmitted infections.

TABLE 16.4	Relative STI Risk of Sexual Activities

Dry Closed-Mouth Kissing, Hugging, Massage, Self-Masturbation

Except for kissing if you come into contact with an infected herpes sore.

Except for massage if lice and scabies are present.

Safer Sex Techniques: Avoid kissing when open cuts or sores are present in the mouth.

Deep French Kissing

A few STIs may be present in the mouth/throat of infected persons.

Safer Sex Techniques: Kiss with the mouth closed, or kiss other parts of the body that have clean skin, not sexual areas or open cuts and sores.

Performing Oral Sex

Several STIs live in semen and vaginal fluids and mucosa linings.

Several STIs can be transmitted through open cuts and sores in the genital area.

Receiving Oral Sex

Several STIs can live in saliva and other body fluids.

Several STIs can be transmitted through open cuts and sores in your mouth.

Safer Sex Techniques: Use commercially available flavored condoms or unlubricated condoms, which do not contain a spermicidal for use during oral sex on a man. Use commercially available dental dams, or create a latex square from an unlubricated condom for use during oral sex on a woman.

Vaginal Intercourse

Most STIs are spread through infected body fluids including semen, pre-cum fluids, vaginal secretions, and blood.

Because one genital is inside the other and there is an exchange of body fluids, it is always important to use protection.

Safer Sex Techniques: Use a condom or a female condom. Birth control protects against pregnancy, not STIs.

Anal Intercourse

Most STIs are spread through infected body fluids, such as semen, pre-cum fluids, vaginal secretions, and blood.

Because one genital is inside the other, there is an exchange of body fluids, and the skin inside the anus mucosa is easily damaged, it is important to use protection.

Safer Sex Techniques: Use lubricated latex condoms with lots of lube to make things go smoother.

SOURCES: Table by Kotecki, J. E., (2012). *BSU Peer Health Educator Training Manual;* Data from National Prevention Information Network, Centers for Disease Control and Prevention. STD Prevention Today. Online: http://www.cdcnpin.org/scripts/std/prevent.asp; and U.S. National Library of Medicine and the National Institutes of Health. MedlinePlus Encyclopedia: Safe Sex. Online: http://www.nlm.nih.gov/medlineplus/ency/article/001949.htm. Accessed April 13, 2012.

likely to dodge the topic of STIs. Prevention would be enhanced if sexually active individuals developed an open attitude about talking about STIs (and other aspects of sex) and acquired the necessary communication skills.

Some barriers to safer sex include the following:

- *Denying that there is a risk.* Many people assume that STIs happen only to "dirty," "promiscuous," and "immoral" people and, because they have sex only with people who are "clean" and "nice," getting an STI is impossible. Another form of denial is to tell yourself "I eat right. I exercise. I can't get an STI."

- *Believing that the campus community is somehow insulated from STIs.* The truth is that about half of college students are sexually active before they enter college. As a result, students can arrive on campus already infected. Also, on many campuses, students in the same living groups and student organizations have sex with one another. One infected person can lead to a whole chain of infections.

- *Feeling guilty and uncomfortable about being sexual.* This prevents individuals from planning sex, carrying condoms, and talking about possible risks with new partners.
- *Succumbing to social and peer pressure to be sexual.* These pressures encourage people to be sexual in situations that are potentially risky, such as one-night stands and brief relationships that are sexual virtually from the beginning. The risk of infection is lessened when individuals resist peer pressure to have sex with a relative stranger and instead ask themselves, "Is this the right relationship?" "Is this the right partner?" and "Am I going to feel OK about this afterward?"

Regular Medical Check-ups

Any sexually active person should have regular medical check-ups, at least once yearly, to check for the presence of infections and to diagnose and treat any signs and symptoms of STIs. STIs can cause serious health problems if left untreated. You should not feel afraid to discuss with your health care provider your sexual practices or to request STI tests. The CDC National STI and AIDS Hotline can help by offering reliable information in a friendly, nonthreatening, nonjudgmental atmosphere. For answers to your STI/AIDS-related questions, referrals to local test sites and treatment centers, or other services, call (800) 227-8922.

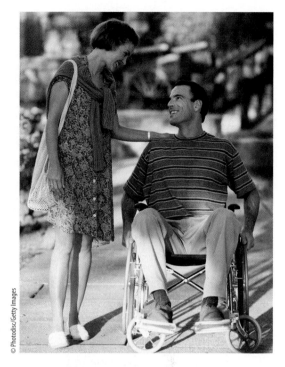

FIGURE 16.11 **Safer Sex.** Everyone has a responsibility to practice safer sex.

Physical Activity and Health Connection

Sexual behavior is an instinctive form of physical intimacy. It is most often performed for the purpose of expressing affection and enjoying yourself. When we decide to have sexual contact, we want it to be satisfying for ourselves and our partner. Regular physical activity makes us feel more energized and makes us look and feel better about ourselves—which has a positive influence on our sex lives. We also need to understand what responsibilities our sexual behavior entails for both ourselves and our partner when it comes to our physical health. Looking after our physical health involves behaving in ways that reduce or eliminate the possibility of being infected with a sexually transmitted infection.

concept connections

1. **A pathogen or infectious agent is a biological agent that causes disease or illness to its host.** Because of their small size, pathogens are sometimes called microorganisms or microbes. Of the many microbes found in nature, only a relatively small proportion cause disease in humans. There are five major types of pathogenic microbes: bacteria, viruses, fungi, protozoa, and helminths. In addition, a new class of infectious agents, the prions, has recently been recognized. An infection results when a pathogen invades and begins growing within a host. Disease results only if and when, as a consequence of the invasion and growth of a pathogen, tissue function is impaired.

2. **Sexually transmitted infections are infections that are spread primarily through person-to-person sexual contact.** More than 25 different infectious bacteria, viruses, and parasites are transmitted through semen, vaginal fluid, blood, or other body fluids during sexual activity. The most common conditions they cause are trichomoniasis, genital warts, chlamydia, herpes, gonorrhea, hepatitis B, syphilis, and HIV/AIDS. STIs can be serious and painful and may have long-term effects, especially if left undetected and untreated.

3. **There are many reasons for the high rates of sexually transmitted infections in the United States.** Not informing your partner that you have an STI, having multiple sexual partners, not practicing safer sex precautions, not recognizing STI symptoms, not treating an STI, having impaired judgment because of alcohol or other drugs, and counting on the sense of security that "I won't get an STI" or that there is a cure for an STI if one is contracted all are reasons for the high rates of STIs in the United States.

4. **Abstinence from sexual activity is the most effective behavior for eliminating your risk of contracting a sexually transmitted infection.** College students choose to abstain from sex for many reasons including waiting for the right partner, waiting until they are ready for a sexual relationship, and wanting to focus on school.

5. *Safer sex* **is a general term used to describe methods for reducing the chance that you will contract or spread sexually transmitted infections.** Using a condom every time you have sexual intercourse is an example of safer sex. Safer sex also involves talking with your partner. The stigma associated with STIs is a great hindrance to prevention efforts. Viewing STIs in moral terms—that is, associating them with dirtiness and immorality—makes people reluctant to think and talk about them.

Terms

Chain of infection, 356
Chancre, 370
Chlamydia, 369
Defense mechanisms, 358
Direct transmission, 357
Epididymitis, 369
Genital herpes, 367
Genital warts, 368
Gonorrhea, 369
Hepatitis B virus, 368
Host, 358
Human immunodeficiency virus (HIV), 365

Human papillomavirus (HPV), 368
Indirect transmission, 357
Infection, 356
Infectious disease, 356
Infectivity, 356
Pathogen, 356
Pathogenicity, 356
Pelvic inflammatory disease (PID), 369
Portals of entry, 357
Portals of exit, 357
Pubic lice, 371

Reservoir, 357
Retrovirus, 366
Safer sex, 373
Scabies, 371
Sexually transmitted infection (STI), 361
Syphilis, 370
Trichomonas vaginalis, 371
Vehicles, 357
Virulence, 356
Zoonoses, 357

making the connection

Jeremy and Christina both realize, after a number of heart-to-heart talks, that sexual intimacy does not necessarily need to include sexual intercourse. In deciding whether to engage in intimate sexual relations, including intercourse, they understand that they must consider psychological as well as physical factors. They have learned that many people choose to abstain from sexual intercourse and that they can choose among varying levels of sexual intimacy. When they decide to become sexually intimate it will be a big step in their relationship, especially because having sex involves an emotional commitment as well as a physical one. Furthermore, the decision to become sexually intimate with one another must also be considered in light of HIV and the other sexually transmitted infections that are prevalent among college students; many times infections may be asymptomatic, so someone may transmit the disease to another person unknowingly.

Critical Thinking

1. Jeremy and Christina have chosen to abstain from sexual intercourse. Describe the pros and cons of sexual abstinence. Have you been able to discuss your thoughts about a possible sexual relationship with your current partner?

2. As more and more people become infected with HIV, more students attending universities and colleges are infected with HIV. Many universities have residence halls with living quarters that accommodate two to four people of the same gender. Is it necessary for universities to notify students in a residence hall if a person living there is HIV-positive? If so, why? If not, why not?

3. Herpes is a sexually transmitted infection that lasts a lifetime; however, herpes can be managed with medication. Explain, in detail, how you would go about telling your new partner that you have the herpes infection.

4. You and your best college friend are talking, and your friend confides to you that about 2 months ago he had sexual intercourse with someone who could be HIV-positive, but your friend is not having any symptoms. What advice would you give him?

References

Centers for Disease Control and Prevention. (1999). CDC Guidelines for National Human Immunodeficiency Virus Case Surveillance, Including Monitoring for Human Immunodeficiency Virus Infection and Acquired Immunodeficiency Syndrome. *Morbidity and Mortality Weekly Report* 48(RR13):1–29.

Centers for Disease Control and Prevention. (2011a). Condom fact sheet in brief. Online: http://www.cdc.gov/condomeffectiveness/brief.html.

Centers for Disease Control and Prevention. (2011b). Ten ways STDs impact women differently from men. Online: http://www.cdc.gov/nchhstp/newsroom/docs/STDs-Women-042011.pdf.

Centers for Disease Control and Prevention. (2012a). HIV in the United States: At a glance, 2010. Online: http://www.cdc.gov/hiv/resources/factsheets/us.htm.

Centers for Disease Control and Prevention. (2012b). Trends in reportable sexually transmitted infections in the United States, 2010. Online: http://www.cdc.gov/std/stats10/default.htm.

Herbeck, J.T., Muller, V., Maust, B.S., Ledergerber, B., Torti, C., Di Giambenedetto, S., Gras, L., Gunthard, H., Jacobson, L.P., Mullins, J.I., & Gottlieb, G.S. (2012). Is the virulence of HIV changing? A meta-analysis of trends in prognostic markers of HIV disease progression and transmission. *AIDS* 26(2):193–205.

Injury Care and Prevention

A

Exercise-Related Injuries

Most exercise-related injuries do not threaten life, nor are they severe. However, exercise-related injuries demand that you make a decision about the proper care for an injury.

This section helps in such decision making with its decision table (If . . . , then . . .) format. Decision tables not only help identify what may be wrong (the *If* column) but also help determine what action to take (the *Then* column).

This appendix does not cover life-threatening conditions requiring rescue breathing and cardiopulmonary resuscitation (CPR) or many other injuries and conditions that a quality first aid course would cover. To find a quality first aid course, go to the American Academy of Orthopedic Surgeons/American College of Emergency Physicians Emergency Care and Safety Institute website— http://www.ECSInstitute.org—to locate a training center near you. Many colleges and universities use the AAOS/ACEP first aid, CPR, and automated external defibrillator (AED) program.

How to Examine for an Injury

See TABLE A.1. Signs of an exercise-related injury may include the following:

- Loss of use. "Guarding" occurs when movement produces pain; the person refuses to use the injured part.
- A grating sensation (crepitus) can be felt—and sometimes even heard—when the ends of a broken bone rub together.

TABLE A.1	How to Examine for an Injury

What to Do	How to Do It
Determine the location the problem.	Ask yourself or the injured person, "What's wrong?" or "Where do you hurt?"
Find out if an injury exists.	Look and feel the area for one or more of the following signs of injury: deformity, open wounds, tenderness, and swelling. The mnemonic "DOTS" can help you remember the signs of an injury: • **Deformities** occur when bones are broken, causing an abnormal shape. Deformity might not be obvious. Compare the injured part with the uninjured part on the other side of the body. • **Open** wounds break the skin and there is bleeding. • **Tenderness** (pain) means sensitive when touched or pressed. It is commonly found only at the injury site. The person usually will be able to point to the site of the pain. • **Swelling** is the body's response to injury that makes the area larger than usual. It appears later and is the result of fluid from inflammation and/or bleeding.

- For extremity (arms and legs) injuries, check blood flow and nerves. Use the mnemonic CSM (circulation, sensation, movement) as a way of remembering what to do.
  - *Circulation:* For an arm injury, feel for the radial pulse (located on the thumb side of the wrist). For a leg injury, feel for the posterior tibial pulse (located between the inside ankle bone and the Achilles tendon). An arm or leg without a pulse requires immediate surgical care.
  - *Sensation:* Lightly touch or squeeze one of the victim's fingers or toes and ask the victim what he or she feels. Loss of sensation is an early sign of nerve damage.
  - *Movement:* Inability to move develops later. Check for nerve damage by asking the victim to wiggle his or her fingers or toes. If the fingers or toes are injured, do not have the victim try to move them.

A quick nerve and circulatory check is very important. The tissues of the arms and legs cannot survive for more than 3 hours without a continuous blood supply. If you note any disruption in the nerve and blood supply, seek immediate medical care.

RICE Procedures

RICE is the acronym—rest, ice, compression, and elevation—for the treatment of all bone, joint, and muscle injuries. The steps taken in the first 48 to 72 hours after such an injury can help to relieve, and even prevent, aches and pains.

Treat all extremity bone, joint, and muscle injuries with the RICE procedures. In addition to RICE, fractures and dislocations should be stabilized against movement.

R: Rest

Injuries heal faster if rested. Rest means to stay off the injured part and avoid moving it. Using any part of the body increases the blood circulation to that area, which can cause more swelling of an injured part.

I: Ice

An ice pack should be applied to the injured area for 20 to 30 minutes every 2 or 3 hours during the first 24 to 48 hours. Skin treated with cold passes through four stages: cold, burning, aching, and numbness. When the skin becomes numb, usually in 20 to 30 minutes, remove the ice pack. After removing the ice pack, compress the injured part with an elastic bandage and keep it elevated (the C and E of RICE).

Cold constricts the blood vessels to and in the injured area, which helps reduce the swelling and inflammation. Cold should be applied as soon as possible after the injury—healing time often is directly related to the amount of swelling that occurs. Heat has the opposite effect when applied to fresh injuries: it increases circulation to the area and greatly increases both the swelling and the pain.

Put crushed ice (or cubes) into a double plastic bag or commercial ice bag. Place the ice pack directly on the skin, and then use an elastic bandage to hold the ice pack in place. Ice bags can conform to the body's contours.

C: Compression

Compressing the injured area may squeeze some fluid and debris out of the injury site. Compression limits the ability of the skin and of other tissues to expand and reduces internal bleeding. Apply an elastic bandage to the injured area, especially the foot, ankle, knee, thigh, hand, or elbow. Fill the hollow areas with padding, such as a sock or washcloth, before applying the elastic bandage.

Start the elastic bandage several inches below the injury and wrap in an upward, overlapping spiral with an even, slightly tight pressure. Pale skin, pain, numbness, and tingling are signs that the bandage is too tight. If any of these appear, immediately remove the elastic bandage. Rewrap later when the symptoms disappear.

For a bruise or strain, place a pad between the injury and the elastic bandage.

E: Elevation

Elevating the injured area, in combination with ice and compression, limits circulation to an area, helps limit internal bleeding, and minimizes swelling.

Returning to Physical Activity After an Injury

Returning to physical activity is generally permissible once an injury is fully healed. Fully healed means the following:

- No pain
- No swelling
- No limping, favoring, or instability

Full rehabilitation means the following:

- Return of full range of motion and flexibility
- Muscle strength and endurance in the affected extremity (arm or leg) equal to that of the unaffected extremity
- Resumption of preinjury endurance levels
- Good balance and coordination

Sometimes, clearance to return to exercising should come from a physician (e.g., after surgery).

Definitions

- *Contusions:* Bruising of tissue.
- *Strains:* Muscles are stretched or torn.
- *Sprains:* Tearing or stretching of the joints that causes mild to severe damage to the ligaments and joint capsules.
- *Dislocations:* Bones are displaced from their normal joint alignment, out of their sockets, or out of their normal positions.
- *Tendonitis:* Inflammation of a tendon from overuse.

Specific Injuries

Foot

Foot injuries are common among exercisers because of the foot's role in bearing weight. Careless treatment can have consequences that may include lifelong disability. See TABLE A.2 .

Ankle

Most ankle injuries are sprains. About 85 percent of sprains involve the ankle's outside (lateral) ligaments and are caused by having the foot turned or twisted inward. If not treated properly, a sprained ankle becomes chronically susceptible to future injuries. See TABLE A.3 for symptoms and treatment.

Lower Leg

The two bones of the lower leg are the tibia (shin bone) and fibula. Most shin injuries are "shin splints," which are strains from overuse. Occasionally, a bone is fractured from overuse. See TABLE A.4 .

TABLE A.2	Determining and Treating Foot Injuries

If	Then
Pain is at top of the heel (over the Achilles tendon). Pain is aggravated by activity—worse at beginning of activity and improved with warm-up.	Suspect *Achilles tendonitis*: • Apply ice to decrease inflammation and pain. • Reduce or stop activity until no more pain occurs while either walking or resting. • Elevate heel with a heel cup or pads in the shoe. • Calf muscles should be stretched after warm-up and cooldown.
Pain is at back of the heel. Injury resembles Achilles tendonitis.	Suspect *retrocalcaneal bursitis*: • Treat the same as for Achilles tendonitis.
Pain, often disabling, is at bottom of the heel.	Suspect *plantar fasciitis*: • Apply ice for 20–30 minutes after activity and 3–4 times daily. • Use a heel cup in the shoe and shoes with good support. • Reduce or stop activity and avoid going barefoot.
Pain is in fifth metatarsal bone, possibly with swelling.	Suspect *fracture* (Jones fracture): • Apply ice. • Stop activity. • Seek medical care.
Pain is on ball of foot between second and third toes or sometimes actually between second and third toes.	Suspect *Morton's neuroma*: • Wear wider, more supportive, softer shoes. • If there is no improvement, surgery may be required.
Pain is on ball of foot at the big toe.	Suspect *sesamoiditis* or a *stress fracture*: • Apply ice for 20–30 minutes, 3–4 times daily. • Rest. • If pain persists, seek medical care.
Area on skin has a "hot spot" (not very painful, red area) from rubbing.	Suspect a *blister*: • Cool the hot spot with an ice pack. AND/OR • Tape several layers of moleskin, which are cut into a doughnut shape to fit around the blister. OR • Apply duct tape over the painful area.
Blister is broken and fluid is seeping out.	• Leave the "roof" on for protection. • Clean with soap and water. • Tape several layers of moleskin, cut into a doughnut shape to fit around the blister. • Apply an antibiotic ointment in the hole over the blister. • Cover with an uncut gauze pad and tape in place.
Blister on foot is very painful, affects walking, and is not broken.	• Drain the blister by puncturing the roof with several holes. • Leave the "roof" on for protection. • Clean with soap and water. • Tape several layers of moleskin, cut into a doughnut shape to fit around the blister. • Apply an antibiotic ointment in the hole over the blister. • Place gauze pad over the moleskin and tape in place.

TABLE A.3	Determining and Treating Ankle Injuries (Ottawa Ankle Rules)

If	Then
Ankle is able to bear weight. The individual is able to take four steps immediately after the injury and an hour later. No tenderness or pain is felt when you push on the ankle knob bone.	Suspect *ankle sprain*: • Use RICE procedures. • For the compression part of RICE, apply an elastic bandage over any soft pliable material (e.g., sock, T-shirt) placed in a U shape around the ankle knob with the curved part down. • If pain and swelling do not decrease within 48 hours, seek medical care.
Ankle is unable to bear weight. The individual is unable to take four steps immediately after the injury and an hour later. Tenderness and pain is felt when you push on the ankle knob bone.	Suspect *ankle fracture*: • Use RICE procedures. • For the compression part of RICE, apply an elastic bandage over any soft pliable material (e.g., sock, T-shirt) placed in a U shape around the ankle knob with the curved part down. • Stabilize ankle against movement. • Seek medical care.

TABLE A.4	Determining and Treating Lower Leg Injuries

If	Then
Shin aches during activity, but ache subsides significantly after activity stops, ache is result of increase in workout routine (e.g., running longer, jogging on hills). Shin is tender when pressed.	Suspect *shin splints* (medial tibial stress syndrome): • Apply ice before activity and for 30 minutes after activity. • Stop activity until pain free. • Stretch calves several times daily.
Leg receives direct hit that produces deformity, open wound, tenderness, and/or swelling.	Suspect *fracture* or *bruise*: • Use RICE procedures. • Control any bleeding. If fracture is suspected: • Stabilize leg against movement. • Seek medical care.
The individual feels a pop or sudden, sharp, burning pain in calf muscle while running or jumping.	Suspect a *muscle strain* (e.g., tear, pull): • Use RICE procedures.
The individual feels a pop while running or jumping, causing pain just above the heel. Leg is tender when pressed. He/she is unable to bear weight on injured leg. He/she has difficulty with controlling foot (flops around).	Suspect a *torn Achilles tendon*: • Use RICE procedures. • Seek medical care.
A muscle (most often the calf muscle) goes into an uncontrolled spasm and contraction, resulting in severe pain and restriction or loss of movement.	Suspect a *muscle cramp*: • Gently stretch the affected muscle OR • Relax the muscle by applying pressure to it. • Apply ice to the muscle. • Drink lightly salted cool water (dissolve ¼ teaspoon salt in a quart of water). Do not give salt tablets.

Knee

Knee injuries are among the most serious joint injuries (TABLE A.5). Their severity is difficult to determine; thus, you should seek medical care.

Thigh

The thigh consists of a single bone, the femur, which is surrounded and protected by heavy muscle. The muscle group on the front of the thigh is the quadriceps. Most thigh injuries are from direct hits. As with other leg muscles, a quadriceps strain can happen. See TABLE A.6 .

TABLE A.5	Determining and Treating Knee Injuries

If

Immediate swelling occurs after injury. Knee locks. Knee gives way. Pain occurs below kneecap. Pain occurs under the kneecap when climbing stairs.

Examining for an acute injury (not overuse type of injury).

Then

Suspect *knee injury* (acute and/or chronic):
- Use RICE procedures.
- Stabilize knee against movement.
- Seek medical care.

Pittsburgh Knee Rules:
- Any blunt trauma or fall-type injury and one of the following present:
  - Age younger than 12 years or older than 50 years
  - Inability to walk four weight-bearing steps

    OR

Ottawa Knee Rules:
- Age older than 55 years
- Tenderness at the patella (kneecap)
- Tenderness at head of fibula (bony knob on outside of knee)
- Inability to flex knee to 90° angle
- Inability to bear weight and take four steps immediately after injury and later

Suspect *serious knee injury:*
- Use RICE procedures.
- Stabilize knee against movement.
- Seek medical care.

If

Deformity obvious, with the kneecap (patella) usually on the outside (lateral side) of the knee. Compare it with the other kneecap.

Then

Suspect a *dislocated kneecap:*
- Apply ice.
- Stabilize against movement.
- Seek medical care.

TABLE A.6	Determining and Treating Thigh Injuries

If

Pain at front of thigh.

Pain at back of thigh.

Then

Suspect a *bruise:*
- Use RICE procedures.

Suspect a *muscle strain* (pulled hamstring):
- Use RICE procedures.

Hip

See TABLE A.7 for information on how to determine and treat hip injuries.

Finger

Most finger injuries are not severe. In rare cases, a finger can dislocate, producing a grotesque deformity that requires immediate medical care. See TABLE A.8.

Elbow

More often than not, elbow injuries are nagging nuisances. Occasionally, an elbow is more seriously injured. Rarely does an elbow dislocate. See TABLE A.9.

TABLE A.7	Determining and Treating Hip Injuries
If	**Then**
Pain is in groin.	Suspect *muscle strain*: • Use RICE procedures.
Pain is on upper hip.	Suspect *hip pointer*: • Use RICE procedures.
Pain is on outer thigh to knee.	Suspect *muscle strain* or *bursitis*: • Use RICE procedures.

TABLE A.8	Determining and Treating Finger Injuries
If	**Then**

Finger is deformed.
Finger is tender/painful.
Finger is swollen.
	Suspect a *possible fracture* and/or *dislocation*:
	• Test for a finger fracture:
	  • If possible, straighten the fingers and place them flat on a hard surface.
	  • Tap the tip of the injured finger toward the hand. Pain lower down in the finger or into the hand can indicate a fracture.
	• Do not try to realign a dislocation.
	• Apply ice.
	• Stabilize finger against movement by "buddy" taping for support. *OR* Keeping hand and fingers in cupping shape as though holding a baseball with extra padding in the palm; secure the hand, fingers, and arm to a rigid board or folded newspapers.
	• Seek medical care.

TABLE A.9	Determining and Treating Elbow Injuries
If	**Then**
Severe elbow pain after fall on arm.	Suspect *dislocation* or *fracture*: • Apply ice. • Stabilize against movement. • Seek medical care.
Elbow pain on inside (medial).	Suspect *"little league, golf, or racquetball" elbow*: • Use RICE procedures. • Gently stretch by placing palms together in front of face, and slowly lowering. • Seek medical care if pain persists.
Elbow pain on outside (lateral).	Suspect *"tennis" elbow*: • Use RICE procedures. • Seek medical care if pain persists.
Elbow with tenderness/pain and swelling.	Suspect a *bruise:* • Use RICE procedures. • Seek medical care if tingling and/or weakness continues for 24 hours (can be serious because of possible nerve injury).

Shoulder

Shoulder injuries can range from mild to those that pose medical emergencies (TABLE A.10). A dislocated shoulder usually occurs during contact sports and requires immediate medical care. A shoulder dislocation can be confused with a shoulder separation. The key difference is that in separation the shoulder joint and upper arm remain mobile. In dislocation, the mobility is lost.

Muscle

See TABLE A.11 for information on how to determine and treat muscle injuries.

Chest

See TABLE A.12 for symptoms and treatment of chest injuries.

Breathing Difficulty

See TABLE A.13 for information on how to determine and treat breathing difficulty.

TABLE A.10	Determining and Treating Shoulder Injuries
If	**Then**
Pain is on top of shoulder after a fall or being hit.	Suspect a *separation:* • Apply ice. • Seek medical care.
Extreme pain is at front of shoulder after a fall. The individual holds upper arm away from the body, supported by the uninjured arm. Arm cannot be brought across the chest to touch the opposite shoulder. The individual describes a history of previous dislocations.	Suspect a *dislocation:* • Apply ice. • Stabilize shoulder against movement and immediately seek medical care.
Burning pain is felt down arm after twisting neck.	Suspect a *"stinger":* • Apply ice. • Seek medical care.
Arm goes limp.	Suspect a *subluxation:* • Apply ice. • Seek medical care.
Pain is felt when raising arm.	Suspect a *rotator cuff injury:* • Apply ice. • Seek medical care.

TABLE A.11	Determining and Treating Muscle Injuries
If	**Then**
Muscle pain occurs 12 to 72 hours after physical activity.	Suspect *delayed-onset muscle soreness:* • Apply ice (some experts suggest heat). • Perform gentle active motion of the area. • Gently stretch the muscle. • Do not use nonsteroidal medications (e.g., ibuprofen, aspirin).

TABLE A.12	**Determining and Treating Chest Injuries**

If

Sudden, severe central chest pain: can occur at rest; worse when exerting; pain is crushing, vice-like; and may radiate up to the jaws or down the left arm. Nausea. Breathlessness. Sweating. Blueness of lips.

No chest pain, but sudden general tiredness, breathlessness as a new symptom, and sudden worsening of existing breathlessness.

Then

Suspect a *heart attack:*
- Give one aspirin to chew (not any other analgesic, only aspirin).
- Seek medical care immediately—usually by calling 9-1-1.
- Monitor for possible cardiac arrest requiring CPR.
- Help the individual into least painful position—usually sitting with legs bent at the knees.
- Ask if he or she is taking a medication known as nitroglycerin; if so, help person take it.

Suspect a *silent heart attack:*
- Treat as you would a heart attack.

TABLE A.13	**Determining and Treating Breathing Difficulty**

If

Coughing. Wheezing, especially when breathing out. Chest feels "tight." Sweating, breathless, rapid pulse. Neck muscles strain in an attempt to increase breathing. As attack worsens, blue lips, tiredness, and drowsiness. Confusion. Coma. Poor response to usual medication.

Then

Suspect *asthma* (asthma can be induced during exercise):
1. Place the individual in a comfortable, upright position to help breathing.
2. Help the individual use medicines (inhaler and/or pills).
3. Give plenty of fluids.
4. Seek medical care if:
   - No improvement within 2 hours after using medications.
   - There are repeated attacks.
   - Attack is severe and prolonged.

How Heat Affects the Body

Human bodies dissipate heat by varying the rate and depth of blood circulation, by losing water through the skin and sweat glands, and—when blood is heated above 98.6°F—by panting. The heart begins to pump more blood, blood vessels dilate to accommodate the increased flow, and the bundles of tiny capillaries threading through the upper layers of skin are put into operation. The body's blood is circulated closer to the skin's surface, and excess heat drains off into the cooler atmosphere. At the same time, water diffuses through the skin as perspiration. The skin handles about 90 percent of the body's heat dissipating function.

Sweating, on its own, does nothing to cool the body, unless the water is removed by evaporation—and high relative humidity retards evaporation. The evaporation process works this way: the heat energy required to evaporate sweat is extracted from the body, thereby cooling it. Under conditions of high temperature (above 90°F) and high relative humidity, the body is doing everything it can to maintain an internal temperature of 98.6°F. The heart is pumping a torrent of blood through dilated circulatory vessels; the sweat glands are pouring liquid—including essential dissolved chemicals, such as sodium and chloride—onto the surface of the skin.

Too Much Heat

Heat disorders generally occur from a reduction or collapse of the body's ability to shed heat by circulatory changes and sweating, or a chemical (salt) imbalance caused by too much sweating. When heat gain exceeds the level the body can remove, or when the body cannot compensate for fluids and salt lost through perspiration, the temperature of the body's inner core begins to rise and heat-related illness may develop.

Heat illnesses include a range of disorders (TABLE A.14). Some of them are common, but only heatstroke is life threatening. Untreated heatstroke victims always die. Ranging in severity, heat disorders share one common feature: the individual has

TABLE A.14 **Determining and Treating Heat-Related Illnesses**	
If	**Then**
Skin is extremely hot when touched— usually dry, but may be moist. Altered mental status, ranging from slight confusion, agitation, and disorientation to unresponsiveness.	Suspect *heatstroke:* Heatstroke is life threatening and must be treated immediately. 　1. Move the individual to a cool place. Monitor ABCs. 　2. Remove clothing down to the individual's underwear. 　3. Keep the individual's head and shoulders slightly raised. 　4. Quickly cool the individual: 　　• Spray the individual with water and vigorously fan. This method does not work well in high humidity. 　　• If ice is available, place ice packs into the armpits, sides of the neck, and groin. 　5. Stop cooling when mental status improves or if shivering occurs. 　6. Evacuate to medical care ASAP. Continue cooling during evacuation.
Sweating. Thirsty. Fatigued. Flu-like symptoms—headache or nausea. Shortness of breath. Rapid pulse.	Differences from *heatstroke:* 　• No altered mental status 　• Skin is not hot, but clammy Suspect *heat exhaustion:* Uncontrolled heat exhaustion can evolve into heatstroke. 　1. Move the individual to a cool place. 　2. Have the individual remove excess clothing. 　3. Have the individual drink cool fluids. 　4. For more severe cases, give lightly salted cool water (dissolve ¼ teaspoon salt in a quart of water). Do not give salt tablets. 　5. Raise the individual's legs 8 to 12 inches (keep legs straight). 　6. Cool the individual, but not as aggressively as for heatstroke. 　7. If no improvement is seen within 30 minutes, seek medical care.
Painful muscle spasms that happen suddenly. Affects muscle in the back of the leg or abdominal muscles. Occurs during or after physical exertion.	Suspect *heat cramp:* Relief may take several hours. 　1. Have the individual rest in a cool area. 　2. Have the individual drink lightly salted cool water (dissolve ¼ teaspoon salt in 1 quart of water) or a commercial sports drink. Do not give salt tablets. 　3. Have the individual stretch the cramped calf muscle or try acupressure method of pinching the upper lip just below the nose.
The individual is dizzy or faints.	Suspect *heat syncope:* 　1. If the individual is unresponsive, check ABCs. Person usually recovers quickly. 　2. If the individual fell, check for injuries. 　3. Have the individual rest and lie down with legs raised in cool area. 　4. Wet skin by splashing water on face. 　5. If not nauseated, have the individual drink lightly salted cool water (dissolve ¼ teaspoon salt in 1 quart of water) or a commercial sports drink. Do not give salt tablets.
Ankles and feet swell. Occurs during first few days in a hot environment.	Suspect *heat edema:* 　1. Have the individual wear support stockings. 　2. Elevate legs.
Itchy rash on skin wet from sweating.	Suspect *prickly heat:* 　1. Dry and cool skin. 　2. Limit heat exposure.

°F	40	45	50	55	60	65	70	75	80	85	90	95	100
110	136												
108	130	137											
106	124	130	137										
104	119	124	131	137									
102	114	119	124	130	137								
100	109	114	118	124	139	136							
98	106	109	113	117	123	128	134						
96	101	104	108	112	116	121	126	132					
94	97	100	101	106	110	114	118	124	129	135			
92	94	96	99	101	105	108	112	116	121	125	131		
90	91	93	95	97	100	103	106	109	113	117	122	127	132
88	88	89	91	93	95	98	100	100	106	110	113	114	121
86	85	87	88	89	91	93	95	97	100	102	105	108	112
84	83	84	85	86	88	89	90	92	94	96	98	100	103
82	81	82	83	84	84	85	86	88	89	90	91	93	95
80	80	80	81	81	82	82	83	84	84	85	86	86	87

Air Temperature — Relative Humidity (%)

Heat Index (Apparent Temperature)

With Prolonged Exposure and/or Physical Activity

Extreme Danger
Heatstroke or sunstroke highly likely

Danger
Sunstroke, muscle cramps, and/or heat exhaustion likely

Extreme Caution
Sunstroke, muscle cramps, and/or heat exhaustion possible

Caution
Fatigue possible

FIGURE A.1 The Heat Index.
SOURCE: National Weather Service, National Oceanic and Atmospheric Adminstration. (2009). Heat index. Online: http://www.crh.noaa.gov/jkl/?n=heat_index_calculator.

been overexposed or has overexercised for his or her age and physical condition in the existing thermal environment.

Studies indicate that, other factors being equal, the severity of heat disorders tends to increase with age—heat cramps in a 17-year-old may be heat exhaustion in a 40-year-old, and heatstroke in a person older than age 60.

Acclimatization concerns adjusting the sweat–salt concentration, among other things. The idea is to lose enough water to regulate body temperature, with the least possible chemical disturbance.

The heat index (or apparent temperature) is how the heat and humidity in the air combine to make us feel (**FIGURE A.1**). Higher humidity plus higher temperatures often combine to make us feel a perceived temperature that is higher than the actual air temperature. The old saying, "It's not the heat, it's the humidity," holds true.

The National Weather Service is using a new "mean heat index" to alert people to the dangers of heat waves. The index, which went into use in May 2002, measures how hot a person will feel over a full day. The idea is the same as the traditional heat index, which shows how hot a particular combination of heat and humidity feels. This index has usually been used to show the danger during the hottest part of the day. The mean heat index averages the heat index from the hottest and coolest parts of a day.

Sunburn

Sunburn, with its ultraviolet radiation burns, can significantly retard the skin's ability to shed excess heat. See TABLE A.15 for information on how to determine and treat sunburns.

Cold-Related Injuries

Hypothermia

Hypothermia happens when the body's temperature (98.6°F/37°C) drops more than 2° (TABLE A.16). Hypothermia does not require subfreezing temperatures. Severe hypothermia is life threatening. Check also for possible frostbite.

TABLE A.15	Determining and Treating Sunburns

If	**Then**
Skin that has been exposed to the sun later becomes red, mildly swollen, and tender and painful.	Suspect *first-degree (superficial) sunburn:* 1. Immerse burned area in cold water or apply a wet, cold cloth until pain free, both in and out of the water (usually 10–45 minutes). If cold water is unavailable, use any cold liquid available. 2. Give ibuprofen (for children, give acetaminophen). 3. Have the individual drink water. 4. Keep burned arm or leg raised. 5. After burn has been cooled, apply aloe vera gel or inexpensive moisturizer.

First-degree burns do not have to be covered. Skin that has been exposed to the sun later becomes blistered, swollen, weeping of fluids, and severely painful.	Suspect *second-degree (partial-thickness) sunburn:*
	• If skin affected is less than 20 percent of the body surface (the individual's palm, not including fingers and thumb, equals 1 percent of body surface area):
	   1. Follow same procedures (steps 1–4) as for a first-degree burn, with these additions:
	      a. After burn has been cooled, apply thin layer of antibacterial ointment (e.g., Bacitracin, Neosporin).
	      b. Cover burn with a dry, nonsticking sterile dressing or clean cloth.
	• If skin has a large second-degree burn over more than 20 percent of the body surface area:
	   1. Follow steps 2–4 of first-degree burn care.
	   2. Seek medical care.
	Do not apply cold because it may cause hypothermia.

TABLE A.16	Determining and Treating Hypothermia

If	**Then**

Shivering uncontrollably. Has the "umbles" (e.g., grumbles, mumbles, fumbles, stumbles). Has cool abdomen when felt with a warm hand.	Suspect *mild hypothermia:*
	1. Stop heat loss:
	   • Get the individual out of the cold.
	   • Handle the individual gently.
	   • Replace wet clothing with dry clothing.
	   • Add insulation (e.g., blankets, towels, pillows, sleeping bags) beneath and around the individual. Cover the individual's head (50–80 percent of body's heat loss is through the head).
	2. Keep in flat (horizontal) position.
	3. Allow the individual to shiver—do not stop the shivering by adding heat. Shivering, which generates heat, rewarms mildly hypothermic victims. DO NOT use the following procedures because they stop shivering:
	   • Warm water immersion
	   • Body-to-body contact
	   • Chemical heat pads
	4. Warm drinks are unable to rewarm sufficiently. However, warm sugary liquids can provide calories for shivering to continue and may provide a psychological boost. DO NOT give alcohol to drink.

Muscles are rigid and stiff. No shivering. Skin feels ice cold and appears blue. Altered mental status. Slow pulse. Slow breathing. The individual appears to be dead.	Suspect *severe hypothermia:* 1. Follow steps 1 and 2 from mild hypothermia for all hypothermic victims. 2. Check ABCs and give CPR as necessary. Check the pulse for 30 to 45 seconds before starting CPR. 3. Gently evacuate victim to medical help for rewarming. Rewarming in a remote location is difficult and rarely effective. However, when the victim is far from medical care, the victim must be warmed by any available external heat source (e.g., body-to-body contact, warm water immersion).

TABLE A.17	Determining and Treating Frostbite

If

Skin color is white, waxy, or grayish yellow. Affected part is cold and numb. Tingling, stinging, or aching sensation is felt. Skin surface feels stiff or crusty, and underlying tissue feels soft when depressed gently.

Then

Suspect *superficial frostbite.*

All frostbite injuries require the same first aid treatment:

1. Get the individual to a warm area.
2. Replace wet clothing or constricting items that could impair blood circulation (e.g., rings).
3. Do not rub or massage the area.
4. For deep frostbite, seek medical care.
5. When you are more than 1 hour from a medical facility, place injured part in warm water (test by pouring some water over the inside of your arm to check whether it is warm, not hot). For ear or face, it is best but may be difficult to apply warm moist cloths, changing them frequently. May have to cover with warm hands. Give pain medication (preferably aspirin or ibuprofen). Rewarming may take 20 to 40 minutes or when parts become soft.

Then

Suspect *deep frostbite.*

If

Affected part feels cold, hard, and solid, and cannot be depressed—feels like a piece of wood or frozen meat. Affected part is pale, and skin may appear waxy. A painfully cold part suddenly stops hurting. Blisters appear after rewarming.

DO NOT:

- Rub or massage part.
- Rewarm with stove, vehicle's tailpipe exhaust, or over a fire.
- Break blisters.
- Allow the individual to smoke or drink alcohol.
- Rewarm if there is any possibility of refreezing.
- Allow thawed part to refreeze.

After thawing:

- Place dry, sterile gauze between toes and fingers to prevent sticking.
- Elevate part to reduce pain and swelling.
- Give aspirin or ibuprofen for pain and inflammation. Do not give to children.
- Apply thin layer of aloe vera over area.
- Seek medical care.

Frostbite and Frostnip

Frostbite happens only in below-freezing temperatures (less than 32°F). Mainly, the feet, hands, ears, and nose are affected. The most severe results are gangrene requiring surgical amputation. See TABLE A.17 for symptoms and treatment. Check for hypothermia because it may also be present. Frostnip is caused when water on the skin's surface freezes (TABLE A.18).

The effect that wind has on our perception of cold is called the *wind chill factor.* The greater the wind speed, the faster we lose body heat. The wind chill temperature always is lower than the air temperature (FIGURE A.2).

TABLE A.18	Determining and Treating Frostnip

If

Skin appears red and sometimes swollen. Painful.

Then

Suspect *frostnip* (it is difficult to tell the difference between frostnip and frostbite):

1. Gently warm area against a warm body part (e.g., armpit, stomach, bare hands) or by blowing warm air on the area.
2. Do not rub area.

Calm	5	10	15	20	25	30	35	40	45	50	55	60
40	36	34	32	30	29	28	28	27	26	26	25	25
35	31	27	25	24	23	22	21	20	19	19	18	17
30	25	21	19	17	16	15	14	13	12	12	11	10
25	19	15	13	11	9	8	7	6	5	4	4	3
20	13	9	6	4	3	1	0	−1	−2	−3	−3	−4
15	7	3	0	−2	−4	−5	−7	−8	−9	−10	−11	−11
10	1	−4	−7	−9	−11	−12	−14	−15	−16	−17	−18	−19
5	−5	−10	−13	−15	−17	−19	−21	−22	−23	−24	−25	−26
0	−11	−16	−19	−22	−24	−26	−27	−29	−30	−31	−32	−33
−5	−16	−22	−26	−29	−31	−33	−34	−36	−37	−38	−39	−40
−10	−22	−28	−32	−35	−37	−39	−41	−43	−44	−45	−46	−48
−15	−28	−35	−39	−42	−44	−46	−48	−50	−51	−52	−54	−55
−20	−34	−41	−45	−48	−51	−53	−55	−57	−58	−60	−61	−62
−25	−40	−47	−51	−55	−58	−60	−62	−64	−65	−67	−68	−69
−30	−46	−53	−58	−61	−64	−67	−69	−71	−72	−74	−75	−76
−35	−52	−59	−64	−68	−71	−73	−76	−78	−79	−81	−82	−84
−40	−57	−66	−71	−74	−78	−80	−82	−84	−86	−88	−89	−91
−45	−63	−72	−77	−81	−84	−87	−89	−91	−93	−95	−97	−98

Temperature (°F)

Wind (mph)

Note: Frostbite occurs in 15 minutes or less.

$$\text{Wind chill (°F)} = 35.74 + 0.6215T - 35.75(V^{0.16}) + 0.4275T(V^{0.16})$$

Where   T = air temperature (°F)
V = wind speed (mph)

FIGURE A.2 **Wind Chill Chart.** SOURCE: National Weather Service, National Oceanic and Atmospheric Adminstration. (2009). Meteorological tables. Online: http://www.erh.noaa.gov/er/iln/tables.htm.

Dietary Reference Intakes (DRIs)

B

The Food and Nutrition Board of the National Academy of Sciences determines recommended nutrient intakes that apply to healthy individuals. Beginning in 1997, the Food and Nutrition Board (with the involvement of Health Canada) began releasing updated recommendations under a new framework called the Dietary Reference Intakes (DRIs). In these revisions, target intake levels for healthy individuals in the United States and Canada are listed as either Adequate Intake (AI) levels or Recommended Dietary Allowances (RDAs). Also, the DRI values include a set of Tolerable Upper Intake Levels (ULs) which are levels of nutrient intake that should not be exceeded due to the potential for adverse effects from excessive consumption.

Dietary Reference Intakes (DRIs)

Life stage group	Vitamin A (µg/d)[1]	Vitamin D (IU/d)[2]	Vitamin E (mg/d)[3]	Vitamin K (µg/d)	Thiamin (mg/d)	Riboflavin (mg/d)	Niacin (mg/d)[4]	Pantothenic Acid (mg/d)	Biotin (µg/d)	Vitamin B$_6$ (mg/d)	Folate (µg/d)[5]	Vitamin B$_{12}$ (µg/d)	Vitamin C (mg/d)	Choline (mg/d)	Sodium (g/d)
Infants															
0–6 mo	400*	400*	4*	2.0*	0.2*	0.3*	2*	1.7*	5*	0.1*	65*	0.4*	40*	125*	0.12*
6–12 mo	500*	400*	5*	2.5*	0.3*	0.4*	4*	1.8*	6*	0.3*	80*	0.5*	50*	150*	0.37*
Children															
1–3 y	300	600	6	30*	0.5	0.5	6	2*	8*	0.5	150	0.9	15	200*	1.0*
4–8 y	400	600	7	55*	0.6	0.6	8	3*	12*	0.6	200	1.2	25	250*	1.2*
Males															
9–13 y	600	600	11	60*	0.9	0.9	12	4*	20*	1.0	300	1.8	45	375*	1.5*
14–18 y	900	600	15	75*	1.2	1.3	16	5*	25*	1.3	400	2.4	75	550*	1.5*
19–30 y	900	600	15	120*	1.2	1.3	16	5*	30*	1.3	400	2.4	90	550*	1.5*
31–50 y	900	600	15	120*	1.2	1.3	16	5*	30*	1.3	400	2.4	90	550*	1.5*
51–70 y	900	600	15	120*	1.2	1.3	16	5*	30*	1.7	400	2.4[7]	90	550*	1.3*
>70 y	900	800	15	120*	1.2	1.3	16	5*	30*	1.7	400	2.4[7]	90	550*	1.2*
Females															
9–13 y	600	600	11	60*	0.9	0.9	12	4*	20*	1.0	300	1.8	45	375*	1.5*
14–18 y	700	600	15	75*	1.0	1.0	14	5*	25*	1.2	400[6]	2.4	65	400*	1.5*
19–30 y	700	600	15	90*	1.1	1.1	14	5*	30*	1.3	400[6]	2.4	75	425*	1.5*
31–50 y	700	600	15	90*	1.1	1.1	14	5*	30*	1.3	400[6]	2.4	75	425*	1.5*
51–70 y	700	600	15	90*	1.1	1.1	14	5*	30*	1.5	400	2.4[7]	75	425*	1.3*
>70 y	700	800	15	90*	1.1	1.1	14	5*	30*	1.5	400	2.4[7]	75	425*	1.2*
Pregnancy															
≤18 y	750	600	15	75*	1.4	1.4	18	6*	30*	1.9	600	2.6	80	450*	1.5*
19–30 y	770	600	15	90*	1.4	1.4	18	6*	30*	1.9	600	2.6	85	450*	1.5*
31–50 y	770	600	15	90*	1.4	1.4	18	6*	30*	1.9	600	2.6	85	450*	1.5*
Lactation															
≤18 y	1,200	600	19	75*	1.4	1.6	17	7*	35*	2.0	500	2.8	115	550*	1.5*
19–30 y	1,300	600	19	90*	1.4	1.6	17	7*	35*	2.0	500	2.8	120	550*	1.5*
31–50 y	1,300	600	19	90*	1.4	1.6	17	7*	35*	2.0	500	2.8	120	550*	1.5*

This table presents Recommended Dietary Allowances (RDAs) and Adequate Intakes (AIs). An asterisk (*) indicates AI. RDAs and AIs may both be used as goals for individual intake.

[1] As retinol activity equivalents (RAE).

[2] As cholecalciferol.

[3] As α-tocopherol.

[4] As niacin equivalents (NE).

[5] As dietary folate equivalents (DFE).

[6] In view of evidence linking folate intake with neural-tube defects in the fetus, it is recommended that all women capable of becoming pregnant consume 400 µg of folic acid from supplements or fortified foods in addition to intake of food folate from a varied diet.

[7] Because 10 to 30% of older people may malabsorb food-bound vitamin B$_{12}$, it is advisable for those older than 50 years to meet their RDA mainly by consuming foods fortified with vitamin B$_{12}$ or a supplement containing vitamin B$_{12}$.

[8] The AI for water represents total water from drinking water, beverages, and moisture from food.

Life stage group	Potassium (g/d)	Chloride (g/d)	Calcium (mg/d)	Phosphorus (mg/d)	Magnesium (mg/d)	Iron (mg/d)	Zinc (mg/d)	Selenium (µg/d)	Iodine (µg/d)	Copper (µg/d)	Manganese (mg/d)	Fluoride (mg/d)	Chromium (µg/d)	Molybdenum (µg/d)	Water (L/d)[8]
Infants															
0-6 mo	0.4*	0.18*	200*	100*	30*	0.27*	2*	15*	110*	200*	0.003*	0.01*	0.2*	2*	0.7*
6-12 mo	0.7*	0.57*	260*	275*	75*	11	3*	20*	130*	220*	0.6*	0.5*	5.5*	3*	0.8*
Children															
1-3 y	3.0*	1.5*	700	460	80	7	3	20	90	340	1.2*	0.7*	11*	17	1.3*
4-8 y	3.8*	1.9*	1,000	500	130	10	5	30	90	440	1.5*	1*	15*	22	1.7*
Males															
9-13 y	4.5*	2.3*	1,300	1,250	240	8	8	40	120	700	1.9*	2*	25*	34	2.4*
14-18 y	4.7*	2.3*	1,300	1,250	410	11	11	55	150	890	2.2*	3*	35*	43	3.3*
19-30 y	4.7*	2.3*	1,000	700	400	8	11	55	150	900	2.3*	4*	35*	45	3.7*
31-50 y	4.7*	2.3*	1,000	700	420	8	11	55	150	900	2.3*	4*	35*	45	3.7*
51-70 y	4.7*	2.0*	1,000	700	420	8	11	55	150	900	2.3*	4*	30*	45	3.7*
>70 y	4.7*	1.8*	1,200	700	420	8	11	55	150	900	2.3*	4*	30*	45	3.7*
Females															
9-13 y	4.5*	2.3*	1,300	1,250	240	8	8	40	120	700	1.6*	2*	21*	34	2.1*
14-18 y	4.7*	2.3*	1,300	1,250	360	15	9	55	150	890	1.6*	3*	24*	43	2.3*
19-30 y	4.7*	2.3*	1,000	700	310	18	8	55	150	900	1.8*	3*	25*	45	2.7*
31-50 y	4.7*	2.3*	1,000	700	320	18	8	55	150	900	1.8*	3*	25*	45	2.7*
51-70 y	4.7*	2.0*	1,200	700	320	8	8	55	150	900	1.8*	3*	20*	45	2.7*
>70 y	4.7*	1.8*	1,200	700	320	8	8	55	150	900	1.8*	3*	20*	45	2.7*
Pregnancy															
≤18 y	4.7*	2.3*	1,300	1,250	400	27	12	60	220	1,000	2.0*	3*	29*	50	3.0*
19-30 y	4.7*	2.3*	1,000	700	350	27	11	60	220	1,000	2.0*	3*	30*	50	3.0*
31-50 y	4.7*	2.3*	1,000	700	360	27	11	60	220	1,000	2.0*	3*	30*	50	3.0*
Lactation															
≤18 y	5.1*	2.3	1,300	1,250	360	10	13	70	290	1,300	2.6*	3*	44*	50	3.8*
19-30 y	5.1*	2.3	1,000	700	310	9	12	70	290	1,300	2.6*	3*	45*	50	3.8*
31-50 y	5.1*	2.3	1,000	700	320	9	12	70	290	1,300	2.6*	3*	45*	50	3.8*

SOURCES: Data compiled from *Dietary Reference Intakes for Calcium, Phosphorus, Magnesium, Vitamin D, and Fluoride*. Washington, DC: National Academies Press; 1997. *Dietary Reference Intakes for Thiamin, Riboflavin, Niacin, Vitamin B₆, Folate, Vitamin B₁₂, Pantothenic Acid, Biotin, and Choline*. Washington, DC: National Academies Press; 1998. *Dietary Reference Intakes for Vitamin C, Vitamin E, Selenium, and Carotenoids*. Washington, DC: National Academies Press; 2000. *Dietary Reference Intakes for Vitamin A, Vitamin K, Arsenic, Boron, Chromium, Copper, Iron, Manganese, Molybdenum, Nickel, Silicon, Vanadium, and Zinc*. Washington, DC: National Academies Press; 2000. *Dietary Reference Intakes for Water, Potassium, Sodium, Chloride, and Sulfate*. Food and Nutrition Board. Washington, DC: National Academies Press; 2005. *Dietary Reference Intakes for Calcium and Vitamin D*. Washington, DC: National Academies Press; 2011. These reports may be accessed via http://nap.edu.

Tolerable Upper Intake Levels (ULs[1])

Life stage group	Vitamin A[2] (μg/d)	Vitamin D (μg/d)	Vitamin E[3,4] (mg/d)	Niacin[4] (mg/d)	Vitamin B$_6$ (mg/d)	Folate[4] (μg/d)	Vitamin C (mg/d)	Choline (g/d)	Calcium (g/d)	Phosphorus (g/d)	Magnesium[5] (mg/d)	Sodium (g/d)
Infants												
0-6 mo	600	25	ND[7]	ND	ND	ND	ND	ND	ND	ND	ND	ND
7-12 mo	600	25	ND	ND	ND	ND	ND	ND	ND	ND	ND	ND
Children												
1-3 y	600	50	200	10	30	300	400	1.0	2.5	3	65	1.5
4-8 y	900	50	300	15	40	400	650	1.0	2.5	3	110	1.9
Males, females												
9-13 y	1,700	50	600	20	60	600	1,200	2.0	2.5	4	350	2.2
14-18 y	2,800	50	800	30	80	800	1,800	3.0	2.5	4	350	2.3
19-70 y	3,000	50	1,000	35	100	1,000	2,000	3.5	2.5	4	350	2.3
>70 y	3,000	50	1,000	35	100	1,000	2,000	3.5	2.5	3	350	2.3
Pregnancy												
≤18 y	2,800	50	800	30	80	800	1,800	3.0	2.5	3.5	350	2.3
19-50 y	3,000	50	1,000	35	100	1,000	2,000	3.5	2.5	3.5	350	2.3
Lactation												
≤18 y	2,800	50	800	30	80	800	1,800	3.0	2.5	4	350	2.3
19-50 y	3,000	50	1,000	35	100	1,000	2,000	3.5	2.5	4	350	2.3

Life stage group	Iron (mg/d)	Zinc (mg/d)	Selenium (μg/d)	Iodine (μg/d)	Copper (μg/d)	Manganese (mg/d)	Fluoride (mg/d)	Molybdenum (μg/d)	Boron (mg/d)	Nickel (mg/d)	Vanadium[6] (mg/d)	Chloride (g/d)
Infants												
0-6 mo	40	4	45	ND	ND	ND	0.7	ND	ND	ND	ND	ND
7-12 mo	40	5	60	ND	ND	ND	0.9	ND	ND	ND	ND	ND
Children												
1-3 y	40	7	90	200	1,000	2	1.3	300	3	0.2	ND	2.3
4-8 y	40	12	150	300	3,000	3	2.2	600	6	0.3	ND	2.9
Males, females												
9-13 y	40	23	280	600	5,000	6	10	1,100	11	0.6	ND	3.4
14-18 y	45	34	400	900	8,000	9	10	1,700	17	1.0	ND	3.6
19-70 y	45	40	400	1,100	10,000	11	10	2,000	20	1.0	1.8	3.6
>70 y	45	40	400	1,100	10,000	11	10	2,000	20	1.0	1.8	3.6
Pregnancy												
≤18 y	45	34	400	900	8,000	9	10	1,700	17	1.0	ND	3.6
19-50 y	45	40	400	1,100	10,000	11	10	2,000	20	1.0	ND	3.6
Lactation												
≤18 y	45	34	400	900	8,000	9	10	1,700	17	1.0	ND	3.6
19-50 y	45	40	400	1,100	10,000	11	10	2,000	20	1.0	ND	3.6

[1] UL = The maximum level of daily nutrient intake that is likely to pose no risk of adverse effects. Unless otherwise specified, the UL represents total intake from food, water, and supplements. Due to lack of suitable data, ULs could not be established for vitamin K, thiamin, riboflavin, vitamin B$_{12}$, pantothenic acid, biotin, or carotenoids. In the absence of ULs, extra caution may be warranted in consuming levels above recommended intakes.

[2] As preformed vitamin A (retinol) only.

[3] As α-tocopherol; applies to any form of supplemental α-tocopherol.

[4] The ULs for vitamin E, niacin, and folate apply to synthetic forms obtained from supplements, fortified foods, or a combination of the two.

[5] The ULs for magnesium represent intake from a pharmacological agent only and do not include intake from food and water.

[6] Although vanadium in food has not been shown to cause adverse effects in humans, there is no justification for adding vanadium to food and vanadium supplements should be used with caution. The UL is based on adverse effects in laboratory animals and these data could be used to set a UL for adults but not children or adolescents.

[7] ND = Not determinable due to lack of data on adverse effects in this age group and concern with regard to lack of ability to handle excess amounts. Source of intake should be from food only to prevent high levels of intake.

SOURCES: Data compiled from *Dietary Reference Intakes for Calcium, Phosphorus, Magnesium, Vitamin D, and Fluoride*. Washington, DC: National Academies Press; 1997. *Dietary Reference Intakes for Thiamin, Riboflavin, Niacin, Vitamin B$_6$, Folate, Vitamin B$_{12}$, Pantothenic Acid, Biotin, and Choline*. Washington, DC: National Academies Press; 1998. *Dietary Reference Intakes for Vitamin C, Vitamin E, Selenium, and Carotenoids*. Washington, DC: National Academies Press; 2000. Institute of Medicine, Food and Nutrition Board. *Dietary Reference Intakes for Vitamin A, Vitamin K, Arsenic, Boron, Chromium, Copper, Iron, Manganese, Molybdenum, Nickel, Silicon, Vanadium, and Zinc*. Washington, DC: National Academies Press, 2000. *Dietary Reference Intakes for Water, Potassium, Sodium, Chloride, and Sulfate*. Washington, DC: National Academies Press; 2005. These reports may be accessed via http://nap.edu.

Daily Values for Food Labels

The Daily Values are standard values developed by the Food and Drug Administration (FDA) for use on food labels.

Nutrient	Amount
Protein[1]	50 g
Thiamin	1.5 mg
Riboflavin	1.7 mg
Niacin	20 mg
Pantothenic Acid	10 mg
Biotin	300 µg
Vitamin B$_6$	2 mg
Folate	400 µg
Vitamin B$_{12}$	6 µg
Vitamin C	60 mg
Vitamin A[2]	5,000 IU
Vitamin D[2]	400 IU
Vitamin E[2]	30 IU
Vitamin K	80 µg
Chloride	3,400 mg
Calcium	1,000 mg
Phosphorus	1,000 mg
Magnesium	400 mg
Iron	18 mg
Zinc	15 mg
Selenium	70 µg
Iodine	150 µg
Copper	2 mg
Manganese	2 mg
Chromium	120 µg
Molybdenum	75 µg

[1] The Daily Values for protein vary for different groups of people: pregnant women, 60 g; nursing mothers, 65 g; infants under 1 year, 14 g; children 1 to 4 years, 16 g.

[2] The Daily Values for fat-soluble vitamins are expressed in International Units (IU), an old system of measurement.

Food Component	Amount	Calculation Factors
Fat	65 g	30% of kcalories
Saturated fat	20 g	10% of kcalories
Cholesterol	300 mg	Same regardless of kcalories
Carbohydrate (total)	300 g	60% of kcalories
Fiber	25 g	11.5 g per 1000 kcalories
Protein	50 g	10% of kcalories
Sodium	2,400 mg	Same regardless of kcalories
Potassium	3,500 mg	Same regardless of kcalories

Note: Daily Values were established for adults and children over 4 years old. The values for energy-yielding nutrients are based on 2,000 kcalories a day.

Dietary Reference Intakes (DRIs) for Carbohydrates, Fiber, Fat, Fatty Acids, and Protein

Life stage group	Carbohydrate (g/d)	Fiber (g/d)	Fat (g/d)	Linoleic Acid (g/d)	a-Linolenic Acid (g/d)	Protein[1] (g/d)
Infants						
0-6 mo	60*	ND[2]	31*	4.4*	0.5*	9.1*
7-12 mo	95*	ND	30*	4.6*	0.5*	11
Children						
1-3 y	130	19*	ND	7*	0.7*	13
4-8 y	130	25*	ND	10*	0.9*	19
Males						
9-13 y	130	31*	ND	12*	1.2*	34
14-18 y	130	38*	ND	16*	1.6*	52
19-30 y	130	38*	ND	17*	1.6*	56
31-50 y	130	38*	ND	17*	1.6*	56
51-70 y	130	30*	ND	14*	1.6*	56
> 70 y	130	30*	ND	14*	1.6*	56
Females						
9-13 y	130	26*	ND	10*	1.0*	34
14-18 y	130	26*	ND	11*	1.1*	46
19-30 y	130	25*	ND	12*	1.1*	46
31-50 y	1ss30	25*	ND	12*	1.1*	46
51-70 y	130	21*	ND	11*	1.1*	46
> 70 y	130	21*	ND	11*	1.1*	46
Pregnancy						
≤ 18 y	175	28*	ND	13*	1.4*	71
19-30 y	175	28*	ND	13*	1.4*	71
31-50 y	175	28*	ND	13*	1.4*	71
Lactation						
≤ 18 y	210	29*	ND	13*	1.3*	71
19-30 y	210	29*	ND	13*	1.3*	71
31-50 y	210	29*	ND	13*	1.3*	71

This table presents Recommended Dietary Allowances (RDAs) and Adequate Intakes (AIs). An asterisk (*) indicates AI. RDAs and AIs may both be used as goals for individual intake.

[1] Based on 1.52 g/kg/day for infants 0-6 mo, 1.2 g/kg/day for infants 7-12 mo, 1.05 g/kg/day for 1-3 y, 0.95 g/kg/day for 4-13 y, 0.85 g/kg/day for 14-18 y, 0.8 g/kg/day for adults, and 1.3 g/kg/day for pregnant women (using pre-pregnancy weight) and lactating women.

[2] ND = Not determinable due to lack of data on adverse effects in this age group and concern with regard to lack of ability to handle excess amounts. Source of intake should be from food only to prevent high levels of intake.

SOURCE: Data compiled from *Dietary Reference Intakes for Energy, Carbohydrate, Fiber, Fat, Fatty Acids, Cholesterol, Protein, and Amino Acids.* Food and Nutrition Board. Washington, DC: National Academies Press; 2005. This report may be accessed via http://nap.edu.

Glossary

Acceptable Micronutrient Distribution Range (AMDR) A range of intakes for a particular energy source that is associated with reduced risk of chronic disease while providing adequate intakes of essential nutrients. An AMDR is expressed as a percentage of total energy intake.

Actin Thin protein filament found in muscle; plays an important role in muscle contraction and relaxation.

Action Stage of change in which the desired level of the new behavior has been reached and is consistently adhered to, although the individual has been doing it for less than 6 months.

Active stretching Requires you to apply force to a stretch.

Adaptation A long-term change in reaction to regular exposure to a stimulus (e.g., lower resting heart rate with increased aerobic fitness).

Added sugars Sugars and syrups added when foods or beverages are processed or prepared.

Adenosine triphosphate A high-energy phosphate that is the only usable form of energy in the human body.

Adipostat Brain mechanism that establishes a set point for a fixed amount of body fat.

Administrative complaint An action that brings about a formal proceeding; much like a court trial, it takes place before an administrative law judge.

Aerobic physical activity Any activity that uses the body's larger muscle groups in a rhythmic manner for a sustained period of time and enhances the body's need for oxygen.

Agonist Muscle that acts as the prime mover; the muscle most responsible for a movement.

Alarm reaction Immediate response to a stressor that is triggered by any threat to our physical or emotional well-being.

Allostatic load The ongoing level of demand for adaptation in an individual.

Amenorrhea Absence of menstrual periods.

Amino acid Complex chemical structure of protein, containing atoms of carbon, hydrogen, oxygen, and nitrogen.

Anaerobic training Metabolic process that does not rely on oxygen.

Anemia Deficiency in red blood cells.

Angina pectoris Main symptom of coronary heart disease; characterized by severe chest pain.

Anorexia nervosa Eating disorder in which individuals incorrectly believe they are overfat; resultant excessive dieting leads to health problems.

Antagonist Muscle that resists the agonist; helps to maintain joint stability.

Anxiety Normal response when a fear-eliciting situation arises.

Anxiety disorders Mental disorders caused by heightened arousal or fear over a sustained period of time.

399

Aorta Large artery that receives blood from the heart's left ventricle and distributes it to the body.

Arteries Blood vessels that carry oxygenated blood from the heart to the body.

Arterioles Small, muscular branches of arteries; when they contract, they increase resistance to blood flow, and blood pressure increases.

Arteriosclerosis A slow, progressive disease process by which the blood vessels' ability to dilate (widen) is restricted, limiting blood flow; also called hardening of the arteries.

Atherosclerosis A slow, progressive disease process by which the blood vessels become damaged through an increasing narrowing and hardening of the inner walls.

Atrophy Decrease in cell size, usually in reference to muscle or fat.

Autonomic nervous system The part of the nervous system that controls smooth muscle, cardiac muscle, and glands; subdivided into sympathetic and parasympathetic.

Autoregulation Self-regulation.

Ball and socket joint A joint that allows one body part to rotate at almost any angle with respect to another.

Ballistic stretching A form of dynamic stretching that utilizes a bouncing motion to move a muscle beyond its normal range of motion.

Basal metabolic rate (BMR) Basic energy requirement necessary to sustain life.

Benign Not cancerous; does not invade nearby tissue or spread to other parts of the body.

Bicarbonate ions (HCO$_3$) As a buffer, they prevent a change in blood pH.

Binge drinking A pattern of drinking that brings a person's blood alcohol concentration to 0.08 percent or above.

Bioelectrical impedance Technique to measure body fat percentage that passes a harmless, low-level, single-frequency electrical current through the body using electrodes placed on the wrist and ankle.

Bisexual individuals People who are attracted to members of both genders.

Blood alcohol concentration (BAC) The amount of alcohol in the blood.

Blood clot Blood that has been converted from a liquid state to a solid state; also called a thrombus.

Blood pressure A measure of the force pushing against the walls of arteries as blood travels through the circulatory system.

Blood pressure cuff (sphygmomanometer) Instrument that measures blood pressure.

Body composition The ratio of fat and fat-free matter (muscle, bone, organs, water) in the body.

Body image The picture you have of your body, what it looks like to you, and how you think it looks to others.

Bone mineral density (BMD) Usually expressed as the amount of mineralized tissue in the scanned area; a risk factor for fractures.

Breasts Network of milk glands and ducts in fatty tissue; secondary sex characteristic.

Bulimia nervosa Eating disorder in which individuals binge eat and then force themselves to vomit.

Calorie Amount of heat it takes to raise the temperature of 1 gram of water by 1° Celsius.

Cancer A complex group of diseases characterized by the uncontrolled growth and spread of abnormal cells. There are at least one hundred different types of cancer.

Cancer screening Checking for cancer in people who have no symptoms of the disease.

Cancer susceptibility gene The type of genes involved in cancer.

Capillaries Tiny blood vessels that circulate blood to all the body's cells.

Carbohydrates Organic compounds that contain carbon, hydrogen, and oxygen and that are an important energy source for many body functions.

Carbon monoxide One of the most abundant and poisonous gases in cigarette smoke.

Carcinogen Chemical that damages cells and causes cancer.

Carcinogenesis Process by which normal cells are transformed into cancer cells.

Cardiac output The amount of blood ejected from the heart each minute; calculated by multiplying heart rate by stroke volume.

Cardiometabolic risk Measure of your risk for developing diabetes and CVD and a good gauge of overall health.

Cardiorespiratory endurance The ability of the circulatory and respiratory systems to supply oxygen and fuel to the body during sustained physical activity.

Cardiovascular disease (CVD) A group of different illnesses that affect your heart and blood vessels.

Cartilage Semirigid tissue that provides support.

Cease-and-desist order A legal order informing a company that it must no longer advertise or market a product.

Cerebral embolism Blood clot formed in one part of the body and then carried by the bloodstream to the brain, where it blocks an artery.

Cerebral hemorrhage Bleeding within the brain that results from a ruptured aneurysm or a head injury.

Cerebral thrombosis Blood clot in an artery that supplies the brain.

Cervix The lower and narrow end of the uterus.

Chain of infection Describes how disease is transmitted from one living organism to another.

Chancre The primary lesion of syphilis, which appears as a hard, painless sore or ulcer, often on the penis or vaginal tissue; pronounced "shanker."

Chlamydia Sexually transmitted infection caused by the bacterium *Chlamydia trichomatis*.

Cholesterol Waxy substance that circulates naturally in the bloodstream; when levels are too high, it forms deposits in the walls of blood vessels.

Chronic diseases Illnesses that can develop early in life and last for many years.

Circuit weight training A system of weight training in which you set up a series of stations where you perform different exercises.

Circumcision A surgical procedure to remove the foreskin from the penis.

Clitoris Small, sensitive female organ located in front of the vaginal opening; center of sexual pleasuring.

Coagulation Process by which a blood clot forms.

Collagen The principal substance connecting fibers and tissues and in bones.

Complex carbohydrates Polysaccharides; these link three or more sugar molecules.

Compliance Ease with which a material is elongated or stretched; the opposite of stiffness.

Compound sets Consecutive performance of two sets of exercises that stimulate the same muscle group.

Concentric muscle action Muscle movement in which the muscle shortens while under tension.

Condyloid joint A joint that allows the head to nod and the fingers to bend.

Consent order An agreement bringing about voluntary compliance without a judicial ruling.

Contemplation Stage of change that begins when the individual starts to think seriously about intending to make a long-term change in the near future (within 6 months).

Copulation Sexual intercourse.

Coronary heart disease (CHD) Disease of the heart caused by atherosclerotic narrowing of the coronary arteries.

Cowper's glands Small glands in a male that secrete drops of alkalinizing fluid into the urethra.

Creatine phosphate Fuel source used in the body to replenish ATP; stored in small amount; it is depleted rapidly.

Decisional balance An individual's relative weighing of the pros and cons of changing.

Degeneration A gradual decrease in function.

Deoxygenated blood Blood returned to the heart to be replenished with oxygen in the lungs.

Depressant A drug that produces a slowing of mental and physical activities.

Depression A mental disorder notable for negative alteration in mood.

Depressive reactions Normal depressed feelings such as sadness and hopelessness.

Diabetes A group of diseases marked by high levels of blood glucose resulting from defects in insulin production, insulin action, or both.

Diastolic pressure The lowest blood pressure measured in the arteries; occurs when the heart muscle is relaxed between beats.

Dietary fiber Diverse carbohydrate polysaccharides of plants that cannot be digested by the human stomach or small intestine.

Dietary Reference Intakes (DRIs) Umbrella term that includes Estimated Average Requirement, Recommended Dietary Allowance, Adequate Intake, and Tolerable Upper Intake Level.

Dietary supplement A product taken by mouth in tablet, capsule, powder, gelcap, or other nonfood form that contains one or more of the following: vitamins, minerals, amino acids, herbs, enzymes, metabolites, or concentrates.

Digestion Metabolizing of food through a series of complex mechanical and chemical reactions.

Direct transmission Immediate transfer of the disease agent between the infected and susceptible individuals by direct contact, such as touching, kissing, sexual intercourse, or by direct droplet spread by sneezing, coughing, or spitting from a distance of one meter or less.

Disaccharide Two-sugar molecule.

Disease Consequence of impaired tissue function.

Distress Harmful or bad stress.

Drug Any absorbed substance, other than food, that changes or enhances any physical or psychological function in the body.

Drug abuse The deliberate use of a substance for other than its intended purpose, in a manner that can damage health or ability to function.

Drug dependence A chronic, progressive, and relapsing disorder that applies to all situations in which drug users develop either a psychological or physical reliance on a drug.

Drug misuse The taking of a substance for its intended purpose, but not in the appropriate amount, frequency, strength, or manner.

Drug therapeutics The proper use of drugs in treating and preventing diseases and preserving health.

Drug use The taking of a drug for its intended purpose in an appropriate amount, frequency, strength, and manner.

Dynamic constant external resistance (DCER) Also known as isotonic training; resistance training exercises in which the external resistance or weight does not change and both a lifting (concentric) and lowering (eccentric) phase occur during each repetition; also known as isotonic resistance training.

Dynamic resistance exercise Exercise that involves muscular actions in which the length of the muscle does change and there is visible movement at the joint.

Dysthymia Chronic form of depression.

Eating disorder A term that refers to a wide range of harmful eating behaviors some individuals use in an attempt to lose weight or achieve a lean appearance.

Eccentric muscle action Muscle movement in which the muscle lengthens while under tension.

Ectomorph A somatotype (body type) that is on the slender side and typically has a genetic predisposition to being skinny.

Elasticity The degree to which a material resists deformation and quickly returns to its normal shape.

Emotional health Encompasses mental states that include feelings or subjective experiences in response to changes in our environment.

Empty calories Measurement of the digestible energy present in high-energy foods with poor nutritional profiles, with most of the energy typically coming from processed carbohydrates, fats, or alcohol.

Endocardium Thin, inner layer that lines the heart.

Endocrine system The hormone-secreting cells of the body; this system is influenced in part by the nervous system.

Endomorph A somatotype (body type) that is genetically geared toward carrying extra body fat and is typically known for having a rounder body shape.

Endorphins Body chemicals responsible for enhancing emotions and providing pain relief.

Environmental engineering Stress management approach that attempts to avoid stress in the first place.

Epidemiology The study of factors affecting the health and illness of populations and that serves as the basic science for public health and preventive medicine.

Epididymitis Inflammation of the epididymis (structure that connects the vas deferens and the testes).

Epinephrine The "fear hormone," which helps supply glucose for increased muscle and nervous system activity.

Ergogenic aid Any substance or phenomenon that enhances performance.

Ergolytic A substance that has a detrimental effect on performance.

Essential amino acids The nine amino acids that the body cannot make.

Essential body fat Fat that is required for normal healthy functioning.

Essential fatty acids Substances that support immune responses, form cell structures, regulate blood pressure, affect blood lipid concentration, and promote clot formation; must be obtained from food.

Essential nutrients Nutrients that the body cannot make for itself; must be obtained from food.

Ethyl alcohol A direct central nervous system depressant that causes a decreased level of consciousness and decreased motor function; the common psychoactive ingredient in all alcoholic beverages.

Eustress Helpful or good stress.

Exercise A subset of physical activity that is a planned, structured, repetitive, and purposeful attempt to improve or maintain physical fitness.

Fallopian tubes A pair of tube-like structures that transport ova from the ovaries to the uterus; the usual site of fertilization.

Fat-soluble vitamins Vitamins A, D, E, and K; must travel with dietary fats in the bloodstream to reach the cells.

Fats Members of a family of compounds called lipids.

Feedback Receiver response to a message that lets the sender know the message was received and what the message was.

Fertilization The fusion of a sperm cell and an ovum.

Fibrous plaque An advanced form of atherosclerosis that occurs from a chronic inflammatory response in the walls of arteries.

Fight-or-flight response Reaction to stressors that challenge the body to respond physically.

FITT formula A basic set of rules of what is necessary to gain a training effect from an exercise program. FITT stands for frequency, intensity, time, and type.

Flexibility The ability to move a joint or a group of joints through its complete range of motion.

Foreskin A fold of skin covering the tip of the penis.

Fraud Intentional act perpetrated to be deceptive in order to gain something of value.

Frequency How often you exercise, which is most often expressed as the number of days per week.

Functional foods Foods that contain significant levels of biologically active components that provide health benefits beyond basic nutrition.

Gametes Sex cells, either sperm or ova, that fuse at fertilization; gametes carry a complete set of genetic information from each parent that is passed on to the child.

Gardnerella vaginalis Bacterium that causes vaginal infection; symptoms of infection include vaginal irritation.

Gay man A man who is physically, romantically, and/or emotionally attracted to other men.

Gender Socialized qualities associated with masculinity or femininity.

Gender identity Awareness and acceptance of being male or female.

Gender roles Complex group of behaviors expected of males and females in a given culture.

General adaptation syndrome (GAS) The body's response to stress and the adaptability of the body to maintain homeostasis.

Generalized anxiety disorder (GAD) Experiencing exaggerated worrying, inability to relax, and insomnia for 6 months or more.

Genital herpes An infection caused by the herpes simplex virus, or HSV.

Genital warts Hard, cauliflowerlike growths that appear in men on the penis, in women on the external genitals and cervix, and in both sexes in the anal region.

Gliding joint A joint that allows two flat bones to slide over each other.

Glucocorticoids Chemicals responsible for speeding up the body's metabolism and increasing access to energy storage.

Glycogen Storage form of sugar energy for humans and animals.

Golgi tendon organs Sense receptors sensitive to rapid forceful contractions that cause a reflexive relaxation to occur within the muscle.

Gonorrhea Sexually transmitted infection caused by the bacterium *Neisseria gonorrhoeae*.

Health Considered less of an abstract state and more as a means to an end, which can be expressed in functional terms as a resource that permits people to lead an individually, socially, and economically productive life. Health is a resource for everyday life, not the object of living. It is a positive concept emphasizing social and personal resources as well as physical capabilities.

Health fraud Deceptive promotion, advertising, distribution, or sale of a product represented as being effective to prevent, diagnose, treat, cure, or lessen an illness or condition, or to provide another beneficial effect on health but that has not been scientifically proven safe and effective for such purposes.

Health habit A health-related behavior that is firmly established and often performed automatically, without thought.

Health literacy Degree to which individuals have the capacity to obtain, process, and understand basic health information and services needed to make appropriate health decisions.

Health-related fitness How well the systems of your body work and contribute to developing optimum health, preventing the onset of chronic disease, or reversing an established chronic disease process associated with inactivity.

Healthy lifestyle A recurring pattern of health-promoting and disease-preventing behaviors undertaken to achieve wellness.

Heart failure A life-threatening condition in which the heart's function as a pump to deliver oxygen-rich blood to the body is inadequate to meet the body's needs. Also called congestive heart failure.

Heart rate The frequency at which the heart beats (contracts).

Heart rate reserve The difference between maximum heart rate and resting heart rate.

Heavy or high-risk drinking Consumption of more than 3 drinks on any day or more than 7 per week for women and more than 4 drinks on any day or more than 14 per week for men.

Hemoglobin The oxygen-carrying pigment of the red blood cells.

Hemorrhage strokes Strokes caused by blood seeping from a hole in the wall of a blood vessel.

Hepatitis B virus A virus that is transmitted sexually and in blood, similar to HIV transmission.

Hereditary cancers Cancers that develop as a result of inheriting a cancer-causing mutation from parents. Also known as a cancer susceptibility gene.

Heritability The amount by which genetics determines the differences between people.

Herpes Sexually transmitted infection caused by herpes simplex virus, or HSV.

Heterosexual individuals People who are attracted to people of the opposite gender.

High blood pressure (HBP) Blood pressure that stays elevated over time. Also known as hypertension.

High-density lipoprotein (HDL) Known as "good" cholesterol because it gives some protection against atherosclerosis by carrying excess cholesterol back to the liver for processing, where it can be removed from the body.

Hinge joint A joint that allows for movement in only one plane so that the body parts can bend and straighten.

Homosexuals People who are attracted to people of the same gender.

Hormones Substances secreted by the glands of the endocrine system that regulate cellular function.

Host An uninfected person who can become infected.

Human immunodeficiency virus (HIV) The virus that causes AIDS; it causes a defect in the body's immune system by invading and then multiplying within the white blood cells.

Human papillomavirus (HPV) Genus of viruses including those causing papillomas (small nipple-like protrusions of the skin or mucous membrane) and warts.

Hyperextension Moving beyond a normal extended position at a joint.

Hyperflexion Moving beyond a normal flexed position at a joint.

Hyperglycemia The medical term for elevated levels of glucose (sugar) in the blood.

Hyperlipidemia The medical term for elevated levels of fats (lipids) in the blood.

Hyperstress Too much stress; the body begins to decrease in its level of performance.

Hypertension Blood pressure that stays elevated over time. Also known as high blood pressure.

Hypertrophy Increase in cell size.

Hypoglycemia Not enough blood sugar.

Hypostress Too little stress or stimulation.

Immunization Process whereby a person is made immune or resistant to an infectious disease.

Incidence The frequency of occurrence of a particular disease; the number of new cases of a disease.

Indirect transmission Travel of infectious agents by means of nonhuman materials and are of three types—airborne, vehicleborne, or vectorborne.

Infection Results when a pathogen invades and begins growing within a host.

Infectious disease Results only if and when, as a consequence of the invasion and growth of a pathogen, tissue function is impaired.

Infectivity The ability of a pathogen to establish an infection or the minimum number of infectious particles to cause disease.

Insoluble fibers Dietary fibers not soluble in water or metabolized by the intestines; these make feces bulkier and softer, promoting decreased passage time.

Insulin A hormone secreted by the pancreas and needed by muscle, fat, and the liver to metabolize glucose.

Insulin resistance A generalized metabolic condition in which the body can't use insulin efficiently.

Intensity How hard you exercise.

Intrinsic motivation Performing a behavior (being active) because you want to rather than because some outside influence is motivating you to do it.

Ischemia Decreased blood flow to an organ, usually resulting from constriction or obstruction of an artery.

Ischemic strokes Strokes caused by clots.

Isokinetic resistance training Form of resistance training in which the speed of movement is fixed and the resistance varies with the force exerted.

Isometric Form of resistance training that involves muscular actions in which the length of the muscle does not change and there is no visible movement at the joint. Also known as static resistance exercise.

Isotonic Form of resistance training that involves muscular actions in which the length of the muscle does change and there is visible movement at the joint. Also known as dynamic resistance exercise.

I-statements Statements beginning with "I"; positive communication skill.

Labia majora A pair of fleshy folds that cover the labia minora.

Labia minora A pair of fleshy folds that cover the vagina.

Lactovegetarian A vegetarian who includes milk in the diet.

Lesbian woman A woman who is attracted physically, romantically, and/or emotionally to other women.

Lipoprotein Lipid (a fatty insoluble substance in blood) surrounded by a protein; the protein makes it soluble in blood.

Literal message Message that is conveyed by symbols.

Low-density lipoprotein (LDL) Carrier of harmful cholesterol in the blood; "bad" cholesterol.

Macronutrients Raw fuel, in the form of protein, carbohydrates, and fats, for biological and mechanical energy requirements.

Maintenance Stage of change in which the behavioral practice is becoming habit.

Major depression Serious condition that leads to inability to function and possibly suicide.

Major minerals Mineral requirements that exceed 100 mg per day.

Malignant Cancerous tumor that is fast growing and that can be fatal; has a tendency to invade and destroy nearby tissue and spread to other parts of the body.

Mental health A "state of successful performance of mental function, resulting in productive activities, fulfilling relationships with other people, and the ability to adapt to change and to cope with adversity" (U.S. Department of Health and Human Services, 1999).

Mental illness Diagnosable mental disorders that change our thinking, mood, or behavior and lead to impaired functioning.

Mesomorph A somatotype (body type) that is naturally geared toward being muscular, which therefore makes it relatively easy for these body types to make gains in the muscle-building process.

Metabolic syndrome A term used to describe a cluster of specific disorders that, when they occur together, may significantly increase a person's risk of developing cardiovascular disease or type 2 diabetes.

Metabolism Process whereby the body takes in energy, converts it to a usable form, stores what is needed, and eliminates what is not.

Meta-message The way the message is interpreted between sender and receiver.

Metastasis The spread of cancer from one part of the body to another. Cells in the metastic (secondary) tumor are the same as those in the original (primary) tumor.

Micronutrients Nutrients required in small amounts; includes vitamins and minerals.

Mind engineering Stress management approach concerned with reducing the intensity of our emotional responses to stressors.

Minerals Inorganic substances vital to many body functions.

Misinformation Information that is not factual but that is passed off as being factual.

Moderate drinking Drinking that causes no problems, either for the drinker or for society; quantified as no more than one drink a day for most women, and no more than two drinks a day for most men.

Monosaccharide One-sugar molecule.

Motor unit A single nerve and all the corresponding muscle fibers it innervates.

Muscle spindles Sense receptors sensitive to rapid, forceful stretching that cause a reflexive contraction of the muscle.

Muscular endurance The ability of a muscle or muscle group to exert repeated force against a resistance or to sustain a muscular contraction for a given period of time.

Muscular strength The amount of force a muscle or muscle group can exert with a single maximum effort.

Mutation Damage to the genes involved in cell division.

Myocardial infarction Medical term for heart attack. The death of heart muscle tissue from a lack of blood supply. An infarct is an area of dead or dying tissue.

Myocardium Muscular middle layer that surrounds the heart.

Myosin Thick protein filament found in muscle; plays an important role in muscle movement.

Myotonia Muscle tension.

Neuroendocrine system The hormone-secreting cells of the body; this system is influenced in part by the nervous system.

Neuromuscular adaptations Changes in the function of the nervous and muscular systems brought on by exposure to regular resistance training. These changes include the ability to recruit motor units selectively, to synchronize the recruitment of these units, and to maintain a state of equilibrium throughout the movement.

Neutralizer Muscle that prevents unwanted activity in muscles not directly involved in performing a movement.

New host An uninfected person who can become infected.

Nicotine A dynamic psychoactive stimulant.

Nonessential nutrients Nutrients made by the body from the foods we eat.

Nonspecific mechanisms The body's primary defense against infectious disease.

Norepinephrine The "anger hormone"; helps speed the heart rate and raises blood pressure to provide more oxygen for the body.

Nutrient-dense foods Those foods and beverages that provide substantial amounts of vitamins, minerals, and other substances that provide many positive health effects with relatively few calories.

Nutrients Elements in foods that are required for energy, growth, and repair of tissues and regulation of body processes.

Nutrition Facts label Mandated food labeling designed to help consumers make appropriate choices.

Obesity A weight that exceeds the threshold of a health criterion standard to a greater degree than overweight.

Omentum A large fold of visceral peritoneum that hangs down from the stomach.

Organ system A collection of specialized tissues that provide an important body function (e.g., musculoskeletal, cardiovascular).

Orgasm The climax of sexual responses and the release of physiological and sexual tensions.

Osteoblasts Bone-forming cells.

Osteoclasts Cells in developing bone concerned especially with the breaking down of unnecessary bone parts.

Osteocytes Bone cells responsible for the maintenance and turnover of the mineral content of surrounding bone.

Osteogenesis imperfecta A disease caused by abnormalities in the collagen matrix within the bone, resulting in a weak structure and the potential for multiple fractures.

Osteopenia Low bone mass.

Osteoporosis Literally means "porous bones"; a metabolic disease resulting in bone loss and bones that fracture easily.

Ova, ovum Eggs, egg.

Ovaries A pair of almond-shaped organs in the female abdomen that produce egg cells (ova) and female sex hormones (estrogen and progesterone).

Overfat Having body fat levels above recommended levels for good health.

Overload principle A greater than normal load or intensity on the body system is required for training adaptation or improved function to take place.

Overuse syndrome Exercising at a level well beyond your current state of fitness that results in symptoms of fatigue, lethargy, depression, and feelings of being overwhelmed.

Overweight A weight that exceeds the threshold of a health criterion standard.

Ovolactovegetarian A vegetarian who eats both eggs and milk products.

Ovovegetarian A vegetarian who includes eggs in the diet.

Ovulation Release of an egg (ovum) from the ovary.

Oxygenated blood Blood leaving the heart that is oxygen-rich.

Paget's disease A disease whose precise cause is unknown but that is a consequence of both genetic and environmental factors, such as a viral infection that triggers the osteoblasts to try to repair the damage (infection) by forming new bone. However, the new formation is disrupted, leading to weakness and deformities in the bone.

Parasympathetic nervous system The counterpart to the sympathetic nervous system.

Passive stretching Requires the assistance of a device or a trained partner to apply the force to the stretch.

Pathogen A biological agent that causes disease or illness to its host. Also known as an infectious agent.

Pathogencity The ability of microbe to induce disease.

Pathogenesis The origination and development of a disease.

Peer-reviewed research Research articles and presentations in which experts in the field of study review material for accuracy and validity before it is disseminated to the public.

Pelvic inflammatory disease (PID) Infection of the female reproductive organs, specifically the uterus, fallopian tubes, and pelvic cavity.

Penis The male organ of copulation and urination.

Pericardium Thin, closed outer sac that surrounds the heart.

Periodization Form of resistance training in which a training program is subdivided into sections, or periods; the focus of training in each period varies, allowing for a greater overall adjustment to occur.

Peripheral arterial disease A blood vessel disease that affects any of the blood vessels outside the heart and brain.

Pharmacology The study of drugs, their sources, how they enter the body, how the body reacts to them, and their short-term and long-term effects on the body.

Phospholipids Lipids made by the body and therefore not considered essential fatty acids.

Physical activity Any bodily movement produced by the contraction of skeletal muscle that increases energy expenditure above a basal (resting) level.

Physical dependence The body's biological adaptation to a drug, in which the drug has become necessary to maintain a balance in certain body processes.

Physical engineering Stress management approach using regular exercise to optimize stress responses.

Physical fitness A set of attributes a person has or achieves that relate to his or her ability or capacity to perform specific types of physical activity efficiently and effectively.

Pituitary-adrenal axis The first pattern of the fight-or-flight response.

Placebo effect A physical or emotional change that is not due to properties of an administered substance. The change reflects participants' expectations.

Plaque A fatty deposit on the inner lining of the artery wall.

Plyometrics Form of resistance training that uses a rapid, dynamic eccentric contraction and stretching of muscles followed by a rapid, dynamic concentric contraction.

PNF stretching Proprioceptive neuromuscular facilitation; utilization and integration of the nervous and muscular systems to enhance flexibility.

Portal of entry How pathogens enter the body.

Portal of exit Any body opening on an infected person that allows a pathogenic agent to leave their reservoir such as mouth, nose, eyes, mucus membranes, and an open wound of the skin.

Precontemplation Stage of change during which individuals are not intending to make a long-term lifestyle change in the foreseeable future (usually the next 6 months).

Pre-diabetes A condition in which an individual's blood glucose is higher than normal but not high enough to be classified as type 2 diabetes.

Prehypertension A blood pressure elevated above normal but not to the level considered to be hypertensive.

Preparation Stage of change in which the individual intends to take action in the immediate future (usually in the next month).

Prevalence The predominance of a disease; the number of people who have the disease at one given point in time.

Primary care provider (PCP) A health care practitioner who sees patients with common medical problems.

Primary hypertension Hypertension where the cause is unknown.

Primary prevention Actions that keep the disease process or health condition from becoming established in the first place by elimination of causes of the disease (reducing known risk factors) or increasing resistance to the disease.

Principle of individual differences A principle that states that we all vary in our ability to develop fitness in each of our fitness components. These differences have to do with genetics, age, body size and shape, chronic conditions, injuries, and gender.

Principle of overload States that a greater than normal load or intensity on the body system is required for training adaptation or improved function to take place.

Principle of progression A principle that states that, to ensure safety and effectiveness, the training overload on the body system must be applied in a systematic and logical fashion over an extended period of time.

Principle of recovery A principle that states that physical activity, no matter how structured, requires a period of rest to permit the body to be restored to a state where it can be exercised once more.

Principle of reversibility A principle that states that changes occurring from physical activity are reversible and that if a person stops being active for an extended period of time, the body will decondition and revert back to its pretraining condition.

Principle of specificity A principle that states that to develop a particular fitness component, activities must be performed to develop the various body parts or body systems for that fitness component.

Problem drinking The consumption of alcohol that results in significant risk of health consequences, social problems, or both.

Processes of change The mechanisms through which different techniques influence a person's behavior change.

Progression stage Stage in which you stress your body so as to develop greater levels of conditioning and fitness. This stage is short because of high levels of stress on the body. Optimal levels of fitness are obtained.

Proprioceptors Sense receptors that provide feedback to our central nervous system.

Prostate gland Gland at the base of the male bladder that provides seminal fluid.

Protein An essential nutrient that the body uses in more ways than any other nutrient.

Protein filaments Strands of protein (actin and myosin) that give muscle its structure and functional ability.

Psychoactive drug A chemical substance that alters your thinking, perceptions, feelings, and behavior.

Psychological dependence Craving for a drug for primarily psychological or emotional reasons.

Psychological factor Factors related to your state of mind that affect your adherence to an activity program.

Psychosomatic disease Bodily symptoms caused by mental or emotional disturbance.

Pubic lice Small insects that live in hair in the genital–rectal region.

Pulmonary system Pertaining to the lungs; includes pulmonary arteries and veins.

Pyramiding A gradual increase in the weight being lifted with a corresponding reduction in the number of repetitions until the one-repetition maximum is reached; this is followed by a gradual decrease in the resistance being lifted and an increase in the number of repetitions, until the exerciser returns to the initial load.

Quackery Overpromotion of a product in the field of health.

Quality of life A subjective measure that reflects our levels of fulfillment, satisfaction, happiness, and feeling good about ourselves despite any limitations we may have.

Relaxation response The opposite of the fight-or-flight response to stressful or threatening situations.

Remodeling The ongoing dual processes of bone formation and bone resorption after cessation of growth.

Repetition One complete movement through an exercise. Also known as reps.

Reservoir Principal habitat where a specific infectious agent lives and multiplies and from which it may spread to cause disease.

Resistance training Any exercise that causes the muscles to contract against an external resistance with the expectation of increases in strength, endurance, tone, and/or mass.

Resorption The loss of substance (bone, in this case) through physiologic or pathologic means.

Response A short-term change in reaction to a stimulus (e.g., increased breathing rate after moving from inactive to active state).

Resting metabolic rate (RMR) Your rate of energy use at rest.

Retrovirus A type of virus (such as the one that causes AIDS) that can invade cells and integrate its own genetic information into chromosomes.

Rickets A deficiency of vitamin D (usually seen in children) that causes weak bones and deformation resulting from overgrowth of cartilage at the ends of the bones. In adults, this condition advances to softening of the bone, leading to fracture and deformity.

Risk factor An exposure that is statistically related in some way to a health outcome; for example, smoking is a risk factor for developing lung cancer.

Saddle joint A joint that allows for the thumb to touch any other finger.

Safer sex General term used to describe methods for reducing the chance that you will contract or spread sexually transmitted infections.

Salutogenesis An approach focusing on factors that support human health and well-being, rather than on factors that cause disease.

Sarcomere The functional unit of a muscle. The site where muscle movement takes place.

Scabies Infestation of the skin by microscopic mites (insects).

Scrotum The sac of skin that contains the testes.

Secondary hypertension Hypertension arising from another physical condition, such as kidney disease.

Secondary prevention Preventative methods aimed at early detection of asymptomatic disease through preventive screenings and tests.

Secondary sex characteristics Anatomic features appearing at puberty that distinguish males from females.

Secondhand smoke Exhaled mainstream smoke and sidestream smoke from another person's cigarette, cigar, or pipe. Also known as environmental tobacco smoke (ETS).

Self-changers Individuals who can manage and control their own lives.

Self-disclosure The sharing of private information.

Self-efficacy The confidence you have in your ability to perform specific behaviors in specific situations.

Semen A whitish, creamy fluid containing sperm.

Seminal vesicles Sac-like structures that secrete a fluid that activates the sperm.

Semivegetarian A vegetarian who may eat fish and poultry but not red meat.

Set point Level of resting metabolism that your body naturally prefers. Some research suggests that our metabolic rate will return to its set point even if we try to change our metabolism through modifying our diet.

Set point theory A theory that proposes that a regulatory system exists in the human body that is designed to maintain body weight at some fixed level.

Sets A group of repetitions.

Sex (1) An individual's classification as male or female based on anatomic characteristics, (2) a set of behaviors, and (3) the experience of erotic pleasure.

Sexual Characterized by, or having, sex; as opposed to asexual.

Sexual orientation Attraction toward and interest in members of one or both genders.

Sexual relationship A relationship in which two people mutually consent to become physically intimate and participate in sexual acts such as kissing, caressing, stroking, rubbing, or penetrative behaviors (penile–vaginal intercourse, anal intercourse, or oral sex).

Sexuality A person's sense of self, which is used to create sexual experiences.

Sexually healthy relationship A relationship that is consensual, nonexploitative, honest, mutually pleasurable, safe, and protected from unwanted pregnancy, STIs, and other harm (National Guidelines Task Force, 2004).

Sexually transmitted infections (STIs) Infections that are spread primarily through person-to-person sexual contact.

Simple carbohydrates Either one-sugar or two-sugar molecules.

Sinoatrial node The natural pacemaker of the heart.

Skill-related fitness Ability to perform a particular sport or athletic activity.

Skinfold technique Measure of subcutaneous fat at various body sites using special calipers.

Smegma A foul-smelling, pasty accumulation of skin cells and sebum that collects in moist areas of the genitalia, especially in uncircumcised males.

Social drinking Use of alcohol that consists of an occasional drink or two in the company of friends.

Social health Feelings of being loved, valued, and respected in relationships; includes notions of giving and receiving assistance.

Social support Closeness felt and derived from a variety of relationships, including family, friends, acquaintances, work/school colleagues, and Internet-based relationships.

Soft tissues Include muscles, tendons, ligaments, joint cartilage, fat, and skin.

Solid fats Fats that are solid at room temperature, like beef fat, butter, and shortening.

Soluble fibers Dietary fibers soluble in water and metabolized in the large intestine; assist in removing cholesterol from the body.

Specific immune mechanisms Enables the body to target particular pathogens and pathogen-infected cells for destruction via the immune system.

Sphygmomanometer Instrument that measures blood pressure.

Spiral model of change A relapse model that demonstrates that individuals move back and forth along the change continuum a number of times before attaining their behavioral goal and therefore views setbacks as positive because changers are learning something new every time they change.

Sporadic cancers Cancers that develop because of complex interactions between our bodies, our lifestyles, our environment, and our genetic makeup.

Stages of change A variable process that is organized in a continuum according to the decision-making process that is required to effect change.

Starches Storage form of carbohydrates for plants.

Static contraction Form of resistance training that involves muscular actions in which the length of the muscle does not change and there is no visible movement at the joint. Also known as *isometric contraction*.

Static stretching Slowly elongating a muscle to the point of slight tension or mild discomfort (not to a point of pain), and then holding it at that position.

Stimulants Drugs that increase central nervous system activity.

Storage fat Body fat, above essential levels, that accumulates in adipose tissue.

Stress Response that includes both a mental reaction (stressor) and a physical reaction (stress response).

Stressor The demand or stimulus that elicits the general adaptation syndrome.

Stretch receptors Primary proprioceptors located within the thick center portion (belly) of the muscle that detect stretching in the muscle.

Stretch reflex Reflexive contraction of the muscle as the result of forceful rapid stretching.

Stroke A rapid loss of brain functions resulting from a loss of oxygen-rich blood flow to the brain. Also known as a brain attack.

Stroke volume The amount of blood ejected with each contraction of the heart.

Subarachnoid hemorrhage Bleeding from a blood vessel on the surface of the brain into the space between the brain and the skull.

Substance abuse The deliberate use of a substance for other than its intended purpose in a manner that can damage health or ability to function.

Substance dependence A chronic, progressive, and relapsing disorder that applies to all situations in which drug users develop either a psychological or physical reliance on a drug.

Substance misuse The taking of a substance for its intended purpose, but not in the appropriate amount, frequency, strength, or manner.

Substance use The taking of a drug for its intended purpose in an appropriate amount, frequency, strength, and manner.

Supersets Consecutive performance of two sets of exercises that stress one muscle group and its antagonist without a rest period separating the sets.

Sympathetic nervous system Part of the autonomic nervous system; helps prepare the body for physical activity.

Sympathoadrenal system The second pattern of the fight-or-flight response.

Synergists Muscles that assist the agonist.

Syphilis Sexually transmitted infection caused by spirochete bacteria (*Treponema pallidum*).

Systolic pressure The pressure as the heart beats or contracts, or the higher number when blood pressure is measured in the arteries.

Talk test A simple way to measure relative aerobic intensity.

Tars The yellowish-brown solid, sticky materials that are inhaled as part of tobacco smoke.

Termination Stage of change in which the individual's former problem behavior represents no threat or temptation; it denotes the concept of exiting the stages of change or the cycle of change.

Tertiary prevention Treatment after a person is already ill; typically offered by medical specialists.

Testes A pair of male reproductive organs that produce sperm cells and male sex hormones.

Thermic effect of activity (TEA) The energy expended in skeletal muscle contraction and relaxation.

Thermic effect of food (TEF) The energy expended by our bodies to eat and process (digest, transport, metabolize, and store) food.

Time How long you exercise.

Tolerance Adaptation of the body to a drug in such a way that repeated exposure to the same dose results in less effect on the body.

Trace minerals Minerals that are required in quantities of less than 100 mg per day.

Trans fats Unsaturated fatty acids formed when vegetable oils are processed (hydrogenation) and made more solid.

Transmission The mechanism by which an infectious agent is spread through the environment to another person.

Transsexual individual An individual whose gender identity does not match his or her biological sex.

Transtheoretical model of health behavior change (TTM) A behavior change model based on a time or temporal dimension, the stages of change, to integrate processes and principles of change using well-established psychological theories of behavior interventions.

Trichomonas vaginalis A protozoan that causes trichomoniasis, symptoms of which include a foul-smelling, foamy white or yellow-green discharge that irritates the vagina.

Triglycerides Fatty acids that provide the body's largest energy store, act as insulation, transport fat-soluble vitamins, and contribute to satiety.

Tri-sets Consecutive performance of three sets of exercises that stress the same muscle group.

Tumors An abnormal mass of tissue that results from excessive cell division. Tumors perform no useful body function and can be benign or malignant.

Type Dictates what kind of exercise you should choose to achieve the appropriate training response for the type of fitness you are trying to improve.

Type 1 diabetes Once known as juvenile diabetes or insulin-dependent diabetes, it is a chronic (lifelong) disease in which the pancreas produces little or no insulin to properly control blood sugar levels.

Type 2 diabetes Once known as adult-onset or non-insulin-dependent diabetes, in this condition the body produces sufficient amounts of insulin, but the body's cells have developed a resistance to it.

Underfat Having body fat levels below what is recommended for good health.

Underwater weighing Technique to measure body fat percentage that requires weighing a person underwater as well as on land.

Underweight Having a body weight below levels recommended for a certain height.

Use and disuse Dictates that, although rest periods are necessary for recovery after workouts, extensive rest intervals (more than a week or two) lead to a gradual loss of fitness.

Uterus The female organ in which a fetus develops.

Vagina Female organ of copulation, and the exit pathway for the fetus at birth.

Valsalva maneuver Condition that occurs when you hold your breath and exert force (grunting action); causes elevated blood pressure that increases the risk for stroke, heart attack, or hemorrhage.

Variability The differences among people.

Vasocongestion Engorgement of blood vessels in particular body parts in response to sexual arousal.

Vegan A strict vegetarian who eats no animal products.

Vehicles Nonliving things like water, food and soil also can be reservoirs for infectious agents.

Veins Blood vessels that return deoxygenated blood to the heart.

Venous return Blood returning through the veins to the heart.

Virulence The seriousness or severity of the disease.

Visceral fat Located inside the peritoneal cavity, packed in between internal organs.

Vitamins Essential organic substances needed by the body to perform highly specific metabolic processes in the cells.

Water-soluble vitamins Vitamins that can be transported throughout the body by a watery medium.

Wellness A complex interaction and integration of the seven dimensions of health, each based on a dynamic level of functioning, oriented toward maximizing your potential based on self-responsibility.

Withdrawal illness Recognizable physical signs and symptoms that result from withdrawing from drug use.

Yerkes–Dodson law A law that predicts an inverted U-shaped function between stress and performance.

You-statements Statements beginning with "you"; negative communication skill.

Zoonoses Diseases for which reservoir resides in animals.

References

National Guidelines Task Force. (2004). *Guidelines for Comprehensive Sexuality Education: Kindergarten–12th Grade*, 3rd ed. New York: Sexuality Information and Education Council of the United States.

U.S. Department of Health and Human Services. (1999). *Mental Health: A Report of the Surgeon General*. Rockville, MD: Author.

Index